Quality of Care for
Children
and Adolescents

A Review of Selected Clinical Conditions and Quality Indicators

Elizabeth A. McGlynn • Cheryl L. Damberg
Eve A. Kerr • Mark A. Schuster

Editors

RAND Health

Supported by the Health Care Financing Administration,
U.S. Department of Health and Human Services

Principal funding for this report was provided by a cooperative agreement from the Health Care Financing Administration, U.S. Department of Health and Human Services.

ISBN: 0-8330-2922-3

RAND is a nonprofit institution that helps improve policy and decisionmaking through research and analysis. RAND® is a registered trademark. RAND's publications do not necessarily reflect the opinions or policies of its research sponsors.

Published 2000 by RAND
1700 Main Street, P.O. Box 2138, Santa Monica, CA 90407-2138
1200 South Hayes Street, Arlington, VA 22202-5050
RAND URL: http://www.rand.org/
To order RAND documents or to obtain additional information, contact Distribution Services: Telephone: (310) 451-7002;
Fax: (310) 451-6915; Internet: order@rand.org

PREFACE

This report is one of a series of volumes describing the QA Tools, a comprehensive, clinically based system for assessing care for children and adults. The quality indicators that comprise these Tools cover 46 clinical areas and all 4 functions of medicine—screening, diagnosis, treatment, and follow-up. The indicators also cover a variety of modes of providing care, including history, physical examination, laboratory study, medication, and other interventions and contacts.

Development of each indicator was based on a review of the literature. Each volume documents the literature on which the indicators were based, explains how the clinical areas and indicators were selected, and describes what is included in the overall system.

The QA Tools were developed with funding from public and private sponsors—the Health Care Financing Administration, the Agency for Healthcare Research and Quality, the California HealthCare Foundation, and the Robert Wood Johnson Foundation.

The other four volumes in this series are:

Quality of Care for General Medical Conditions: A Review of the Literature and Quality Indicators. Eve A. Kerr, Steven M. Asch, Eric G. Hamilton, and Elizabeth A. McGlynn, eds. MR-1280-AHRQ, 2000.

Quality of Care for Oncologic Conditions and HIV: A Review of the Literature and Quality Indicators. Steven M. Asch, Eve A. Kerr, Eric G. Hamilton, Jennifer L. Reifel, and Elizabeth A. McGlynn, eds. MR-1281-AHRQ, 2000.

Quality of Care for Cardiopulmonary Conditions: A Review of the Literature and Quality Indicators. Eve A. Kerr, Steven M. Asch, Eric G. Hamilton, and Elizabeth A. McGlynn, eds. MR-1282-AHRQ, 2000.

Quality of Care for Women: A Review of Selected Clinical Conditions and Quality Indicators. Elizabeth A. McGlynn, Eve A. Kerr, Cheryl L. Damberg, and Steven M. Asch, eds. MR-1284-HCFA, 2000.

These volumes should be of interest to clinicians, health plans, insurers, and health services researchers. At the time of publication, the QA Tools system was undergoing testing in managed care plans, medical groups, and selected communities. For more information about the QA Tools system, contact RAND_Health@rand.org.

CONTENTS

TABLES

FIGURES

ACKNOWLEDGMENTS

Funding for this work was provided by a Cooperative Agreement (No. 18-C-90315/9-02, "Development of a Global Quality Assessment Tool") from the Health Care Financing Administration, U.S. Department of Health and Human Services. We appreciate the continued and enthusiastic support of our project offer, Beth Benedict, Ph.D.

We are indebted to our expert panelists:

David A. Bergman, M.D. (Chair)
Lucile Salter Packard Children's Hospital
Palo Alto, California
Clinical Associate Professor
Stanford University
Palo Alto, California

Yi-Chuan Ching, M.D.
Kaiser Permanente
Honolulu, Hawaii
Associate Professor
University of Hawaii
Honolulu, Hawaii

John B. Coombs, M.D.
Associate Vice President
Associate Dean
Professor
University of Washington
Seattle, Washington

Arthur B. Elster, M.D.
American Medical Association, Department of Adolescent Health
Chicago, Illinois

Caroline Breese Hall, M.D.
Professor
University of Rochester School of Medicine and Dentistry
Rochester, New York

Katherine S. Lobach, M.D.
New York City Health and Hospitals Corporation
New York, New York
Clinical Professor
Albert Einstein College of Medicine
Bronx, New York

Thomas K. McInerney, M.D.
Panorama Pediatric Group
Rochester, New York
Clinical Professor, Pediatrics
University of Rochester School of Medicine and Dentistry
Rochester, New York

Eric M. Wall, M.D., M.P.H.
QualMed Health Plans of Oregon
Portland, Oregon

Charles J. Wibbelsman, M.D.
Kaiser Foundation Hospital
San Francisco, California
Assistant Clinical Professor of Pediatrics
University of California San Francisco
San Francisco, California

We are also indebted to the project staff:

Landon Donsbach
Tamara Majeski
Paul Murata, M.D.
Eve Schenker, M.P.H.

INTRODUCTION

Developing and implementing a valid system of quality assessment is essential for effective functioning of the health care system. Although a number of groups have produced quality assessment tools, these tools typically suffer from a variety of limitations. Information is obtained on only a few dimensions of quality, the tools rely exclusively on administrative data, they examine quality only for users of services rather than the population, or they fail to provide a scientific basis for the quality indicators.

Under funding from public and private sponsors, including the Health Care Financing Administration (HCFA), the Agency for Healthcare Research and Quality (AHRQ), the California HealthCare Foundation, and the Robert Wood Johnson Foundation (RWJ), RAND has developed and tested a comprehensive, clinically based system for assessing quality of care for children and adults. We call this system QA Tools.

In this introduction, we discuss how the clinical areas were selected, how the indicators were chosen, and what is included in the overall system. We then describe in detail how we developed the indicators for children and adolescents.

ADVANTAGES OF THE QA TOOLS SYSTEM

QA Tools is a comprehensive, clinically based system for assessing the quality of care for children and adults. The indicators cover 46 clinical areas and all four functions of medicine including screening, diagnosis, treatment, and follow-up. The indicators also cover a variety of modes of providing care, such as history, physical examination, laboratory study, medication, and other interventions and contacts. Initial development of indicators for each clinical area was based on a review of the literature.

The QA Tools system addresses many limitations of current quality assessment tools by offering the following:

- They are clinically detailed rather than just relying exclusively on data from administrative records.

- They examine quality for a population-based sample rather than for a more restricted sample of those who use care or have insurance.
- They document the scientific basis for developing and choosing the indicators.
- The QA Tools system is designed to target populations vulnerable to underutilization.
- Because of the comprehensiveness of the system, it is difficult for health care organizations to focus on a few indicators to increase their quality scores.
- QA Tools is a system that can be effective for both internal and external quality reviews. Health plans can use the system in order to improve the overall quality of the care provided.
- Because of the simple summary scores that will be produced, it will be an important tool for purchasers and consumers who are making choices about health care coverage and which provider to see.

Given its comprehensiveness, the QA Tools system contrasts with *leading indicators*, the most common approach to quality measurement in use today. Under the leading indicators approach, three to five specific quality measures are selected across a few domains (for example, rates of mammography screening, prevalence of the use of beta blockers, and appropriateness of coronary angioplasty).

Leading indicators may work well for drawing general conclusions about quality when they correlate highly with other similar but unmeasured interventions and when repeated measurement and public reporting does not change the relationship of those indicators to the related interventions. However, to date no real evaluation of the utility of leading indicators in assessing health system performance has been done. We also do not know whether the selected indicators currently in use consistently represent other unmeasured practices.

By contrast, a comprehensive system can represent different dimensions of quality of care delivery by using a large number of measures applied to a population of interest and aggregated to produce index scores to draw conclusions about quality. A comprehensive system works well when evidence exists of variability within and between the diagnosis and management of different conditions and when the question being asked is framed at a high level (for instance, how well is the health system helping the population stay healthy, or how much of a problem does underuse present?).

In the 46 clinical areas they encompass, the QA Tools adequately represent scientific and expert judgment on what constitutes quality care. However, both the science and the practice of medicine continue to evolve. For the QA Tools to remain a valid tool for quality assessment over time, the scientific evidence in each area needs to be reviewed annually to determine if the evidence warrants modifying the indicators and/or clinical areas included in the system.

SELECTING CLINICAL AREAS FOR THE QA TOOLS

We reviewed Vital Statistics, the National Health Interview Survey, the National Hospital Discharge Survey, and the National Ambulatory Medical Care Survey to identify the leading causes of morbidity and mortality and the most common reasons for physician visits in the United States. We examined statistics for different age and gender groups in the population (0-1, 1-5, 6-11, 12-17, 18-50 [men and women], 50-64, 65-75, over 75).

We selected topics that reflected these different areas of importance (death, disability, utilization of services) and that covered preventive care as well as care for acute and chronic conditions. In addition, we consulted with a variety of experts to identify areas that are important to these various populations but that may be underrepresented in national data sets (for example, mental health problems). Finally, we sought to select enough clinical areas to represent a majority of the health care delivery system.

Table I.1 lists the 46 clinical areas included in the QA Tools system by population group; 20 include indicators for children and 36 for adults. The clinical areas, broadly defined, represent about 55 percent of the reasons for ambulatory care visits among children, 50 percent of the reasons for ambulatory care visits for the entire population, and 46 percent of the reasons for hospitalization among adults.

Note: Table I.1 reflects the clinical areas that were included in the system currently being tested. Several clinical areas (e.g., lung cancer, sickle cell disease) for which indicators were developed were not incorporated into the current tool due to budgetary constraints.

Table I.1

Clinical Areas in QA Tools System By Covered Population Group

Clinical Areas	Children	Adults
Acne	X	
Adolescent preventive services	X	
Adult screening and prevention		X
Alcohol dependence		X
Allergic rhinitis	X	
Asthma	X	X
Atrial fibrillation		X
Attention deficit/hyperactivity disorder	X	
Benign prostatic hyperplasia		X
Breast cancer		X
Cataracts		X
Cerebrovascular disease		X
Cervical cancer		X
Cesarean delivery	X	X
Chronic obstructive pulmonary disease		X
Colorectal cancer		X
Congestive heart failure		X
Coronary artery disease		X
Depression	X	X
Developmental screening	X	
Diabetes Mellitus	X	X
Diarrheal disease	X	
Family planning and contraception	X	X
Fever of unknown origin	X	
Headache		X
Hip fracture		X
Hormone replacement therapy		X
Human immunodeficiency virus		X
Hyperlipidemia		X
Hypertension		X
Immunizations	X	X
Low back pain		X
Orthopedic conditions		X
Osteoarthritis		X
Otitis media	X	
Pain management for cancer		X
Peptic ulcer disease & dyspepsia		X
Pneumonia		X
Prenatal care and delivery	X	X
Prostate cancer		X
Tuberculosis	X	X
Upper respiratory tract infections	X	
Urinary tract infections	X	X
Uterine bleeding and hysterectomy		X
Vaginitis and sexually transmitted diseases	X	X
Well child care	X	
Total number of clinical areas	**20**	**36**

SELECTING QUALITY INDICATORS

In this section, we describe the process by which indicators were chosen for inclusion in the QA Tools system. This process involved RAND staff drafting proposed indicators based on a review of the pertinent clinical literature and expert panel review of those indicators.

Literature Review

For each clinical area chosen, we reviewed the scientific literature for evidence that effective methods of prevention, screening, diagnosis, treatment, and follow-up existed (Asch et al., 2000; Kerr et al., 2000a; Kerr et al., 2000b; McGlynn et al., 2000). We explicitly examined the continuum of care in each clinical area. RAND staff drafted indicators that

- addressed an intervention with potential health benefits for the patient
- were supported by scientific evidence or formal professional consensus (guidelines, for example)
- can be significantly influenced by the health care delivery system
- can be assessed from available sources of information, primarily the medical record.

The literature review process varied slightly for each clinical area, but the basic strategy involved the following:

- Identify general areas in which quality indicators are likely to be developed.
- Review relevant textbooks and summary articles.
- Conduct a targeted MEDLINE search on specific topics related to the probable indicator areas.

The levels of evidence for each indicator were assigned to three categories: randomized clinical trial; nonrandomized controlled trials, cohort or case analysis, or multiple time series; and textbooks, opinions, or descriptive studies. For each proposed indicator, staff noted the highest level of evidence supporting the indicator.

Because of the breadth of topics for which we were developing indicators, some of the literature reviews relied exclusively on textbooks and review articles. Nonetheless, we believe that the reviews adequately summarize clinical opinion and key research at the time that they were conducted. The literature reviews used to develop quality indicators for children and adolescents, and for women, were conducted between January and July 1995. The reviews for general medical conditions, oncologic conditions, and cardiopulmonary conditions were conducted between November 1996 and July 1997.

For each clinical area, we wrote a summary of the scientific evidence and developed tables of the proposed indicators that included the level of evidence, specific studies in support of the indicator, and the clinical rationale for the indicator. Because the organization of care delivery is changing so rapidly, we drafted indicators that were not in most cases inextricably linked to the place where the care was provided.

Types of Indicators

Quality of care is usually determined with three types of measures:

- *Structural measures* include characteristics of clinicians (for instance, board certification or years of experience), organizations (for instance, staffing patterns or types of equipment available), and patients (for instance, type of insurance or severity of illness).
- *Process measures* include the ways in which clinicians and patients interact and the appropriateness of medical treatment for a specific patient.
- *Outcomes measures* include changes in patients' current and future health status, including health-related quality of life and satisfaction with care.

The indicators included in the QA Tools system are primarily process indicators. We deliberately chose such indicators because the system was designed to assess care for which we can hold providers responsible. However, we collect data on a number of intermediate outcomes measures (for example, glycosylated hemoglobin, blood pressure, and cholesterol) that could be used to construct intermediate clinical outcomes indicators. In many instances, the measures included in the QA

Tools system are used to determine whether interventions have been provided in response to poor performance on such measures (for instance, whether persons who fail to control their blood sugar on dietary therapy are offered oral hypoglycemic therapy).

The Expert Panel Process

We convened expert panels to evaluate the indicators and to make final selections using the RAND/UCLA Appropriateness Method, a modified Delphi method developed at RAND and UCLA (Brook 1994). In general, the method quantitatively assesses the expert judgment of a group of clinicians regarding the indicators by using a scale with values ranging from 1 to 9.

The method is iterative with two rounds of anonymous ratings of the indicators by the panel and a face-to-face group discussion between rounds. Each panelist has equal weight in determining the final result: the quality indicators that will be included in the QA Tools system.

The RAND/UCLA Appropriateness Method has been shown to have a reproducibility consistent with that of well accepted diagnostic tests such as the interpretation of coronary angiography and screening mammography (Shekelle et al., 1998a). It has also been shown to have content, construct, and predictive validity in other applications (Brook, 1994; Shekelle et al., 1998b; Kravitz et al., 1995; Selby et al., 1996).

Approximately six weeks before the panel meeting, we sent panelists the reviews of the literature, the staff-proposed quality indicators, and separate rating sheets for each clinical area. We asked the panelists to examine the literature review and rate each indicator on a nine-point scale on each of two dimensions: validity and feasibility.

A quality indicator is defined as valid if:

1. Adequate scientific evidence or professional consensus exists supporting the indicator.

2. There are identifiable health benefits to patients who receive care specified by the indicator.

3. Based on the panelists' professional experience, health professionals with significantly higher rates of adherence to an indicator would be considered higher-quality providers

4. The majority of factors that determine adherence to an indicator are under the control of the health professional (or are subject to influence by the health professional—for example, smoking cessation).

Ratings of 1-3 mean that the indicator is not a valid criterion for evaluating quality. Ratings of 4-6 mean that the indicator is an uncertain or equivocal criterion for evaluating quality. Ratings of 7-9 mean that the indicator is clearly a valid criterion for evaluating quality.

A quality indicator is defined as feasible if:

1. The information necessary to determine adherence is likely to be found in a typical medical record.

2. Estimates of adherence to the indicator based on medical record data are likely to be reliable and unbiased.

3. Failure to document relevant information about the indicator is itself a marker for poor quality.

Ratings of 1-3 mean that it is not feasible to use the indicator for evaluating quality. Ratings of 4-6 mean that there will be considerable variability in the feasibility of using the indicator to evaluate quality. Ratings of 7-9 mean that it is clearly feasible to use the indicator for evaluating quality.

The first round of indicators was rated by the panelists individually in their own offices. The indicators were returned to RAND staff and the results of the first round were summarized. We encouraged panelists to comment on the literature reviews, the definitions of key terms, and the indicators. We also encouraged them to suggest additions or deletions to the indicators.

At the panel meeting, participants discussed each clinical area in turn, focusing on the evidence, or lack thereof, that supports or refutes each indicator and the panelists' prior validity rankings. Panelists had before them the summary of the panel's first round ratings and a confidential reminder of their own ratings.

The summary consisted of a printout of the rating sheet with the distribution of ratings by panelists displayed above the rating line (without revealing the identity of the panelists) and a caret (^) marking the individual panelist's own rating in the first round displayed below the line. An example of the printout received by panelists is shown in Figure I.1.

panelist _; round 1; page 1   **September 14, 1997**

Chapter 1
ASTHMA   Validity   Feasibility

DIAGNOSIS

3. Spirometry should be measured in patients   1   1 2 3 1 1   3 4 2
with chronic asthma at least every 2 years.   1 2 3 4 5 6 7 8 9   1 2 3 4 5 6 7 8 9   (1- 2)
                                                              ^   ^

TREATMENT

7. Patients requiring chronic treatment with
systemic corticosteroids during any 12 month
period should have been prescribed inhaled
corticosteroids during the same 12 month   1 6   2   2 3 4
period.   1 2 3 4 5 6 7 8 9   1 2 3 4 5 6 7 8 9   (3- 4)
                                                              ^   ^

10. All patients seen for an acute asthma
exacerbation should be evaluated with a
complete history including all of the
following: 2 2 2   3   2 2   1 1 3
    a. time of onset   1 2 3 4 5 6 7 8 9   1 2 3 4 5 6 7 8 9   (5- 6)
                                                              ^   ^

                                                      4 1 4   3 1 5
    b. all current medications   1 2 3 4 5 6 7 8 9   1 2 3 4 5 6 7 8 9   (7- 8)
                                                              ^   ^

    c. prior hospitalizations and emergency   5 1 3   5 1 3
       department visits for asthma   1 2 3 4 5 6 7 8 9   1 2 3 4 5 6 7 8 9   (9-10)
                                                              ^   ^

    d. prior episodes of respiratory   1 1 3 2 2   1   2   3 1 2
       insufficiency due to asthma   1 2 3 4 5 6 7 8 9   1 2 3 4 5 6 7 8 9   (11-12)
                                                              ^   ^

Scales: 1 = low validity or feasibility; 9 = high validity or feasibility

Figure I.1 Sample Panelist Summary Rating Sheet

Panelists were encouraged to bring to the discussion any relevant published information that the literature reviews had omitted. In a few cases, they supplied this information which was, in turn, discussed. In several cases, the indicators were reworded or otherwise clarified to better fit clinical judgment.

After further discussion, all indicators in each clinical area were re-ranked for validity. These final round rankings were analyzed in a manner similar to past applications of the RAND/UCLA Appropriateness Method (Park et al., 1986; Brook, 1994). The median panel rating and measure of dispersion were used to categorize indicators on validity.

We regarded panel members as being in *disagreement* when at least three members of the panel judged an indicator as being in the highest tertile of validity (that is, having a rating of 7, 8, or 9) and three members rated it as being in the lowest tertile of validity (1, 2, or 3) (Brook, 1994). Indicators with a median validity rating of 7 or higher without disagreement were included in the system.

We also obtained ratings from the panelists about the feasibility of obtaining the data necessary to score the indicators from medical. This was done to make explicit that failure to document key variables required for determining eligibility or scoring of an indicator would be treated as though the recommended care was not provided.

Although we do not intend for quality assessment to impose significant additional documentation burdens, we wanted the panel to acknowledge that documentation itself is an element of quality particularly when patients are treated by a team of health professionals. Because of the variability in documentation patterns and the opportunity to empirically evaluate feasibility, indicators with a median feasibility rating of 4 and higher were accepted into the system. Indicators had to satisfy both the validity and feasibility criteria.

Five expert panels were convened on the topics of children's care, care for women 18-50, general medicine for adults, oncologic conditions and HIV, and cardiopulmonary conditions.

The dates on which the panels were conducted are shown in Table I.2.

Table I.2

Dates Expert Panels Convened

Children	October 1995
Women	November 1995
Cardiopulmonary	September 1997
Oncology/HIV	October 1997
General Medicine	November 1997

Tables I.3 through I.6 summarize the distribution of indicators by level of evidence, type of care (preventive, acute, chronic), function of medicine (screening, diagnosis, treatment, follow-up, continuity), and modality (for example, history, physical examination, laboratory test, medication) (Malin et al., 2000; Schuster et al., 1997).

The categories were selected by the research team and reflect terminology commonly used by health services researchers to describe different aspects of health service delivery. The categories also reflect the areas in which we intend to develop aggregate quality of care scores. However, a significant benefit of the QA Tools system is its adaptability to other frameworks.

Note: In the following tables, the figures in some columns may not total exactly 100 percent due to the rounding of fractional numbers.

Table I.3

Distribution of Indicators (%) by Level of Evidence

Level of Evidence	Children	Women	Cancer/HIV	Cardio-pulmonary	General Medicine
Randomized trials	11	22	22	18	23
Nonrandomized trials	6	16	37	4	17
Descriptive studies	72	59	26	71	57
Added by panel	12	4	15	7	4
Total	100	100	100	100	101

Table I.4

Distribution of Indicators (%) by Type of Care

Type of Care	Children	Women	Cancer/HIV	Cardio-pulmonary	General Medicine
Preventive	30	11	20	3	18
Acute	36	49	7	26	38
Chronic	34	41	74	71	44
Total	100	101	101	100	100

Table I.5

Distribution of Indicators (%) by Function of Medicine

Function of Medicine	Children	Women	Cancer/HIV	Cardio-pulmonary	General Medicine
Screening	23	18	9	3	12
Diagnosis	31	30	27	54	41
Treatment	36	43	53	36	41
Follow-up	10	12	10	8	6
Total	100	103	99	101	100

Table I.6

Distribution of Indicators (%) by Modality

Modality	Children	Women	Cancer/HIV	Cardio-pulmonary	General Medicine
History	19	18	4	11	23
Physical	19	10	5	21	15
Lab/Radiology	21	23	24	23	18
Medication	25	29	25	25	26
Other	17	19	42	20	17
Total	101	99	100	100	99

DEVELOPING QUALITY INDICATORS FOR CHILDREN AND ADOLESCENTS

We now describe in more detail the process by which we developed quality indicators for children and adolescents.

Selecting Clinical Areas

We began by examining national data sources to identify the leading causes of mortality, morbidity, and functional limitation among children and adolescents. The principal data sources for this review were Vital Statistics, the National Health Interview Survey (NHIS), the National Ambulatory Medical Care Survey (NAMCS), and the National Hospital Discharge Survey (NHDS). From the leading causes of morbidity and mortality, we selected areas that would be representative of primary, secondary, and tertiary care.

We completed literature reviews and proposed quality of care criteria for the following children's health conditions (in alphabetical order):

- Acne
- Adolescent preventive services
- Allergic rhinitis
- Asthma
- Attention deficit/hyperactivity disorder
- Cesarean delivery*
- Depression*
- Developmental screening
- Diabetes mellitus*
- Diarrheal disease
- Family planning/contraception*
- Fever without source of infection in children under 3 years of age
- Headache*
- Immunizations
- Otitis media
- Prenatal care*
- Sickle cell screening and select topics in prevention of complications
- Tuberculosis screening
- Upper respiratory infections*
- Urinary tract infections
- Vaginitis and sexually transmitted diseases*

- Well child care[*]

The system is designed to evaluate services for a substantial portion of the ambulatory care received by the population. In order to determine the percentage of ambulatory care visits the indicator system would cover, we classified the 1993 NAMCS data ICD-9 codes for children 0 to 18 years of age into the 21 conditions for which we developed quality indicators (see Table I-7).

Table I.7 takes a fairly broad approach to categorizing an area as "included" in the quality indicators. The diagnoses with the highest frequency include upper respiratory tract infections, well child care, and allergic rhinitis. By developing indicators for the 21 pediatric clinical areas listed in the table, we will capture more than one-half (55 percent) of all the diagnoses in the 1993 NAMCS data.

---

[*] The indicators for these clinical areas were originally developed for the women's health panel and then modified to apply to adolescents (defined for the study as age 13 or older).

Table I.7

**Estimated Proportion of Ambulatory Care Conditions to be Evaluated
in the QA Tools Indicator System, Based on 1993 NAMCS Data**

Clinical Area*	Frequency of Visits	Percentage of Total
Acne (11-18)	151	2.7
Adolescent Preventive Services (11-18)	115	2.1
Allergic Rhinitis (2-18)	344	6.2
Asthma (0-18)	333	6.0
Attention Deficit Hyperactivity Disorder (3-18)	175	3.1
Depression (11-18)	48	0.9
Developmental Screening (0-12)	95	1.7
Diabetes Mellitis (11-18)	2	0.0
Diarrheal Disease, Acute (0-2)	26	0.5
Family Planning/Contraception (11-18)	6	0.1
Fever without Source (0-2)	14	0.3
Headache (11-18)	28	0.5
Immunizations (0-18)	19	0.3
Medication Allergies (0-18)	0	0.0
Otitis Media (1-3)	247	4.4
Sickle Cell Disease (0-5)	1	0.0
Tuberculosis (0-18)	3	0.1
Upper Respiratory Tract Infections (2-18)	740	13.2
Urinary Tract Infections (0-12)	28	0.5
Vaginitis and STDs (12-18)	63	1.1
Well Child Care (0-12)	578	10.3
Visits with codes applicable to more than one clinical area	58	1.0
Total Included	3,074	55.0
Overall Total	5,592	

*Includes covered age range expressed in years.

Developing Indicators

In each clinical area, we developed indicators to define the
explicit criteria by which quality of care in managed care plans would
be evaluated. Indicators were developed for screening, diagnosis,
treatment, and follow-up.

The indicator tables at the end of each chapter of this book

- note the population to which the indicators apply

- define the indicator itself
- provide a "grade" for the quality of the scientific evidence that supports the indicator
- list the specific literature used to support the indicator
- provide a statement of the health benefits of complying with the indicator
- give comments to further explain the purpose or reasoning behind the indicator.

The indicators were developed by the research staff person(s) responsible for summarizing the literature. Every indicator table was then reviewed by Drs. Kerr and McGlynn for content, consistency, and the likely availability of information necessary to score adherence to the indicator from the medical record.

Selecting Panel Participants

We requested nominations for expert panel participants from the American Academy of Pediatrics, the American Academy of Family Practice, the Ambulatory Pediatrics Association, and the Society for Adolescent Medicine. RAND research staff also made a few supplemental recommendations. We received 70 nominations from the professional societies.

We sent each nominee a letter summarizing the purpose of the project and what group recommended them. Interested candidates were asked to return a curriculum vitae and calendar with available dates for a two-day panel meeting. We received 53 positive responses from potential panelists. The quality of the recommended panelists was excellent.

We sought to assemble a panel that was diverse with respect to type of practice (academic, solo community practice, managed care organizational practice), geographic location, and specialty. Because of the wide variety of medical conditions that would be considered by the panel, we decided on a specialty distribution of four general pediatricians, two family practitioners, two adolescent medicine specialists, and one pediatric infectious disease specialist. A general pediatrician (Dr. Bergman) chaired the panel.

Selecting the Final Indicators

The expert panel process was conducted as described earlier in this Introduction.

The panelists' ratings sheet for each condition is shown in Appendix B. For example, Figure I.2 shows the ratings sheet for adolescent preventive services. The chapter number and clinical condition is shown in the top left margin. The rating bar is numbered from 1 to 9, indicating the range of possible responses. The number shown above each of the responses in the rating bar indicates how many panelists provided that particular rating for the indicator. Below the score distribution, in parentheses, the median and the mean absolute deviation from the median are listed. Each dimension is assigned an A (for "Agreement"), D (for "Disagreement"), or an I (for "Indeterminate") based on the score distribution.

We recommend caution when reviewing the ratings for each indicator. The overall median does not tell us anything about the extent to which these indicators occur in clinical practice. To determine that, actual clinical data to assess the indicators must be collected and analyzed.

Staff proposed 572 indicators for panel evaluation. Before final scoring by the panel, 82 indicators were removed from the set or merged with others in the set and 67 were added or split (19 of the additions were made at the panel meeting). In addition, 98 indicators underwent substantial change (for instance, change of time frame or logic). Among the 557 pediatric indicators available for final scoring, 453 (81 percent) were retained. Eighty-seven indicators were removed for low validity, 1 for low feasibility, 5 for substantial disagreement on validity or feasibility scores, and 11 by consensus.

A crosswalk table including the original indicators proposed by staff, the modified indicators (based on panel input), and comments explaining any changes (additions, deletions, or modifications) to the indicators as well as their final disposition is provided in Appendix C. This table is useful for tracking the progress of indicator development and selection.

Because the quality indicators are designed to produce aggregate scores, it is useful to examine the distribution of indicators by

- type of care (preventive, acute, and chronic)
- function of medical care (screening, diagnosis, treatment, and follow-up)
- modality of care delivery (history, physical examination, laboratory study, medication, other intervention such as counseling, education, procedure, psychotherapy, surgery, and other contact such as general follow-up, referral to subspecialist, or hospitalization).

Indicators are assigned to one type of care, but can have up to two functions or three modalities.

panelist 10; round 2; page 3   Mon Mar 25 14:22:10 1996

Chapter 2
QUALITY INDICATORS FOR ADOLESCENT PREVENTIVE SERVICES

                                                          Validity   Feasibility

(SCREENING)

General

1. Between the ages of 11 and 18 years, all adolescents should have an
annual visit at which risk assessment/preventive services were discussed.
    Validity: 1 1   1 2 1 3 / 1 2 3 4 5 6 7 8 9   (7.0, 2.0, I)
    Feasibility: 1   3 4 / 1 2 3 4 5 6 7 8 9   (8.0, 1.4, A)
    (1- 3)

2. Confidentiality should be discussed and documented by age 14
or at the first visit afterwards.
    Validity: 1   1 1 5 / 1 2 3 4 5 6 7 8 9   (8.0, 1.6, I)
    Feasibility: 1 1 1 3 1 1 / 1 2 3 4 5 6 7 8 9   (5.0, 1.4, I)
    (4- 6)

2. Weight and height should be measured at least once a year and
plotted on a growth chart.
    Validity: 1 1   1 6 / 1 2 3 4 5 6 7 8 9   (9.0, 1.1, A)
    Feasibility: 1 5 3 / 1 2 3 4 5 6 7 8 9   (8.0, 0.4, A)
    (7- 9)

Substance Abuse Screening

3. Documentation of discussion of substance use (tobacco, alcohol,
marijuana, other illicit drugs, anabolic steroids) or of the
adolescent's history should occur annually.
    Validity: 1 1 1   1 5 / 1 2 3 4 5 6 7 8 9   (9.0, 1.8, I)
    Feasibility: 1   2   2 2 2 / 1 2 3 4 5 6 7 8 9   (7.0, 1.9, I)
    (10- 12)

3. There should be documentation that the risks of anabolic
steroid use were discussed or a history of anabolic steroid use
was taken for adolescent males participating in team sports or
weight-training at least once a year.
    Validity: 1 2 3 4 5 6 7 8 9   (,)
    Feasibility: 1 2 3 4 5 6 7 8 9   (,)
    (13- 15)

Sexually Transmitted Diseases and HIV Prevention

4. Documentation of discussion of sexual activity and risk
reduction should occur annually.
    Validity: 1   1   3 4 / 1 2 3 4 5 6 7 8 9   (8.0, 1.6, A)
    Feasibility: 1 1   2 4 / 1 2 3 4 5 6 7 8 9   (8.0, 2.1, I)
    (16- 18)

5. Patients for whom the medical records indicate that they have
ever been sexually active should be asked the following
questions: if they currently have a single sexual partner; if
they have had more than 2 sexual partners in the past 6 months;
and if they have had a history of any STDs.
    Validity: 1 1   1 2 1 3 / 1 2 3 4 5 6 7 8 9   (7.0, 1.8, I)
    Feasibility: 1 2 1 1 1 1 2 / 1 2 3 4 5 6 7 8 9   (5.0, 2.1, D)
    (19- 21)

Injury Prevention

7. Documentation of discussion of injury prevention should occur
annually.
    Validity: 1   2 3 4 / 1 2 3 4 5 6 7 8 9   (8.0, 1.7, A)
    Feasibility: 1 1   2 3 1 / 1 2 3 4 5 6 7 8 9   (7.0, 2.0, I)
    (22- 24)

8. Patients should receive counseling regarding the use of seat
belts annually.
    Validity: 1 1 1 1 1 2 1 / 1 2 3 4 5 6 7 8 9   (6.0, 2.2, I)
    Feasibility: 1 2   2 1 2 1 / 1 2 3 4 5 6 7 8 9   (4.0, 1.7, I)
    (25- 27)

Hyperlipidemia Screening

9. Documentation of parental history of hypercholesterolemia
should be sought.
    Validity: 2 3 2   1 / 1 2 3 4 5 6 7 8 9   (3.0, 1.6, I)
    Feasibility: 2 3   2 1 / 1 2 3 4 5 6 7 8 9   (2.0, 1.8, I)
    (28- 30)

10. Adolescents whose parents have a serum cholesterol level
greater than 240 mg/dl should receive a total blood cholesterol
screen.
    Validity: 2 4   2 1 / 1 2 3 4 5 6 7 8 9   (3.0, 2.2, D)
    Feasibility: 2   1 1 2 1 / 1 2 3 4 5 6 7 8 9   (4.0, 2.4, D)
    (31- 33)

11. Documentation of parents' or grandparents' history of coronary artery
disease (CAD), peripheral vascular disease (PVD), cerebrovascular disease
or sudden cardiac death at age 55 or younger should occur annually.
    Validity: 1 3   1 2 1 1 / 1 2 3 4 5 6 7 8 9   (4.0, 2.0, I)
    Feasibility: 1 1 1 2 1 1 1 / 1 2 3 4 5 6 7 8 9   (4.0, 1.9, I)
    (34- 36)

Scales: 1 = low validity or feasibility;   9 = high validity or feasibility.

Figure I.2 - Sample Rating Results Sheet

Analyzing the Final Set of Indicators

As indicated in Table I.8, of the final set of 453 indicators, 30 percent are considered preventive care, 36 percent acute care, and 34 percent chronic care. When categorized by function, two-thirds of the indicators fell into the diagnosis and treatment categories. Finally, there was a fairly even distribution of indicators by modality, with 19 percent each in the history and physical examination categories, 21 percent in the laboratory or radiologic study category, 25 percent in medications, and the remainder in other interventions and contacts.

Table I.8

**Distribution of Final Set of Pediatric Indicators by
Type of Care, Function, and Modality**

Category	Pediatric Indicators (%) (n=453)
Clinical Area	
Preventive	30
Acute	36
Chronic	34
Function	
Screening	23
Diagnosis	31
Treatment	36
Follow-up	10
Modality	
History	19
Physical Examination	19
Laboratory or Radiologic Study	21
Medication	25
Other Intervention	8
Other Contact	9

Note: Percentages may not add to 100% due to rounding.

As noted earlier (see Table I.3), each indicator was assigned a strength of evidence code of I (randomized controlled trial [RCT]), II (nonrandomized controlled trial, cohort or case-control study, multiple time series), or III (expert opinion or descriptive study). Table I.9 outlines the distribution of the indicators by strength of evidence for the original indicators proposed by staff, the indicators that were voted on by panelists, and the final set of indicators.

The majority (72 percent) of the final set of 453 indicators was based on expert opinion or descriptive studies. Nine percent of the indicators were based on RCTs and 6 percent on nonrandomized controlled trials. However, it is interesting to note that panelists were more likely to retain indicators based on RCTs or nonrandomized controlled trials than on expert opinion or descriptive studies.

Table I.9

Distribution of Pediatric Indicators by Strength of Evidence

Strength of Evidence*	Original % (n)		Voted On % (n)		After Vote % (n)	
I	10	(60)	10	(57)	11	(52)
II	5	(29)	5	(28)	6	(28)
III	84	(483)	76	(418)	72	(327)
N/A			10	(54)	12	(46)
Total**	100	(572)	100	(557)	100	(453)

*I indicates randomized controlled trial; II nonrandomized controlled trial, cohort or case-control study, multiple time series; III expert opinion or descriptive study; NA, indicator for which strength of evidence is not available because it was added after literature reviews were completed.

**Percentages may not total 100% due to rounding.

ORGANIZATION OF THIS DOCUMENT

The rest of this volume is organized as follows:

- Each chapter summarizes
  - results of the literature review for one condition
  - provides a table of the staff recommended indicators based on that review
  - lists the cited studies.
- *Appendix A* provides definitions of terms used in the indicator tables.

- *Appendix B* contains the panel rating sheets for each condition.
- *Appendix C* shows the original proposed definition of each indicator, notes any modifications resulting from the panel process, and provides additional comments, including whether the panel adopted or rejected the indicator.

REFERENCES

Asch, S. M., E. A. Kerr, E. G. Hamilton, J. L. Reifel, E. A. McGlynn (eds.), *Quality of Care for Oncologic Conditions and HIV: A Review of the Literature and Quality Indicators,* Santa Monica, CA: RAND, MR-1281-AHRQ, 2000.

Brook, R. H., "The RAND/UCLA Appropriateness Method," *Clinical Practice Guideline Development: methodology perspectives,* AHCPR Pub. No. 95-0009, Rockville, MD: Public Health Service, 1994.

Kerr E. A., S. M. Asch, E. G. Hamilton, E. A. McGlynn (eds.), *Quality of Care for Cardiopulmonary Conditions: A Review of the Literature and Quality Indicators,* Santa Monica, CA: RAND, MR-1282-AHRQ, 2000a.

Kerr E. A., S. M. Asch, E. G. Hamilton, E. A. McGlynn (eds.), *Quality of Care for General Medical Conditions: A Review of the Literature and Quality Indicators,* Santa Monica, CA: RAND, MR-1280-AHRQ, 2000b.

Kravitz R. L., M. Laouri, J. P. Kahan, P. Guzy, et al., "Validity of Criteria Used for Detecting Underuse of Coronary Revascularization," *JAMA* 274(8):632-638, 1995.

Malin, J. L., S. M. Asch, E. A. Kerr, E. A. McGlynn. "Evaluating the Quality of Cancer Care: Development of Cancer Quality Indicators for a Global Quality Assessment Tool," *Cancer* 88:701-7, 2000.

McGlynn E. A., E. A. Kerr, C. Damberg, S. M. Asch (eds.), *Quality of Care for Women: A Review of Selected Clinical Conditions and Quality Indicators,* Santa Monica, CA: RAND, MR-1284-HCFA, 2000.

Park R. A., Fink A., Brook R. H., Chassin M. R., et al., "Physician Ratings of Appropriate Indications for Six Medical and Surgical Procedures," *AJPH* 76(7):766-772, 1986.

Schuster M. A., S. M. Asch, E. A. McGlynn, et al., "Development of a Quality of Care Measurement System for Children and Adolescents: Methodological Considerations and Comparisons With a System for Adult Women," *Archives of Pediatrics and Adolescent Medicine* 151:1085-1092, 1997.

Selby J. V., B. H. Fireman, R. J. Lundstrom, et al., "Variation among Hospitals in Coronary-Angiography Practices and Outcomes after Myocardial Infarction in a Large Health Maintenance Organization," *N Engl J Med* 335:1888-96, 1996.

Shekelle P. G., J. P. Kahan, S. J. Bernstein, et al., "The Reproducibility of a Method to Identify the Overuse and Underuse of Medical Procedures," *N Engl J Med* 338:1888-1895, 1998b.

Shekelle P. G., M. R. Chassin, R. E. Park, "Assessing the Predictive
Validity of the RAND/UCLA Appropriateness Method Criteria for
Performing Carotid Endarterectomy," *Int J Technol Assess Health
Care* 14(4):707-727, 1998a.

1. ACNE

Lisa Schmidt, M.P.H., and Eve A. Kerr, M.D.

Approach

The general approach to summarizing the key literature on acne in adolescents and adult women was to review two adolescent health text books (Vernon and Lane, 1992; Paller et al., 1992) and two articles chosen from a MEDLINE search of all English language articles published between the years of 1990 and 1995 on the treatment of acne.

IMPORTANCE

Acne is the most common skin disorder seen during adolescence. Forty percent of children between the ages of 8 and 10 develop early acne lesions, and eventually 85 percent of adolescents develop some degree of acne (Vernon and Lane, 1992; Paller et al., 1992). Acne can persist into mid-adulthood in some persons, and can also present initially in adulthood. It is estimated that 40 to 50 percent of adult women are affected by a low-grade persistent form of acne (Nguyen et al., 1994). Overall, acne affects approximately 10 percent of the U.S. population (Glassman et al., 1993). Acne was the most common reason for visits to dermatologists over the two-year period from 1989 to 1990, accounting for 16.6 percent of all visits (Nelson, 1994). Although acne is not associated with severe morbidity, mortality, or disability it can produce psychological effects. For instance, it has been reported that some adolescents with acne avoid social situations or athletic activities (Brook et al., 1980). Furthermore, in severe cases, acne can lead to physical scarring which may exacerbate the emotional effects of the disease.

EFFICACY AND/OR EFFECTIVENESS OF INTERVENTIONS

Screening

There is no role for screening for acne.

Diagnosis

Common acne is a disorder of the pilosebaceous glands and is characterized by follicular occlusion and inflammation (Paller et al., 1992). Acne occurs primarily on the face, but it can occur on the back, chest, and shoulders. Four factors contribute to the development of acne: 1) the sebum excretion rate, 2) sebaceous lipid composition, 3) bacteriology of the pilosebaceous duct, and 4) obstruction of the pilosebaceous duct. The anaerobic bacterium *Propionibacterium acnes* appears to play an important role in the pathogenesis of acne (Paller et al., 1992). *P. acnes* is capable of releasing lipolytic enzymes that convert the triglycerides in sebum into irritating fatty acids and glycerol, which may contribute to inflammation (Paller et al., 1992).

There are six types of acne lesions: comedones, papules, pustules, nodules, cysts, and scars. Individual patients may have one or more predominant type of lesion or a mixture of many lesions (Paller et al., 1992).

Vernon and Lane (1992) and Glassman et al. (1993) recommend the following in diagnosing acne:

Documentation of the acne history including:

- age at onset of acne;
- location (face, back, neck, chest);
- aggravating factors (stress, seasons, cosmetics, cremes);
- menstrual history and premenstrual worsening of acne;
- previous treatments;
- family history of acne; and
- medications and drug use.

The physical examination should include:

- location of acne;
- types of lesions present;
- severity of disease (numbers of each type of lesion and intensity of inflammation); and
- complications (extent and severity of hyperpigmentation and scarring).

Treatment

Medical treatment of acne is determined by the extent and severity of disease, prior treatments, and therapeutic goals. Each regimen must be followed for a minimum of 4 to 6 weeks before determining whether it is effective (Vernon and Lane, 1992). Table 1.1 lists guidelines to be used in the treatment of acne.

Table 1.1

Guidelines for the Treatment of Acne

Clinical Appearance	Treatment
Comedonal Acne - no inflammatory lesions	Topical tretinoin *or* benzoyl peroxide
Mild to Moderate Inflammatory Acne - red papules, few pustules	Topical tretinoin *and* benzoyl peroxide *and/or* topical antibiotic If acne is resistant to above therapy, add oral antibiotic.
Moderate to Severe Inflammatory Acne - red papules, many pustules	Topical tretinoin; topical antibiotic *or* benzoyl peroxide; *and* oral antibiotics
Severe Nodulocystic Acne - red papules, pustules, cysts and nodules	Topical tretinoin; benzoyl peroxide *or* topical antibiotic; oral antibiotics; *and* consider isotretinoin

Adapted from: Weston and Lane, 1991; Vernon and Lane 1992; Nguyen, 1994; Taylor, 1991.

Tretinoin and Benzoyl Peroxide

Topical keratolytic therapy is recommended as the primary treatment for comedonal acne to prevent new acne lesions as well as to treat preexisting ones (Paller et al., 1992). Two classes of keratolytics, tretinoin (retin A) and benzoyl peroxide, can be used alone or in combination with each other and will control 80 to 85 percent of acne (Taylor, 1991; Weston and Lane, 1991; Nguyen, 1994). Cream preparations of both tretinoin and benzoyl peroxide should be used because they are less irritating to the skin than gel forms. Tretinoin has a propensity to severely irritate the skin if used incorrectly. To avoid irritation, a low strength (0.025 percent) cream should be applied every other night for one week and then nightly. In addition, because skin treated with tretinoin is more sensitive to sun exposure, sunscreen should be used.

Tretinoin should be avoided during pregnancy because of the potential of photoisomerization to isotretinoin (a teratogen) (Weston and Lane, 1991; Vernon and Lane, 1992).

Improvement of acne after treatment of tretinoin can take six to twelve weeks and flare-ups of acne can occur during the first few weeks due to surfacing of the lesions onto the skin (Nguyen, 1994). Benzoyl peroxide is available over-the-counter in various strengths and applications (gels, creams, lotions, or soaps). All concentrations seem to be therapeutically equivalent (Nguyen, 1994). Mild redness and scaling of the skin may occur during the first week of use.

Topical Antibiotics

Topical antibiotics decrease the quantity of *P. acnes* in the hair follicles. However, they are less effective than oral antibiotics because of their low solubility and consequent difficulty in penetrating sebum-filled follicules (Nguyen, 1994). Topical erythromycin and clindamycin are similar in efficacy and can be used once or twice a day (Weston, and Lane, 1991; Nguyen, 1994). Some percutaneous absorption may rarely occur with clindamycin, resulting in diarrhea and colitis (Weston and Lane, 1991; Nguyen, 1994). Topical antibiotics are frequently used in combination with keratolytics and are most useful for maintenance therapy if improvement after 1 to 2 months of oral antibiotics is observed (Weston and Lane, 1991).

Oral Antibiotics

Patients with moderate to severe inflammatory acne will require oral antibiotics in addition to topical therapy. Tetracycline and erythromycin are the most commonly used systemic antibiotics. Because tetracycline can cause enamel hyperplasia and tooth discoloration it should not be used in pregnant women or in children under 12 years of age (Nguyen, 1994). Minocycline is very effective for many adolescents who have used tetracycline without success (Weston and Lane, 1991). The cost of minocycline, however, limits its use to those patients with severe or recalcitrant acne. When tetracycline is prescribed for female patients, pregnancy status must be monitored since tetracycline is teratogenic (Glassman et al., 1993). There is the potential for broad-spectrum antibiotics to alter the absorption of oral contraceptives (OCs); therefore, it may be prudent for women on OCs to use an alternate method of birth control when possible.

Isotretinoin

The oral retinoid isotretinoin has been very efficacious in nodulocystic acne resistant to standard therapeutic regimens. In appropriate regimens, isotretinoin has resulted in long-term remission of acne in approximately 60 percent of patients treated (Weston and Lane, 1991). However, it is not recommended as the drug of first choice because of its severe teratogenicity. Current recommendations for women of child-bearing age are: to obtain informed consent; to perform pregnancy tests throughout treatment; to postpone initiating therapy until the menstrual cycle begins; and, to use two effective birth control methods from the month before treatment to one month after discontinuing treatment (Weston and Lane, 1991). Side effects of isotretinoin include dryness and scaliness of the skin, dry lips and occasionally dry eyes and nose. It can also cause decreased night vision, hypertriglyceridemia, abnormal liver function, electrolyte imbalance, and elevated platelet count. Glassman et al. (1993) recommend monthly liver function tests to monitor potential for liver toxicity. Up to 10 percent of patients experience mild hair loss, but the effect is reversible (Weston and Lane, 1991).

Follow-up

Follow-up visits for acne should be scheduled initially every 4 to 6 weeks. Ideal control is defined as no more than a few new lesions every two weeks (Weston and Lane, 1991).

RECOMMENDED QUALITY INDICATORS FOR ACNE

The following criteria apply to adolescents ages 13-18.

Diagnosis

	Indicator	Quality of evidence	Literature	Benefits	Comments
1.	For all patients presenting with acne, the following history should be documented in their chart: • location of lesions (back, face, neck, chest) • aggravating factors (stress, seasons, cosmetics, creams) • menstrual history and premenstrual worsening of acne • previous treatments • medications and drug use	III	Paller et al., 1992; Vernon and Lane, 1992	Improve acne; decrease psychological effects of acne; and, decrease potential physical scarring.	An adequate history is necessary to determine any potential causes or exacerbating factors of the acne and to document severity and response to treatments.

Treatment

	Indicator	Quality of evidence	Literature	Benefits	Comments
2.	If oral antibiotics are prescribed, there must be documentation of moderate to severe acne (papules and pustules).	III	Vernon and Lane, 1992; Glassman et al., 1993; Weston and Lane, 1991	Improve acne; decrease psychological effects of acne; and, decrease potential physical scarring.	If only comedones are present, antibiotics should not be prescribed since they are not effective for comedones and have potential toxicities.
3.	Tetracycline should not be prescribed for adolescents less than 12 years of age.	III	Nguyen, 1994	Prevent tooth discoloration.	
4.	If tetracycline is prescribed, there must be documentation of the last menstrual period or a negative pregnancy test for all girls who have reached puberty.	III	Vernon and Lane, 1992	Prevent birth defects.	Tetracycline is a known teratogen.
5.	If isotretinoin is prescribed, there must be documentation of severe acne (papules, pustules, cysts and nodules) and failure of previous therapy.	III	Vernon and Lane, 1992; Glassman et al., 1993; Weston and Lane, 1991; Nguyen, 1994	Improve acne; decrease psychological effects of acne; and, decrease potential physical scarring.	Isotretinoin has severe teratogenic effects and potential for liver toxicity. Its use should be restricted to those with severe, recalcitrant nodulocystic acne.

32

Indicator	Quality of evidence	Literature	Benefits	Comments
6. If isotretinoin is prescribed, a negative serum pregnancy test should be obtained within two weeks of start of therapy.	III	Vernon and Lane, 1992; Glassman et al., 1993; Weston and Lane, 1991	Prevent teratogenic effects to fetus.	Isotretinoin has severe teratogenic effects.
7. If isotretinoin is prescribed, there should be documentation that counseling regarding use of an effective means of contraception (including abstinence) was provided.	III	Weston and Lane, 1991	Prevent teratogenic effects to fetus.	Isotretinoin has severe teratogenic effects.

Follow-up

Indicator	Quality of evidence	Literature	Benefits	Comments
8. If isotretinoin is prescribed, monthly serum pregnancy tests should be performed.	III	Vernon and Lane, 1992; Glassman et al., 1993; Weston and Lane, 1991	Prevent teratogenic effects to fetus.	Isotretinoin has severe teratogenic effects.
9. If isotretinoin is prescribed, monthly liver function tests should be performed.	III	Glassman et al., 1993	Prevent liver disease.	Isotretinoin has the potential effects on the liver such as toxicity or failure.

Quality of Evidence Codes:

I: RCT
II-1:   Nonrandomized controlled trials
II-2:   Cohort or case analysis
II-3:   Multiple time series
III: Opinions or descriptive studies

REFERENCES - ACNE

Brook, RH, KN Lohr, GA Goldberg, et al. 1980. *Conceptualization and Measurement of Physiologic Health for Adults: Acne*. RAND, Santa Monica, CA.

Glassman, PA, D Garcia, and JP Delafield. 1993. *Outpatient Care Handbook*. Philadelphia, PA: Hanley and Belfus, Inc.

Nelson, C. 10 March 1994. Office visits to dermatologists: National Ambulatory Medical Care Survey, United States, 1989-90. *Advance Data*. National Center for Health Statistics. U.S. Department of Health and Human Services, Hyattsville, MD.

Nguyen QH, YA Kim, RA Schwartz, et al. July 1994. Management of acne vulgaris. *American Family Physician* 50 (1): 89-96.

Paller AS, EA Abel, and IJ Frieden. 1992. Dermatologic problems. In *Comprehensive Adolescent Health Care*. Editors Friedman SB, M Fisher, and SK Schonberg, 584-64. St. Louis, MO: Quality Medical Publishing, Inc.

Taylor MB. June 1991. Treatment of acne vulgaris. *Postgraduate Medicine* 89 (8): 40-7.

Vernon HJ, and AT Lane. 1992. Skin disorders. In *Textbook of Adolescent Medicine*. Editors McAnarney ER, RE Kreipe, DP Orr, et al., 272-82. Philadelphia, PA: W.B. Saunders Company.

Weston WL, and AT Lane. 1991. Acne. In *Color Textbook of Pediatric Dermatology*. 15-25. St. Louis, MO: Mosby-Year Book, Inc.

2. ADOLESCENT PREVENTIVE SERVICES
Mark Schuster, M.D., Ph.D.

Because the topic of adolescent preventive services has been considered by several expert panels, we relied on their findings in developing our recommendations. Specifically, we reviewed: (1) the AMA Guidelines for Adolescent Preventive Services (GAPS) (Elster and Kuznets, 1994), (2) the American Academy of Pediatrics (AAP) Guidelines for Health Supervision II (AAP, 1988), (3) Bright Futures (Green, 1994), and (4) the Guide to Clinical Preventive Services (USPSTF, 1989).

This review does not cover every aspect of adolescent preventive services that is recommended by these sources. Rather, we have covered topics that lend themselves to the development of quality indicators and are likely to have broad support from clinicians. Many recommended components of preventive services are the product of expert opinion and have not been evaluated using rigorous research designs. This is particularly true for the frequency and timing of certain aspects of the physical examination, topics for counseling, and tests.

Immunizations and tuberculosis screening are addressed in Chapters 14 and 18, respectively.

GENERAL TOPICS IN ADOLESCENT PREVENTIVE SERVICES

Routine Health Visit

GAPS recommends an annual routine health visit for all adolescents (defined by the AMA as ages 11 to 21). Each of these 11 visits should cover education and counseling; three should include physical examinations (though GAPS recommends certain aspects of the physical examination be done annually, e.g., blood pressure measurement) (Elster and Kuznets, 1994). Bright Futures recommends an annual visit between 11 and 21 years of age, with more frequent visits for adolescents considered at high risk for health and social problems (Green, 1994). In 1995, the American Academy of Pediatrics increased the recommendation of one visit every two years in its Guidelines for Health Supervision II (AAP, 1988) to one visit every year (AAP, 1995). The Guide to Clinical

Preventive Services recommends one visit between 13 and 18 years of age (USPSTF, 1989).

Guarantee of Confidentiality

The various guidelines recommend a discussion of the scope and limits of confidential care (AAP, 1989; AAP, 1990; American Academy of Family Physicians [AAFP], 1988; AAFP, 1994; ACOG Technical Bulletin, 1986; Elster and Kuznets, 1994; SAM, 1991; SAM, 1992; USPSTF, 1989). Adolescents want confidential care and say they will be inhibited if it is not offered (Cheng et al., 1993). While this finding is not surprising, we are not aware of any studies that show a negative effect on outcomes if confidentiality is ignored. Confidentiality laws vary by state, so it is difficult to create indicators that are specific to the content of such discussions. However, given the broad support for such discussions, it seems reasonable to expect that clinicians will address the topic, even if only to say that they do not provide confidential care. Discussions about confidentiality may be poorly documented, but they should be documented for the protection of the physician and adolescent.

Anticipatory Guidance

Essentially all guidelines for adolescents recommend education and counseling on a variety of topics (AAP, 1988; Elster and Kuznets, 1994; Green, 1994; USPSTF, 1989), though there is not much evidence about the effectiveness of clinician counseling. For sensitive topics (e.g., drug use, sex, contraception), documentation is likely to vary widely. Recommendations on such issues have two components: (a) counseling about risks and prevention and (b) an inquiry into the adolescent's experience with the pertinent topic. While both are typically recommended, many clinicians may not document the latter because of the risk of breaching the adolescent's confidentiality. Therefore, it may only be feasible to expect documentation that the topic was discussed (without expecting documentation that the adolescent had experience with it). Though some clinicians may not routinely document anticipatory guidance (whether the topic is sensitive or not), it seems particularly important to document anticipatory guidance for adolescent patients, who may seek care erratically, and in managed care settings where patients may not see the same provider at each visit. An expectation that anticipatory guidance be documented may prompt more clinicians to provide it.

SPECIFIC TOPICS IN PREVENTION

Substance Use Screening and Cigarette Use Counseling
Steven Asch, M.D., M.P.H., and Mark Schuster, M.D., Ph.D.

We relied on Chapter 48 of the Guide to Clinical Preventive Services published by the U.S. Preventive Services Task Force (USPSTF, 1989) to construct quality indicators for prevention of smoking and screening for and treatment of cigarette use. When this core reference cited studies to support individual indicators, we have referenced the original source. We also performed narrow MEDLINE literature searches for articles from 1990 to 1995 to update the literature support for the proposed indicators.

Importance

Cigarette Use. Sixteen percent of adolescents smoke, and 22 percent of adolescent males use smokeless tobacco (Elster and Kuznets, 1994). The interval between use of tobacco and development of nicotine addiction is about two years, so there is a window of opportunity after the start of tobacco use for smoking cessation intervention. The long-term consequences of cigarettes and passive smoking include coronary artery disease, lung cancer, and chronic obstructive pulmonary disease. Smoking is responsible for 1 in 6 adult deaths in the United States and is the single most preventable cause of death. The use of smokeless tobacco causes oral cancer, gingivitis, periodontal disease, and other problems. There is evidence that office-based physician counseling can be effective in reducing tobacco use among adults. Community and school-based programs have been found to be effective for adolescents (Elster and Kuznets, 1994).

Alcohol Use. Thirty to 44 percent of high school seniors, 23 to 36 percent of 10th graders, and 10 percent of 8th graders report a recent episode of binge drinking (five or more drinks at one time). Among adolescents 12 to 17 years old, 15 percent have used marijuana, 8 percent have used an inhalant psychoactive substance, 3 to 6 percent have used cocaine, and 3 percent have used a hallucinogen. From 5 to 11 percent of high school students have used anabolic steroids (Elster and Kuznets, 1994).

The leading cause of death in adolescence is motor vehicle crashes, half of which are related to the use of alcohol by adolescent drivers. Alcohol is a factor in 50 percent of homicides, 30 percent of suicides, and 24 percent of fatal pedestrian or bicycle accidents among adolescents.

Inappropriate anabolic steroid use can affect hepatic, gonadal, and psychological function, as well as serum lipids and blood pressure (Elster and Kuznets, 1994).

Efficacy and/or Effectiveness of Interventions

Screening

There is some evidence that suggests that clinical intervention may be effective in preventing substance use, particularly when the intervention is reinforcing messages provided by teachers, parents, and other adults (Elster and Kuznets, 1994).

GAPS recommends asking adolescents annually about their use of tobacco products, including cigarettes and smokeless tobacco; alcohol; and other abusable substances. It also recommends annual counseling to promote avoidance of tobacco, alcohol, and abusable substances (Elster and Kuznets, 1994). The AAP suggests bringing tobacco, alcohol, and other abusable substances into the history and anticipatory guidance as early as 10 years old and throughout the rest of adolescence, with the level of detail and specificity changing with the age of the adolescent (AAP, 1988). The USPSTF recommends both screening and counseling on these topics during the 13 to 18 year old age period (USPSTF, 1989). Bright Futures recommends that physicians discuss these topics starting with the 11th-year visit (Green, 1994).

Most patients begin smoking as adolescents and tobacco usage has been rising in this age group. As a result, the Surgeon General and the USPSTF have recommended that clinicians counsel their adolescent patients to avoid starting smoking. We found no randomized clinical trials that specifically address clinician-based programs for adolescents, though the preponderance of controlled trials support the effectiveness of similar school-based programs (Perry, 1987; Perry and Silvis, 1987; Elder et al., 1993; Elders et al., 1994; Sussman et al., 1993; Murray et al., 1992).

Treatment for Cigarette Use[1]

Once a patient has been identified as a smoker, providers have modest but definite impact in helping them quit (Russell et al., 1979; Ewart et al., 1983; Wilson et al., 1982; Wilson et al., 1988). A meta-analysis of 39 controlled trials found that counseling yielded an 8.4 percent (95 percent CI +/- 2.8 percent) reduction in the number of smokers at six months and a 5.8 percent (95 percent CI +/- 2.6 percent) reduction at one year (Kottke et al., 1988). While most of the individual trials did not demonstrate an effect, the 95 percent confidence limits after pooling the subjects exclude zero for both time points (Kottke et al., 1988).

A broad-based program to stop smoking appears to be most effective. The most successful trials were more likely to employ both group and individual counseling, teams of physicians and nonphysicians, multiple reinforcement sessions, and face-to-face advice. Multivariate analysis of the attributes of successful trials showed that the number of interventions was strongly associated with the smoking cessation rate (Table 2.1) (Kottke et al., 1988).

Adding nicotine replacement therapy may increase the success rate of counseling alone by up to one-third, particularly in heavy smokers. A meta-analysis of 14 randomized trials of nicotine gum compared to placebo gum found that more patients who used nicotine gum had quit smoking at 6 months (27 percent vs. 18 percent, n=734) and 12 months (23 percent vs. 13 percent), although this study occurred in the setting of specialized smoking cessation clinics (Lam et al., 1987). The meta-analysis found lower rates of effectiveness when the treatment occurred in general medical clinics, however. Placebo controlled trials in general practice did not demonstrate an effect, though uncontrolled trials show that nicotine replacement had a modest effect at 6 months

---

[1]From the Women's Quality of Care Review.

(17 percent vs. 13 percent; n=2238) and 12 months (9 vs. 5 percent) in general practice. Given its questionable efficacy in the setting of general practice, we propose that nicotine replacement be prescribed as second line therapy after counseling alone has failed (Lam et al., 1987).

There are several contraindications for nicotine replacement therapy. Nicotine replacement is contraindicated in the settings of pregnancy and nursing because it crosses the placenta and is excreted in the breast milk. Patients with temporomandibular joint disease may experience symptomatic worsening. If the patient continues to smoke, the potential toxicities of nicotine replacement become much more likely. Nicotine gum may not be as effective in the absence of counseling; all the controlled studies combined gum with some form of advice (Lam et al., 1987; Oster et al., 1986; Russell et al., 1983; Benowitz, 1988; Wilson et al., 1988; Fagerström, 1984).

Follow-up

The above-mentioned meta-analysis of 39 clinical trials of smoking cessation counseling showed that one of the common attributes of successful programs is reinforcement through follow-up appointments. Both the number of subject contacts with the program and the number of months duration of the program were positively correlated with the cessation rate (Table 2.1). We propose that the medical record should indicate a plan for such reinforcement either by adding tobacco abuse to the patient's problem list or through addressing the problem during at least one subsequent visit.

Table 2.1

Descriptors for Interventions (Continuous Variables) Reporting Results 12 Months After Initiation of Intervention

Descriptors	Range	Mean ± SD	Correlation With Cessation Rate
No. of intervention modalities	1-6	2.1 ± 0.9	.48*
Participant drop-out rate	0%-51%	13.8% ± 12.0%	.05
No. of subject contacts with program	1-15	3.8 ± 4.6	.38*
Months subject in contact with program	0-12	1.1 ± 2.1	.55*
No. of participants	32-8189	608.2 ± 948.6	.20
No. of times smoking status was assessed	1-18	4.0 ± 4.5	.13
Months from first contact to last verification	0-12	7.6 ± 11.8	.16
No. of times cessation claims were validated	0-6	0.9 ± 1.2	.09
Subjective rating of study quality	0-5	3.2 ± 1.0	-.23

*p<.01.
Source: Kottke et al., 1988.

Sexually Transmitted Diseases and HIV Prevention
Eve Kerr, M.D., M.P.H., and Mark Schuster, M.D., Ph.D.

The primary references for the review done for adults were the Guide to Clinical Preventive Services of the U.S. Preventive Services Task Force and the Healthy People 2000 National Health Promotion and Disease Prevention Objectives. For adolescents, we also reviewed GAPS (Elster and Kuznets, 1994) and guidelines from various specialty societies (AAP et al., 1989; AAP, 1990; AAFP, 1988; AAFP, 1994; ACOG Technical Bulletin, 1986; SAM, 1991; SAM, 1992).

Importance

An estimated 1-1.5 million people are infected with the human immunodeficiency (HIV) virus (USPSTF, 1989). Within 10 years of infection with HIV, approximately 50 percent of persons develop AIDS and another 40 percent or more develop other clinical illnesses associated with HIV infection (USDHHS, 1991). Persons with AIDS can develop severe opportunistic infections, malignancies, and multiple-system medical complications. In a study performed before the licensure of AZT, the five-year survival rate was only 15 percent (USPSTF, 1989). The economic consequences of AIDS are enormous; it is estimated that the annual cost of treating AIDS is $2.2 billion (USPSTF, 1989).

Almost 12 million cases of sexually transmitted diseases occur annually (USDHHS, 1991). Each year there are about 3-4 million cases of chlamydia, 2 million cases of gonorrhea, over 35,000 cases of primary and secondary syphilis, and 270,000 primary episodes of genital herpes (USPSTF, 1989). These diseases are associated with considerable morbidity. Chlamydia and gonorrhea produce mucopurulent cervicitis and pelvic inflammatory disease (PID) in women. PID is an important risk factor for ectopic pregnancy and infertility; approximately 1 million cases of PID are reported annually in the United States (USPSTF, 1989). Syphilis produces ulcers of the genitalia, pharynx, and rectum and can progress to secondary and tertiary syphilis if left untreated (USPSTF, 1989). Genital herpes causes painful vesicular and ulcerative lesions and recurrent infections due to latent infection (USPSTF, 1989). The total societal costs of STDs is estimated to be $3.5 billion annually (USDHHS, 1991).

Over 50 percent of females and over 60 percent of males ages 15 to 19 years have had sexual intercourse. Over one million adolescents conceive each year, with 40 percent having elective abortions. Adolescents account for an estimated 3 to 6 million cases of sexually transmitted diseases each year. It is not known whether clinical counseling has an impact, though school-based interventions have been found to effect behavior change (Elster and Kuznets, 1994).

Efficacy and/or Effectiveness of Interventions

The most efficacious means of reducing the risk of acquiring AIDS and other STDs through sexual contact is either abstinence from sexual relations or maintenance of a mutually monogamous sexual relationship with an uninfected partner (USPSTF, 1989). In addition, the use of latex condoms and spermicides may reduce the risk of infection with HIV or other STDs (USPSTF, 1989). Intravenous drug use and unsterilized needles should be avoided to reduce the risk of HIV infection. The prevalence of HIV infection in heterosexual partners of persons in high-risk categories may be as high as 11 percent and as many as 60 percent of heterosexual partners of HIV-infected individuals may be seropositive (USPSTF, 1989).

The primary purposes of HIV and STD counseling are to prevent further spread of infection (USDHHS, 1991). Physicians can play an important role in preventing infection in asymptomatic persons by reinforcing and clarifying educational messages, providing literature and community resource references for additional information, and dispelling misconceptions about unproved modes of transmission (USPSTF, 1989). Although it has not been proven that physicians can change the sexual behavior of patients, there is evidence that the frequency of high-risk behaviors can be reduced in response to information provided through public education (USPSTF, 1989). A survey of primary care physicians found that only 10 percent asked new patients questions specific enough to identify those at risk of exposure to HIV (USPSTF, 1989).

GAPS recommends annual counseling about sexual risk and prevention. It also recommends an annual inquiry about involvement in sexual behaviors that may result in unintended pregnancy and STDs, including HIV infection (Elster and Kuznets, 1994). Bright Futures recommends providing age-appropriate sexuality education starting in childhood and asking the child about his/her own sexual experiences starting with the 10 year old visit (though it includes vague questions that might prompt a response about sexual activity or sexual abuse at an earlier age) (Green, 1994). The USPSTF recommends screening of sexual practices and counseling about them between ages 13 and 18 (USPSTF, 1989). Other guidelines also generally recommend taking a sexual history and providing counseling about preventing sexually transmitted diseases and pregnancy, though the recommendations do not specify the frequency (AAP et al., 1989; AAP, 1990; AAFP, 1988; AAFP, 1993; ACOG Technical Bulletin, 1986; SAM, 1991; SAM, 1992).

The indicators require documentation of counseling about sexual activity. If a sexual history is recorded, it will serve as presumptive evidence that counseling was provided.

The need to protect confidentiality raises troubling issues both for policies for recording information in medical records and for the development of quality of care indicators. For example, the USPSTF (1989) recommends a Pap smear every 1 to 3 years for sexually-active females between the ages of 13 and 18. However, if the adolescent's positive history of vaginal intercourse is not recorded in the chart, then the provider who sees her at the next visit may not know to obtain a Pap smear (unless a prior Pap smear result appears in the chart), making it difficult to assess whether the adolescent is receiving quality care (i.e., whether she needs and receives a Pap smear). The same applies to testing for STDs, for which GAPS recommends annual screening of sexually active adolescents.

Injury Prevention and Seat Belt Use Counseling
Lisa Schmidt, M.P.H.

The primary references for this review were the Guide to Clinical Preventive Services of the U.S. Preventive Services Task Force and the Healthy People 2000 National Health Promotion and Disease Prevention Objectives. The major focus of this section will be on injury prevention through seat belt use counseling.

Importance

Almost 70 percent of deaths among 10- to 19-year-olds are due to injuries, and 70 percent of these deaths are from unintentional injuries (Elster and Kuznets, 1994).

Injuries are the fourth leading cause of death in the United States and the leading cause of death in persons under age 45. Motor vehicle injuries account for about one-half of these deaths (USPSTF, 1989). In 1986, nearly 48,000 Americans died in motor vehicle crashes, and each year several million suffer nonfatal injuries (USPSTF, 1989). Although males and persons aged 15-24 account for one-third of all deaths from motor vehicle accidents (MVA), a significant number of women and children are killed or injured in MVAs each year. Many of these deaths and injuries are preventable with use of a safety restraint. However, only 46 percent of Americans used seat belts in 1988, up from 13 percent in 1978 (USPSTF, 1989).

Efficacy and/or Effectiveness of Interventions

The effectiveness of safety belts has been demonstrated in a variety of study designs that include laboratory experiments (using human volunteers, cadavers, and anthropomorphic crash dummies), post-crash comparisons of injuries sustained by restrained and unrestrained occupants, and post-crash judgments by crash analysts regarding the probable effects of restraints had they been used (USPSTF, 1989). It has been estimated on the basis of such evidence that the proper use of lap and shoulder belts can decrease the risk of moderate to serious injury to front seat occupants by 45 to 55 percent and can reduce crash mortality by 40 to 50 percent (USPSTF, 1989). When brought to the hospital, crash victims who are wearing safety belts at the time of the crash have less severe injuries, are less likely to require admission, and have lower hospital charges (USPSTF, 1989).

The USPSTF recommends that clinicians regularly urge their patients to use safety belts whenever driving or riding in an automobile. In addition, they should be counseled regarding the dangers of operating a motor vehicle while under the influence of alcohol or other drugs, as well as on the risks of riding in a vehicle operated by someone who is under the influence of these substances (USPSTF, 1989). A number of other organizations have issued recommendations on physician counseling of patients on seat belt use, including the American Medical Association, the American College of Physicians, the American Academy of Family Physicians and the National Highway Traffic Safety Administration (USPSTF, 1989). In addition, the American College of Obstetricians and Gynecologists has issued recommendations for the use of passenger restraints by pregnant women (USPSTF, 1989). Lastly, the Healthy People 2000 objectives include a risk-reduction objective to increase the use of occupant protection systems to at least 85 percent of motor vehicle occupants (Healthy People 2000, 1991).

It is not known, however, how effectively clinicians can alter behaviors regarding seat belt use. In one questionnaire survey, patients claimed to have increased their use of safety belts as a result of a brief statement by their physician during a routine office visit, but the study lacked controls and the patients were carefully selected (USPSTF, 1989). Other measures that have been proven successful in motivating people to use safety belts, such as community educational programs and intensive psychological strategies, may not be generalizable to the clinical practice setting (USPSTF, 1989).

GAPS recommends annual health guidance to promote reduction of intentional and unintentional injuries (e.g., not using alcohol or other substances while driving; using seat belts, helmets, etc.) (Elster and Kuznets, 1994). The AAP recommends anticipatory guidance on bicycle and vehicle safety, wearing a seat belt, and not riding in a car with a driver who has been using alcohol or drugs (AAP, 1988). Bright Futures recommends anticipatory guidance for a long list of injury and violence prevention throughout adolescence (Green, 1994). The USPSTF recommends addressing injury prevention with 13- to 18-year-olds (USPSTF, 1988).

Hyperlipidemia and Hypertension Screening
Steven Asch, M.D., M.P.H., and Mark Schuster, M.D., Ph.D.

Importance

Identifying high blood pressure in asymptomatic patients allows modifications of an important risk factor for coronary artery disease, the leading cause of death in the United States (Reed, 1987). The MRFIT trial found that patients with a cholesterol in the highest quintile (>246 mg/dl) were 3.4 times as likely to die from coronary heart disease as those in the lowest quartile (<181) (Martin et al., 1986). Several other major observational cohorts including Framingham and Whitehall have demonstrated the same risk relationship between cholesterol (particularly low density lipoprotein subcomponent and cardiovascular mortality) and most have found a synergistic relationship between cholesterol and other cardiovascular risk factors like hypertension and smoking (Littenberg et al., in Eddy, 1991; Rose and Shipley, 1986; and Kannel et al., 1971). The relationship between serum cholesterol and *total* mortality appears to be J-shaped; those with very low cholesterol die more frequently from cancer. Most experts believe that the higher mortality rates in patients with very low cholesterol derive from occult malignancies or other serious illnesses rather than low cholesterol inducing those conditions (Littenberg et al., in Eddy, 1991). The relationship between hypertriglyceridemia and coronary artery disease is less certain, but recent studies tend to confirm the suspected relationship (AHA, 1993). The American Heart Association estimates that cardiovascular disease costs the US about $80 billion each year (AHA, 1993).

Efficacy and/or Effectiveness of Interventions

The tests for total cholesterol, HDL cholesterol and LDL cholesterol, and triglycerides are inexpensive and safe. The accuracy of the test varies somewhat by laboratory. The American College of Pathology found a range of 197 to 379 mg/dl in 5000 samples with a known concentration of 262 mg/dl mailed to labs throughout the country (Laboratory Standardization Panel, 1988). The same study found similar problems with the measurement of triglycerides, HDL and LDL. Serum cholesterol varies somewhat with recent dietary fat intake. So do serum triglycerides, which also vary greatly with a number of other noncardiac conditions including liver disease, pancreatitis and hyperthyroidism. Despite this, there is no strong evidence that fasting lipids are any more predictive of coronary artery disease than nonfasting lipids. Perhaps more importantly for the current study, cholesterol measurements in younger patients are highly predictive of elevations later in life (Gillum et al., 1982). Like in hypertension, while the screening test itself poses little risk to the patient's health, incorrectly labeling a patient as having hyperlipidemia may impose some risk of unnecessary side effects of pharmacologic therapy. The subgroup of patients with the highest mortality are those with familial hyperlipidemia (National Cholesterol Education Program, 1991).

About 1 percent of adolescents have sustained hypertension, defined as a consistent blood pressure (BP) over the 95th percentile for age and gender. Even mild hypertension has subtle cardiovascular effects during adolescence, and hypertension is one of the major preventable risk factors that contribute to the development of cardiovascular disease (Elster and Kuznets, 1994).

There is evidence that blood pressure can be reduced in adolescents with hypertension and there is some evidence that this reduction will decrease future cardiovascular disease. Effective nonpharmacologic treatment includes weight reduction for obese adolescents, physical exercise, and dietary modification. Antihypertensive medications are effective in adolescents with hypertension unresponsive to other treatments. Some adolescents will have treatable underlying conditions causing their hypertension, such as renal or cardiac disease (Elster and Kuznets, 1994).

The National Heart, Lung, and Blood Institute (NHLBI) Second Task Force on Blood Pressure Control in Children recommends an annual screen for hypertension among adolescents, and GAPS incorporates this recommendation (Elster and Kuznets, 1994). Bright Futures also recommends annual blood pressure screening (Green, 1994). The AAP recommends the blood pressure be checked at each recommended biannual adolescent visit (AAP, 1988). Annual measurement of blood pressure would be difficult to implement given that an annual clinical visit has not become part of routine care for adolescents. However, given the inconsistency with which adolescents currently visit physicians, it is reasonable to expect documentation of blood pressure at each well visit or at least once a year if visits occur more than once a year.

GAPS recommends that adolescents with either systolic or diastolic BP at or above the 90th percentile for gender and age have BP readings repeated at three different times within one month under similar physical conditions to confirm baseline values. It also recommends that adolescents with baseline BP values greater than the 95th percentile have a complete evaluation. Adolescents with BP values between the 90th and 95th percentiles should be assessed for obesity and have their BP monitored every six months (Elster and Kuznets, 1994).

Cervical Cancer Screening[1]
Deidre Gifford, M.D.

The following guidelines are based primarily on the US Preventive Services Task Force's review of "Screening for Cervical Cancer" (USPSTF, 1989). This document addresses the questions of which populations should be screened and at what interval, but does not address follow-up of abnormal testing. In addition, we performed a review of the English language literature between 1990 and 1995. Articles were obtained using

---

[1]Originally prepared for the Women's Quality of Care Panel.

a MEDLINE search with the search terms cervix dysplasia, cervix neoplasms, and vaginal smears.

Importance

There are approximately 13,000 new cases of cervical cancer diagnosed each year in the United States, and about 7,000 deaths annually from the disease (CDC, 1992a). The annual incidence of invasive cervical cancer is estimated to be 20 per 100,000, and the lifetime probability of developing cervical cancer was estimated in 1985 to be 0.7 percent (Eddy, 1990). Five-year survival for women with advanced disease is about 40 percent, whereas it is about 90 percent for women with localized cancer (USPSTF, 1989). Cervical cancer is a good candidate for screening programs because it has a long preinvasive stage during which the disease can be detected and cured.

Effectiveness of Intervention

The Pap smear is the primary method of screening for cervical cancer. Pap smears can detect early cell changes which are precursors to invasive disease. Women in whom such abnormalities are detected can then have further diagnostic testing and treatment with interventions such as colposcopy and biopsy, cervical conization, and local excision, which can prevent further progression of the disease.

Evidence of the effectiveness of screening programs comes from observational studies showing decreases in cervical cancer mortality following the introduction of population screening programs. Such decreases have been observed in the United States and Canada, as well as in several European countries (USPSTF, 1989). For example, data from Iceland demonstrated a rising cervical cancer mortality during the 1960s. Screening was introduced in 1964, and by 1970 the annual mortality rate began to decline. By 1974 it had fallen significantly, decreasing from 23 per 100,000 in 1965-1969 to about 15 per 100,000 in 1970-74 (Johannesson et al., 1978). Further evidence comes from Canada, where the reduction in cervical cancer mortality has been noted to correlate with the proportion of the population screened with Pap tests (Eddy, 1990). In addition to this evidence, several case control studies have noted a marked decrease in risk of cervical cancer in women screened with Pap smears when compared to unscreened women. Such studies indicate that screening for cervical cancer with Pap smears is highly effective, decreasing the occurrence of invasive cancer by 60-90 percent (Eddy, 1990).

The effectiveness of cervical cancer screening appears to increase with decreasing screening intervals. This evidence also comes from case control studies, which demonstrated decreased relative risks of invasive disease in women with shorter screening intervals (Eddy, 1990). However, there is also evidence that annual screening may produce only a minimally lower risk of invasive disease than screening every two to three years (USPSTF, 1989; Eddy, 1990). According to one study of eight cervical cancer screening programs in Europe and Canada, the incidence of cervical cancer can be reduced by 64.1 percent with a screening interval of ten years, by 83.6 percent with a five-year interval, and by 90.8 percent, 92.5 percent and 93.5 percent with intervals of three, two and one years, respectively (IARC Working Group, 1986).

Several important risk factors have been identified for cervical cancer (Eddy, 1990). These include:

1) race/ethnicity, with blacks and Hispanics having a two-fold increased risk;

2) early age at first sexual intercourse;

3) number of sexual partners;

4) smoking;

5) human immunodeficiency virus (HIV) infection; and

6) human papillomavirus (HPV) infection.

There is also some evidence that long-term use of oral contraceptives may predispose a woman to cervical neoplasia. There has been debate in the literature about whether or not women with such risk factors should be screened more frequently than the general population of women. Published recommendations leave room for physician discretion in screening such women. A consensus recommendation has been adopted by the American Cancer Society, the National Cancer Institute, the American College of Obstetricians and Gynecologists, the American Medical Association, the American Nurses Association, the American Academy of

Family Physicians and the American Medical Women's Association (Fink, 1988). This guideline recommends annual Pap smears for all women who are or have been sexually active, or who are at least 18 years of age. After three normal annual smears, and *if recommended by the physician*, less frequent testing is permitted. The U.S. Preventive Services Task Force (1989) makes similar recommendations about the onset of testing and about annual testing until three normal tests have been obtained. They add that "...pap tests are appropriately performed at an interval of one to three years, to be recommended by the physician on the basis of risk factors (e.g., early onset of sexual intercourse, history of multiple sexual partners, low socioeconomic status). Women who have never been sexually active or who have had a total hysterectomy for benign indications with previously normal screening do not need regular Pap smears because they are not at risk for cervical cancer.

Treatment and Follow-up

Although there is generally less consensus about appropriate treatment and follow-up of abnormal pap smears than there is about their effectiveness as a screening technique, reductions in cervical cancer mortality are dependent on follow-up and treatment of women who have positive screening exams.

The classification of abnormal smears is variable, with different systems for reporting abnormalities (Table 2.2).

Table 2.2

Cytopathology Reporting Systems for Pap Smears

Class system	World Health Organization System	Cervical Intraepithelial Neoplasia System	Bethesda System
I	Normal	Normal	Within normal limits
II	Inflammation		Other Infection Reactive and reparative
III	Dysplasia		Squamous intraepithelial lesions
	Mild	CIN-1	
	Moderate	CIN-2	Low grade
	Severe		High grade
IV	Carcinoma in situ	CIN-3	
V	Invasive squamous cell carcinoma Adenocarcinoma	Invasive squamous cell carcinoma Adenocarcinoma	Squamous cell carcinoma Adenocarcinoma

Source: Miller et al., 1992

The Bethesda system was introduced to replace the previous Pap classifications and to facilitate precise communication between cytopathologists and clinicians. There is not universal agreement that it is superior to the CIN designations (Kurman et al., 1991), nor any evidence that it has been widely adopted.

Recommendations for follow-up of abnormal smears have been summarized by the report of a Canadian National workshop on screening for cancer of the cervix (Miller et al., 1991). First, they stress that screening recommendations (as summarized above) apply only to women with normal screening exams, and that women with abnormal smears should be screened and treated differently. This group recommends that women with so-called "benign atypia," mild dysplasia (CIN I, low grade SIL) or HPV infection without dysplasia should be rescreened at intervals of 6 to 12 months, and referred for colposcopy if the abnormality persists at 24 months past the original smear. This is based on the finding that many of these lesions will regress spontaneously without intervention (Montz et al., 1992); however, some have argued that the inconvenience, distress, and possibly the cost of this strategy are excessive, and that all women with abnormal smears should be referred immediately for colposcopic evaluation (Soutter, 1992; Wright et al., 1995). ACOG suggests that women with these low grade lesions may either be followed at six-month intervals or referred for colposcopy. They recommend colposcopic evaluation eventually for all women with "persistent" lesions.

There is not disagreement about management of women with more dysplastic lesions on pap smear. Women with Pap smears read as "moderate dysplasia," "severe dysplasia," "carcinoma in-situ," CIN II or greater, high grade squamous intraepithelial lesions, squamous cell carcinoma or adenocarcinoma should be referred for colposcopic evaluation. Further, the presence of a visible cervical lesion, even with a normal Pap smear, requires colposcopy because of the possibility of a false negative screening test (Miller et al., 1991; ACOG, 1993).

Eating Disorders
Mark Schuster, M.D., Ph.D.

Anorexia is estimated to occur in 0.5 percent of adolescents and is most common among white females. Bulimia is estimated to occur in 2 to 20 percent of females and 1 to 5 percent of males. Among adolescents, obesity is estimated to occur in about 20 percent of white males, 13 percent of black males, 26 percent of white females, and 25 percent of black females; excessive obesity is estimated to occur in 8, 5, 11, and 12 percent of these groups (USDHHS, 1991). In addition to discussing dietary patterns and satisfaction with weight, following weight and body mass index (BMI) are the screening tools to use for early signs of eating disorders. The BMI is also useful in screening for obesity (Elster and Kuznets, 1994).

GAPS recommends annual measurement of weight and height (Elster and Kuznets, 1994). The USPSTF recommends weight and height be measured between ages 13 and 18 but does not state how often (USPSTF, 1989). The AAP recommends height and weight be checked at each recommended biannual adolescent visit (AAP, 1988). Based on these recommendations, it is reasonable to expect weight and height to be measured at every visit or once a year, whichever occurs less often. While it would be ideal for the BMI to be recorded for each adolescent, it is certainly unnecessary for the many adolescents who are visibly neither too thin nor obese or who are visibly much too thin or obese.   Therefore, the BMI will not be incorporated into an indicator.

RECOMMENDED QUALITY INDICATORS FOR PREVENTIVE SERVICES FOR ADOLESCENTS

The following criteria apply to adolescents ages 13 to 18.

Screening

	Indicator	Quality of evidence	Literature	Benefits	Comments
	General				
1.	Between the ages of 13 and 18 years, all adolescents should have at least one clinician visit.	III	USPSTF, 1989	To detect treatable health problems (e.g., STDs, hypertension).	There is no consensus among experts regarding the frequency of well visits for adolescents. The least restrictive recommendation was selected.
2.	Confidentiality should be discussed and documented by age 14 or at the first visit afterwards.	III	Elster and Kuznets, 1994; USPSTF, 1989	To prevent problems related to sensitive topics (e.g., STDs, illicit substance use).	An age cut-off is not described in the literature.
	Substance Abuse Screening				
3.	Documentation of discussion of substance use (tobacco, alcohol, marijuana, other illicit drugs, anabolic steroids) or of the adolescent's history should occur by age 14 or the first well visit afterwards.	III	AAP, 1988; Elster and Kuznets, 1994; Green, 1994; USPSTF, 1989	To prevent and reduce substance use. To treat addiction.	There is limited evidence that clinical interventions reduce risk behaviors.
	Sexually Transmitted Diseases and HIV Prevention				
4.	Documentation of discussion of sexual activity and risk reduction or the adolescent's sexual history should occur by age 14 or the first well visit afterwards.	III	AAP, 1988; Elster and Kuznets, 1994; Green, 1994; USPSTF, 1989	To prevent and treat STDs, to prevent unwanted pregnancies, and to detect pregnancies.	There is limited evidence that clinical interventions reduce risk behaviors.
5.	Patients for whom the medical records indicate that they have ever been sexually active should be asked the following questions: if they currently have a single sexual partner; if they have had more than 2 sexual partners in the past 6 months; and if they have had a history of any STDs.	III	USPSTF, 1989	Prevent HIV; Prevent STDs.**	Non-monogamous relationships, more than 2 sexual partners in the past 6 months and past history of STDs are risk factors for HIV and/or other STDs.
6.	Patients for whom the medical records indicate that they are sexually active and not in a monogamous relationship, have had more than 2 sexual partners in the past six months, have a history of STDs, or have used intravenous drugs, should be counseled regarding the prevention and transmission of HIV and other STDs.	III	USPSTF, 1989	Prevent HIV; Prevent STDs.**	Persons with risk factors for HIV or other STDs should receive appropriate counseling

55

#	Recommendation	Grade	Citation	Purpose	Comment
Injury Prevention					
7.	Documentation of discussion of injury prevention should occur by age 14 or the first well child visit afterwards.	III	AAP, 1988; Elster and Kuznets, 1994; Green, 1994; USPSTF, 1989	To prevent serious morbidity or death from unintentional injuries.	There is limited evidence that clinical interventions reduce risk behaviors.
8.	Patients should receive counseling regarding the use of seat belts on at least one occasion.	III	USPSTF, 1989	Prevention of motor vehicle injuries and fatalities.	In practice, it is not known how effecctively physicians can alter this behavior.
Hyperlipidemia Screening					
9.	Adolescents whose parents have a serum cholesterol level greater than 240 mg/dl should receive a total blood cholesterol screen.	III	Elster and Kuznets, 1994	Prevention of coronary heart disease.	These adolescents have an increased risk of hyperlipidemia.
10.	Documentation of parental history of hypercholesteremia should occur by 14 years of age or the first well visit afterwards.	III	Elster and Kuznets, 1994	Prevention of coronary heart disease.	These adolescents have an increased risk of hyperlipidemia.
11.	Documentation of parents' or grandparents' history of coronary artery disease (CAD), peripheral vascular disease (PVD), cerebrovascular disease, or sudden cardiac death at age 55 or younger should occur by 14 years of age or the first well visit afterwards.	III	Elster and Kuznets, 1994	Prevention of CAD, PVD, and cerebrovascular disease.	A family history of these diseases increases one's risk of getting them.
12.	Adolescents whose parents or grandparents have a positive history of CAD, PVD, cerebrovascular disease or sudden cardiac death at age 55 or younger should have a fasting lipoprotein analysis.	III	Elster and Kuznets, 1994	Prevention of CAD, PVD, and cerebrovascular disease.	A family history of these diseases increases one's risk of getting them.
Hypertension Screening					
13.	Blood pressure should be measured at least once a year or at every visit, if visits occur less frequently than once a year.	III	Elster and Kuznets, 1994	To treat hypertension (and in some cases underlying causes of hypertension).	The blood pressure measurement not only screens for hypertension but also provides a baseline to compare with future readings.
14.	If a patient has 3 or more blood pressure readings above the 95th percentile for age, a full work-up for hypertension should be conducted.	III	Elster and Kuznets, 1994	To treat hypertension and prevent future cardiovascular disease.	Care should be taken to avoid overdiagnosing hypertension in adolescents.
Cervical Cancer Screening					
15.	The medical record should contain the date and result of the last Pap smear for all females under 18 years of age, for whom there is documentation of a history of vaginal intercourse, if it has been at least one year since they first had vaginal intercourse.	II-2	USPSTF, 1989	Prevent cervical cancer morbidity and mortality.* Prevent cervical cancer.	The appropriate timing of the next Pap smear is determined by the time elapsed since the last smear, and the result of the last smear.

No.	Recommendation		Reference	Goal	Notes
16.	All females under 18 years of age, for whom there is documentation of a history of vaginal intercourse, who have not had 3 consecutive normal smears and who have not had a Pap smear within the last year should have one performed.	III	USPSTF, 1989	Prevent cervical cancer morbidity and mortality.* Prevent cervical cancer.	A normal Pap smear is defined as one without atypia, dysplasia, CIS or invasive carcinoma. If there is no documentation of the actual pathology/cytology reports (i.e., because previous Pap smears were done at another facility) but there is documentation that all previous Paps were normal in the history, then the appropriate screening interval may be regarded as three years.
17.	All females under 18 years of age, for whom there is documentation of a history of vaginal intercourse, who have had three consecutive normal smears and subsequently have not had a Pap smear within the last 3 years should have one performed.	II-2	USPSTF, 1989	Prevent cervical cancer morbidity and mortality.* Prevent cervical cancer.	The maximum interval for all women with intact uteri is every three years. The incidence of cervical cancer is increased when screening intervals exceed 3 years.
18.	All females under 18 with a history of cervical dysplasia or carcinoma-in-situ who have not had a Pap smear within the last year should have one performed.	III	Miller et al., 1991; ACOG, 1993	Prevent cervical cancer morbidity and mortality.* Prevent cervical cancer.	These women are at increased risk for cervical disease, and should not be returned to 3-year screening intervals.
19.	Adolescent girls presenting for contraception who have not previously had a Pap test should have one.	III	Wilson and Jaffe, 1988	Prevent cervical cancer morbidity and mortality.*	Presentaton for contraception may provide presumptive evidence of sexual activity.
	Eating Disorders				
20.	Weight and height should be measured at least once a year or at every visit, if visits occur less frequently.	III	AAP, 1988; Green, 1994; Elster and Kuznets, 1994; USPSTF, 1989;	To identify and treat anorexia nervosa, bulimia, obesity, or other diseases affecting growth (e.g., hypothyroidism).	These measurments not only screen for abnormalities but also allow tracking growth trends over time.

57

Treatment

Indicator	Quality of evidence	Literature	Benefits	Comments
Cigarette Use Counseling—Treatment				
21. All current smokers should receive counseling to stop smoking.‡	I	Kottke et al., 1988	Decrease smoking-related morbidity and mortality.†	Meta-analysis of 39 trials of counseling showed 8% decrease in smoking rate at six months and 6% at one year.
22. If counseling alone fails to help the patient quit smoking, the patient should be offerred nicotene replacement therapy (gum or patch).	I-II	Lam et al., 1987	Decrease smoking-related morbidity and mortality.†	Meta-analysis of RCTs of nicotine replacement therapy demonstrated efficacy in setting of specialized smoking clinics; adding nicotine replacement may increase cessation rate by one third. Weaker evidence in general practice. For adolescent girls, the provider may consider whether the risk of unprotected sex and attendant risk to fetus overrides this approach to smoking cessation.
23. Nicotine replacement should only be prescribed in conjunction with counseling.‡	I	Lam et al., 1987	Avert potential side effects of nicotine therapy in patients who will not benefit without concomitant counseling. Decrease smoking-related morbidity and mortality.†	All controlled trials of nicotine replacement combine it with some form of counseling.
24. Nicotine replacement should not be prescribed if the patient: 1) is pregnant or nursing 2) has temporomandibular joint disease 3) continues to smoke	I-II	Benowitz, 1988	Avert premature births, birth defects, potential harm to nursing newborns, ischemic events.	Nicotine crosses placenta and is excreted into breast milk. It can worsen symptoms of temporomandibular joint disease. Continuing to smoke makes side effects of nicotine replacement much more likely.
Cervical Cancer Screening—Follow-up				
25. All adolescents with severely abnormal Pap smear should have colposcopy performed.***	III	Miller et al., 1991	Prevent cervical cancer morbidity and mortality.*	Appropriate follow-up for abnormal findings is key in preventing progression to cervical cancer or disease progression.
26. If an adolescent has a Pap smear that is not normal but is not severely abnormal,*** then one of the following should occur within 1 year of the initial Pap: 1) repeat Pap smear; or 2) colposcopy.	III	Miller et al., 1991	Prevent cervical cancer morbidity and mortality.*	Patients with intermediate findings should be monitored closely. In many cases, abnormal findings resolve spontaneously, so follow-up with Pap smears or immediate colposcopy are both appropriate.
27. All adolescents with a Pap smear that is not "normal" but is not severely abnormal*** and who have had the abnormality documented on at least 2 Pap smears in a 2-year period should have colposcopy performed.	III	Miller et al., 1991	Prevent cervical cancer morbidity and mortality.*	Patients with intermediate findings should be monitored closely since some portion of these may represent preinvasive disease, or progress to a high-grade SIL. If findings persist, colposcopy should be performed. This may be difficult to operationalize for women who have not been enrolled in the same plan for two years or more.

Cigarette Use Counseling—Follow-up				
28.	Tobacco abuse should be added to the problem list of all current smokers or addressed during at least one subsequent visit.	Kottke et al., 1988; Wilson et al., 1988	I	Decrease smoking-related morbidity and mortality.†	One of the common characteristics of successful counseling in the Kottke meta-analysis is reinforcement at subsequent visits.

*Morbidity of cervical cancer includes postsurgical and chemotherapeutic complications, infertility, incontinence, and pain from metastases.

**HIV causes fatigue, diarrhea, neuropathic symptoms, fevers, and opportunistic infections (OIs). OIs cause a wide variety of symptoms, including cough, shortness of breath, and vomiting. Average life expectancy after HIV infection is less than 10 years. Other STDs include gonorrhea, syphilis, and chlamydia. They cause a wide variety of symptoms, including dysuria, genital ulcers, infertility, rashes, neurologic and cardiac problems and rarely contribute to mortality. Preventing HIV and STDs has the added benefit of interrupting the spread of disease and preventing morbidity and mortality in those who thus avoid infection.

***Severly abnormal Pap smear: "moderate dysplasia," "severe dysplasia," "carcinoma in situ," CIS, CIN II, CIN III, "high grade SIL," squamous cell carcinoma, or adenocarcinoma.

†Smoking has been associated with increased risk of cancer of the lung, trachea, bronchus, lip, oral cavity, pharynx, larynx, esophogus, kidney, bladder, stomach, and pancreas. Smoking also causes or exacerbates COPD, asthma, bronchitis, cerebrovascular accidents and coronary heart disease. Smoking while pregnant is a contributing factor in low birthweight, shortened gestation, and sudden infant death syndrome. Each of these conditions causes a wide range of morbid symptoms and most increase mortality.

‡We plan a broad operationalization of counseling to include everything from from pamphlets and brief advice in the primary care setting to specialized structured programs.

Quality of Evidence Codes:

I: RCT
II-1:   Nonrandomized controlled trials
II-2:   Cohort or case analysis
II-3:   Multiple time series
III: Opinions or descriptive studies

REFERENCES - ADOLESCENT PREVENTIVE SERVICES

American Academy of Family Physicians. 1994. Adolescent health care. *1993-1994 Compendium of AAFP Positions on Selected Health Issues*. American Academy of Family Physicians, Kansas City, MO.

American Academy of Pediatrics. 1989. Confidentiality in adolescent health care. *AAP News*, (RE9151), 101.

American Academy of Pediatrics, Committee on Practice and Ambulatory Medicine. 1995. Recommendations for preventive health care. *AAP News* 11(8):insert.

American Academy of Pediatrics, and Committee on Adolescence. July 1990. Contraception and adolescents. *Pediatrics* 86 (1): 134-8.

American Academy of Pediatrics, and Committee on Psychosocial Aspects of Child and Family Health, 1985-1988. 1988. *Guidelines for Health Supervision II*, Second ed.Elk Grove Village, Illinois: American Academy of Pediatrics.

American College of Obstetricians and Gynecologists. July 1986. The adolescent obstetric-gynecologic patient. *ACOG Technical Bulletin* 94: 1-5.

American College of Obstetricians and Gynecologists. August 1993. Cervical cytology: Evaluation and management of abnormalities. *ACOG Technical Bulletin* 183: 1-8.

Benowitz NL. 1988. Toxicity of nicotine: Implications with regard to nicotine replacement therapy. In *Nicotine Replacement: A Critical Evaluation*. Editors Pomerleau OF, and CS Pomerleau, 187-217. New York, NY: Alan R. Liss, Inc.

Cheng TL, JA Savageau, AL Sattler, et al. 17 March 1993. Confidentiality in health care: A survey of knowledge, perceptions, and attitudes among high school students. *Journal of the American Medical Association* 269 (11): 1404-7.

Eddy DM. 1 August 1990. Screening for cervical cancer. *Annals of Internal Medicine* 113 (3): 214-26.

Elder JP, M Wildey, C de Moor, et al. September 1993. The long-term prevention of tobacco use among junior high school students: Classroom and telephone interventions. *American Journal of Public Health* 83 (9): 1239-44.

Elders MJ, CL Perry, MP Eriksen, et al. April 1994. The report of the Surgeon General: Preventing tobacco use among young people. *American Journal of Public Health* 84 (4): 543-7.

Elster, AB, and NJ Kuznets. 1994. *AMA Guidelines for Adolescent Preventive Services (GAPS): Recommendations and rationale*. Chicago, IL: American Medical Association.

Ewart CK, VC Li, and TJ Coates. June 1983. Increasing physicians' antismoking influence by applying an inexpensive feedback technique. *Journal of Medical Education* 58: 468-73.

Fagerstrom K. 1984. Effects of nicotine chewing gum and follow-up appointments in physician-based smoking cessation. *Preventive Medicine* 13: 517-27.

Fink DJ. March 1988. Change in American Cancer Society checkup guidelines for detection of cervical cancer. *Cancer Journal for Clinicians* 38 (2): 127-128.

Green, M. 1994. *Bright Futures: Guidelines for Health Supervision of Infants, Children, and Adolescents*. Arlington, VA: National Center for Education in Maternal and Child Health.

IARC Working Group on Evaluation of Cervical Cancer Screening Programmes. 13 September 1986. Screening for squamous cervical cancer: Duration of low risk after negative results of cervical cytology and its implication for screening policies. *British Medical Journal* 293: 659-64.

Kottke TE, RN Battista, GH DeFriese, et al. 20 May 1988. Attributes of successful smoking cessation interventions in medical practice: A meta-analysis of 39 controlled trials. *Journal of the American Medical Association* 259 (19): 2883-9.

Kurman RJ, GD Malkasian, A Sedlis, et al. May 1991. From Papanicolaou to Bethesda: The rationale for a new cervical cytologic classification. *Obstetrics and Gynecology* 77 (5): 779-82.

Lam W, PC Sze, HS Sacks, et al. 4 July 1987. Meta-analysis of randomised controlled trials of nicotine chewing-gum. *Lancet* 2 (8549): 27-30.

Littenberg B, AM Garber, and HC Sox. 1991. Screening for hypertension. In *Common Screening Tests*. Editor Eddy DM, 22-47 &397. Philadelphia, PA: American College of Physicians.

Miller AB, G Anderson, J Brisson, et al. 15 November 1991. Report of a national workshop on screening for cancer for the cervix. *Canadian Medical Association Journal* 145 (10): 1301-25.

Miller KE, DP Losh, and A Folley. January 1992. Evaluation and follow-up of abnormal pap smears. *American Family Physician* 45: 143-50.

Montz F, BJ Monk, JM Fowler, et al. September 1992. Natural history of the minimally abnormal papanicolaou smear. *Obstetrics and Gynecology* 80 (3): 385-8.

Murray DM, CL Perry, G Griffin, et al. 1992. Results from a statewide approach to adolescent tobacco use prevention. *Preventive Medicine* 21: 449-72.

---- 1991. *Report of the Expert Panel on Blood Cholesterol Levels in Children and Adolescents*. National Cholesterol Education Program. National Institutes of Health, National Heart, Lung and Blood Institute, Bethesda.

Oster G, DM Huse, TE Delea, GA Colditz. 1986. Cost-effectiveness of nicotine gum as an adjunct to physician's advice against cigarette smoking. *JAMA* 256(10):1315-1318.

Perry CL. 1987. Results of prevention programs with adolescents. *Drug and Alcohol Dependence* 20: 13-9.

Perry CL, and GL Silvis. May 1987. Smoking prevention: Behavioral prescriptions for the pediatrician. *Pediatrics* 79 (5): 790-9.

Russell MA, R Merriman, J Stapleton, et al. 10 December 1983. Effect of nicotine chewing gum as an adjunct to general practitioners' advice against smoking. *British Medical Journal* 287: 1782-5.

Russell MAH, C Wilson, C Taylor, et al. 28 July 1979. Effect of general practitioners' advice against smoking. *British Medical Journal* 2: 231-5.

Society for Adolescent Medicine. 1992. Access to health care for adolescents: A position paper of the Society for Adolescent Medicine. *Journal of Adolescent Health* 13: 162-70.

Society of Adolescent Medicine. 1991. Society of Adolescent Medicine Position Paper on Reproductive Health Care for Adolescents. *Journal of Adolescent Health* 12: 649-61.

Soutter WP. 23 May 1992. Conservative treatment of mild/moderate cervical dyskaryosis. *Lancet* 339: 1293.

Sussman S, CW Dent, AW Stacy, et al. September 1993. Project towards no tobacco use: 1-year behavior outcomes. *American Journal of Public Health* 83 (9): 1245-50.

U.S. Preventive Services Task Force. 1989. *Guide to Clinical Preventive Services: An Assessment of the Effectiveness of 169 Interventions*. Baltimore, MD: Williams and Wilkins.

Wilson DM, W Taylor, R Gilbert, et al. 16 September 1988. A randomized trial of a family physician intervention for smoking cessation. *Journal of the American Medical Association* 260 (11): 1570-4.

Wilson D, G Wood, N Johnston, et al. 15 January 1982. Randomized clinical trial of supportive follow-up for cigarette smokers in a family practice. *Canadian Medical Association Journal* 126: 127-9.

Wright TC, XW Sun, and J Koulos. February 1995. Comparison of management algorithms for the evaluation of women with low-grade cytologic abnormalities. *Obstetrics and Gynecology* 85: 2.

3. ALLERGIC RHINITIS
Eve Kerr, M.D., M.P.H.

We conducted a MEDLINE search of review articles on rhinitis between the years of 1990-1995 and selected articles pertaining to allergic rhinitis. We also performed a MEDLINE search of randomized controlled trials on allergic rhinitis patients between January 1990 and May 1995. Identified studies tended to use investigative therapies or compare new formulations of nasal steroids or antihistamines to previously used formulations. Since the general approach to treatment of allergic rhinitis is currently not controversial, these were not separately reviewed.

IMPORTANCE

Allergic rhinitis ranks thirteenth among the principal diagnoses rendered by physicians, based on the 1991 National Ambulatory Medical Care Survey (Vital and Health Statistics, Series 13, No. 116), accounting for over 11 million visits to the physician in that year. In fact, allergic rhinitis affects about 20 percent of the American population (Bernstein, 1993). Allergic rhinitis results in limitation of daily activities, and time lost from school and work (Bernstein, 1993). Complications of allergic rhinitis include serous otitis media (especially in children) and bacterial sinusitis (Kaliner and Lemanske, 1992).

EFFICACY/EFFECTIVENESS OF INTERVENTIONS

Diagnosis

The history is the fundamental diagnostic tool in allergic rhinitis. Symptoms include sneezing, itching of the nose, eyes, palate or pharynx, nasal stuffiness, rhinorrhea and post-nasal drip (Kaliner and Lemanske, 1992). A careful history of allergen exposure may reveal exacerbating allergies. In addition, one should inquire as to use of medications, especially nose drops or sprays. On physical exam, pale, edematous nasal turbinates and clear secretions are characteristic.

Temperature elevation, purulent nasal discharge, or cervical adenopathy should indicate the possibility of sinusitis, otitis, pharyngitis, or bronchitis (Kaliner and Lemanske, 1992).

Selected skin testing with appropriate allergens is the least time-consuming and expensive diagnostic modality, when confirmation of allergen sensitivity is necessary. Specific serum IgE determinations, although more expensive, may also be employed. Results need to be interpreted in the context of the patient's history. Total IgE levels and peripheral eosinophil counts are neither sensitive nor specific. Nasal smears from eosinophils are not specific for allergic rhinitis (Kaliner and Lemanske, 1992).

Treatment

Treatment rests with allergen avoidance, use of pharmaceutical agents and, when indicated, immunotherapy. Careful counseling regarding allergen avoidance is the mainstay of treatment (Naclerio, 1991). If it is unclear which allergen causes symptoms, skin testing should be performed (Naclerio, 1991). In addition, oral antihistamines (first- or second-generation H1-antagonistic drugs) are appropriate first-line agents, and decrease local and systemic symptoms of allergic rhinitis (Kaliner and Lemanske, 1992; Bernstein, 1993). Antihistamines may also be used in combination with decongestants for symptomatic relief. Topical nasal decongestants should be used for a maximum of four days. Nasal cromolyn sodium can be useful as a single agent, but requires regular, frequent dosing for optimal benefit (Bernstein, 1993). Topical nasal corticosteroids are effective in treating allergic rhinitis, but have no effect on ocular symptoms. Local burning, irritation, epistaxis and, very rarely, nasal septal perforation, are the reported side effects. Currently, both antihistamines and topical steroids have been advocated as first-line agents (Kaliner and Lemanske, 1992).

Immunotherapy should be considered if symptoms are present more than a few weeks of the year and medication and avoidance measures are ineffective (Naclerio, 1991). Allergy injections are reported to reduce symptoms in more than 90 percent of patients (Bernstein, 1993). Reported toxicities, although uncommon, include hives, asthma and hypotension. The duration of treatment for optimal effect and maintenance of benefits after treatment cessation are unclear (Creticos, 1992).

RECOMMENDED QUALITY INDICATORS FOR ALLERGIC RHINITIS

The following criteria apply to children ages 2 to 18.

Diagnosis

	Indicator	Quality of evidence	Literature	Benefits	Comments
1.	If a diagnosis of allergic rhinitis is made, the search for a specific allergen by history should be documented in the chart (for initial history).	III	Kaliner and Lemanske, 1992; Naclerio, 1990	Decrease nasal congestion, rhinorrhea, and itching.	Allergen avoidance is the mainstay of treatment
2.	If a diagnosis of allergic rhinitis is made, history should include whether the patient uses any topical nasal decongestants.	III	Bernstein, 1993	Decrease nasal congestion, rhinorrhea, and itching.	Chronic use of topical nasal decongestants can cause rhinitis medicamentosa and may mimic allergic rhinitis

Treatment

	Indicator	Quality of evidence	Literature	Benefits	Comments
3.	Treatment for allergic rhinitis should include at least one of the following: antihistamine, nasal steroids, nasal cromolyn.	I-III	Naclerio, 1991; Kaliner and Lemanske, 1992	Decrease nasal congestion, rhinorrhea, and itching.	These have proven efficacy in allergic rhinitis
4.	If nasal decongestants are prescribed, duration of treatment should be for no longer than 4 days.	II	Stanford et al., 1992; Barker, 1991	Decrease nasal congestion, rhinorrhea, and itching.	Longer treatment may cause rebound congestion.

Quality of Evidence Codes:

I: RCT
II-1:   Nonrandomized controlled trials
II-2:   Cohort or case analysis
II-3:   Multiple time series
III: Opinions or descriptive studies

66

REFERENCES - ALLERGIC RHINITIS

Bernstein JA. 1 May 1993. Allergic rhinitis: Helping patients lead an unrestricted life. *Postgraduate Medicine* 93 (6): 124-32.

Creticos PS. 25 November 1992. Immunotherapy with allergens. *Journal of the American Medical Association* 268 (20): 2834-9.

Kaliner M, and R Lemanske. 25 November 1992. Rhinitis and asthma. *Journal of the American Medical Association* 268 (20): 2807-29.

Naclerio RM. 19 September 1991. Allergic rhinitis. *New England Journal of Medicine* 325 (12): 860-9.

National Center for Health Statistics. 1994. *National Ambulatory Medical Care Survey: 1991 summary*. U.S. Department of Health and Human Services, Hyattsville, MD.

4. ASTHMA

Cheryl Damberg, Ph.D., And Caren Kamberg, M.P.H.

Approach

The National Asthma Education Program (NAEP) *Guidelines for the Diagnosis and Management of Asthma* (NAEP, 1991) served as the primary source of information for constructing quality indicators for asthma in children. An expert panel convened by the coordinating committee of the National Asthma Education Program developed the guidelines.[1] In addition, we conducted a MEDLINE search to identify all English language review articles published on childhood asthma for the years 1990-1995. Selected articles identified from reviews were also examined.

IMPORTANCE

Asthma is a complex syndrome of reversible airway obstruction, airway inflammation, and bronchial hyperirritability that occurs following exposure to stimuli (triggers) such as allergens, viral respiratory infections, vigorous exercise, cold air, cigarette smoke, and air pollutants (American Academy of Pediatrics [AAP], 1994; NAEP, 1991; Weiss, 1994). It is one of the most common chronic conditions in children.

The 1988 Child Health Supplement of the National Health Interview Survey (NHIS) reported an asthma prevalence rate of 4.3 percent among children younger than 18 years of age (Taylor and Newacheck, 1992). Between 1981 and 1988 the prevalence of childhood asthma increased 39 percent and the death rate increased 46 percent (Weitzman et al., 1992). Asthma among adults and children is responsible for 6.5 million office visits per year, and asthma-related health expenditures exceeded $6 billion in the United States in 1990 (Barach, 1994; Weiss et al., 1992). Asthma is associated with increased lost school days and is one of the major reasons for hospitalization among children. Approximately 30

---

[1] The recommendations are based upon review of the scientific evidence, expert judgment, and the collective opinion of the panel members.

percent of children with asthma have some activity limitation compared to 5 percent of non-asthmatic children. Furthermore, children with asthma have almost twice the risk of having a learning disability as do well children (Taylor and Newacheck, 1992).

Although it is difficult to disentangle the effects of race, socioeconomic status, poverty, environmental factors, and drug management, the fact remains that prevalence, morbidity, and mortality are higher among black and Hispanic children in every study that addresses this issue (Lang and Polansky, 1994; Wood et al., 1993; Gerstman et al., 1993; Weitzman et al., 1992; Crain et al., 1994; Weiss and Wagener, 1990). Hospital admissions for asthma are two-to-five times higher among non-white than white children (Halfon and Newacheck, 1986; Carr et al., 1992). Moreover, Huss et al. (1994) found that only about one-third of black urban children receive the maximally beneficial medication regimen for the control of their asthma and Bosco et al. (1993) determined that black children obtain fixed-combination drugs (bronchodilator, adrenergic, sedative) more often and steroids less often than other groups of children. Finkelstein et al. (1995) found that Hispanic children were less likely than white children to have taken beta$_2$-agonists before their admission, and that both Hispanics and blacks were less likely to have taken anti-inflammatory medications. Blacks and Hispanics were also less likely to be prescribed a nebulizer for home use.

Diagnosis

Diagnosis of asthma is based on patient medical history, physical examination, lung function measures, and laboratory tests (see Table 4.1). Symptoms include wheezing, shortness of breath, coughing, exercise intolerance, chest tightness and sputum production. Precipitating and/or aggravating factors may include viral respiratory infections, exposure to environmental allergens, irritants, cold air, drugs (e.g., aspirin), exercise, and endocrine factors.

Table 4.1

Diagnosis of Asthma

Medical History	Symptoms and patterns of symptoms (e.g., seasonal, at night) Precipitating factors (e.g., respiratory infection, exposure to environmental allergens) Household conditions (age of house, type of heating) Age and progress of disease Activity limitations (e.g., school days lost) Exercise tolerance Nocturnal asthma Life-threatening events Family's and patient's perception of the illness Family smoking history Other family history
Physical Examination	Presence of rhinitis and/or sinusitis, nasal polyps Evidence of hyperinflation of the lungs Quality of breath sounds Flexural eczema
Lung Function Measures	Forced Expiratory Volume 1 Second (FEV$_1$)[a] Peak Expiratory Flow Rate (PEFR)[b] Forced Vital Capacity (FVC)[c] Maximum midexpiratory Flow Rate (MMEF)[d] Bronchoprovocation (with methacholine, histamine) or exercise challenge
Laboratory Tests	Complete blood count Chest x-ray Sputum examination and stain for eosinophilia Nasal secretion and stain for eosinophils Determination of specific IgE antibodies to common inhalant allergens Rhinoscopy Sinus x-rays Evaluation of pH for gastroesophageal reflux

Sources: NAEP, 1991; Stempel and Szefler, 1992.
[a]The volume of air expired in one second from maximum expiration.
[b]The maximum flow rate that can be generated during a forced expiration starting with fully inflated lungs.
[c]Total volume of air expired as rapidly as possible.
[d]The slope of line between 25 and 75 percent of the forced expiratory volume.

Severity of disease ranges widely, with some patients having infrequent symptoms and others experiencing severe limitation of daily activities with frequent exacerbations. Severity may be measured in terms of clinical characteristics (e.g., type and frequency of symptoms such as cough, shortness of breath, or wheezing), pulmonary function measurements (e.g., peak expiratory flow rate), functional impairment (e.g., the number of school days lost due to asthma), and health care utilization (e.g., drug regimens or use of urgent care). Approximately 10 percent of children with asthma have severe disease as measured by functional limitations and self- or parent report about the frequency in which they are bothered by symptoms (Wertzman et al., 1992).

The measurement of severity is not straightforward. An assessment of severity based on the number of medications may be confounded because a greater number of medications may indicate more severe disease or more intense care; the latter may be inappropriate. Also, measuring severity is confounded by the time of day the evaluation occurs (it is often worse at night), the time of year (worse in the winter), or the age of the child (better in older children). Finally, children with more severe disease may live in an environment that contains more allergens or other asthma triggers.

Table 4.2 contains assessment criteria for different levels of asthma severity, including symptoms, lung function measures, and functional ability (NAEP, 1991).

Table 4.2

Classification of Asthma by Severity of Disease

Clinical Characteristics (Symptoms)	Lung Function Assessment*	Functional Ability
Mild Asthma Exacerbations of cough and wheezing no more often than 1-2 times/week	PEFR>80% of baseline/predicted Variability**<20%	Good exercise tolerance but not vigorous exercise; nocturnal asthma <1-2 times per month; good school attendance
Moderate Asthma Symptoms 1-2 times/week; exacerbations that may last several days; emergency care < 3 times/year	PEFR 60-80% of baseline/predicted; Variability** 20-30%	Diminished exercise tolerance; nocturnal asthma 2-3 times per week; school work may be affected
Severe Asthma Daily wheezing, limited activity level, frequent exacerbations that are often severe; frequent nocturnal symptoms, hospitalization (>2 times/year) and emergency treatment (>3 times/year)	PEFR <60% of baseline/predicted; Variability**>30%	Very poor exercise tolerance with marked activity limitation; almost nightly sleep interruption; poor school attendance

Source: NAEP, 1991. *FEV_1 or PEFR. **Variability refers to the difference between either a morning and evening measure or among morning peak flow measurements each day for a week.

Stempel and Szefler (1992), as shown in Table 4.3, proposed a similar four-level staging of asthma severity based on (1) frequency, severity, and duration of symptoms; (2) limitations in daily activities; (3) functional abilities (e.g., exercise ability); and (4) results of pulmonary function tests.

Table 4.3

Four-Level Staging of Asthma Severity

Clinical Classification (Symptoms)	Lung Function Assessment	Functional Ability
Stage 1: Intermittent symptoms triggered by acute respiratory infection or allergen exposure; wheezing with vigorous exercise; a few episodes of acute asthma requiring multiple medication intervention	Normal lung function when asymptomatic	Wheezing with vigorous exercise
Stage 2: Symptoms many days of the month; some exertional dyspnea; more than once-a-day use of inhaled bronchodilator; cough variant asthma included; several flare-ups during year	Baseline forced expiratory flow 25-75% may be depressed with normal or near normal FEV_1 or FVC	Wheezing with exercise
Stage 3: Frequent exacerbations	Forced expiratory flow 27-75% abnormal with some depression of FEV_1	Significant impact on routine activity, sleep if not on therapy
Stage 4: Deteriorating pulmonary function, persistent symptoms, frequent flare-ups	Abnormal forced expiratory flow 25-75%, FEV_1, FVC	Daily activities limited

Source: Stempel and Szefler, 1992.

Studies show that physicians underestimate the presence and severity of asthma, especially if based on the presence and degree of physical symptoms such as wheezing (Barach, 1994). A wheeze that occurs only with a respiratory infection is often dismissed as bronchitis or pneumonia although the symptoms are compatible with asthma. Pneumonia was the initial inpatient diagnosis in 25 percent of children with asthma at a study conducted at the Kaiser Permanente Hospital in Honolulu (Roth, 1993). If the diagnosis of asthma is based on medical history taking and physical examination, other causes of obstruction need to be ruled out (e.g., foreign body, vascular rings, viral bronchiolitis, pulmonary edema). If asthma is suspected, then the history and physical examination should be followed by objective measures--such as lung function and laboratory tests--to both diagnose and make appropriate therapeutic recommendations.

Indications for lung function testing associated with pediatric asthma include: recurrent wheezing, unexplained dyspnea, chronic cough (particularly nocturnal), exercise intolerance or induced coughing, recurrent pneumonia, coughing or wheezing induced by cold air exposure or weather changes, and slow resolution of or recurrent bronchitis (Mueller and Eigen, 1992).

Lung function tests can include formal spirometry (for measurement of FEV_1) or peak expiratory flow rate (PEFR) using a hand-held peak flow meter. A pulmonary function test is done to document the severity of airflow obstruction and to establish acute bronchodilator responsiveness. PEFR only measures large airway function; therefore, patients with mild asthma linked to small airway obstruction will be underdiagnosed unless spirometry is used (NAEP, 1991). Consequently, spirometry should be performed in the medical setting at the initial assessment of all patients for whom the diagnosis of asthma is being considered, and periodically thereafter as appropriate (NAEP, 1991). The results of spirometry should demonstrate an obstructive process. Additional laboratory testing, such as chest x-rays, complete blood count, sputum examination, complete pulmonary function studies, and determination of specific IgE antibodies to common allergens should be considered, but need only be performed when appropriate for the clinical situation (NAEP, 1991).

Spirometry can be performed reliably by many, but not all, children by age 5 or 6 (Mueller and Eigen, 1992). Spirometry equipment chosen for children should have low inertia and be responsive to small volumes and low flows. A device that provides a graph of the breathing maneuver is essential in children so patient effort can be assessed. Infant pulmonary function testing is available in specialized laboratories. The testing requires that the child be asleep, often with sedation (Mueller and Eigen, 1992).

PEFR, using a portable, hand-held peak flow meter, has become the standard tool for assessing asthma severity, particularly day-to-day changes (Barach, 1994). PEFR is the greatest flow velocity that can be obtained during a forced expiration starting with fully inflated lungs. Children as young as age 5 can perform PEFR. Daily measurement of PEFR is useful for monitoring and assessing variations in lung function and providing information about allergens, environmental factors, or asthma triggers, such as exercise. Because the standard deviation of the PEFR is large, serial assessments are more accurate than single values (Mueller and Eigen, 1992). PEFR correlates well with forced expiratory volume at 1 second (FEV_1) measured by spirometry (NAEP, 1991). Measurement of PEFR is useful both in the medical and home setting. The NAEP Expert Panel suggests the guidelines summarized in Table 4.4 for measuring PEFR in children.

Table 4.4

Guidelines for Measuring PEFR in Children in Different Settings

---

Clinician's Office/Emergency Department:

Chronic Asthma

1. Measure PEFR in all patients > 5 years of age at each office visit for therapeutic judgments (i.e., changes in medication).

2. Measure to confirm exercise-induced asthma as a diagnostic tool.

Acute Exacerbations

1. Measure PEFR during all acute exacerbations in patients > 5 years of age as a means to judge how far the patient is from baseline measurements and to make decisions regarding management.

2. Measure PEFR after beta$_2$-agonist inhalation to judge response.

3. Measure PEFR just prior to discharge from emergency department. This will help determine need for a steroid taper.

Hospital

1. Measure 2-4 times/day for all hospitalized patients > 5 years of age to follow course of asthma therapy and plan discharge.

Home

1. Consider measuring in all patients > 5 years of age with moderate or severe asthma to monitor course of asthma.

2. Measure diagnostically before and after exposure to allergens.

3. Measure during acute exacerbations to monitor course of exacerbation and response to therapy.

Source: NAEP, 1991.

When using PEFR measurements to judge response to treatment or severity of exacerbation, it is useful to compare the measurement to patient "baseline." This baseline is usually regarded as the norm or personal best PEFR for the individual patient. The personal best value should be re-evaluated at least yearly to account for growth in children and progression of the disease. Alternately, comparisons can be made to standard PEFR measurements based on height, as shown in Table 4.5.

Table 4.5

Predicted Average Peak Expiratory Flow for Normal Children and Adolescents

Height (inches)	Males & Females
43	147
44	160
45	173
46	187
47	200
48	214
49	227
50	240
51	254
52	267
53	280
54	293
55	307
56	320
57	334
58	347
59	360
60	373
61	387
62	400
63	413
64	427
65	440
66	454
67	467

Source: NAEP, 1991.

EFFICACY AND/OR EFFECTIVENESS OF INTERVENTIONS

Asthma therapy has several components: patient education, environmental control, pharmacologic therapy, and the use of objective measures to monitor severity of disease and the course of therapy (NAEP, 1991). In this section, we also discuss vaccine recommendations, care for acute exacerbations, and care in the hospital.

Patient Education

Patient education is one of the most important modalities in asthma control (NAEP, 1991; Larsen, 1992) and is associated with improved patient outcomes. Health education designed to promote self-management of asthma has been shown to reduce emergency room visits and hospitalizations, improve school attendance, reduce episodes of wheezing, and improve self-image and family adjustment (Bailey et al., 1992; Hughes et al., 1991). Education should focus on (1) home use of a portable peak flow meter to monitor the disease, (2) awareness of early signs of upper respiratory infections, (3) antimicrobial therapy at the first sign of bacterial infections, (4) elimination of a known allergen or trigger (e.g., cold air, animal dander, tobacco smoke), (5) prophylactic treatment during seasonal exposures, and (6) treatment of cough. Patients should be instructed in and asked to demonstrate their use of peak flow meters during office visits. Because the performance and adequacy of education is not easily assessed from the medical record, the review and the indicators that follow will not focus on the patient-education component of care.

Pharmacologic Therapy

Most of the recent change in the management of chronic asthma has resulted from the increased recognition of the importance of the inflammatory component in the pathogenesis of asthma (Podell, 1992; Stempel and Szefler, 1992). As a result, anti-inflammatory treatments are now considered the first-line step in the pharmacologic management of chronic asthma. Anti-inflammatory drugs such as cromolyn sodium and inhaled corticosteroids, with or without chronic $beta_2$-agonist therapy, interrupt the development of bronchial inflammation. Bronchodilators (e.g., $beta_2$-adrenergic agonists, methylaxanthines) act to relieve the symptoms of the disease. Side effects seen in adults for all anti-asthma drugs are likely to be seen to a greater degree in children (Selcow, 1994).

The NAEP Guidelines state that "only the mildest, intermittent cases of asthma severity can be managed with an inhaled short-acting $beta_2$-agonist given alone as needed. As the frequency or severity of the asthma increases, inhaled corticosteroids, inhaled cromolyn, or inhaled nedocromil should be added to the treatment regimen" (Bergner and Bergner, 1994).

For young children, the use of a nebulizer at home is an effective delivery route for inhaled asthma medications. However, a nebulizer is difficult to transport and therefore children under 5 may have to use a nebulizer at home and take oral medication when they are away from home. Children older than 5 years of age can usually use a metered-dose inhaler (MDI) to administer their medication. A spacer is used for those who have trouble with the MDI and can be used in children as young as 3 years of age to permit inhalation therapy. Some recommend that physicians test children on their use of the MDI during office visits (Smith, 1993).

However, if patients use inhaled $beta_2$-agonists more than 3 to 4 times per day (NAEP, 1991), have more than 8 inhalations per day (practice parameters), or use inhaled $beta_2$-agonists on a daily basis, additional daily therapy may be indicated.

Corticosteroids

Corticosteroids, the most effective (and most potent) anti-inflammatory drugs for the treatment of reversible airway obstruction, can be administered orally (to treat flare-ups) or by inhalation (to prevent flare-ups). Their use has been associated with decreased need for emergency department visits and hospitalizations (NAEP, 1991). There is some evidence that corticosteroids increase the effectiveness of $beta_2$-agonists (Larsen, 1992). Inhaled corticosteroid therapy is considered a safe and effective treatment for asthma, with minimal side effects, but a trial of cromolyn sodium should be tried first.

Inhaled corticosteroids are recommended for patients over 5 years of age who are taking cromolyn sodium but who continue to need a $beta_2$-agonist more than 3-4 times daily or who continue to have nocturnal symptoms. After the patient stabilizes on the corticosteroid (2-4 weeks), the cromolyn therapy may be discontinued. Oral corticosteroids are usually reserved for treatment of acute exacerbations and for patients with severe disease due to significant adverse side effects. In any patient requiring chronic treatment with oral corticosteroids, a trial of inhaled corticosteroids should first be attempted in an effort to reduce or eliminate oral steroids. In patients on long-term oral corticosteroids, pulmonary function tests should be used to objectively assess efficacy.

Inhaled corticosteroids are being utilized more frequently as primary therapy for patients with moderate and severe asthma, and some investigators feel that they are appropriate as first-line therapy in patients with mild asthma (Haahtela et al., 1991). However, the use of inhaled steroids is controversial. Kelly (1993) and Zora et al. (1986) found that chronic administration of large doses of inhaled steroids in children was associated with adrenal suppression and growth retardation. Starfield et al. (1994) state that a child taking this medication should be monitored for growth patterns regularly. Others have concluded that prophylactic steroids are effective in childhood asthma when taken in conventional doses (Gustafsson et al., 1993; Volovitz et al., 1994; Price, 1993). Adverse effects of inhaled corticosteroids can be reduced or prevented by administering the agent with a chamber or spacer and by rinsing the mouth after each use (NAEP, 1991).

Cromolyn sodium

Cromolyn sodium is a nonsteroidal anti-inflammatory agent that is used prophylactically to prevent asthma flare-ups. It produces only minimal side effects such as occasional coughing (O'Brien, 1994; NAEP, 1991; Stempel and Szefler, 1992). Because of its safety record and anti-inflammatory actions, cromolyn is an agent of choice for the initial treatment of children with chronic moderate asthma (NAEP, 1991). Cromolyn sodium delivered by MDI can be used by most children over 5 years of age. Children under age 5 who cannot master the use of an MDI (with spacer) must use a nebulizer. Because there is no way to predict reliably who will respond to cromolyn sodium therapy, a 4-6 week trial is recommended to determine efficacy in individual patients (NAEP, 1991).

Beta$_2$-agonists

Inhaled beta$_2$-agonists remain the first-line therapy for the emergency treatment of asthma and for the prophylaxis of exercise-induced asthma in children, with other treatments used for preventive therapy (Larsen, 1992). Their primary advantage is their rapid onset of effect in the relief of acute bronchospasm (Stempel and Szefler, 1992). However, prolonged use of beta$_2$-agonists has been associated with diminished control of asthma, such that the recommended dosage is not to exceed three to four administrations per day. Patients who regularly use inhaled beta$_2$-agonists should be re-evaluated to assess bronchial reactivity. Some asthma experts discourage the routine use of beta$_2$-agonists because of evidence of worsening pulmonary functions when patients are maintained on bronchodilators without anti-inflammatory medications (O'Brien, 1994; Larsen, 1992). There appears to be some consensus in the medical community that regular use of beta$_2$-agonists (i.e., 4 times/day) should be discouraged in favor of anti-inflammatory treatment (Executive Committee of the American Academy of Allergy and Immunology, 1993).

Inhaled administration of the agent is comparable to oral administration in providing bronchodilation; however, inhalation therapy is preferable since it causes fewer systemic adverse effects, has a faster onset of action, and achieves desired results at lower dosages (NAEP, 1991). The correct use of metered-dose inhalers is critical, which may limit the use of inhaled beta$_2$-agonists in very young children.

Theophylline

Theophylline, which is used in some patients primarily for its bronchodilator effects, has the major disadvantages of variable clearance from the body and potential for multiple toxicities. It is eliminated from the body rapidly, especially in children, so sustained-release preparations are needed for chronic therapy. Life-threatening events (seizures, cardiac arrhythmias) have been observed (Larsen, 1992) as well as nervousness, headache, and upset stomach (O'Brien, 1994). Although it has been reported to cause deficits in cognitive functioning and school performance, Lindgren et al. (1992) found academic achievement to be unaffected by appropriate doses of theophylline, if the child's medical care is closely monitored. Monitoring serum theophylline concentrations at initiation of therapy and subsequently at least yearly is therefore useful (NAEP, 1991). Theophylline levels should also be checked for patients who do not exhibit the expected bronchodilator effect or who develop an exacerbation while on their usual dose (NAEP, 1991). Theophylline may be particularly useful for nocturnal asthma. The NAEP guidelines recommend that theophylline not be used in patients with mild asthma. It can be used with inhaled beta$_2$-agonists in patients with moderate asthma and with beta$_2$-agonists and corticosteroids in those with severe asthma.

Diagnosis and Treatment of Allergic Asthma

Allergy may have a significant role in the symptoms of asthma for some persons. A determination of an allergic component may be made in persons whose asthma worsens when they are exposed to allergens (e.g., dust mites, animal allergens) or who have seasonal worsening of symptoms. A careful history plays the most critical role in patients suspected of having allergic asthma. In such patients, determination of specific IgE antibodies, skin testing, and/or a referral to an immunologist, may be useful (NAEP, 1991).

Once it is determined through history and/or ancillary testing that allergy plays a role in the person's asthma, allergen avoidance should be the first recommendation (NAEP, 1991). However, when avoidance is not possible and appropriate medication fails to control symptoms of allergic asthma, immunotherapy should be considered (NAEP, 1991). Several randomized controlled studies show that immunotherapy can reduce symptoms in asthma patients (NAEP, 1991). Immunotherapy should only be administered in a physician's office where facilities and trained personnel are available to treat potentially life-threatening reactions.

Routine Monitoring

The NAEP guidelines (1991) recommend that PEFR or spirometry be used at each office visit to monitor the disease and therapy effectiveness. In children older than five years of age with moderate to severe asthma, peak flow should be monitored at home twice a day until the asthma is controlled and then daily or twice a day, two to three times a week. Starfield et al. (1994) recommend that routine office visits occur twice a year unless acute exacerbations occur, and that changes in medication be followed-up at three weeks. The NAEP guidelines (1991) call for physician visits at one- to three-month intervals after therapy control is achieved.

Bacterial otitis and sinusitis may be associated with asthma in all age groups. Antibiotic therapy for 10 days to 3 weeks can hasten control of asthma.

Vaccine Recommendations

The U.S. Preventive Services Task Force (USPSTF, 1989) recommends pneumococcal vaccination and regular influenza vaccination for those with chronic cardiac or pulmonary disease. The NAEP (1991) guidelines state that "influenza vaccinations and pneumococcal vaccine should be considered for patients with moderate or severe asthma in order to avoid aggravation of asthma."

Care of an Acute Asthma Exacerbation

The NAEP Expert Panel has outlined five general principles of treatment for asthma exacerbations:

- written action plans to help patient/family co-manage asthma exacerbation;
- early recognition of indicators (worsening PEFR or FEV_1);
- prompt communication between patient and health care provider;
- appropriate intensification of anti-asthma medications (treatment can begin at home); and
- removal of the allergen or irritant, if one or the other triggered the exacerbation.

Patients at high risk of death from exacerbations should be counseled to seek immediate medical care rather than initiate home therapy. High risk patients include those with a history of:

- prior intubation;
- ≥2 hospitalizations for asthma in past year;
- ≥3 emergency care visits for asthma in the past year;
- hospitalization or emergency care visit within the past month;
- current use of systemic corticosteroids or recent withdrawal from systemic corticosteroids;
- past history of syncope/hypoxic seizure due to asthma;

- prior admission for asthma to hospital-based intensive care unit; or

- serious psychiatric or psychosocial problems.

In general, patients who do not have a good response to home inhaled beta$_2$-agonist treatment should contact their health care provider. Severe symptoms at rest, such as breathlessness, speech fragmented by rapid breathing and inability to walk 100 feet without stopping to rest, that do not improve within 30 minutes, indicate a visit to the emergency department.

All patients presenting with an acute exacerbation should be evaluated with a complete history including:

- length of current exacerbation;

- severity of symptoms;

- all current medication, including use of systemic corticosteroids;

- prior hospitalizations and emergency department visits for asthma;

- prior episodes of respiratory insufficiency due to asthma; and

- significant prior cardiopulmonary disease.

All patients presenting with an acute exacerbation should be evaluated with at least one measurement of airflow obstruction:

- peak expiratory flow rate measured with a peak flow meter; or

- one-second forced expired volume (FEV$_1$) determined by spirometry.

In general, all patients with an acute exacerbation should receive initial treatment with inhaled beta$_2$-agonists (McFadden and Hejal, 1995; NAEP, 1991). Albuterol is specifically recommended for treating children in the emergency department or other urgent care setting and can be delivered by nebulizer, preferably with oxygen. Nebulized treatments should be given every 20 minutes for one hour and the patient should be continually assessed (McFadden and Hejal, 1995). Patients should be re-evaluated at least three times within 90 minutes of treatment. For infants and children, corticosteroids should be given very early in the course of a severe asthma exacerbation and should be started if the infant/child fails to respond completely to two albuterol treatments. Patients with a good response to inhaled beta$_2$-agonist treatment should be observed for 30-60 minutes after the last treatment to ensure stability prior to discharge.

Patients who have persistent symptoms, diffuse wheezes audible on chest auscultation, and a PEFR or FEV$_1$ <40 percent of predicted or baseline should be admitted to the hospital.

The following are recommended steps for follow-up care once a patient has been stabilized following an acute exacerbation:

1) Treatment regimen should be given for at least three days.

2) Treatment regimen should include oral corticosteroids for all patients with an FEV$_1$ or PEFR <70 percent of baseline at discharge, and for all patients at increased risk for potential life-threatening deterioration.

3) A follow-up medical appointment should occur within 48 to 72 hours of discharge.

Care of Patients Hospitalized for Asthma

Patients whose airflow obstruction does not respond to intensive bronchodilator treatment require close attention in the hospital. These patients should be followed with lung function measurement (PEFR or spirometry) at least twice per day, before and after bronchodilator therapy (NAEP, 1991). Patients who are admitted to the intensive care unit or who have had multiple hospital admissions should consult an asthma specialist.

All asthma patients admitted to the hospital should receive systemic corticosteroids (preferably intravenously) and beta$_2$-agonists. The NAEP guidelines also recommend that all hospitalized patients, including children, be administered oral or intravenous methylaxanthines (e.g., theophylline or aminophylline). Oxygen should be given to all patients with an oxygen saturation less than 90-92 percent. Measurement of oxygen saturation by oximetry is recommended. Hydration therapy may be warranted in infants and young children who may become dehydrated as

a result of increased respiratory rates and decreased oral intakes. In
these young age groups, assessment of fluid status (e.g., urine output,
electrolytes) should be made and appropriate corrections provided.
Chest physical therapy has not been found to be helpful for most
patients. Use of mucolytics (e.g., acetylcysteine, potassium iodide)
and sedation (i.e., with anxiolytics and hypnotic drugs) should be
strictly avoided. Antibiotics should be reserved for those patients
with purulent sputum and/or fever since bacterial and myoplasmal
respiratory infections are thought to rarely contribute to severe asthma
exacerbations.

Patients with PEFR or FEV_1 <25 percent of baseline or predicted
should receive an arterial blood gas measurement to evaluate pCO_2. If
pCO_2 is greater than 40 mm Hg, the patient will require repeated
arterial blood gas measurement to evaluate their response to treatment,
preferably in an intensive care setting.

Children ages 5 or older who are discharged from the hospital
should either be on an oral prednisone taper and $beta_2$-agonist therapy
administered by MDI, a dry powder inhaler, or a compressor-driver
nebulizer. In general, the PEFR should be 70 percent of predicted or
personal best baseline value. The NAEP guidelines (1991) recommend
close medical follow-up during the tapering period, but do not specify a
follow-up interval.

RECOMMENDED QUALITY INDICATORS FOR ASTHMA

The following criteria apply to children with chronic asthma and exclude patients with exercise-induced asthma.

Diagnosis

	Indicator	Quality of evidence	Literature	Benefits	Comments
1.	All patients age 5 or older with the diagnosis of asthma should have baseline spirometry performed (within six months of diagnosis).	III	NAEP, 1991	Decrease baseline shortness of breath.	By documenting the diagnosis with spirometry, one can initiate the appropriate therapy, minimize inappropriate use of medications, and document future worsening or improvement. Spirometry will identify small airway obstruction, unlike PEFR which only measures large airway obstruction. Children > 5 can reliably perform spirometry.
2.	All patients with the diagnosis of asthma should have had a historical evaluation of asthma triggers (e.g., environmental exposures, exercise, allergens) within six months (before or after) of the initial diagnosis.	III	NAEP, 1991	Decrease baseline shortness of breath. Improve exercise tolerance. Decrease steroid toxicity.[1] Decrease number of exacerbations.[2]	This may result in improved control of asthma and less need for medications such as steroids, which have undesirable toxicities.[1]
3.	PEFR should be measured in all patients > 5 years of age with chronic asthma (except for those with only exercise-induced asthma) at least annually in an office visit in which asthma is evaluated.	III	NAEP, 1991	Decrease baseline shortness of breath. Improve exercise tolerance.	Sequential measurement of PEFR is useful for assessing severity of condition and making appropriate therapeutic decisions. Interpretations obtained in children ≤5 are often not valuable. The personal best PEFR measurement should be re-evaluated yearly in children to account for growth and the progression of the disease. No randomized trial has been conducted to provide evidence of improved outcomes among patients who receive PEFR in the office.

88

Indicator	Quality of evidence	Literature	Benefits	Comments
4. All patients > 5 years of age with the diagnosis of asthma should have been prescribed a beta₂-agonist inhaler for symptomatic relief of exacerbations.	III	NAEP, 1991	Decrease shortness of breath. Prevent need for emergency room treatment.	Beta₂-agonists are the first line therapy for asthma exacerbations. All asthmatics should have ready access to this therapy.
5. Patients <= 5 years of age should be prescribed a nebulizer (for administering asthma medications).	III	NAEP, 1991	Decrease shortness of breath.	Nebulized beta₂-agonist is more effective and has fewer side effects and thus is preferred over oral routes of administration among those with infrequent exacerbations.
6. Patients who report using a beta₂-agonist inhaler more than 3 times per day on a daily basis should be prescribed a longer acting bronchodilator (theophylline) and/or an anti-inflammatory agent (inhaled corticosteroids, cromolyn).	II, III	NAEP, Executive Committee of the American Academy of Allergy and Immunology, 1993	Decrease baseline shortness of breath. Improve exercise tolerance.	This recommendation is somewhat controversial since some clinicians are still advocating chronic treatment with beta₂-agonists; however, chronic use of beta₂-agonists appears to increase bronchial reactivity and may contribute to asthma mortality. A trial of cromolyn sodium should precede the use of inhaled corticosteroids.
7. Patients with asthma should not receive beta-blocker medications (e.g., atenolol, propanalol).	III	NAEP, 1991	Prevent worsening of shortness of breath.	Beta-blockage promotes airway reactivity.
8. In any patients requiring chronic treatment with oral corticosteroids a trial of inhaled corticosteroids should have been attempted.	III	NAEP, 1991	Reduce toxicities of chronic systemic steroid use.[1]	Inhaled steroids have lower toxicities than oral steroids. It is unclear if it would be useful to attempt a trial every year or so, or if a single attempt is sufficient. This may be difficult to operationalize.
9. Any child with asthma who takes high doses of inhaled corticosteroids should have growth patterns monitored annually.	III	Starfield et al., 1994	Prevent growth retardation.	There is limited evidence that high-dose steroid treatment in children may affect growth patterns.
10. Patients who require frequent bursts of prednisone (2-3 trials of 5-day therapy with oral corticosteroids after an exacerbation of asthma within the past 6 months) who are not already on inhaled corticosteroids or chromolyn sodium should be started on them.	III	NAEP, 1991	Decrease steroid toxicity.[1]	Inhaled corticosteroids have fewer systemic toxicities and regular use prevents exacerbations.
11. Patients on theophylline should have at least one theophylline level determination per year.	III	NAEP, 1991	Decrease shortness of breath. Improve exercise tolerance. Prevent theophylline toxicity.	Regular evaluation should occur to monitor possible low or high levels, since clearance of theophylline is variable. Patients may therefore become subtherapeutic or toxic on doses that were previously therapeutic. Toxicities include tremulousness and agitation, nausea, vomiting, and cardiac arrhythmias.

Indicator	Quality of evidence	Literature	Benefits	Comments
12. Patients with the diagnosis of asthma that is moderate to severe who are at least six months of age should have a documented flu vaccination in the fall/winter of the previous year (September-January).	III	NAEP, 1991; CDC, 1993	Prevent secondary pneumonia. Prevent asthma exacerbation.[2]	Influenza can precipitate exacerbations and lead to secondary pneumonia in patients with asthma. Studies indicate that fewer than 10 percent of children at risk are immunized (Hall, 1987; Carter et al., 1986).
13. Patients with the diagnosis of asthma that is moderate to severe should have a pneumoccal vaccination documented in the chart.	III	USPSTF, 1989; Zimmerman & Burns, 1994	Prevent pneumonia.	Pneumonia is more life-threatening in persons with asthma.

Treatment of exacerbations

Indicator	Quality of evidence	Literature	Benefits	Comments
14. All patients > 5 years of age presenting to the physician's office with an asthma exacerbation or historical worsening of asthma symptoms should be evaluated with PEFR or FEV1.	III	NAEP, 1991	Decrease shortness of breath.	Objective measurements are useful for treatment decisions. They help intitate appropriate level of theraputic intervention, whether that be with beta$_2$-agonists, steroids, or hospitalization.
15. At the time of exacerbation, symptomatic patients on theophylline should have a theophylline level measured.	III	NAEP, 1991	Decrease shortness of breath.	Theophylline clearance may vary to a great degree even in the same individual. Subtherapeutic levels in persons on chronic treatment may add to exacerbations.
16. A physical exam of the chest should be performed in all patients presenting with an asthma exacerbation.	III	NAEP, 1991; McFadden & Hejal, 1995	Prevent mortality due to asthma.	Silent chest may predict more severe asthma. Physical exam helps guide therapy by evaluating severity.
17. All patients presenting to the physician's office or emergency department with an FEV1 or PEFR<=70 percent of baseline (or predicted) should be treated with beta$_2$-agonists before discharge.	III	NAEP, 1991; McFadden & Hejal, 1995	Decrease shortness of breath.	The percentage cut-off for this and the next three indicators are achieved through expert opinion; 70 percent is generally felt to be a cut-off for moderately severe exacerbations. It is generally agreed, however, that beta$_2$-agonists are first-line drugs in an exacerbation. Lack of improvement indicates the need for additional therapy.
18. Patients who receive treatment with beta$_2$-agonists for FEV1<70 percent in the physician's office or emergency department (ED) should have and FEV1 or PEFR repeated prior to discharge.	III	NAEP, 1991	Decrease shortness of breath.	Repeat measure documents response (or lack thereof) to therapy.
19. Patients with an FEV1 or PEFR <=70 percent of baseline (or predicted) after treatment for an asthma exacerbation in the physician's office should be placed on an oral corticosteroid taper.	III	NAEP, 1991; McFadden & Hejal, 1995	Decrease shortness of breath.	Steroids have been shown to improve recovery, but little objective data exists to back-up the appropriate cut-off. If patients do not improve significantly with beta$_2$-agonist alone, then the severity of exacerbation warrants steroid treatment.

	Quality of evidence	Literature	Benefits	Comments
20. Patients who have persistent symptoms, diffuse wheezes on chest auscultation, or a PEFR or FEV1 $\leq$40 percent of baseline (or predicted) after treatment with beta$_2$-agonist should be admitted to the hospital.	III	NAEP, 1991; McFadden & Hejal, 1995	To prevent mortality from asthma.	This defines a severe asthma exacerbation; these patients require close supervision to prevent mortality.

Hospital Treatment

Indicator	Quality of evidence	Literature	Benefits	Comments
21. All patients admitted to the hospital for asthma exacerbation should have oxygen saturation measured.	III	NAEP, 1991	Prevent mortality. Prevent cardiac ischemia. Decrease shortness of breath.	Oxygen saturation identifies patients who are hypoxic and for whom oxygen therapy should be initiated.
22. All hospitalized patients with PEFR or FEV1 < 25 percent of predicted or personal best should receive arterial blood gas measurement.	III	NAEP, 1991	Prevent mortality from extreme exacerbation.	Arterial blood gases identify acidosis and hypercarbia, which indicate potential need for intubation.
23. All hospitalized patients should receive systemic (IV) or oral steroids.	III	NAEP, 1991	Prevent mortality. Decrease shortness of breath.	Steroids improve recovery from severe asthma exacerbation.
24. All hospitalized patients should receive treatment with beta$_2$-agonists.	III	NAEP, 1991	Prevent mortality. Decrease shortness of breath.	Initial treatment should include the use of selective beta$_2$-agonist (e.g., albuterol); these are first-line agents for treatment of bronchoconstriction.
25. All hospitalized patients should receive treatment with methylxanthines.	III	NAEP, 1991	Prevent mortality. Decrease shortness of breath.	This area is controversial and not well supported by RCTs.
26. All hospitalized patients with oxygen saturation less than 92 percent should receive supplemental oxygen.	III	NAEP, 1991	Prevent mortality. Prevent cardiac ischemia. Decrease shortness of breath.	
27. All hospitalized patients with pCO$_2$ of greater than 40 should receive at least one additional blood gas measurement to evaluate response to treatment.	III	NAEP, 1991	Decrease shortness of breath. Prevent mortality.	CO$_2$ retention indicates poor gas exchange and fatigue, and these patients should be monitored closely for treatment response.
28. Hospitalized patients with pCO$_2$ of greater than 40 should be monitored in an intensive care setting.	III	NAEP, 1991	Prevent mortality.	CO$_2$ retention indicates poor gas exchange and fatigue, and these patients should be monitored closely for treatment response.
29. Patients with 2 or more hospitalizations for asthma exacerbation in the previous year should receive (or should have received) consultation with an asthma specialist.	III	NAEP, 1991	Improve quality of life. Decrease shortness of breath.	Among other things, hospitalization is a marker for severity and poor control. Patients with frequent hospitalizations may benefit from evaluation by an expert.
30. Hospitalized patients should not receive sedative drugs (e.g., benzodiazapines).	III	NAEP, 1991	Prevent worsening of shortness of breath.	Sedation may worsen exacerbation.

Follow-up

	Indicator	Quality of evidence	Literature	Benefits	Comments
31.	Patients with the diagnosis of asthma should have at least 2 visits within a calendar year.	III	NAEP, 1991; Starfield et al., 1994	Decrease baseline shortness of breath.	Minimum visit intervals have not been well specified or studied. However, follow-up visits should serve to optimize treatment regimen.
32.	Patients whose asthma medication is changed (new medication added, current dose decreased/increased) during one visit should have a follow-up visit within 3 weeks.	III	NAEP, 1991	Decrease shortness of breath. Minimize medication toxicity.	If medication regimen is altered, a change in symptoms is expected. Follow-up should indicate if new medication regimen is working appropriately. However, the time interval is arbitrary and this may not take into account telephone follow-up.
33.	Patients on chronic oral corticosteroids should have follow-up visits at least 4 times in a calendar year.	III	NAEP, 1991	Decrease toxicities of oral steroids.[2]	Minimum follow-up intervals have not been defined. Patients on chronic oral steroids have severe asthma and should be monitored more closely. This is important in children to assess normal growth patterns.
34.	Patients seen in the emergency department with an asthma exacerbation should have a follow-up reassessment within 72 hours.	III	NAEP, 1991	Prevent exacerbation recurrence.	NAEP recommends that treatment be given for 3 days and then patient be reassessed. Worsening of an exacerbation usually occurs in this time period.
35.	Patients with a hospitalization for an asthma exacerbation should receive outpatient follow-up within 14 days.	III	NAEP, 1991	Prevent exacerbation recurrence.	NAEP recommends follow-up but does not state a time interval. Two weeks seems reasonable since a taper off steroids is usually for approximately 2 weeks. Four weeks would be the least restrictive criterion that is acceptable.

[1] Toxicities of glucocorticoid therapy include fluid/electrolyte disturbances, peptic ulcer disease, ulcerative esophagitis, diabetes mellitus, glaucoma, psychosis, myopathy, osteoporosis, pancreatitis, impaired wound healing, adrenal atrophy, cataracts, and increased susceptibility to infections (Barker et al., 1991).

[2] An asthma exacerbation is characterized by acute obstruction to airflow. Exacerbations may be inititated through exposure to allergens and irritants, influenza, pneumonia, as well as other unidentified factors. Patients become acutely short of breath, tachycardic, and if severe, use accessory muscles of respiration. Exacerbation could lead to death if improperly treated. Treatment for an exacerbation should begin at home with beta$_2$-agonists. Physicians need to evaluate the severity of the exacerbation in order to inititate appropriate treatment.

Quality of Evidence Codes:

I:	RCT
II-1:	Nonrandomized controlled trials
II-2:	Cohort or case analysis
II-3:	Multiple time series
III:	Opinions or descriptive studies

REFERENCES - ASTHMA

American Academy of Pediatrics. January 1994. Practice parameter: The office management of acute exacerbations of asthma in children. *Pediatrics* 93 (1): 119-26.

Bailey WC, DM Higgins, BM Richards, et al. September 1992. Asthma severity: A factor analytic investigation. *American Journal of Medicine* 93: 263-9.

Barach EM. February 1994. Asthma in ambulatory care: Use of objective diagnostic criteria. *Journal of Family Practice* 38 (2): 161-5.

Bergner A, and RK Bergner. 1994. The International Consensus report on diagnosis and treatment of asthma: A call to action for US practitioners. *Clinical Therapeutics* 16 (4): 694-706.

Bosco LA, BB Gerstman, and DK Tomita. December 1993. Variations in the use of medication for the treatment of childhood asthma in the Michigan Medicaid population, 1980 to 1986. *Chest* 104 (6): 1727-32.

British Thoracic Society. 1993. Chronic asthma in adults and children. *Thorax* 48 (Suppl.): S1-S24.

Carr W, L Zeitel, and K Weiss. January 1992. Variations in asthma hospitalizations and deaths in New York City. *American Journal of Public Health* 82 (1): 59-65.

Crain EF, KB Weiss, PE Bijur, et al. September 1994. An estimate of the prevalence of asthma and wheezing among inner-city children. *Pediatrics* 94 (3): 356-62.

Executive Committee of the American Academy of Allergy and Immunology. 1993. Inhaled beta-2-adrenergic agonists in asthma. *Journal of Allergy and Clinical Immunology* 91: 1234-7.

Finkelstein JA, RW Brown, LC Schneider, et al. March 1995. Quality of care for preschool children with asthma: The role of social factors and practice setting. *Pediatrics* 95 (3): 389-94.

Gertsman BB, LA Bosco, and DK Tomita. April 1993. Trends in the prevalence of asthma hospitalization in the 5- to 14-year-old Michigan Medicaid population, 1980-1986. *Journal of Allergy and Clinical Immunology* 91 (4): 838-43.

Gustafsson P, J Tsanakas, M Gold, et al. 1993. Comparison of the efficacy and safety of inhaled fluticasone propionate 200 micrograms/day with inhaled beclomethasone dipropionate 400 micrograms/day in mild and moderate asthma. *Archives of Disease in Childhood* 69: 206-11.

Haahtela T, M Jarvinen, T Kava, et al. 8 August 1991. Comparison of a beta-2-agonist, terbutaline, with an inhaled corticosteroid, budesonide, in newly detected asthma. *New England Journal of Medicine* 325 (6): 388-92.

Halfon N, and PW Newacheck. November 1986. Trends in the hospitalization for acute childhood asthma, 1970-84. *American Journal of Public Health* 76 (11): 1308-11.

Hughes DM, M McLeod, B Garner, et al. January 1991. Controlled trial of a home and ambulatory program for asthmatic children. *Pediatrics* 87 (1): 54-61.

Huss K, CS Rand, AM Butz, et al. February 1994. Home environmental risk factors in urban minority asthmatic children. *Annals of Allergy* 72: 173-7.

Kelly HW. October 1993. Current controversies in asthma treatment. *American Pharmacy* NS33 (10): 48-54.

Lang DM, and M Polansky. 8 December 1994. Patterns of asthma mortality in Philadelphia from 1969 to 1991. *New England Journal of Medicine* 331 (23): 1542-6.

Larsen GL. 4 June 1992. Asthma in children. *New England Journal of Medicine* 326 (23): 1540-5.

Lindgren S, B Lokshin, A Stromquist, et al. 24 September 1992. Does asthma or treatment with theophylline limit children's academic performance? *New England Journal of Medicine* 327 (13): 926-30.

McFadden ER, and R Hejal. 13 May 1995. Asthma. *Lancet* 345: 1215-20.

Mueller GA, and H Eigen. December 1992. Pediatric pulmonary function testing in asthma. *Pediatric Clinics of North America* 39 (6): 1243-58.

National Asthma Education Program. August 1991. *Guidelines for the diagnosis and management of asthma*. U.S. Department of Health and Human Services, Hyattsville, MD.

O'Brien, KP. 1994. *The Prudential Asthma Program: The physician manual*. The Prudential Insurance Company of America, Roseland, NJ.

Podell RN. October 1992. National guidelines for the management of asthma in adults. *American Family Physician* 46 (4): 1189-96.

Price JF. 1993. The use of inhaled steroids in young children. *Agents and Actions Supplements* 40: 201-10.

Roth A. December 1993. Hospital admissions of young children for status asthmaticus in Honolulu, Hawaii, 1986 to 1989. *Annals of Allergy* 71: 533-6.

Selcow JE. 1994. Safety of bronchodilator therapy in pediatric asthma patients. *Clinical Therapeutics* 16 (4): 622-33.

Smith L. August 1993. Childhood asthma: diagnosis and treatment. *Current Problems in Pediatrics* 23: 271-305.

Starfield B, NR Powe, JR Weiner, et al. 28 December 1994. Costs vs quality in different types of primary care settings. *Journal of the American Medical Association* 272 (24): 1903-8.

Stempel DA, and SJ Szefler. December 1992. Management of chronic asthma. *Pediatric Clinics of North America* 39 (6): 1293-1310.

Taylor WR, and PW Newacheck. November 1992. Impact of childhood asthma on health. *Pediatrics* 90 (5): 657-62.

U.S. Preventive Services Task Force. 1989. *Guide to Clinical Preventive Services: An Assessment of the Effectiveness of 169 Interventions.* Baltimore, MD: Williams and Wilkins.

Volovitz B, J Amir, H Malik, et al. 1994. Administration of half-dose theophylline together with ketotifen to asthmatic children--a double blind, placebo-controlled study. *Journal of Asthma* 31 (1): 27-34.

Weiss KB, PJ Gergen, and TA Hodgson. 26 March 1992. An economic evaluation of asthma in the United States. *New England Journal of Medicine* 326 (13): 862-6.

Weiss KB, and DK Wagener. 1990. Geographic variations in US asthma mortality: Small-area analyses of excess mortality, 1981-1985. *American Journal of Epidemiology* 132 (1): S107-S115.

Weiss ST. 1994. The origins of childhood asthma. *Monaldi Archives of Chest Diseases* 49 (2): 154-8.

Weitzman M, SL Gortmaker, AM Sobol, et al. 18 November 1992. Recent trends in the prevalence and severity of childhood asthma. *Journal of the American Medical Association* 268 (19): 2673-7.

Wood PR, HA Hidalgo, TJ Prihoda, et al. 1993. Hispanic children with asthma: Morbidity. *Pediatrics* 91: 62-9.

Zimmerman RK, and IT Burns. December 1994. Childhood immunization guidelines: Current and future. *Primary Care* 21 (4): 693-715.

Zora JA, D Zimmerman, T Carey, et al. 1986. Hypothalamic-pituitary-adrenal axis suppression after short-term, high-dose glucocorticoid therapy in children with asthma. *Journal of Allergy and Clinical Immunology* 77: 9-13.

5. ATTENTION DEFICIT/HYPERACTIVITY DISORDER
Glenn Takata, M.D., M.S., and May Lau, M.D.

The recommendations on the evaluation and management of attention deficit/hyperactivity disorder (ADHD) in children were developed by summarizing the guidelines and recommendations of review articles (Pliszka, 1991; Voeller, 1991; Kelly and Aylward, 1992; Reiff et al., 1993; Culbert et al., 1994; Vinson, 1994; Searight et al., 1995) and a textbook (Mercugliano, in Schwartz, 1990). The review articles were selected from a MEDLINE literature search on the key phrase "attention deficit disorder," looking for articles in the English language published between the years 1985 and 1995. Focused assessment of the literature with respect to specific areas of importance or disagreement among the reviews were then conducted to further clarify those issues.

IMPORTANCE

Attention deficit/hyperactivity disorder (ADHD) or attention deficit disorder or attentional disorder is a common and important problem among children. About 3 to 5 percent of school-age children have characteristics consistent with the clinical presentation of ADHD (Kelly and Aylward, 1992; Reiff et al., 1993). ADHD occurs about six times more frequently among boys than girls in clinical studies (Reiff et al., 1993) and three times more frequently in population-based studies (Searight et al., 1995). These disorders have serious effects on a child's functioning in our society.

Though not explicitly documented in any of the reviews, it is evident that the core symptoms of ADHD, inattention and impulsivity/hyperactivity, may lead to secondary morbidity for the child, the child's family, and society. The child may suffer from insult to the affect such as poor self-esteem as well as more tangible negative outcomes such as greater risk of accidents, cigarette or alcohol use, drug abuse, criminal activity, and poor school performance and subsequent failure in the adult work force (Searight et al., 1995).

The child's family may suffer dysfunction in trying to deal with a child with an attentional disorder. Society suffers the disruption of classrooms by children with ADHD in addition to the costs associated with the specific effects on the child and family and the costs to society of an unemployed adult.

ADHD is one of the most common chronic neurobehavioral problems of childhood. As noted below present studies indicate that the appropriate diagnosis and treatment of these disorders may lead to short-term and perhaps long-term benefits to the child, the child's family, and society. Inappropriate diagnosis and treatment will lead to unwarranted or inappropriate use of scarce mental health resources and possible adverse side effects from pharmacologic interventions.

EFFICACY AND/OR EFFECTIVENESS OF INTERVENTIONS

Screening and Prevention

Though health care providers do not specifically screen for the presence of ADHD among children, they should in the course of routine health supervision inquire and provide guidance with regard to the child's temperament and behavior and in the areas of parenting and discipline (American Academy of Pediatrics Committee on Psychosocial Aspects of Child and Family Health, 1988). By identifying earlier the child with the potential for ADHD, the health care provider might expect to circumvent secondary morbidity to the child and the family, such as low self esteem and family dysfunction, though not the attention deficit itself.

Diagnosis

ADHD comprises a constellation of clinical symptoms. It has been defined as a disorder where "Children ... exhibit core symptoms of inattention, impulsivity and overactivity that are inappropriate for their developmental level and interfere with their optimal functioning (Reiff et al., 1993).

The symptoms characterizing the syndrome of ADHD have been formalized into diagnostic criteria in the Diagnostic and Statistical Manual of Mental Disorders IV (DSM-IV) (American Psychiatric Association

[APA], 1994). All 5 criteria must be met for diagnosis. In this
classification, ADHD is divided into three subtypes (see Table 5.1).

Table 5.1

Diagnostic Criteria for Attention-Deficit/Hyperactivity Disorder

A. Six or more of the following symptoms of inattention and six or more of the following symptoms of hyperactivity/ impulsivity have persisted for at least 6 months to a degree that is maladaptive and inconsistent with developmental level in either of the following categories:

1. **Inattention**
   - often fails to give close attention to details or makes careless mistakes in schoolwork, work, or other activities
   - often has difficulty sustaining attention in tasks or play activities
   - often does not seem to listen when spoken to directly
   - often does not follow through on instructions and fails to finish schoolwork, chores, or duties in the workplace
   - often has difficulty organizing tasks and activities
   - often avoids, dislikes, or is reluctant to engage in tasks that require sustained mental effort (such as schoolwork or homework)
   - often loses things necessary for tasks or activities (e.g., toys, school assignments, pencils, books or tools)
   - is often easily distracted by extraneous stimuli
   - is often forgetful in daily activities

2. **Hyperactivity-impulsivity**
   Hyperactivity
   - often fidgets with hands or feet or squirms in seat
   - often leaves seat in classroom or in other situations in which remaining seated is expected
   - often runs about or climbs excessively in situations in which it is inappropriate (in adolescents or adults, may be limited to subjective feelings of restlessness)
   - often has difficulty playing or engaging in leisure activities quietly
   - is often "on the go" or often acts as if "driven by a motor"
   - often talks excessively
   Impulsivity
   - often blurts out answers before questions have been completed
   - often has difficulty waiting turn
   - often interrupts or intrudes on others (e.g., butts into conversations or games)

B. Some hyperactive-impulsive or inattentive symptoms that caused impairment were present before age 7 years

C. Some impairment from the symptoms is present in two or more settings (e.g., at school/work and at home).

D. There must be clear evidence of clinically significant impairment in social, academic, or occupational functioning.

E. The symptoms do not occur exclusively during the course of a Pervasive Developmental Disorder, Schizophrenia, or other Psychotic Disorder and are not better accounted for by another mental disorder.

Types

ADHD, Combined Type: if criteria 1 and 2 are met

ADHD, Predominantly Inattentive Type: if criteria 1 only is met

ADHD, Predominantly Hyperactive-Impulsive Type: if criteria 2 only is met

ADHD, Not Otherwise Specified: if prominent symptoms of inattention or hyperactivity-impulsivity are present but do not meet criteria for ADHD.

Source: Diagnostic and Statistical Manual of Mental Disorders IV, 1994.

The distinguishing feature of these subtypes is degree of hyperactivity-impulsivity. In ADHD predominantly hyperactive-impulsive type, the children are more disruptive, irresponsible, messy and immature. They usually have more problems with peer relationships than their ADHD primarily inattentive type counterparts. In addition, family members of this former group of children have been found to be more aggressive, with greater tendency towards substance abuse and lower incidence of Learning Disability and anxiety than the group with ADHD-inattentive type (APA, 1994).

In contrast, the group of children with ADHD predominantly inattentive type tend to function with a slower cognitive speed and appear more confused and apathetic. Forty percent of girls who present with ADHD are found to have the ADHD-inattentive type. This subgroup of children tend to be diagnosed at a later age when academic difficulties escalate (Reiff et al., 1993).

Children may also have ADHD-combined type, fulfilling the criteria for both inattention and hyperactivity-impulsivity. The last category is ADHD-Not Otherwise Specified, in which the diagnostic criteria are not fully met. The importance of differentiating clinical subtypes has implications for treatment strategies.

Prior to the formulation of DSM-IV, the diagnosis of ADHD by DSM-III-R was based on a 14-item list of symptoms of inattention, impulsivity and hyperactivity. The presence of 8 or more of the listed symptoms would be consistent with a diagnosis of ADHD. There was no diagnostic distinction between the clinical subtypes.

Both DSM-III and DSM-IV stipulate that onset of symptoms must occur before 7 years of age, that symptoms be present for greater than 6 months and are not accounted for by other mental disorders.

The developmental level of each child must be considered when presented with parental concerns of hyperactivity and inattention. Preschool children may exhibit these symptoms, but the level of activity and attention may be appropriate for their age and developmental level. Many will not go on to be diagnosed with ADHD (APA, 1994). In fact, some authors have proposed changing the criteria for preschool children by extending the duration of symptoms to 12 months and increasing the number of criteria behaviors to 10 of the 14 listed in DSM-III-R (Reiff et al., 1993). One may also consider the degree of dysfunction caused by the symptoms in a preschool setting as a criterion for diagnosis (Reiff et al., 1993).

The symptoms of inattention and hyperactivity are nonspecific and may be a manifestation of many medical, neurological, or psychiatric disorders. The challenge of making an accurate diagnosis of ADHD is compounded by the fact that many of the entities in the list of differential diagnosis may co-exist with ADHD. In one report, Learning Disability and Language Disorder may occur in 30-60 percent of children with ADHD. Anxiety Disorder occurs in 25 percent and other mood disorders may be present in 30 percent of the ADHD children. Oppositional Defiant Disorder may occur as often as 40-65 percent while Conduct Disorder may occur in 21-50 percent in children with ADHD (Reiff et al., 1993). In another series of consecutive referrals to a tertiary university based behavioral neurology clinic, only 4 out of 63 children with ADHD had the single diagnosis. Eighty-three percent of the children also had Learning Disability and 73 percent fulfilled the criteria for depression (Weinberg and Emslie, 1991). Making the correct diagnosis and identifying the comorbid disorders are important in determining the appropriate treatment.

Specific diagnoses to be considered as differential diagnoses and comorbid conditions are (Weinberg and Emslie, 1991; Reiff et al., 1993):

1. Affective Disorders: Depression, Anxiety, Mania
2. Learning Disorders: Mental Retardation, Specific Learning Disabilities
3. Language Disorders
4. Disorders of Disruptive Behaviors: Oppositional Defiant Disorder, Conduct Disorder
5. Thought Disorder
6. Sleep Disorders: Narcolepsy, Obstructive Sleep Apnea
7. Poor environmental fit
8. Underlying medical or neurological problem: Hyperthyroidism, Seizures, Tourettes' Syndrome, Sensory Impairments

Because ADHD represents a clinical syndrome with multiple etiologies and comorbidities, the evaluation should involve investigation into all aspects of the child's life including developmental, psychological, psychosocial and psychoeducational components (Reiff et al., 1993). Ideally, such a broad scope of evaluation necessitates a multidisciplinary team approach to diagnosis and treatment. The practitioner has two options when a child presents with attentional problems: 1) refer the child to a multidisciplinary clinic specializing in developmental/behavioral problems, or 2) serve as a central coordinator who obtains information from various sources and consultants and synthesizes the information to reach a diagnosis and treatment plan.

In either case, a comprehensive evaluation of the child with attentional problems as conceptualized by Reiff et al. (1993) includes four components:

1. Medical
2. Psychological
3. Psychosocial
4. Psychoeducational

This component of the evaluation may be considered the initial work-up to establish working diagnoses. The objective is to differentiate symptoms through the interview, examination and screening tests.

A careful history obtained from the caretaker should be the first step. A description of the symptoms and behaviors of concern, the time of onset, preceding events and duration are essential. Questions should focus on the ruling in or out differential diagnoses. While not clearly stated in the DSM-IV (APA, 1994), the diagnosis of ADHD can be made based solely on the history obtained from the caretakers (Shaywitz, 1991). The DSM-IV does stipulate that the symptoms of inattention and impulsivity/hyperactivity be present in more than two settings (APA, 1994). It also suggests that the practitioner obtain information on the child's behavior in a variety of settings. Other authors recommend obtaining input specifically from the child's caretaker and teacher(s) as well as the child (Weinberg and Emslie, 1991; Kelly and Aylward, 1992; Reiff et al., 1993).

The child's developmental history is important to support the finding of subaverage intellectual functioning (Kelly and Aylward, 1992). A review of the current medications may reveal some that affect attention and learning (Mercugliano, in Schwartz, 1990; Voeller, 1991). Documenting the past medical history, including the birth history may suggest an underlying medical problem. Family history of ADHD, Learning Disorder, mental retardation, neurologic and psychiatric illnesses should be elicited.

The physical examination should include identifying dysmorphic features which may indicate a further work-up and the presence of physical findings suggesting an underlying medical condition. Hearing and vision should be a routine part of the evaluation to rule out sensory impairment as a contributing cause of decreased attention (Kelly and Aylward, 1992; Reiff et al., 1993). A thorough neurological examination is necessary to rule out static or progressive neurological deficits. This includes a mental status examination, assessment of cranial nerves, motor, sensory and cerebellar functions. Soft neurological signs such as dysdiadokinesis, dysgraphesthesia and motor incoordination may be present, but are not diagnostic of ADHD (Kelly and Aylward, 1992).

Further information may be obtained through screening tests in the practitioner's office, behavior rating scales, or through consultants and schools (see below). The practitioner should obtain the following information regarding the child:

1. Level of cognition
2. Behavior and performance at school
3. Behavior and function at home
4. Social environment
5. Affective state

After reviewing all the information, the practitioner can formulate the diagnosis and treatment plan.

The practitioner may use different methods to assess a child's affective and behavioral state. The assessment should include both the child's and adults' perspectives.

Behavioral rating scales have been widely used. They are an efficient means of obtaining input from various sources regarding a child's behaviors (Mercugliano, in Schwartz, 1990; Reiff et al., 1993). Rating scales are available for teachers and parents. Some assess single specific behaviors (unidimensional) and others a series of behaviors (multidimensional). The most widely used are the Conners Scales for parents and teachers. These are standardized for children from age 3 to 17 years old and contains scales for conduct problem, learning problem, psychosomatic symptoms, impulsivity-hyperactivity, and anxiety (Kelly and Aylward, 1992). A shorter index assessing just the impulsivity-hyperactivity symptoms has been used to assess medication efficacy (Kelly and Aylward, 1992). Other commonly used scales that can be used to evaluate a range of behaviors include the Child Behavior Checklist and the Yale Children's Inventory, Aggregate Neurobehavioral Student Health and Education Review (ANSER), and Attention Deficit Disorder with Hyperactivity Comphrehensive Teacher Rating Scale (AcTERS); each evaluates a specific complex of behaviors and the child's current functioning (Reiff et al., 1993). Other scales are used to assess for affective symptomatology such as the Children's Depression

Inventory and the Revised Children's Manifest Anxiety Scale (Reiff et al., 1993), both of which are completed by the child.

The pitfall of rating scales is that they are nonspecific and are subject to the "halo-effect" where the child's behavior is either rated as all good or all bad (Searight et al., 1995). Often there is a discrepancy between a teacher's and parent's perception of the child's behavior. Evidence tends to support giving greater weight to the teacher's evaluation of the child's behavior because the teacher is observing the child's behavior in a structured and task-oriented setting which tends to accentuate the attentional and behavioral problems (Pliszka, 1991).

The child's perspective on his difficulties can be obtained through an interview with the child. This interaction also allows the practitioner to observe the child's behavior and affect, assess language skills and cooperation. The interview itself may disclose the child's perception of the problems, himself and his environment, the presence of a thought disorder, and indications of affective disorders. Other methods that can be used to elicit information from the child are drawings, sentence completion, and rating scales for symptoms such as anxiety and depression. Referral to a psychiatrist is indicated if any psychopathology is suspected.

Only 20 percent of children with ADHD will exhibit behaviors of inattention, hyperactivity, and impulsivity while at a doctor's office. The lack of observed behavior in a clinical setting does not rule out ADHD (Pliszka, 1991).

Objective measures of attention may assist in the diagnosis of attentional disorders but should not be used in isolation. One widely used test is the Continuous Performance Task. However, this test is affected by age and intelligence and has a variable but high false negative rate of 15-35 percent (Kelly and Aylward, 1992). This test also can be used to monitor medication response. Other specific tests for inattention have yet to be proven in validity (Kelly and Aylward, 1992).

The practitioner should obtain information about the child's environment including home, school, and daycare center (Kelly and

Aylward, 1992). Delineation of the family constellation is important to assess the level of stability and support that is available. The functional status of the family should also be assessed in terms conflict resolution, coping strategies and degree of stressors (Reiff et al., 1993). Parental expectations for the child should be explored to evaluate the appropriateness for that particular child (Voeller, 1991; Reiff et al., 1993).

Psychoeducational testing involves establishing the child's cognitive function and academic achievements. Psychoeducational testing may also provide supporting evidence of attentional difficulties and identify the presence of a learning disability (Kelly and Aylward, 1992). The testing situation allows the clinician to observe the child's behaviors and can be a valuable source of information in making the diagnosis (Kelly and Aylward, 1992; Reiff et al., 1993).

An assessment of the child's cognitive functioning is needed to rule out mental retardation. For screening purposes, neurodevelopmental assessment using standardized tests such as the Pediatric Examination of Educational Readiness (PEER), the Pediatric Early Elemental Examination (PEEX), and the Pediatric Examination of Educational Readiness at Middle Childhood (PEERAMID) may be used to look for deficits in language, cognition, and visual-motor functioning (Kelly and Aylward, 1992; Reiff et al., 1993). One author has formulated a Mental Status Exam for the same purpose (Searight et al., 1995).

A full evaluation of a child's cognitive functioning can be obtained using the Weschlers Scales of Intelligence, the Stanford-Binet, and the Kaufman Assessment Battery for Children. Subtests in the Weschler Intelligence Scales may provide supporting evidence for attention deficits (Kelly and Aylward, 1992). The Kaufman ABC likewise yields simultaneous processing and sequential scores which are sensitive to attention deficits (Kelly and Aylward, 1992). Other tests are available to distinguish ADHD from other learning disorders and processing problems (Kelly and Aylward, 1992).

The Woodcock-Johnson Psychoeducational Battery Tests of Achievement is widely used to assess the child's academic level in subjects such as math, reading, written language, knowledge and skills clustering (Reiff et al., 1993). Kelly and Aylward (1992) suggest that tests of academic achievement should be routinely incorporated into the evaluation of ADHD.

The full psychoeducational assessment battery may be obtained through the school as an evaluation for an Individualized Education Plan, or through a consulting psychologist. Voeller (1991) suggests that psychoeducational testing be done prior to the recommendation of starting medication. Searight et al. (1995) suggest that formal psychoeducational testing be done in cases where clinical evidence for diagnosis of ADHD is equivocal, where comorbid conditions are suspected and where medical treatment meets with poor response.

Speech and language evaluation by a speech pathologist is indicated if screening reveals deficits in this area. Neuropsychological assessment is another option if screening reveals specific neurological defects (Mercugliano, in Schwartz, 1990; Reiff et al., 1993).

In summary, ADHD is a clinical diagnosis based on fulfilling the DSM-IV criteria. The evaluation involves obtaining a detailed history, physical and neurologic examination, neurodevelopmental assessment, vision/hearing screen, assessment of social/emotional status as well as environmental factors in both school and home (Kelly and Aylward, 1992; Reiff et al., 1993). In addition, specific evaluation of attention, behavior and cognitive functioning is necessary (Kelly and Aylward, 1992). Using a unidimensional scale with environmental descriptors is the minimum assessment recommended for diagnosis (Kelly and Aylward, 1992). In addition, Reiff et al. (1993) stress that interviews with teachers, parents and child are essential to the evaluation. Additional evaluations may be indicated if during the initial work-up, the possibility of comorbid disorders arise.

Treatment

Though the evidence is not overwhelming, most agree that the treatment of ADHD should be multidisciplinary and is dependent, to some extent, on cormorbid conditions (Voeller, 1991; Kelly and Aylward, 1992; Culbert et al., 1994). Though studied inadequately, the few treatment plans for ADHD that have shown any long-term benefit have involved the use of multiple modalities incorporating medical, psychological, psychosocial, and educational interventions (Culbert et al., 1994). Vinson (1994) notes that long-term outcome cannot be predicted (Klein and Mannuzza, 1991). Some suggest that, in a subset of children with minimal ADHD, that psychological and behavioral therapies alone may be sufficient and medical therapy may not be needed (Voeller, 1991). The goals of treatment are normal development and reduction of problem behaviors such as poor self-esteem and dysfunctional parent-child and peer-child relationships (Culbert et al., 1994).

Following the diagnosis of ADHD, the first responsibility of the health care provider is to educate the family and child about the disorder (Kelly and Aylward, 1992; Culbert et al., 1994). Parents should be assured that they are not to blame for the presence of the attention deficit in their child. Another function of education is for the health care provider to point out the child's personal strengths (Kelly and Aylward, 1992; Culbert et al., 1994).

Psychological and behavioral therapies combined to meet the characteristics of the child, family, and school are thought by some to be essential to appropriate management of children with ADHD (Culbert et al., 1994). In addition, behavioral intervention may enhance stimulant therapy (Pelham and Murphy, in Hersen, 1986), though Culbert et al. (1994) state that such evidence is difficult to document (despite the fact that they recommend multimodal therapy as the standard of care). On the other hand, Pliszka (1991), a psychiatrist, states quite strongly that behavioral or psychologic or psychiatric therapy is not a substitute for stimulant pharmacotherapy but may be helpful if the child does not respond to stimulant therapy, if a disciplinary issue arises, such as aggression or stealing, or in the presence of an oppositional or antisocial behavior.

The goals of psychological and behavioral therapies are to target cognitive problems and behavioral deficits, treat comorbid problems such as oppositional defiant behavior and conduct disorders, enhance competencies, and increase family and school involvement in the child's treatment (Culbert et al., 1994). Psychological and behavioral therapies include (Culbert et al., 1994):

1. behavioral parent training

2. behavioral family therapy

3. classroom contingency management procedures

4. self-instructional problem-solving training

5. anger management training

6. group social skills training

Such therapies are provided by developmental/behaviorists, psychologists, and/or psychiatrists.

Kelly and Aylward (1992) divide behavior therapies into home interventions and classroom interventions involving environmental modifications in those respective milieus. Providing parents written information about behavioral techniques is minimally effective (Vinson, 1994; Long et al., 1993). Family therapy may decrease parent-child conflict (Vinson 1994; Barkley et al., 1992) and reduce delinquency in children when applied in conjunction with stimulant therapy (Satterfield et al., 1987). Behavior modification in the classroom setting may aid the child's behavior when coupled with low-dose methylphenidate, but not to a greater degree than with a higher dose of methylphenidate alone (Vinson 1994; Carlson et al., 1992; Pelham et al., 1993). Self-control techniques based on social learning theory may add little benefit to methylphenidate therapy (Vinson 1994; Horn et al., 1991; Ialongo et al., 1993).

Despite the general recommendation to provide psychological and behavioral therapy to children with ADHD, there are few studies that support their use (Gittleman and Abikoff, 1989), though these few are described as promising by Culbert et al. (1994). Vinson (1994) indicates that psychological and social therapies are at best modest in their effects and are extremely labor intensive. Any positive effects are not curative, but rather help the child, family, and the teacher cope with the difficulties of the attentional disorder, utilizing the strengths of all involved (Culbert et al., 1994). Psychotherapy may be helpful in individual cases; there is little evidence that cognitive therapy is useful (Kelly and Aylward, 1992; Abikoff, 1991).

Psychoeducational intervention is also required (Culbert et al., 1994). Each school-age child with ADHD should have an Individual Education Plan (IEP) formulated by the school system that takes into account the child's information processing and production capabilities (Culbert et al., 1994). The IEP may be requested by the parent, teacher, or health care provider. The IEP and its implementation are mandated by federal Public Law 94-142 when learning disabilities or emotional disturbances, as well as other medical conditions, are impeding the education of a child (American Academy of Pediatrics Committee on Children with Disabilities, 1992). Speech or language disorders are among the many psychoeducational issues that must be addressed (Culbert et al., 1994).

Pharmacologic treatment may lead to improved short-term abatement of the core symptom complex of inattention, impulsivity, and overactivity compared to nonpharmacologic or no treatment (Kavale, 1982; Culbert et al., 1994; Vinson, 1994; Pelham et al., 1990). By increasing attention and decreasing impulsivity, the child may have fewer disruptive behaviors (Pelham et al., 1990) and show additional effects such as an improvement in handwriting (Culbert et al., 1994) and enhanced academic performance (Kavale, 1982; Kelly and Aylward, 1992; Pelham et al., 1990). Medication has not been shown to lead to long-term removal of these symptoms (Fox and Rieder, 1993; Culbert et al., 1994; Barkley et al., 1990; Horn et al., 1991; Ialongo et al., 1993; Brown et al., 1986a; Brown et al., 1986b). Long-term benefits occur only while medication is still being administered; this also appears to be the case for behavioral therapy (Vinson, 1994; Firestone et al., 1986). As mentioned above, a favorable response to pharmacologic intervention should not be used as confirmation of the diagnosis of ADHD since many children without ADHD show a positive response to medication as well (Voeller, 1991; Culbert et al., 1994; Rapoport et al., 1980; Ullman and Sleator, 1986). The health care provider must educate the child, the family, and the teacher about the risks and benefits of pharmacologic treatment, including side effects.

Unlike the narrative reviews of other authors, a rigorous meta-analytic review of 135 studies by Kavale (1982) showed quite convincingly that stimulant therapy is efficacious for the treatment of short-term outcomes in ADHD. Studies with findings amenable to meta-analysis that looked at hyperactivity as a primary symptom and that had a comparison group were included. Outcomes were then partitioned into behavior, cognitive, and physiologic groups. He found that stimulant therapy had positive effects on behavioral and cognitive outcomes and some negative effects on physiologic outcomes. The average child with hyperactivity treated with stimulant therapy had better behavioral outcomes than 72 percent of control subjects in the areas of general ratings, activity level, attention and concentration, and behavior characteristics, though not for anxiety. Although the effects were not as large, the average hyperactive child treated with stimulants scored higher than 69 percent of control subjects on measures of intelligence, achievement, perception, motor skills, and memory. Most psychophysiologic outcomes revealed a negative effect of stimulant therapy such as effects on the cardiorespiratory system and on weight and height; positive effects were found on galvanic skin response, average evoked potential, electroencephalogram, and sleep variables. He also found that methyphenidate, dextroamphetamine, pemoline, levoamphetamine, and benzedrine were all effective while caffeine was not. In addition, he tempered his analysis by analyzing issues of study variables, subject variables, and design variables, but still came to the conclusion that stimulant pharmacotherapy was efficacious in the treatment of ADHD. Kavale (1982) then closed his meta-analytic review with a call to "debate the ethical questions concerning the use of stimulant drugs with hyperactive children."

The most commonly used medications for the treatment of ADHD are the stimulants methylphenidate (Ritalin), dextroamphetamine (Dexedrine), and pemoline (Cylert) (Voeller, 1991; Kelly and Aylward, 1992; Fox and Rieder, 1993; Culbert et al., 1994; Searight et al., 1995). Pliszka (1991) reports that the stimulants have a rapid onset of action (i.e., within a few days to two weeks). The stimulants lead to an improvement in at least 75 percent of children with attention deficit disorders and appear to be efficacious from childhood through adulthood (Culbert et al., 1994). Stimulant therapy is not recommended for children less than

three years of age (Barkley, 1989). Improved outcomes include measures
of: attention and vigilance, short-term memory, fine motor output in
the laboratory, behavior in the classroom, interpersonal interactions,
teacher and peer perceptions of the child, and academic achievement
(Culbert et al., 1994; Tannock et al., 1989; Vyse and Rapport, 1989;
DuPaul and Rapport, 1993; Evans and Pelham, 1991; Dalby et al., 1989;
Klorman et al., 1988; Barkley et al., 1989; Klorman et al., 1990; Kaplan
et al., 1990). The stimulants are safe and of low cost (Culbert et al.,
1994). Searight (1995) states an unreferenced opinion that stimulants
appear in general to be more effective in treating ADHD compared to
other medications.

Methylphenidate is the most commonly prescribed stimulant for
treatment of ADHD. Culbert et al. (1994) recommend that the use of
methylphenidate in a child begin with a double-blind placebo-controlled
trial in which 0.3 and 0.5 milligram per kilogram doses and placebo are
tested over a three-week period using teacher, parent, and child ratings
to assess response on a weekly basis. Voeller (1991), Kelly and Aylward
(1992), Vinson (1994) and Searight et al. (1995) make similar
recommendations for a double-blind placebo trial (McBride, 1988; Porrino
et al., 1983; Fine and Jewesson, 1989; DiTraglia, 1991; Ullmann et al.,
1986; Barkley et al., 1988). Standard dosing of methylphenidate is 0.3
to 0.5 milligram per kilogram per dose at four-hour intervals, two to
three times per day (Culbert et al., 1994). Voeller (1991) states that
doses as high as 1.0 milligram per kilogram per dose may be permissible
in certain children. Symptoms of inattention and impulsivity respond to
lower doses whereas symptoms of overactivity respond to higher doses but
decrease cognitive performance (Voeller, 1991; Kelly and Aylward, 1992;
Culbert et al., 1994; Tannock et al. 1989; Barkley et al., 1991; Sprague
and Sleator, 1977; Rapport et al., 1988; Swanson and Kinsbourne, 1988).
Methylphenidate efficacy is usually evident within one to two weeks
(Searight et al., 1995). The sustained release form of methyphenidate
does not seem to be as effective as the standard form (Voeller, 1991;
Kelly and Aylward, 1992; Searight et al., 1995; Fitzpatrick et al.,
1992; Pelham et al., 1987; Pelham et al., 1990).

Dextroamphetamine may be used in children who do not respond to methylphenidate (Culbert et al., 1994). The dose for dextroamphetamine is half that for methylphenidate (Culbert et al., 1994). Kelly and Aylward (1992) raise concerns of abuse potential and side effects with dextroamphetamine but also acknowledge that at the time of their publication it was the only stimulant approved for use among children less than six years of age. It is evident from the literature, however, that dextroamphetamine is not the only stimulant used in that age group.

Pemoline is another stimulant alternative. Pemoline may be given once per day (Searight et al., 1995). Searight et al. (1995) recommend an initial dose of 37.5 milligrams increased by 18.75 milligrams every three to five days until a change in behavior is noted. A positive response with pemoline may not be apparent for several weeks (Fox and Rieder, 1993). Children on pemoline must be monitored for possible liver toxicity (Pratt and Dubois, 1990; Nehra et al., 1990) and should have baseline liver function tests performed (Kelly and Aylward, 1992; Searight et al., 1995). Dextroamphetamine and pemoline are equal in effectiveness to methylphenidate (Kavale, 1982; Vinson 1994; Pelham et al., 1990).

The use of stimulant therapy should be preceded by collection and evaluation of the following data (Culbert et al., 1994):

1. blood pressure
2. weight and height

The presence of tics or Tourette disorder is a relative contraindication to the use of stimulant therapy (Voeller, 1991; Culbert et al., 1994). Kelly and Aylward (1992) feel that stimulants may be used in children with Tourette disorder if the morbidity due to the ADHD outweighs that due to Tourette disorder. Seizure disorder is no longer thought to be a contraindication to stimulant therapy (Culbert et al., 1994) particularly with regard to methylphenidate (Voeller, 1991; Kelly and Aylward, 1992).

Culbert et al. (1994) suggest that the following side effects be monitored:

1. tics

2. decreased appetite

3. insomnia

4. headaches

5. stomach aches

6. irritability

7. anxiety

8. excessive sadness or weepiness

9. social withdrawal

10. euphoria

11. dizziness

12. mildly elevated heart rate

13. minor increases in blood pressure

Fox and Rieder (1993) also mention transient psychosis, rash, and eosinophilia as possible side effects of stimulant therapy. Growth delay may occur in children on stimulant therapy; however, catch-up growth may occur once off the medication (Voeller, 1991; Kelly and Aylward, 1992; Vinson, 1994). Barkley et al. (1990) have suggested that side effects should be monitored before and after start of medication therapy.

Tricyclic antidepressants, including imipramine and desipramine, are second-line choices for pharmacologic treatment of children with ADHD (Kelly and Aylward, 1992; Fox and Rieder, 1993; Culbert et al., 1994; Garfinkel et al., 1983; Gualtieri et al., 1991). Double-blind placebo-controlled trials have shown a 60 to 70 percent efficacy rate. The positive effects of the tricyclic antidepressants have been mostly on inattention, impulsivity, and overactivity; cognitive effects are equivocal (Culbert et al., 1994; Vinson, 1994; Searight et al., 1995; Pliszka, 1987; Biederman et al., 1989a; Biederman et al., 1989b; Biederman et al., 1993). Some studies indicate long-term memory may also be improved (Culbert et al.. 1994). The initial dose for imipramine and desipramine is 0.3 milligram per kilogram per day and it is increased every 3 to 4 days to a maximum of 2 to 3 milligrams per kilogram per day. Pre-treatment assessment should include an electrocardiogram (Fox and Rieder, 1993; Vinson, 1994), as cardiac arrhythmias and sudden cardiac death are side effects (Biederman et al., 1989b; Riddle et al., 1991), and drug levels should be monitored as well as follow-up electrocardiograms (Culbert et al., 1994). Other side effects include blurred vision, irritability, drowsiness, dry mouth, dizziness, appetite changes, constipation, tremor, sleep disturbance, and abdominal cramps (Kelly and Aylward 1992; Fox and Rieder 1993).

Clonidine is another alternative pharmacologic treatment for children with attention deficit disorders (Kelly and Aylward, 1992; Culbert et al., 1994). Clonidine is estimated to have an efficacy rate of 70 per cent (Culbert et al., 1994). The effects of clonidine have been on inattention, impulsivity, and overactivity without negative cognitive effects (Culbert et al., 1994; Hunt et al., 1985; Hunt et al., 1986). Clonidine is thought to be particular useful in children who are hyperaroused or aggressive and those with tics or Tourette disorder (Kelly and Aylward, 1992; Culbert et al., 1994). The maximal dose of clonidine is 0.1 to 0.3 milligrams per day after slow increases of 0.05 milligram per day every 3 days (Culbert et al., 1994). Kelly and Aylward (1992) state that the maximal dose of clonidine is four to five micrograms per kilogram per day and that it should not be stopped abruptly because of possible rebound hypertension. The major side effects are somnolence and elevated blood pressure (Culbert et al., 1994).

Other medications used in treatment of attention deficit disorders are thioridazine, lithium, and monoamine oxidase inhibitors, but their use in children is not recommended by Culbert et al. (1994) because of their less than optimal risk-to-benefit ratios, except in specific situations noted below.

The above pharmacologic treatment options for children with isolated ADHD may require modification for those with specific comorbidities. For children with attention deficit without hyperactivity or attention deficit hyperactivity disorder predominantly inattentive type, lower doses of methylphenidate may be required than for those with hyperactivity (Culbert et al., 1994). Children with ADHD associated with oppositional defiant disorder or conduct disorder may respond to stimulant therapy but may respond more favorably to clonidine if they demonstrate episodes of hyperarousal or aggressive behavior (Culbert et al., 1994). One must take care to rule out bipolar or manic-depressive disorder in these children prior to treatment as bipolar children may have better response to lithium (Culbert et al., 1994). If children have depression along with ADHD, a tricyclic antidepressant might be a better medication choice (Culbert et al., 1994; Biederman et al., 1989a). Children who have ADHD with anxiety also may respond well to tricyclic antidepressants (Biederman et al., 1989a) or clonidine (Culbert et al., 1994). For the 60 percent of children with Tourette disorder who have ADHD, clonidine is the medication of choice (Culbert et al., 1994). Those with ADHD and pervasive developmental disorder or autism may benefit from clomipramine or fluoxetine while those with concomitant mental retardation may benefit from the same pharmacologic regimen as those with ADHD alone (Culbert et al., 1994).

Controversial treatments abound in the lay press. Some relate to the role of dietary factors in the etiology of ADHD. The Feingold diet, which purports the etiologic role of food additives in ADHD, has been found ineffective in treatment of ADHD in formal reviews of published studies (Kavale and Forness, 1983; Mattes, 1983; Rimland, 1983).

Follow-up

Children under treatment for ADHD require close follow-up (Kelly and Aylward, 1992; Culbert et al., 1994). At minimum, close phone contact must be maintained with the family during the first several weeks of treatment, particularly if the child is on medication (Mercugliano, in Schwartz, 1990; Culbert et al., 1994). As noted above, if the child is on medication, the child will initially need weekly follow-up to monitor the double-blind placebo-controlled trial of pharmacologic intervention for positive effects, as measured for example by rating scales filled out by both the parents and the teacher, and for side effects (Culbert et al., 1994).

Once the psychological and behavioral baseline therapies are in place, with or without pharmacologic intervention, the next follow-up may be in one month with subsequent follow-up visits at 3- to 4-month intervals (Culbert et al., 1994). Voeller (1991) suggests that the initial follow-up take place one month after the start of medication therapy. Items for review at follow-up visits include (Culbert et al., 1994):

1. the child's understanding of ADHD
2. issues of self esteem and peer-child, parent-child, and teacher-child relationships
3. medication issues (as noted above)
4. the child's personal strengths and accomplishments
5. home behavior management issues
6. school functioning
7. parent advocacy issues
8. anticipatory guidance
9. provision of appropriate reading materials
10. the multimodal treatment plan

Searight et al. (1995) recommend that a mental status examination be repeated every 3 to 6 months. Voeller (1991) emphasizes that treatment of the child with ADHD is a long-term commitment to monitor the child's school environment and progress and other aspects of the child's life and is not limited to the renewal of prescriptions. Some advocate the use of repeated ratings during the course of therapy to assess efficacy (Culbert et al., 1994), while others feel such assessment is required only if the intervention does not seem to be effective (Voeller, 1991).

Sentinel events/adverse outcomes

Adverse outcomes relate to the side effects of pharmacologic intervention and to delay in diagnosis and treatment leading to secondary morbidity for the child and the family, especially in the short term. The side effects of medication therapy are as noted above.

Up to 70 percent of children with ADHD become adults with attentional disorders (Culbert et al., 1994). Though Culbert et al. (1994) believe these long-term outcomes are to some degree dependent on the successful implementation of a multimodal treatment plan, Kelly and Aylward (1992) cite a longitudinal study of 100 children with ADHD whose long-term outcome was affected by intelligence level, academic achievement, conduct problems, social relations, parental psychopathology or family dysfunction, and socioeconomic status and not by therapeutic intervention (Lambert et al., 1987). Culbert et al. (1994) lists the long-term problems in adults as attention problems, "affective lability, difficulty completing tasks, temper problems, impulsivity, and poor stress tolerance." Searight et al. (1995) list as problems among adults with attention deficits poor concentration, cognitive confusion, dysphoric mood, and problems with interpersonal relationships. Vinson (1994) lists in addition drug use disorder and criminality if coupled with antisocial disorder.

RECOMMENDED QUALITY INDICATORS FOR ATTENTION DEFICIT/HYPERACTIVITY DISORDER

These indicators apply to children age 3 to 18.

Diagnosis

Indicator	Quality of evidence	Literature	Benefits	Comments
1. Before making the diagnosis of ADHD, the health care provider should document a history of inattention or impulsivity/hyperactivity, using input from all of the following: • a rating scale by the parent;* • an interview with the parent; • a rating scale by the teacher;** • communication with the teacher (phone or in person); and • physician observation.	III	Atkins et al., 1985; Gordon, 1989; Biederman et al., 1990; Mercugliano, 1990; Schachar et al., 1990; Voeller, 1991; Kelly and Aylward, 1992; Reiff et al., 1993; APA, 1994; Searight et al., 1995	Enhance attention. Decrease impulsivity/hyperactivity. Increase self-esteem. Enhance social function.	Accurate diagnosis of ADHD is important to the treatment of ADHD and requires the presence of the core symptoms. Inattention is one of the core symptoms of ADHD.
2. Before making the diagnosis of ADHD, the health care provider should document: a. that the core symptoms of inattention and impulsivity/hyperactivity happen in more than one setting;	III	APA, 1994	Enhance attention. Decrease impulsivity/hyperactivity. Increase self-esteem. Enhance social function.	Accurate diagnosis of ADHD requires the elimination of a primary or comorbid family dysfunction problem or a problem of poor environmental fit of the family and aspects of the home or school with the child. Alternate settings include home, school, and the doctor's office.
b. that the core symptoms of inattention and impulsivity/hyperactivity have been of >= 6 months duration;	III	APA, 1994	Enhance attention. Decrease impulsivity/hyperactivity. Increase self-esteem. Enhance social function.	Accurate diagnosis of ADHD requires that the child's inattention or impulsivity/hyperactivity is not due to a transient medical, environmental, or psychiatric problem. In those cases, treatment should be directed at those specific underlying problems.
c. that the core symptoms of inattention and impulsivity/hyperactivity had been present prior to 7 years of age;	III	APA, 1994	Enhance attention. Decrease impulsivity/hyperactivity. Increase self-esteem. Enhance social function.	Age of onset is a requirement of DSM IV diagnostic criteria.

120

d. the child's social functioning, especially with regard to Pervasive Developmental Disorder, by evaluating at least one of the following: – impairment of social interaction, – impairment in communication, or – restricted repetitive and stereotyped patterns of behavior, interests, and activities;	III	APA, 1994	Enhance attention. Decrease impulsivity/hyperactivity. Increase self-esteem. Enhance social function.	DSM IV specifically requires the elimination of Pervasive Developmental Disorder as the primary condition.
e. the presence or absence of affective symptoms;***	III	Weinberg and Emslie, 1991; Brent, 1993; Reiff et al., 1993; APA, 1994; Searight et al., 1995	Enhance attention. Decrease impulsivity/hyperactivity. Increase self-esteem. Enhance social function.	DSM IV specifically requires the elimination of a mood disorder as the primary condition. The presence of affective symptoms may point to the presence of depression or some other mood disorder. Whether primary or secondary, any attention disorder will be less problematic to treat if the mood disorder is treated also. It is adequate to specify that no affective symptoms are present.
f. the child's social functioning, especially with regard to: – Oppositional Defiant Disorder† – Conduct Disorder.‡	III	Reiff et al., 1993; APA, 1994	Enhance attention. Decrease impulsivity/hyperactivity. Increase self-esteem. Enhance social function.	Accurate diagnosis of ADHD as the primary or comorbid disorder requires the elimination of a primary disruptive behavior disorder with secondary hyperactivity, such as Oppositional Defiant Disorder or Conduct Disorder. Whether primary or secondary, any attention disorder will be less problematic to treat if any other disruptive disorders are adequately treated.
3. The health care provider should document that past medical history was reviewed, including birth history, and history of accidents.	III	Reiff et al., 1993	Enhance attention. Decrease impulsivity/hyperactivity. Increase self-esteem. Enhance social function.	The health care provider should rule out a medical reason for poor attention. A history of accidents may suggest impulsivity.
4. The health care provider should document that a review of systems was done.	III III	Weinberg and Emslie, 1991; Reiff et al., 1993	Enhance attention. Decrease impulsivity/hyperactivity. Increase self-esteem. Enhance social function.	The health care provider should rule out a medical reason for poor attention and impulsivity/hyperactivity. Though it would be optimal for the health care provider to specifically mention consideration of lead toxicity, thyroid disease, sleep disorders, migraine headache, seizure disorders, and neurodegenerative disease, documentation may only consist of of the notation "ROS—negative" even if the appropriate questions were asked.
5. The health care provider should document the child's overall development. This may be based on parental-reported developmental milestones, such as social, fine motor/adaptive, language, and gross motor.	III	Voeller, 1991; Kelly and Aylward, 1992	Enhance educational achievement and adaptation.	Accurate diagnosis of ADHD requires the elimination of a primary or comorbid developmental problem which may point to a cognitive disorder or specific language disorder. Milestones will be specified as appropriate for age.

121

#	Recommendation	Strength of Evidence	Goals	References	Rationale
6.	The health care provider should document the child's cognitive level and academic achievement levels, including: a. academic performance;†† b. cognitive level,†† c. achievement level (only for school-age children).‡‡	III	Enhance attention. Decrease impulsivity/hyperactivity. Increase self-esteem. Enhance social function.	Lamden, 1990; Mercugliano, 1990; Voeller, 1991; Kelly and Aylward, 1992 Reiff et al., 1993; Searight et al., 1995	Accurate diagnosis of ADHD requires the elimination of a primary or comorbid cognitive disorder or learning disorder. For the child older than three years of age, the health care provider may refer the child to the public school system for an Individual Education Program (IEP) assessment, mandated by federal Public Law 94-142.
7.	The health care provider should document the structure of the family, home environment, and school environment. Such information should include:	III	Enhance attention. Decrease impulsivity/hyperactivity. Increase self-esteem. Enhance social function.	Kelly and Aylward, 1992; Reiff et al., 1993	Accurate diagnosis of ADHD requires the elimination of a primary or comorbid family dysfunction problem or a problem of poor environmental fit of the family and aspects of the home or school with the child. Whether primary or secondary, any attention disorder will be less problematic to treat if the family is well functioning and the environments in which the child functions is structured to aid in modifying the child's behavior. For reasons of confidentiality, environmental stressors may be documented in the medical record simply as "stressor present" or "stressor not present."
	a. Parents or guardians and other household members,				Information on household members should include one or more of the following: age, employment, education, marital relationships, and level of communication.
	b. environmental stressors,				Information on environmental stressors should include: financial status of family, current illnesses, marital difficulties, and stability of living arrangements.
	c. family functioning, and				Information on family functioning should include: parental beliefs about child's behavior, parental expectations for child's behavior, parental explanations for child's behavior, family activities, how family members get along, family members' support of each other, perceived family weaknesses, and parental beliefs about child discipline.
	d. school features.				Information on school features should include: involvement of school official other than teacher, grade level or special education, number of children or teacher-student ratio, locations of child's seat in class, and teacher's beliefs about child discipline.

#	Recommendation		Reference	Outcomes	Literature Review/Rationale

8.	The health care provider should document the presence or absence of any family history of:
	• psychiatric disorder, specifically
	  — depression,
	  — anxiety,
	  — psychosis,
	  — substance abuse, or
	  — antisocial behavior;
	• attention deficit hyperactivity disorder; or
	• learning disorder
		III	Voeller, 1991; Weinberg and Emslie, 1991; Reiff et al., 1993	Enhance attention. Decrease impulsivity/hyperactivity. Increase self-esteem. Enhance social function.	The presence of a family history of learning disorder, behavioral problem, or psychiatric disorder would be significant since such conditions can be familial and are within the differential diagnosis of ADHD and may indicate a source of family stress.

9.	The health care provider should document a family history of medical conditions.	III	Kelly and Aylward, 1992; Reiff et al., 1993	Enhance attention. Decrease impulsivity/hyperactivity. Increase self-esteem. Enhance social function.	Knowledge of family medical conditions will lead to consideration of other primary diagnoses and may indicate source of family stress.
10.	The physical examination should include a neurologic exam and observation of mood and social interactions.	III	Kelly and Aylward, 1992; Reiff et al., 1993	Enhance attention. Decrease impulsivity/hyperactivity. Increase self-esteem. Enhance social function.	Accurate diagnosis of ADHD requires a thorough physical examination to aid in ruling out medical causes of inattention and impulsivity/hyperactivity. Various neurologic and psychiatric conditions need to be considered, such as seizure disorder, migraine headache, neurodegenerative processes, mood disorders, Pervasive Developmental Disorder, etc.
11.	The health care provider should document the child's current medications.	III	Mercugliano, 1990; Voeller, 1991	Enhance attention. Decrease impulsivity/hyperactivity. Increase self-esteem. Enhance social function.	Accurate diagnosis of ADHD requires the elimination of a primary or comorbid pharmacologic side effect problem. Whether primary or secondary, any attention disorder will be less problematic to treat if any problems with substance or medication side effects are treated.
12.	The health care provider should document the presence or absence of alcohol and illicit drug use by the child.	III	Mercugliano, 1990; Voeller, 1991	Enhance attention. Decrease impulsivity/hyperactivity. Increase self-esteem. Enhance social function.	Accurate diagnosis of ADHD requires the elimination of a primary or comorbid substance abuse side effect problem. Whether primary or secondary, any attention disorder will be less problematic to treat if any problems with substance or medication side effects are treated.
13.	If the child is on theophylline, the health care provider should check a theophylline level.	III	Mercugliano, 1990; Voeller, 1991	Enhance attention. Decrease impulsivity/hyperactivity. Increase self-esteem. Enhance social function.	A side effect of theophylline is agitation.
14.	If the theophylline level is high (>15 mg/ml), the dose should be reduced.	III	Mercugliano, 1990; Voeller, 1991	Enhance attention. Decrease impulsivity/hyperactivity. Increase self-esteem. Enhance social function.	A side effect of theophylline is agitation.

No.	Recommendation		Reference	Outcome	Rationale
15.	The health care provider should document a vision screening test.	III	Kelly and Aylward, 1992; Reiff et al., 1993	Enhance attention. Decrease impulsivity/hyperactivity. Increase self-esteem. Enhance social function.	Accurate diagnosis of ADHD requires the elimination of a primary or comorbid vision problem. Whether primary or secondary, any attention disorder will be less problematic to treat if any vision problem is treated.
16.	If a vision problem exists, the health care provider should refer for evaluation and treatment, e.g., ophthalmologic or optometric care.	III	Kelly and Aylward, 1992; Reiff et al., 1993	Enhance attention. Decrease impulsivity/hyperactivity. Increase self-esteem. Enhance social function.	
17.	The health care provider should document a hearing screening test.	III	Kelly and Aylward, 1992; Reiff et al., 1993	Enhance attention. Decrease impulsivity/hyperactivity. Increase self-esteem. Enhance social function.	Accurate diagnosis of ADHD requires the elimination of a primary or comorbid hearing problem. Whether primary or secondary, any attention disorder will be less problematic to treat if any hearing problem is treated.
18.	If a hearing problem exists, the health care provider should refer for evaluation and treatment, e.g., audiologic and/or otolaryngologic care.	III	Kelly and Aylward, 1992; Reiff et al., 1993	Enhance attention. Decrease impulsivity/hyperactivity. Increase self-esteem. Enhance social function.	

Treatment

	Indicator	Quality of evidence	Literature	Benefits	Comments
19.	The health care provider should document efforts to adjust the home and school environments. These adjustments would include: a. at home - predictable schedule for bed time, meal times, play times, and homework, - breakdown of chores into smaller tasks, - predictable acceptable limits of behavior, and - predictable and immediate consequences for inappropriate behavior; and b. at school (any 1) - a seat with minimal distractions, - allow child to get up periodically from seat, - brief instructions, - frequent reminders to stay on task with discrete cues or signs, - predictable and immediate consequences for inappropriate behavior, and - provide opportunities for success.	III	Whalen, 1979; Kelly and Aylward, 1992; Culbert et al., 1994; Vinson, 1994	Reduce risk of medication side effects.	A subset of children with ADHD may respond sufficiently to environmental modifications to forego the need for pharmacotherapy or more intense psychologic intervention.
20.	If the child has isolated ADHD, the health care provider should initiate or refer for behavioral modification including any of the following techniques: • positive reinforcement, • negative consequences, or • response cost.	III	Pelham and Murphy, 1986; Voeller, 1991; Culbert et al., 1994; Searight et al., 1995	Reduce risk of medication side effects. Enhance attention. Decrease impulsivity/hyperactivity. Increase self-esteem. Enhance social function.	A subset of children with ADHD may respond sufficiently to behavioral modification to lessen the need for medication.
21.	If a child has oppositional-defiant disorder or conduct disorder, the child should be referred for psychiatric or psychologic therapy.	III	Pliszka, 1991; Kelly and Aylward, 1992; Culbert et al., 1994	Enhance attention. Decrease impulsivity/hyperactivity. Increase self-esteem. Enhance social function. Decrease disruptive behaviors.	The health care provider must treat any other disruptive behaviors in addition to ADHD.
22.	If the child has a mood disorder, the child should be referred for psychiatric or psychologic therapy.	III	Pliszka, 1991; Kelly and Aylward, 1992; Culbert et al., 1994	Enhance attention. Decrease impulsivity/hyperactivity. Increase self-esteem. Enhance social function. Decrease affective symptoms.	The health care provider must treat the mood disorder in addition to ADHD.
23.	If the child has a learning disorder, the child should receive psychoeducational intervention.	III	Pliszka, 1991; Kelly and Aylward, 1992; Culbert et al., 1994	Enhance attention. Decrease impulsivity/hyperactivity. Increase self-esteem. Enhance social function. Enhance educational achievement.	The health care provider must treat the learning disorder in addition to ADHD.

#	Recommendation	Level	References	Goals	Comments
24.	The health care provider should never prescribe stimulant pharmacotherapy for a child less than three years of age.	III	Barkley, 1989	Reduce risk of medication side effects.	The diagnosis of ADHD is almost impossible to confirm in the child less than three years of age. The risk of side effects is greater in the child less than three years of age.
25.	If the child has ADHD without a comorbidity and is started on pharmacotherapy, the initial medication choice should be a stimulant such as methylphenidate, dextroamphtamine, or pemoline.	III	Kavale, 1982; Voeller, 1991; Kelly and Aylward, 1992; Fox and Rieder, 1993; Culbert et al., 1994; Vinson, 1994; Searight et al., 1995	Improve short-term behavioral outcomes. Reduce serious medication side effects.	Searight et al. (1995) is the only review which states outright that stimulants appear more effective than other classes of medication for treatment of ADHD while the other reviews note that the stimulants are the most commonly prescribed for ADHD and have had the greatest experience of use. Kavale (1982) presents the most convincing review, a meta-analysis based on controlled studies of at least level II-1, demonstrating the effectiveness of stimulant therapy on short-term behavioral outcomes.
26.	If a child has ADHD and oppositional-defiant disorder or conduct disorder and is begun on pharmacotherapy, the child should be started on a stimulant medication, such as methylphenidate, pemoline, or dextroamphetamine.	III	Pliszka, 1991; Kelly and Aylward, 1992; Culbert et al., 1994	Enhance attention. Decrease impulsivity/hyperactivity. Increase self-esteem. Enhance social function.	The pharmacotherapeutic treatment of a child with ADHD and oppositional-defiant disorder or conduct disorder is the same as for isolated ADHD.
27.	If the child has ADHD and Tourette Syndrome or a tic disorder and is begun on pharmacotherapy, the child should be started on clonidine or stimulant medication (methylphenidate, pemoline, or dextroamphetamine).	III	Pliszka, 1991; Kelly and Aylward, 1992; Culbert et al., 1994	Enhance attention. Decrease impulsivity/hyperactivity. Increase self-esteem. Enhance social function.	In children with ADHD and Tourette Syndrome or a tic disorder stimulant medications may exacerbate the tic disorder.
28.	If the child has ADHD and a mood disorder and is begun on pharmacotherapy, the child should be started on a tricyclic antidepressant.	III	Pliszka, 1991; Kelly and Aylward, 1992; Culbert et al., 1994	Enhance attention. Decrease impulsivity/hyperactivity. Increase self-esteem. Enhance social function. Decrease affective symptoms.	In children with ADHD and mood disorder tricyclic antidepressants are more effective than stimulant medications.
29.	If the child has ADHD and a learning disorder and is begun on pharmacotherapy, the child should be started on a stimulant medication, such as methylphenidate, pemoline, or dextroamphetamine.	III	Pliszka, 1991; Kelly and Aylward, 1992; Culbert et al., 1994	Enhance attention. Decrease impulsivity/hyperactivity. Increase self-esteem. Enhance social function. Enhance educational achievement.	The pharmacotherapeutic treatment of a child with ADHD and learning disorder is the same as for isolated ADHD.
30.	If the child is started on pharmacotherapy, the health care provider should document that the risks and benefits have been explained to the child, guardian, and teacher.	III	Voeller, 1991	Optimize positive effects on behavior. Minimize the risk of side effects.	Knowledge of the benefits will aid the child, parent, and teacher in reporting the positive effects of pharmacotherapy in monitoring optimal dosing of medication. Knowledge of the risks will aid the child, parent, and teacher in assisting the health care provider to modify pharmacotherapy.

31.	Before a child is started on stimulant medication such as methylphenidate, dextroamphetamine, or pemoline, the health care provider should document the weight, height, pulse, and blood pressure of the child.	III		Minimize the risk of side effects.	The health care provider will monitor pharmacotherapy in terms of side effects to aid in adjusting medication dosages.
32.	If a child is started on pemoline, the health care provider should document the absence of hepatic disease prior to the start of therapy by history and baseline liver function tests.	III	Barkley, et al., 1990	Avoid hepatic toxicity.	The health care provider should take care not to prescribe pemoline to a child with liver disease.
33.	If a child is started on a tricyclic antidepressant, the health care provider should document the absence of cardiac disease by history and by a baseline electrocardiogram.	III	Kelly and Aylward, 1990; Searight et al., 1995	Avoid cardiac side effects.	Tricyclic antidepressants may cause arrhythmias and cardiac sudden death. The health care provider should take care not to prescribe tricyclic antidepressants to a child with underlying heart disease, especially an arrhythmia. A baseline electrocardiogram will help to rule out the presence of an arrhythmia and, if normal, will provide a baseline against which to compare monitoring electrocardiograms.
34.	The primary health care provider who is not an ADHD specialist should not prescribe for treatment of ADHD medications other than: • methylphenidate, • pemoline, • dextroamphetamine, • clonidine, or • tricyclic antidepressant.	III	Fox and Rieder, 1993; Vinson, 1994	Avoid adverse medication effects.	General pediatricians and family practitioners may not have sufficient ongoing experience with the use of neurotropic medications. Inadequate experience could increase the risk of adverse side effects. Some feel that the primary care provider should not prescribe clonidine or tricyclic antidepressants without consultation of an ADHD specialist.
35.	The primary health care provider should not simultaneously treat a child with ADHD with more than one medication for treatment of ADHD without the consultation of an ADHD specialist, e.g., a psychiatrist, neurologist, or behavioralist.	III		Avoid adverse medication effects.	General pediatricians and family practitioners may not have sufficient ongoing experience with the use of multiple neurotropic medications. Inadequate experience could increase risk of adverse effects.

		Quality of evidence	Literature	Benefits	Comments

36.	The primary health care provider should request consultation from an ADHD specialist (e.g., a multidisciplinary referral center or psychiatrist, neurologist, or behavioralist) if a child fails to respond to separate trials with methylphenidate, dextroamphetamine, pemoline, clonidine, and a single tricyclic antidepressant.	III		Enhance attention. Decrease impulsivity/hyperactivity. Increase self-esteem. Reduce risk of medication side effects.	If the child does not have ADHD, a new diagnosis must be considered so that effective treatment may be implemented. If the child fails to improve on separate courses of multiple drugs felt to be effective in the treatment of ADHD, the diagnosis of ADHD must be reconsidered. Some feel that the primary care provider should not prescribe clonidine or tricyclic antidepressants without consultation of an ADHD specialist.
					
					Failure may be defined as:
					• lack of improvement in:
					  – attention, or
					  – impulsivity/hyperactivity; or
					• presence of side effects
					
					A trial may be defined as failure to respond despite:
					• maximal therapeutic dosage, and
					• of sufficient duration.

Follow-up

	Indicator	Quality of evidence	Literature	Benefits	Comments
37.	During the initial evaluation and treatment, the health care provider coordinating care should maintain at least biweekly contact with the family, either through office visits or by phone, for at least 4 contacts.	III	Mercugliano, 1990; Voeller, 1991; Kelly and Aylward, 1992; Culbert et al., 1994	Enhance attention. Decrease impulsivity/hyperactivity. Increase self-esteem. Enhance social function.	Close follow-up by the coordinating provider early in the course of diagnosis and treatment will assure the timely completion of required diagnostic tests and implementation of interventions. The exact timing of such follow-up is not specified in most references. Some references suggest weekly follow-up initially. The duration of such frequent follow-up is not specified apart from stabilization of the therapeutic regimen which is difficult to define.

#	Recommendation		References	Goals	Comments
38.	During the initial implementation of behavioral or psychologic treatment, the provider of such services should see the child for office visits on a weekly basis for at least 4 visits.	III	Mercugliano, 1990; Voeller, 1991; Kelly and Aylward, 1992; Culbert et al., 1994	Enhance attention. Decrease impulsivity/hyperactivity. Increase self-esteem. Enhance social function.	Though some references suggest weekly follow-up visits in general, specific recommendations for behavioral or psychologic intervention are not available. One would suppose, however, that close follow-up by the provider of behavioral or psychologic intervention early in the course of such treatment may increase the likelihood of compliance with therapy. The duration of such frequent follow-up is not specified apart from stabilization of the therapeutic regimen which is difficult to define. The literature reports the use of rating scales to monitor the effects of therapy.
39.	For children receiving behavior or psychologic treatment, after the initial four visits, the health care provider coordinating care should see the child in the office every four months.	III	Culbert et al., 1994	Enhance attention. Decrease impulsivity/hyperactivity. Increase self-esteem. Enhance social function.	Monitoring of the child will help to identify positive changes and provide positive reinforcement to the child, parent, and teacher to comply with intervention.
40.	During the initial implementation of pharmacotherapy, the provider of such services should maintain biweekly contact with the family, either through office visits or by phone, for at least 4 contacts. Office visits should be at least at monthly intervals until improvement is seen in attention or impulsivity/hyperactivity by parent report or rating scale* and, if in school, teacher report or rating scale.**	III	Mercugliano, 1990; Voeller, 1991; Kelly and Aylward, 1992; Culbert et al., 1994	Enhance attention. Decrease impulsivity/hyperactivity. Increase self-esteem. Enhance social function.	Though some references suggest weekly follow-up visits in general, specific recommendations for pharmacotherapeutic intervention are not available. Based on the half-life of the commonly used medications, one would suppose that biweekly visits would be a suitable compromise. Frequent follow-up early in the course of treatment should be helpful in monitoring for side effects and adjustment of dosage. The duration of such frequent follow-up is not specified apart from stabilization of the therapeutic regimen which is difficult to define. This provider may be the same person as the coordinating provider.
41.	After the initial four visits for pharmacotherapeutic intervention, the provider of such therapy should see the child in the office at least every four months once an improvement is seen in attention or impulsivity/hyperactivity by parent report or rating scale* and, if in school, teacher report or rating scale.**	III	Culbert et al., 1994	Enhance attention. Decrease impulsivity/hyperactivity. Increase self-esteem. Reduce medication side effects	Though this recommendation for follow-up is general and not specific to pharmacotherapeutic intervention, such follow-up would seem necessary to monitor for side effects or diminishing behavioral effects. The literature reports the use of rating scales to monitor the effects of pharmacotherapy. This provider may be the same person as the coordinating provider.

#	Recommendation	Level	References	Objective	Rationale
42.	If a change in therapy has occurred, the health care provider initiating the change must: a. evaluate the effect of the change within two weeks, either by an office visit or by phone contact, and b. inform the provider coordinating care about the change.	III	Mercugliano, 1990; Voeller, 1991; Kelly and Aylward, 1992; Culbert et al., 1994	Enhance attention. Decrease impulsivity/hyperactivity. Increase self-esteem. Enhance social function. Reduce medication side effects.	Close follow-up will allow monitoring of behavioral changes and side effects to allow more effective adjustment of therapy, including medication dosage.
43.	At each follow-up visit, the health care provider should document the child's behavior both at home and at school by parent report or rating scale* and, if in school, teacher report or rating scale.**	III	Winsberg, 1982; Barkley, 1985; Voeller, 1991; Culbert et al., 1994	Enhance attention. Decrease impulsivity/hyperactivity. Increase self-esteem. Enhance social function.	The main effects of therapy appear to be on the core behaviors of inattention and impulsivity/hyperactivity, so those behaviors should be monitored. The literature reports the use of rating scales to monitor the effects of pharmacotherapy.
44.	The health care provider should request and review the child's academic records, such as report cards or interviews with the child's teacher, at least once a year.	III	Voeller, 1991; Culbert et al., 1994	Enhance attention. Decrease impulsivity/hyperactivity. Increase self-esteem. Enhance social function.	Some studies indicate that therapy for ADHD may have positive effects on academic performance, and so academic performance should also be monitored.
45.	If medications have been prescribed, at each follow-up visit the health care provider should document: a. weight, b. height, c. pulse, and d. blood pressure.	III	Klein, 1988; Barkely et al., 1990; Culbert et al., 1994	Avoid continued or more serious side effects of medications.	Monitoring side effects of stimulant therapy will aid the health care provider in monitoring the need for modifications in pharmacotherapy.
46.	If stimulant medications have been prescribed, the health care provider should document at each follow-up visit the presence or absence of side effects.	III	Culbert et al., 1994	Avoid continued or more serious side effects of medications.	Monitoring side effects of pharmacotherapy will aid the health care provider in monitoring the need for modifications in pharmacotherapy. It is sufficient to state "no side effects" or only to mention one side effect. Side effects include any of the following: tics, decreased appetite, insomnia, headaches, or stomach aches.
47.	If a tricyclic antidepressant has been prescribed, the health care provider should document at each follow-up visit the presence or absence of side effects.	III	Kelly and Aylward, 1992; Fox and Rieder, 1993; Searight et al., 1995	Avoid continued or more serious side effects of medications.	Monitoring side effects of tricyclic antidepressant therapy will aid the health care provider in monitoring the need for modifications in pharmacotherapy. In addition to the side effects of dizziness and drowsiness, anticholinergic side effects may be seen. The listed symptoms may indicate an underlying cardiac side effect.
48.	If clonidine has been prescribed, the health care provider should document at each follow-up visit the presence or absence of side effects.	III	Culbert et al., 1994; Searight et al., 1995	Avoid continued or more serious side effects of medications.	Monitoring side effects of clonidine therapy will aid the health care provider in monitoring the need for modifications in pharmacotherapy. The symptoms of dizziness and drowsiness may indicate an underlying cardiac side effect.

49.	If the child is on pemoline, the health care provider should assess liver function every six months.	III	Nehra et al., 1990; Pratt and Dubois, 1990; Culbert et al., 1994	Reduce risk of hepatoxicity.	Since pemoline is hepatoxic, the health care provider must monitor for this complication. None of the references specify the exact frequency of monitoring required.
50.	If the child is on a tricyclic antidepressant, the health care provider should order an electrocardiogram every six months.	III	Fox and Rieder, 1993; Culbert et al., 1994	Avoid continued or more serious side effects of tricyclic medications.	Monitoring side effects of tricyclic antidepressant therapy will aid the health care provider in monitoring the need for modifications in pharmacotherapy. None of the references specify the exact frequency of monitoring required.

*Acceptable parent rating scales include: ADHD Rating Scale; Swanson, Nolan, and Pelham Rating Scale; Child Behavior Check List; Conners Scales; Yale Children's Inventory; or Aggregate Neurobehavioral Student Health and Education Review.

**Acceptable teacher rating scales include: ADHD Rating Scale; Swanson, Nolan, and Pelham Rating Scale; Child Behavior Check List; ADD-H Comprehensive Teacher Rating Scale; Conners Scales; Yale Children's Inventory; or Aggregate Neurobehavioral Student Health and Education Review.

***Affective symptoms include: unexplained somatic complaints; drop in school performance; apathy and loss of interest; social withdrawal; increased irritability or tearfulness; sleep changes; appetite changes; suicidal ideation or behavior; substance use; promiscuous sexual behavior; or risk-taking behavior.

†Oppositional Defiant Disorder symptoms include: negativistic, hostile, and defiant behavior.

‡Conduct Disorder symptoms include: aggression to people and animals, destruction of property, deceitfulness or theft, and serious violations of rules.

††Cognitive level may be measured using the Wechsler Scales of Intelligence-III, Kaufman Assessment Battery for Children, Stanford-Binet, or an alternative measure of cognitive function specified by child's school district.

‡‡Achievement level for school-age children may be measued using the Woodcock-Johnson Psycho-educational Battery or the Wide Range Achievement Test-Revised.

Quality of Evidence Codes:

I:	RCT
II-1:	Nonrandomized controlled trials
II-2:	Cohort or case analysis
II-3:	Multiple time series
III:	Opinions or descriptive studies

REFERENCES - ATTENTION DEFICIT/HYPERACTIVITY DISORDER

Abikoff H. 1991. Cognitive training in ADHD children: Less to it than meets the eye. *Journal of Learning Disabilities* 24: 205-8.

American Academy of Pediatrics, and Committee on Psychosocial Aspects of Child and Family Health, 1985-1988. 1988. *Guidelines for Health Supervision II*, Second ed.Elk Grove Village, Illinois: American Academy of Pediatrics.

American Academy of Pediatrics, and Committee on Children with Disabilities. 1992. Pediatriacian's role in the development and implementation of an individual education plan (IEP) and/or an individual family service plan (IFSP). *Pediatrics* 89 (2): 340-2.

American Psychiatric Association. 1994. *Diagnostic and Statistical Manual of Mental Disorders: DSM-IV*. Washington, DC: American Psychiatric Association.

Barkley RA. 1990. *Attention Deficit Hyperactivity Disorder: A Handbook for Diagnosis and Treatment*.New York, NY: Guilford Press.

Barkley RA, GJ DuPaul, and MB McMurray. 1991. Attention deficit disorder with and without hyperactivity: Clinical response to three dose levels of methylphenidate. *Pediatrics* 87: 519-32.

Barkley RA, M Fischer, RF Newby, et al. 1988. Development of a multimethod clinical protocol for assessing stimulant drug response in children with attention deficit disorder. *Journal of Clinical Child Psychology* 17: 14-24.

Barkley RA, DC Guevremont, AD Anastopoulos, et al. 1992. A comparison of three family therapy programs for treating family conflicts in adolescents with attention-deficit hyperactivity disorder. *Journal of Consulting and Clinical Psychology* 60: 450-62.

Barkley RA, MB McMurray, CS Edelbrock, et al. 1989. The response of agressive and nonaggressive ADHD children to two doses of methylphenidate. *Journal of the American Academy of Child and Adolescent Psychiatry* 28: 873-81.

Barkley RA. 1989. Attention deficit-hyperactivity disorder. In *Treatment of Childhood Disorders*. Editors Mash MF, and RA Barkley, 39-72. New York: Guilford Press.

Biederman J, RJ Baldessarini, V Wright, et al. 1 1989. A double-blind placebo controlled study of desipramine in the treatment of ADD: I. Efficacy. *Journal of the American Academy of Child and Adolescent Psychiatry* 28 (5): 777-84.

Biederman J, RJ Baldessarini, V Wright, et al. 2 1989. A double-blind placebo controlled study of desipramine in the treatment of ADD: II. Serum drug levels and cardiovascular findings. *Journal of the American Academy of Child and Adolescent Psychiatry* 28: 199-204, 903-11.

Biederman J, RJ Baldessarini, V Wright, et al. January 1993. A double-blind placebo controlled study of Desipramine in the treatment of ADD: III. Lack of impact of comorbidity and family history factors on clinical response. *Journal of the American Academy of Child and Adolescent Psychiatry* 32 (1): 199-205.

Brown RT, KA Borden, ME Wynne, et al. 1 1986. Methylphenidate and cognitive therapy with ADD children: A methodological reconsideration. *Journal of Abnormal Child Psychology* 14: 481-97.

Brown RT, ME Wynne, KA Border, et al. 2 1986. Methylphenidate and cognitive therapy in children with attention deficit disorder: A double-blind trial. *Journal of Developmental and Behavioral Pediatrics* 7: 163-74.

Culbert TP, GA Banez, and MI Reiff. 1994. Children who have attentional disorders: Interventions. *Pediatrics in Review* 15 (1): 5-15.

Dalby JT, M Kinsbourne, and JM Swanson. 1989. Self-paced learning in children with attention deficit disorder with hyperactivity. *Journal of Abnormal Child Psychology* 17: 269-75.

DiTraglia J. 1991. Methylphenidate protocol: Feasibility in a pediatric practice. *Clinical Pediatrics* 30: 656-60.

DuPaul GJ, and MD Rapport. 1993. Does methylphenidate normalize the classroom performance of children with attention deficit disorder? *Journal of the American Academy of Child and Adolescent Psychiatry* 32: 190-8.

Evans SW, and WE Pelham. 1991. Psychostimulant effects on academic and behavioral measures for ADHD junior high school students in a lecture format classroom. *Journal of Abnormal Child Psychology* 19: 537-52.

Fine S, and B Jewesson. 1989. Active drug placebo trial of methylphenidate: A clinical service for chidlren with an attention deficit disorder. *Canadian Journal of Psychiatry* 34: 447-9.

Firestone P, D Crowe, JT Goodman, et al. 1986. Vicissitudes of follow-up studies: Differential effects of parent training and stimulant medication with hyperactives. *American Journal of Orthopsychiatry* 5 (6): 184-94.

Fitzpatrick PA, R Klorman, JT Brumaghim, et al. 1992. Effects of sustained-release and standard preparations of methylphenidate on attention deficit disorder. *Journal of the American Academy of Child and Adolescent Psychiatry.* 31: 226-34.

Fox AM, and MJ Rieder. 1993. Risks and Benefits of Drugs Used in the Management of the Hyperactive Child. *Drug Safety* 9 (1): 38-50.

Garfinkel BD, PH Wender, L Sloman, et al. 1983. Tricyclic antidepressant and methylphenidate treatment of attention deficit disorder in children. *Journal of the American Academy of Child and Adolescent Psychiatry* 22: 343-8.

Gittelman KR, and H Abikoff. 1989. The role of psychostimulants and psychosocial treatments in hyperkinesis. In *Attention Deficit Disorder: Clinical and Basic Research.* Editors Sagvolden, and Archer, 167-80. Hillsdale: Lawrence Erlbaum.

Gualtieri CT, PA Keenan, and M Chandler. 1991. Clinical and neuropsychological effects of desipramine in children with attention deficit hyperactivity disorder. *Journal of Clinical Psychopharmacology* 11: 155-9.

Horn WF, NS Ialongo, JM Pascoe, et al. 1991. Additive effects of psychostimulants, parent training, and self-control therapy with ADHD children. *Journal of the American Academy of Child and Adolescent Psychiatry* 30: 233-40.

Hunt RD, RB Minderra, and DJ Cohen. 1985. Clonidine benefits children with attention deficit disorder and hyperactivity: Report of a double-blind placebo-crossover therapeutic trial. *Journal of the American Academy of Child and Adolescent Psychiatry* 24: 617-29.

Hunt RD, B Ruud, MD Minderaa, et al. 1986. The therapeutic effect of clonidine in attention deficit disorder with hyperactivity: A comparison with placebo and methylphenidate. *Psychopharmacology Bulletin* 22: 229-36.

Iolango NS, WF Horn, JM Pascoe, et al. 1993. The effects of a multimodal intervention with attention-deficit hyperactivity disorder children: A 9-month follow-up. *Journal of the American Academy of Child and Adolescent Psychiatry* 32: 182-189.

Kavale K. 1982. The efficacy of stimulant drug treatment for hyperactivity: A meta-analysis. *Journal of Learning Disabilities* 15 (5): 280-9.

Kavale KA, and SR Forness. 1983. Hyperactivity and diet treatment: A meta-analysis of the feingold hypothesis. *Journal of Learning Disabilities* 16 (6): 324-30.

Kelly DP, and GP Aylward. 1992. Attention deficits in school-aged children and adolescents. *Pediatric Clinics of North America* 39 (3): 487-512.

Klein RG, and S Mannuzza. 1991. Long-term outcome of hyperactive children: A review. *Journal of the American Academy of Child and Adolescent Psychiatry* 30: 383-7.

Klorman R, JT Brumaghim, PA Fitzpatrick, et al. 1990. Clinical effects of a controlled trial of methylphenidate on adolescents with attention deficit disorder. *Journal of the American Academy of Child and Adolescent Psychiatry* 29: 702-9.

Klorman R, JT Brumaghim, LF Salzman, et al. 1988. Effects of methylphenidate on attention-deficit hyperactivity disorder with and without aggressive-noncompliant features. *Journal of Abnormal Psychology* 97: 413-22.

Lambert NM, CS Hartsough, D Sassone, et al. 1987. Persistence of hyperactivity symptoms from childhood to adolescence and associated outcomes. *American Journal of Orthopsychiatry* 57: 22-32.

Long N, VI Rickert, and EW Ashcraft. 1993. Bibliotherapy as an adjunct to stimulant medication in the treatment of attention-deficit hyperactivity disorder. *Journal of Pediatric Health Care* 7: 82-8.

Mattes JA. 1983. The Feingold diet: A current reappraisal. *Journal of Learning Disabilities* 16 (6): 319-23.

McBride MC. 1988. An individual doube-blind crossover trial for assessing methylphenidate response in children with attention deficit disorder. *Journal of Pediatrics* 113: 137-45.

Mercugliano M. 1990. Attention deficit-hyperactivity disorder. In *Pediatric Primary Care: A Problem-Oriented Approach*, Second ed. Editor Schwartz MW, 718-23. Chicago, IL: Year Book Medical Publishers, Inc.

Nehra A, F Mullick, KG Ishak, et al. 1990. Pemoline-associated hepatic injury. *Gastroenterology* 99: 1517-9.

Pelham WE, KE Greenslade, M Vodde-Hamilton, et al. 1990. Relative efficacy of long-acting stimulants in children with attention deficit-hyperactivity disorders: A comparison of standard methylphenidate, sustained-release methylphenidate, sustained-release dextroamphetamine and pemoline. *Pediatrics* 86: 226-37.

Pelham WE, and HA Murphy. 1986. Attention-deficit and conduct disorders. In *Pharmacological and Behavioral Treatments: An Integrative Approach*. Editor Hersen A, pp. 108-148. New York, NY: Wiley.

Pelham WE, and SE Sams. 1992. Behavior modification. *Child Adolesc. Psychiatr. Clin. North Am.* 1: 505-19.

Pelham WE, J Sturges, J Hoza, et al. 1987. Sustained release and standard methylphenidate effects on cognitive and social behavior in children with attention deficit disorder. *Pediatrics* 80: 491-501.

Pliszka SR. 1987. Tricyclic antidepressants in the treatment of children with attention deficit disorder. *Journal of the American Academy of Child and Adolescent Psychiatry* 26: 127-32.

Pliszka SR. 1991. Attention-deficit hyperactivity disorder: A clinical review. *American Family Physician* 43 (4): 1267-75.

Porrino LJ, JL Rupoport, D Behar, et al. 1983. A naturalistic assessment of the motor activity of hyperactive boys in comparison with normal controls. *Archives of General Psychiatry* 40: 681-7.

Pratt DS, and RS Dubois. 1990. Hepatotoxicity due to Pemoline (Alert): A report of two cases. *Journal of Pediatric Gastroenterology and Nutrition* 10: 239-41.

Rapoport JL, M Buchsbaum, H Weingartner, et al. 1980. Cognitive and behavioral effects in normal and hyperactive boys and normal adult males. *Archives of General Psychiatry* 37: 933-43.

Rapport MD, G Stoner, GJ DuPaul, et al. 1988. Attention deficit disorder and methylphenidate: A multilevel analysis of dose-response effects on children's impulsivity across settings. *Journal of the American Academy of Child and Adolescent Psychiatry* 27: 60-9.

Reiff MI, GA Banez, and TP Culbert. 1993. Children who have attentional disorders: Diagnosis and evaluation. *Pediatrics in Review* 14 (12): 455-65.

Riddle MA, JC Nelson, CS Kleinman, et al. 1991. Sudden death in children receiving Norpramin: A review of three reported cases and commentary. *Journal of the American Academy of Child and Adolescent Psychiatry* 30: 104-9.

Satterfield JH, BT Satterfield, and AM Schell. 1987. Therapeutic interventions to prevent deliquency in hyperactive boys. *Journal of the American Academy of Child and Adolescent Psychiatry* 26: 56-64.

Searight HR, JE Nahlik, and DC Campbell. 1995. Attention-deficit/hyperactivity disorder: Assessment, diagnosis, and management. *Journal of Family Practice* 40 (3): 270-9.

Shaywitz BA, and SE Shaywitz. 1991. Comorbidity: A critical issue in attention deficit disorder. *Journal of Child Neurology* 6 (Supplement): S13-S20.

Sprague RL, and EK Sleator. 1977. Methylphenidate in hyperkinetic children: Differences in dose effects on learning and social behaviour. *Science* 198: 1274-6.

Swanson JM, and M Kinsbourne. 1979. The cognitive effects of stimulant drugs on hyperactive children. In *Attention and Cognitive Development*. Editors Hale GA, and M Lewis, 249-74. New York, NY: Plenum.

Tannock R, RJ Schachar, RP Carr, et al. 1989. Dose-response effects of methylphenidate on academic performance and overt behavior in hyperactive children. *Pediatrics* 84: 648-57.

Ullman RK, and EK Sleator. 1986. Responders, nonresponders and placebo responders among children with attention deficit disorder. *Clinical Pediatrics* 25: 594-9.

Vinson DC. 1994. Therapy for attention-deficit hyperactivity disorder. *Archives of Family Medicine* 3 (5): 445-51.

Voeller KKS. 1991. Clinical management of attention deficit hyperactivity disorder. *Journal of Child Neurology* 6 (Supplement): S49-S65.

Vyse SA, and MD Rapport. 1989. The effects of methylphenidate on learning in children with ADDH: The stimulus equivalence paradign. *Journal of Consulting and Clinical Psychology* 57: 425-35.

Weinberg WA, and GJ Emslie. 1991. Attention deficit hyperactivity disorder: The differential diagnosis. *Journal of Child Neurology* 6 (Supplement): S23-S34.

6. CESAREAN DELIVERY

The pediatric expert panel agreed to defer scoring and modification of the pediatric cesarean delivery indicators to the women's expert panel. In doing so, the pediatric expert panel agreed to accept any changes (modifications, deletions, additions) the women's expert panel made to the cesarean section indicators.

The literature review and proposed adult women's cesarean section indicators can be found in Chapter 6, "Cesarean Delivery" in the RAND document, *Quality of Care for Women: A Review of Selected Clinical Conditions and Quality Indicators,* DRU-1720-HCFA. The final set of pediatric cesarean section indicators can be found in the indicator crosswalk table in Appendix C of this document. The pediatric and women's cesarean section indicators are identical.

7. DEPRESSION[1]

Eve Kerr, M.D., M.P.H.

We relied on the following sources to construct quality indicators for depression in adult women: the AHCPR Clinical Practice Guideline *Depression in Primary Care (Volumes 1 and 2): Treatment of Major Depression* (Depression Guideline Panel, 1993), as well as selected review and journal articles. We conducted a MEDLINE search of review articles published in English between the years 1985 and 1995.

IMPORTANCE

Major depression is a common condition, affecting more than 10 percent of adults between the ages of 14 and 55 annually (Kessler, 1994). Major depressive disorder is characterized by one or more episodes of major depression without episodes of mania or hypomania. By definition, major depressive episodes last at least two weeks, and typically last much longer. Up to one in eight individuals may require treatment for depression during their lifetime (Depression Guideline Panel, 1993). The common age of onset is in a person's 20's to 30's; however, depression can start at any age.

Approximately 11 million people in the United States suffered from depression in 1990, the disproportionate share of whom were women (7.7 million) (Greenberg et al., 1993). The point prevalence for major depressive disorder in western industrialized nations is 2.3 to 3.2 percent for men and 4.5 to 9.3 percent for women (Depression Guideline Panel, 1993a).[2] Katon and Schulberg (1992) report that among general medical outpatients, the prevalence rate for major depression is between 5 and 9 percent and 6 percent for dysthymia. Consistent with these findings, Feldman et al. (1987) found that the point prevalence of major depressive disorder in primary care outpatient settings ranged from 4.8

---

[1]This review was prepared for the Women's Quality of Care Panel; it is included here to explain the literature supporting the indicators that we propose to apply to adolescents.

[2]For a summary of the prevalence literature, refer to pg. 25, Volume 1, *Depression Guidelines*.

to 8.6 percent. The lifetime risk for developing depression is between 20 and 25 percent for women.

Depression is associated with severe deterioration in a person's ability to function in social, occupational, and interpersonal settings (Broadhead et al., 1990; Wells et al., 1989a). Broadhead et al. (1990) found that patients with major depressive disorder reported 11 disability days per 90-day interval compared to 2.2 disability days for the general population. Roughly one-quarter of all persons with major depressive disorder reported restricted activity or bed days in the past two weeks (Wells et al., 1988). The functioning of depressed patients is comparable with or worse than that of patients with major chronic medical conditions.

The direct costs associated with treating major depressive disorder combined with the indirect costs from lost productivity account for about $16 billion per year in 1980 dollars (Depression Guideline Panel, 1993a). Greenberg et al. (1993) estimate that the total costs of affective disorders are $12.4 billion for direct treatment, $7.5 billion for mortality costs due to suicide, and $23.8 billion in morbidity costs due to reduction in productivity ($11.7 billion from excess absenteeism and $12.1 billion while at work).

Strum and Wells (1994) recently demonstrated the cost-effectiveness of treatment for depression. They found that improved treatment lowers the average cost per improvement in functioning outcomes as compared to no treatment; however, to achieve this gain, total costs of care are higher.

EFFICACY AND/OR EFFECTIVENESS OF INTERVENTIONS

Screening/Detection

The under-diagnosis of depression seriously impedes efforts to intervene on a clinical level. The Depression Guidelines report that only one-third to one-half of all cases of major depressive disorders are properly recognized by primary care and non-psychiatric practitioners (Depression Guideline Panel, 1993a; Wells et al., 1989b). The Medical Outcomes Study (MOS) revealed that approximately 50 percent of patients with depression were detected by general medical clinicians, and among patients in prepaid health plans the rates of detection were much lower than those observed for patients in fee-for-service plans (Wells et al., 1989b).

No definitive screening method exists to detect major depression. Patient self-report questionnaires are available but are non-specific. These questionnaires can be used to supplement the results of direct interview by a clinician (Depression Guideline Panel, 1993a). Burnam et al. (1988) used an eight-item screening questionnaire in the MOS; however, no standard screening questionnaire currently exists for clinical work.

A clinical interview is the most effective method for detecting depression (Depression Guideline Panel, 1993a). Clinicians should especially look for symptoms in patients who are at high risk. Risk factors for depression include (Depression Guideline Panel, 1993a):

1) Prior episodes of depression (one major depressive episode is associated with a 50 percent chance of a subsequent episode; two episodes with a 70 percent chance and three or more with a 90 percent chance of recurrent depression over a lifetime (NIMH Consensus Development Conference, 1985);

2) Family history of depressive disorder;

3) Prior suicide attempts;

4) Female gender;

5) Age of onset under 40;

6) Postpartum period;

7) Medical co-morbidity;

8) Lack of social support;

9) Stressful life events; and,

10) Current alcohol or substance abuse.

Laboratory testing for depression is effective only in identifying underlying physiologic reasons for depression (e.g., hypothyroidism). No laboratory screening test exists for depression per se and thus, laboratory tests should be tailored individually to the patient as part of a diagnostic work-up when indicated. Laboratory testing should especially be considered as part of the general evaluation if:

1) the medical review of systems reveals signs or symptoms that are rarely encountered in depression;

2) the patient is older;

3) the depressive episode first occurs after the age of 40-45; or

4) the depression does not respond fully to routine treatment (Depression Guideline Panel, 1993a).

Diagnosis

The diagnosis of depression is based primarily on DSM-IV criteria. The criteria state that at least five of the following symptoms must be present during the same period to receive a diagnosis of major depression (APA, 1994):

1) depressed mood most of the day, nearly every day;

2) markedly diminished interest or pleasure in almost all activities most of the day, nearly every day;

3) significant weight loss/gain;

4) insomnia/hypersomnia;

5) psychomotor agitation/retardation;

6) fatigue;

7) feelings of worthlessness (guilt);

8) impaired concentration; and,

9) recurrent thoughts of death or suicide.

The symptoms should be present most of the day, nearly daily, for a minimum of two weeks.

Practitioners need to consider the presence of other co-morbidities prior to making a diagnosis of major depression. Other factors that may contribute to the patient's mental health and that the clinician may want to treat first include:

1) substance abuse;

2) medications;

3) general medical disorder;

4) causal, non-mood psychiatric disorder; and/or,

5) grief reaction (Depression Guideline Panel, 1993a).

The clinician should also consider alternative diagnoses by eliciting a proper patient history. Examples of alternative diagnoses include:

1) Bipolar disorder--if the patient manifests prior manic episodes.

2) Dysthymic disorder--chronic mood disturbance (sadness) present most of the time for at least two consecutive years (Depression Guideline Panel, 1993a).

Treatment

Treatment is more effective if provided earlier in the depressive episode, prior to the condition becoming chronic (Bielski and Friedel, 1976; Kupfer et al., 1989). Unless noted otherwise, the recommendations for treatment are drawn from the *Depression Guidelines* (Depression Guideline Panel, 1993b).

Use of anti-depressant medications

Antidepressant medications are the first-line treatments for major depressive disorder. Medications have been shown to be effective in all forms of major depressive disorder (Depression Guideline Panel, 1993b). Anti-depressant medications are highly likely to be of benefit when:

1) the depression is moderate to severe;

2) there are psychotic, melancholic, or atypical symptom features;

3) the patient requests medication;

4) psychotherapy by a trained, competent psychotherapist is not available;

5) the patient has shown a prior positive response to medication; and,

6) maintenance treatment is planned.

The choice of anti-depressant is less important than use of antidepressants at appropriate dosages (Wells et al., 1994). No single antidepressant medication is clearly more effective than another and no single medication results in remission for all patients. Pharmacologic doses are recommended in the *Depression Guidelines* (1993b).

The specific choice of medication could be based on

1) short and long term side-effects;

2) prior positive/negative response to medication;

3) concurrent, nonpsychiatric medical illnesses that may make selected medications more or less risky; and/or

4) the concomitant use of other nonpsychotropic medications that may alter the metabolism or increase the side effects of the antidepressant (Depression Guideline Panel, 1993b).

In general, anti-anxiety agents should not be used (with the possible exception of alprazolam) (Depression Guideline Panel, 1993b).

Use of psychotherapy

Maintenance medication clearly prevents recurrences, while, to date, maintenance psychotherapy does not (Depression Guideline Panel, 1993a). Clinicians should consider psychotherapy alone for major depression as a first-line treatment if the episode is mild to moderate AND the patient desires psychotherapy as the first-line therapy (Depression Guideline Panel, 1993b). If psychotherapy is completely ineffective by 6 weeks of treatment, or if psychotherapy does not result in nearly a fully symptomatic remission within 12 weeks, then a switch to medications is appropriate due to the clear evidence of the efficacy of treatment with medications (Depression Guideline Panel, 1993b).

Medication plus psychotherapy

Clinicians should consider combined treatment initially with medications and psychotherapy if:

1) the depression is chronic or characterized by poor inter-episode recovery;

2) either treatment alone has been only partially effective;

3) the patient has a history of chronic psychosocial problems; or

4) the patient has a history of treatment adherence difficulties.

However, there is little evidence that indicates that primary care patients with major depression require initial psychotherapy in addition to medication. It is recommended that medication be added to (or substituted for psychotherapy) if:

1) there is no response to psychotherapy at 6 weeks;

2) there is only partial response at 12 weeks;

3) the patient worsens with psychotherapy; or;

4) the patient requests medications and symptoms are appropriate (Depression Guideline Panel, 1993b, pg. 88).

Clinicians may add psychotherapy to prescribed medications if:

1) residual symptoms are largely psychological (e.g., low self-esteem); or

2) patient has difficulty with adherence.

Follow-up

Most patients with major depressive disorder respond partially to medication within 2 to 3 weeks and full remission of symptoms is typically seen within 6 to 8 weeks (Depression Guideline Panel, 1993a). Most patients who receive time-limited psychotherapy respond partially by 5 to 6 weeks and fully by 10 to 12 weeks. Office visits or telephone contacts for medication management should occur weekly for the first 3 to 4 weeks to ensure adherence to medication regime, adjust dosage as necessary, and to detect and manage side effects. The depression panel recommends that patients with severe depression be seen weekly for the first 6 to 8 weeks (Depression Guideline Panel, 1993a). Once the depression has resolved, visits every 4 to 12 weeks are reasonable (Depression Guideline Panel, 1993a).

At each visit, clinicians should assess the degree of response/remission and side effects.

Failure to respond to medications

If the patient shows no response to the current medication by six weeks, then the clinician should both reassess adequacy of the diagnosis and reassess adequacy of treatment. Change in diagnosis or treatment plan (e.g., change of medication, referral to mental health specialist) is indicated (Depression Guideline Panel, 1993b).

If the patient exhibits a partial response by six weeks but cognitive symptoms remain, then the clinician should:

- continue treatment;
- reassess response to treatment in six more weeks;
- if reevaluation reveals only a partial response then it is appropriate to increase the dose of current medication or change the medication entirely. Alternately, one could refer to a mental health specialist for addition of psychotherapy. If two attempts at acute-phase medication have failed to resolve symptoms, consultation by a psychiatrist is indicated (Depression Guideline Panel, 1993b).

Continuation of treatment

Unless maintenance treatment is planned, anti-depressant medication should be discontinued at four to nine months (Depression Guideline Panel, 1993b). Patients should be followed for the next several months to ensure that a new depressive episode does not occur. It is unclear from the literature when the optimal time is to discontinue psychotherapy.

Maintenance

Maintenance treatment is designed to prevent new episodes of depression. Patients should be considered for maintenance treatment if they have had:

a) Three or more episodes of major depressive disorder; or
b) Two episodes of major depressive disorder and other circumstance--i.e., family history of bipolar disorder, history of recurrence within one year after previously effective medication was discontinued, family history of recurrent major depression, early onset (prior to age 20) of the first depressive episode, both episodes were severe, sudden, or life-

threatening in the past three years (Depression Guideline Panel, 1993b).

Sentinel Events/Adverse Outcomes

Emergency hospitalization for depression

Suicide attempts

All depressed patients should be asked about their feelings regarding suicide during the diagnostic visit(s) (Depression Guideline Panel, 1993b). Indications that warrant hospitalization for suicidality include:

a) psychosis;

b) suicidal ideation with substance abuse, severe hopelessness, strong impulses to act on the ideas, or specific plans;

c) lack of social support;

d) concurrent medical conditions that make outpatient treatment unsafe;

e) inability to participate in outpatient care.

RECOMMENDED QUALITY INDICATORS FOR DEPRESSION

The following indications apply to adolescents aged 13 to 18.

Diagnosis/Detection

	Indicator	Quality of evidence	Literature	Benefits	Comments
1.	Clinicians should ask about the presence or absence of depression or depressive symptoms* in any person with any of the following risk factors for depression: • divorce in past six months, • unemployment, • history of depression, • death in family in past six months, and • alcohol or other drug abuse.	III	USPSTF, 1989	Alleviate symptoms of depression.*	Risk factors for depression have been relatively well-defined in cross-sectional studies.
2.	If the diagnosis of depression is made, specific co-morbidities should be elicited and documented in the chart: - presence or absence of substance abuse - medication use - general medical disorder(s)	III	Depression Guideline Panel, 1993a & 1993b	Alleviate symptoms of depression.* Prevent complications of substance abuse.**	Certain co-morbidities may contribute to or cause depression. The practitioner should be aware of these co-morbidities when making a treatment plan for depression. Documentation may have occurred on previous visits.

Treatment

	Indicator	Quality of evidence	Literature	Benefits	Comments
3.	If co-morbidity (substance abuse, contributing medication, general medical disorder) is present that contributes to depression, the initial treatment objective should be to remove the comorbidity or treat medical disorder.	III	Depression Guideline Panel, 1993a & 1993b (meta-analysis)	Alleviate symptoms of depression.* Prevent complications of substance abuse.**	Depression may be treated by addressing the co-morbidity. For example, alcoholism should be treated and patients should be taken off of medications that may have CNS depressant properties.
4.	Once diagnosis of major depression has been made, treatment with anti-depressant medication and/or psychotherapy should begin within 2 weeks.	I, II-1, II-2	Depression Guideline Panel, 1993a & 1993b	Alleviate symptoms of depression.* Reduce disability days.	Randomized controlled trials cited in the guidelines (not individually reviewed) substantiate the usefulness of medication and psychotherapy for the treatment of depression. Antidepressant medication therapy is probably more effective as a sole modality. The guidelines recommend "prompt" treatment, but no definition of prompt is given. We suggest two weeks is a reasonable time interval.
5.	Presence or absence of suicidal ideation should be documented during the first or second diagnostic visit.	II-2, III	Depression Guideline Panel, 1993a & 1993b	Prevent death from suicide. Prevent morbidity from suicide attempts.	Presence of suicidality is a marker for severe depression and would argue for instituting therapy with anti-depressants and against psychotherapy alone. Suicidality with psychosis, drug abuse, and/or plan of action warrants hospitalization.
6.	Medication treatment visits or telephone contacts should occur weekly for a minimum of 4 weeks.	III	Depression Guideline Panel, 1993a & 1993b	Alleviate symptoms of depression.* Reduce disability days.	Once treatment is started, the practitioner needs to document improvement. Most patients improve at least partially within 3 weeks. The guidelines advocate weekly follow-up by phone or in person for 4-6 weeks. Our indicator specifies the lower end of the recommendations.
7.	At least one of the following should occur if there is no or incomplete response to therapy for depression at 6 weeks: 1) Referral to psychotherapist if not already seeing one; or 2) Change or increase in dose of medication if on medication; or 3) Addition of medication if only using psychotherapy; or 4) Change in diagnosis documented in chart.	III	Depression Guideline Panel, 1993a & 1993b	Alleviate symptoms of depression.* Reduce disability days.	Almost all clinical depression responds at least partially by 6 weeks. If response is incomplete, the diagnosis needs to be re-evaluated and/or treatment plan changed/augmented.
8.	Anti-depressants should be used at appropriate dosages.	I	Depression Guideline Panel, 1993b; Wells, 1988	Alleviate symptoms of depression.* Reduce disability days.	Only appropriate doses of anti-depressants will be effective in treatment, yet subtherapeutic doses are often used. For example, a patient on 25 mg of amitryptilline at bed time is not on a therapeutic antidepressant dose. We will exclude those with renal and hepatic dysfunction from this indicator.

#	Recommendation		Goal	Comment
9.	Anti-anxiety agents should generally NOT be used (except alprazolam).	I Depression Guideline Panel, 1993b	Alleviate symptoms of depression.* Reduce disability days. Avoid dependance on anti-anxiety agents.	With the possible exception of alprazolam, anti-anxiety agents have not been shown to be of benefit and may be of harm. Foregoing antidepressants in favor of anxiolytics deprives patients of potential benefits of antidepressant treatment.
10.	Persons who have suicidality should be asked if they have specific plans to carry out suicide.	III Depression Guideline Panel, 1993b	Prevent death from suicide. Prevent morbidity from suicide attempts.	If a person has a plan to carry out suicide, the risk of success increases. These persons should be hospitalized.
11.	Persons who have suicidality and have any of the following risk factors should be hospitalized: a. psychosis, b. current alcohol or drug abuse, or c. specific plans to carry out suicide (e.g., obtaining a weapon, putting affairs in order, making a suicide note).	III Depression Guideline Panel, 1993b	Prevent death from suicide. Prevent morbidity from suicide attempts.	Presence of risk factors for successful suicide in a person who admits to suicidality warrants hospitalization.

152

Follow-up

Indicator	Quality of evidence	Literature	Benefits	Comments
12. Once depression has resolved, visits should occur every 16 weeks at a minimum, while patient is still on medication, for the first year of treatment.	III	Depression Guideline Panel, 1993b	Alleviate symptoms of depression.* Reduce disability days. Reduce relapses.	The guidelines recommend visit intervals every 12 weeks for the duration of treatment. Occasionally, patients may be on indefinite treatment. In order to allow variation in follow-up times given patient preferences and long-term duration of treatment, we recommend 16 week intervals visits during the first year of treatment. Even so, it may be difficult to penalize a practitioner whose patients are seeing a psychotherapist in addition to him/herself for not seeing a patient on a frequent basis.
13. At each visit during which depression is discussed, degree of response/remission and side effects of medication should be assessed and documented during the first year of treatment.	III	Depression Guideline Panel, 1993b	Alleviate symptoms of depression.* Reduce toxicities of medication. Reduce relapses.	Even effectively treated patients may relapse or develop toxicities to medications. While most persons will be off of medications after one year, the optimal time to remove medications is still not well established.
14. Persons hospitalized for depression should have follow-up with a mental health specialist or their primary care doctor within two weeks of discharge.	III	Depression Guideline Panel, 1993b	Alleviate symptoms of depression.* Reduce disability days. Prevent death from suicide. Prevent morbidity from suicide attempts.	The guidelines do not specifically address time-interval between discharge and follow-up. However, given severity of disease, longer than two weeks should probably not pass before re-evaluation. If the patient is also seeing a mental health specialist, the two week interval can apply to that specialist instead of the primary care provider.

*Symptoms of depression include depressed mood, diminished interest or pleasure in activities, weight loss/gain, impaired concentration, suicidality, fatigue, feelings of worthlessness and guilt, and psychomotor agitation/retardation.

**Medical complications of substance abuse are numerous and include: for alcohol, blackouts, seizures, delerium, liver failure; for IV drugs of any kind, local infection, endocarditis, hepatitis and HIV, death from overdose; for cocaine and amphetamines, seizures, myocardial infarction, and hypertensive crises.

Quality of Evidence Codes:

I:	RCT
II-1:	Nonrandomized controlled trials
II-2:	Cohort or case analysis
II-3:	Multiple time series
III:	Opinions or descriptive studies

153

REFERENCES - DEPRESSION

American Psychiatric Association. 1994. Substance-related disorders. In *Diagnostic and Statistical Manual of Mental Disorders: DSM-IV*, Fourth ed. 175-205. Washington, DC: American Psychiatric Association.

Bielski RJ, and RO Friedel. December 1976. Prediction of tricyclic antidepressant response: A critical review. *Archives of General Psychiatry* 33: 1479-89.

Broadhead WE, DG Blazer, LK George, et al. 21 November 1990. Depression, disability days, and days lost from work in a prospective epidemiologic survey. *Journal of the American Medical Association* 264 (19): 2524-8.

Burnam MA, KB Wells, B Leake, et al. 1988. Development of a brief screening instrument for detecting depressive disorders. *Medical Care* 26: 775-89.

Depression Guideline Panel. April 1993. *Depression in Primary Care: Volume 1. Detection and Diagnosis. Clinical Practice Guideline, Number 5.* AHCPR Publication No. 93-0550. Rockville, MD: U.S. Department of Health and Human Services, Public Health Service, Agency for Health Care Policy and Research.

Depression Guideline Panel. April 1993. *Depression in Primary Care: Volume 2. Treatment of Major Depression. Clinical Practice Guideline, Number 5.* AHCPR Publication No. 93-0551. Rockville, MD: U.S. Department of Health and Human Services, Public Health Service, Agency for Health Care Policy and Research.

Feldman E, R Mayou, K Hawton, et al. May 1987. Psychiatric disorder in medical in-patients. *Quarterly Journal of Medicine* New Series 63 (241): 405-12.

Greenberg PE, LE Stiglin, SN Finkelstein, et al. November 1993. Depression: A neglected major illness. *Journal of Clinical Psychiatry* 54 (11): 419-24.

Hays RD, KB Wells, CD Sherbourne, et al. January 1995. Functioning and well-being outcomes of patients with depression compared with chronic general medical illness. *Archives of General Psychiatry* 52: 11-9.

Katon W, and H Schulberg. 1992. Epidemiology of depression in primary care. *General Hospital Pscyhiatry* 14: 237-47.

Kessler RC, KA McGonagle, S Zhao, et al. January 1994. Lifetime and 12-month prevalence of DSM-III-R psychiatric disorders in the United States. *Archives of General Psychiatry* 51: 8-19.

Kupfer DJ, E Frank, and JM Perel. September 1989. The advantage of early treatment intervention in recurrent depression. *Archives of General Psychiatry* 46: 771-5.

NIMH Consensus Development Conference. April 1985. Mood disorders: Pharmacologic prevention of recurrences. *American Journal of Psychiatry* 142 (4): 469-76.

Sturm, R, and KB Wells. June 1994. *Can Prepaid Care for Depression Be Improved Cost-Effectively?* RAND, Santa Monica, CA.

Wells KB, JM Golding, and MA Burnam. June 1988. Psychiatric disorder and limitations in physical functioning in a sample of the Los Angeles general population. *American Journal of Psychiatry* 145 (6): 712-7.

Wells KB, RD Hays, MA Burnam, et al. 15 December 1989. Detection of depressive disorder for patients receiving prepaid or fee-for-service care: Results from the medical outcomes study. *Journal of the American Medical Association* 262 (23): 3298-3302.

Wells KB, W Katon, B Rogers, et al. May 1994. Use of minor tranquilizers and antidepressant medications by depressed outpatients: Results from the medical outcomes study. *American Journal of Psychiatry* 151 (5): 694-700.

Wells KB, A Stewart, RD Hays, et al. 18 August 1989. The functioning and well-being of depressed patients: Results from the Medical Outcomes Study. *Journal of the American Medical Association* 262 (7): 914-9.

8. DEVELOPMENTAL SCREENING
Mark Schuster, M.D., Ph.D.

The recommended indicators for developmental screening were derived from (1) textbooks on pediatric medicine (Palmer and Capute, in Oski, 1994) and general pediatrics (Shapiro, in Dershewitz, 1993; Simeonsson and Simeonsson, in Hoekelman, 1992), (2) the American Academy of Pediatrics (AAP) Guidelines for Health Supervision II (American Academy of Pediatrics [AAP], 1988), (3) a policy statement of the AAP's Committee on Children With Disabilities (AAP, 1994), and (4) *Bright Futures: Guidelines for Health Supervision of Infants, Children, and Adolescents* (Green, 1994). A review article by First and Palfrey (1994) was used as well, as were other articles identified from the above list.

IMPORTANCE

Developmental delay has a 10 percent prevalence rate, but early identification is difficult (First and Palfrey, 1994). Early diagnosis of developmental disabilities is important in order to identify etiologic factors, design treatment programs, and provide a prognosis (Shapiro, in Dershewitz, 1993). Assessment of development should be integrated into the pediatric examination. The physician's role in developmental assessment is particularly critical in the preschool years because growth and development are rapid and qualitative developmental indexes such as language and socialization, serve as markers for school readiness (Simeonsson and Simeonsson, in Hoekelman et al., 1992).

Patterns of development in the earliest years of life are sequential and predictable. Development can be viewed as a series of milestones normally achieved at specific ages or a series of critical tasks to be mastered within certain stages of life. Development needs to be assessed repeatedly over time. Observations and assessments should be made on two or more occasions to determine developmental rate. This is particularly necessary to rule out transient deficits resulting from normal variation or from the influence of illness or fatigue (Simeonsson and Simeonsson, in Hoekelman et al., 1992). Though screening of asymptomatic populations has been advocated to detect developmental disability as early as possible, it is unclear whether this significantly improves the detection of developmental disabilities. However, it does focus attention on the development of infants and young children, so that children with disabilities may be identified earlier (Shapiro, in Dershewitz, 1993).

Developmental delay, which is the failure to reach developmental milestones at the expected age range for normal children, may result from biologic factors (e.g., a chromosomal disorder) and environmental factors (e.g., maternal depression). Delay is most often considered the result of the interaction of both biologic and environmental factors. For example, an inattentive mother might be unable to nurture a child with intrauterine growth retardation through each developmental stage, whereas a supportive mother can promote the development of a child with cerebral palsy or Down syndrome (First and Palfrey, 1994).

The AAP's Committee on Children With Disabilities recommends early identification of children with developmental disabilities because (a) treatment is available for some conditions, and (b) for conditions that cannot be cured, there is nonetheless the opportunity to improve the child's condition and help the family both develop strategies for coping and obtain the resources for successful family functioning (AAP, 1994).

There are a number of causes of developmental disability, and they can primarily manifest as an isolated motor handicap, a cognitive handicap, or a specific processing deficit despite globally normal cognition. For example, cerebral palsy is the most common movement disorder of childhood. It results from a static lesion to the immature central nervous system. Another example is mental retardation, which is significantly subaverage intellectual functioning associated with deficits in social/adaptive function. Specific deficits in processing provide another example. They can be subdivided into peripheral disorders of processing, such as deafness and blindness, and central processing disorders, which preclude function at a level predicted by IQ alone. These include autism (without mental retardation), preschool communication disorder, developmental dysphasia, and specific learning disabilities. We do not have a good understanding of the specific neural mechanism of these dysfunctions. Attentional problems, hyperactivity, impulsivity, and emotional lability may be part of abnormal neurologic development and not secondary reactions to disability (Shapiro, in Dershewitz, 1993). The other broad category of developmental disabilities is those attributable to emotional/behavioral disorders that may involve abnormal peer relations and socialization.

Developmental Streams

For decades, pediatricians have separated the complex developmental processes into separate developmental streams for easier evaluation and detection of delay and deviancy. Streams refer to a series of milestones for related skills, such as language skills. Various authors use different names for these streams and some divide them in slightly different ways, but the various classification systems generally cover the same skills (Palmer and Capute, in Oski et al., 1994). Palmer and Capute describe the following streams: language, visuomotor, gross and fine motor, social development, and self-help. Shapiro includes four major categories of milestones: gross motor, language, fine motor/problem solving, and personal/social (Shapiro, in Dershewitz, 1993). First and Palfrey (1994) include fine and gross motor, language, cognitive, and psychosocial development.

Generally, speech, social and emotional behavior (such as smiling), and fine motor coordination, particularly in a young child, have greater prognostic significance than gross motor skills and toileting. The times at which speech and language skills develop are typically the most useful clues in the determination of normality (though this is not the case for high-functioning autistic children). Appropriate social behaviors are the next most important. Delayed or atypical communication and socialization behaviors are highly significant in identifying children at risk in terms of development (Simeonsson and Simeonsson, in Hoekelman et al., 1992).

Gross motor milestones cover independent locomotion, and the recognition of gross motor delay often leads to the diagnosis of cerebral palsy (Shapiro, in Dershewitz, 1993). Most infants with moderate or severe cerebral palsy can be identified in the first 6 to 8 months of life (Palmer and Capute, in Oski et al., 1994).

Language milestones cover the development of symbolic thought. They can be subdivided into expression (that which is said), reception (that which is understood), speech (the manner in which things are said), and visual language (nonverbal communication, e.g., play). Language is the best predictor of cognition (Shapiro, in Dershewitz, 1993). The pediatric assessment of early language relies almost entirely on prelinguistic and linguistic milestones, which are related to later cognitive development. Recognition of early language delay is probably the most sensitive indicator of subsequent mental retardation. Subtle manifestations of language delay or deviancy indicate risk for school-age learning disability and general academic underachievement. Language delay is best identified by determining the child's level of consistent language performance by milestone criteria (Palmer and Capute, in Oski et al., 1994).

Fine motor/visuomotor/problem solving milestones cover visual maturation, hand function, problem solving, and visual motor abilities. They comprise the other major cognitive stream of development, and they form the basis for most of the infant intelligence scales. This area covers visual and fine-motor manipulative tasks. These skills are not easily covered by asking parents (history-taking) about previously attained skills. The clinician usually can only determine a current visuomotor age and development quotient. In global mental retardation, there is broad cognitive delay in language and visuomotor skills. In communication disorders, visuomotor skills tend to be preserved (Palmer and Capute, in Oski et al., 1994; Shapiro, in Dershewitz, 1993).

Personal/social abilities are the end result of multiple streams, including problem solving, motor, and language. They depend on environmental factors but are associated with cognitive thresholds; social dysfunction may be a symptom of neurodevelopmental abnormality as well as environmental problems (Palmer and Capute, in Oski et al., 1994; Shapiro, in Dershewitz, 1993). Shapiro (in Dershewitz, 1993) would include feeding, dressing, and hygiene in this category, though Palmer and Capute (in Oski et al., 1994) separate them out into a self-help category. The latter is described as providing information on how the child integrates the developmental streams into basic daily functioning. Most activities of daily living require a minimum level of motor, language, problem-solving, and attentional maturity (Palmer and Capute, in Oski et al., 1994).

Assessment

Bright Futures (Green, 1994) incorporates developmental assessment and milestone checks throughout the first five years of life. The AAP (1988) covers developmental issues throughout childhood, sometimes referring to them as behavioral assessments.

The clinician should consider the assessment of delay as a matter of ongoing surveillance rather than a screening procedure performed at a particular visit in order to detect more problems (First and Palfrey, 1994).

Assessments can be done by standardized tests or by parental recall of the developmental milestones attained by the child. Formal screening tests are limited by applicability to only certain ages or poor test qualities. Most initial screenings are done by the parents, and can be elicited with a question from the clinician. Clinicians should record milestone attainment data at each well-child examination. Usually four or five questions need to be asked about language, motor, and personal/social development. If concerns arise from the questions, then fine motor/problem solving skills can be elicited. Viewing developmental rates over time allows the detection of degeneration or acceleration (Shapiro, in Dershewitz, 1993).

Though developmental screening tests have been widely used in pediatric practice for years, they are not highly sensitive for developmental abnormalities and they also produce too many false positives. Children with mild disabilities, in particular, tend to be missed. To prevent missing many children, the clinician should take a broader clinical approach to developmental detection rather than solely relying on published screening measures (Palmer and Capute, in Oski et al., 1994).

Several formal screening tests exist for developmental assessment. These are generally too long to conduct on a routine basis for every child at every well child visit, though they are used when there is a concern about possible delay and may be done routinely by some clinicians at particular ages. The Denver Developmental Screening Test (DDST) covers ages 0-6 years and provides an overall assessment of development as well as specific data on personal-social, fine motor, language, and gross motor status. A recently revised version is called DDST II. Revisions include an update in norms, an increase in language items, the addition of speech intelligibility items and a subjective behavior rating scale, the removal or modification of items from the DDST that were difficult to administer or interpret, and a new age scale. The DDST II appears to have a high rate of overall sensitivity, but limited specificity and positive predictive value and thus a high overall referral rate (Dworkin, 1992). Dworkin (1992) points out that the DDST II should not be used in isolation as a basis for referral, diagnosis, or prediction of future functioning. It should not be used as a traditional screening test. Instead, it should help with active developmental surveillance by serving as a developmental chart or inventory. In other words, it should be used in a similar manner to growth charts, which serve to document and compare growth over time (First and Palfrey, 1994).

The Denver Prescreening Developmental Questionnaire (PDQ) and its revised form (R-PDQ) are questionnaires for parents to complete. The R-PDQ includes all the DDST items and uses the same categories, which allows a comparison of a child's achievement with that of the standardization sample. When a clinician uses the PDQ or R-PDQ, verification of the parental report should be obtained by administering the DDST either in full or in part (Simeonsson and Simeonsson, in Hoekelman et al., 1992).

Screening measures with high sensitivity and specificity include: the Minnesota Child Development Inventory (MCDI) (6 months to 6 years), the Early Screening Inventory (ESI) (3 to 6 years), and the Minnesota Preschool Screening Inventory (MPSI) (3.5 to 5.5 years). The Peabody Picture Vocabulary Test (PPVT) (2 years to adult) assesses receptive language in terms of a mental age and an intelligence quotient (IQ) and correlates well with more general measures of intellectual development. The Goodenough-Harris Drawing Test (3 to 15 years) assesses general development and provides an index of self-awareness and social awareness (Simeonsson and Simeonsson, in Hoekelman et al., 1992).

Definition of Delay and Deviancy

Developmental delay is quantified by the developmental quotient (calculated as the developmental age divided by chronologic age, and multiplied by 100). Different streams have different recommended cutoffs for what is considered delay. Recognition of dissociations between rates of development in different streams is essential for the early diagnosis of atypical development within a specific stream (Palmer and Capute, in Oski et al., 1994).

When a child is at least one-third below the expected age level in mental or motor development on the basis of developmental assessment or screening, referral for diagnosis and treatment (to a psychologist, neurologist, or physical therapist, depending on the areas of concern) may be appropriate. The DDST, PPVT, MCDI, MPSI, and ESI may be useful for documenting such delays. The conditions most often associated with such delays are mild to moderate mental retardation and mild forms of cerebral palsy. Some children demonstrate wide gaps in developmental skills. When a discrepancy of one third or more is observed in developmental skills between one area and others, the child should be referred for further assessment and possible intervention by developmental specialists. These discrepancies may signal sensory problems, perceptual or learning disabilities, or minimal brain dysfunction (Simeonsson and Simeonsson, in Hoekelman et al., 1992).

Developmental deviancy is a subtle sign of central nervous system abnormality. It refers to atypical development within a single stream, such as developmental milestones occurring out of normal sequence (Palmer and Capute, in Oski et al., 1994).

Treatment

There is no cure for developmental disorders, so treatment should be viewed as palliative. The broad goals of treatment are to allow the child to function at the maximum level permitted by his/her impairment and to prevent secondary social or biologic dysfunctions (Shapiro, in Dershewitz, 1993).

Early intervention is predicated on three assumptions: the condition can be modified by the intervention; earlier intervention is more effective than later intervention for the primary disorder; and secondary problems may be avoided. Early intervention can be categorized as an intervention designed to offset social disadvantage, biological risk, or developmental disability. The assumptions about early intervention are the least well-proven for developmental disability. While the goal of achieving normal function is unlikely in children with developmental disability, early intervention seeks to assist parental acceptance of the child and to prevent secondary disorders. Also, the Education of the Handicapped Act Amendments of 1986, Public Law 99-457, mandates service to children 3 to 5 years of age who demonstrate developmental delays or who are at risk for such delays (in cognitive, speech/language, motor, self-help, or psychological development). The provision of early intervention services under this law must include a multidisciplinary assessment and a written Individualized Family Service Plan (IFSP). It is anticipated that 5 to 10 percent of children will be eligible for early intervention services under this legislation (Shapiro, in Dershewitz, 1993).

There is evidence that even in the absence of an etiologic explanation, early identification helps both children and their parents (First and Palfrey, 1994). The best chance for effecting developmental change is while the nervous system of the young child is still malleable and responsive. Once one has identified problems, it is important to help parents adjust expectations to the child's developmental stage and provide developmentally appropriate equipment, stimulation, and toys. Early identification allows the family members to feel that they are doing all they can to assist the child and to bolster the child's sense of being appreciated for who he or she is, which helps prevent secondary emotional disability. When there is a diagnosis of a genetic, metabolic, or infectious disease, early identification can prevent further disability. It can also provide the parents information relevant to future pregnancies (First and Palfrey, 1994).

RECOMMENDED QUALITY INDICATORS FOR DEVELOPMENTAL SCREENING FOR CHILDREN

Because of the large number of screening tools and various specific milestones that different clinicians might choose to track, indicators will require documentation that assessment has taken place, but will not require use of any particular tool. It will be sufficient to note that a specific screening tool was used (along with the results) or that specific milestones have or have not been achieved. Furthermore, this review covers routine assessment. It does not cover the specific response to delays that are identified by such assessments. It would be difficult to write indicators that specified at what point referrals or interventions should be made, since developmental assessment frequently requires assessments at multiple time points. Because of the variation in reasonable responses to delay and the dependence of the response on trends, other health conditions, and environmental factors, it would be difficult to develop indicators to evaluate the proper response to developmental delay in the initial phase of this study. Documentation is important both because the same provider may not conduct each assessment and because trends must be examined. It would be unwise to merely document abnormal findings and delay because there is enough variation in what is normal that if one found a delay, one might not be able to determine what milestones had been previously achieved.

RECOMMENDED QUALITY INDICATORS FOR DEVELOPMENTAL SCREENING FOR CHILDREN

The following criteria apply to developmental evaluation for children.

	Indicator	Quality of evidence	Literature	Benefits	Comments
1.	Social/personal development should be documented: a. three times during the first year of life; b. two times during the second year of life; c. one time during the third year of life; d. one time during the fourth year of life; and e. one time during the fifth year of life.	III	AAP, 1988; Green, 1994	Improve social functioning. Improve ability to function with disability. Improve family interactions and coping skills. Improve functioning of autistic children.	Since most physicians would believe that children should be evaluated developmentally at most or all well child visits, these indicators are fairly loose in the number of times per year documentation of developmental assessment is required. Children with severe neurologic devastation who are not expected to improve with age may not have such documentation. However, there should be too few such children to affect the overall quality score for an individual managed care facility. Delay can be due to neurodevelopmental abnormalities or environmental problems.
2.	Fine motor/visuomotor/problem solving development should be documented at least: a. three times during the first year of life; b. two times during the second year of life; c. one time during the third year of life; d. one time during the fourth year of life; and e. one time during the fifth year of life.	III	AAP, 1988; Green, 1994	Improve fine motor and visual functioning. Improve ability to function with disabilities. Improve family interactions and coping skills.	Delay can help in the diagnosis of global mental retardation and visual deficits. Appropriate milestones will be assessed based on age. Documentation of "no deficit" is also adequate to meet this indicator.
3.	Language development should be documented at least: a. three times during the first year of life; b. two times during the second year of life; c. one time during the third year of life; d. one time during the fourth year of life; and e. one time during the fifth year of life.	III	AAP, 1988; Green, 1994	Improve language abilities. Reduce hearing impairment. Improve ability to function with disabilities. Improve family interactions and coping skills.	Language is the best predictor of cognition. Recognition of early language delay is the most sensitive indicator of subsequent mental retardation. Language delay or deviancy can indicate risk of school-age learning disability and academic underachievement. Appropriate milestones will be assessed based on age. Documentation of "no deficit" is also adequate to meet this indicator.
4.	Gross motor development should be documented at least: a. three times during the first year of life; b. two times during the second year of life; c. one time during the third year of life; d. one time during the fourth year of life; and e. one time during the fifth year of life.	III	AAP, 1988; Green, 1994	Improve gross motor functioning. Improve ability to function with disabilities. Improve family interactions and coping skills.	Gross motor delay can be due to cerebral palsy. Appropriate milestones will be assessed based on age. Documentation of "no deficit" is also adequate to meet this indicator.

5.	In children with known developmental delay, referral to a specialist for early intervention should be documented.	III	Simeonsson & Simeonsson, in Hoekelman, 1992	Improve functioning in area of developmental delay. Improve family interactions and coping skills.	Because of the complex needs of children with developmental problems, it is desirable that assessment and management of the developmental problem be integrated into an overall plan for the child's care.
6.	In children with diagnosed language delay, referral to a specialist for speech therapy should be documented.	III	Simeonsson & Simeonsson, in Hoekelman, 1992	Improve language abilities. Improve ability to function with disabilities. Improve family interactions and coping skills.	Because of the complex needs of children with developmental problems, it is desirable that assessment and management of the developmental problem be integrated into an overall plan for the child's care.
7.	In children with gross or fine motor development delay, referral to a specialist for physical therapy should be documented.	III	Simeonsson & Simeonsson, in Hoekelman, 1992	Improve ability to function with disabilities. Improve family interactions and coping skills. Improve gross or fine motor functioning.	Because of the complex needs of children with developmental problems, it is desirable that assessment and management of the developmental problem be integrated into an overall plan for the child's care.

Quality of Evidence Codes:

I:	RCT
II-1:	Nonrandomized controlled trials
II-2:	Cohort or case analysis
II-3:	Multiple time series
III:	Opinions or descriptive studies

REFERENCES - DEVELOPMENTAL SCREENING

American Academy of Pediatrics, and Committee on Psychosocial Aspects of Child and Family Health, 1985-1988. 1988. *Guidelines for Health Supervision II*, Second ed.Elk Grove Village, Illinois: American Academy of Pediatrics.

American Academy of Pediatrics, and Committee on Children With Disabilities. May 1994. Screening infants and young children for developmental disabilities. *Pediatrics* 93 (5): 863-5.

Dworkin PH. 1992. Developmental screening: (Still) expecting the impossible? *Pediatrics* Commentaries: 1253-5.

First LR, and JS Palfrey. 17 February 1994. The infant or young child with developmental delay. *New England Journal of Medicine* 330 (7): 478-83.

Green, M. 1994. *Bright Futures: Guidelines for Health Supervision of Infants, Children, and Adolescents*. Arlington, VA: National Center for Education in Maternal and Child Health.

Palmer FB, and AJ Capute. 1994. Streams of development. In *Principles and Practice of Pediatrics*. Editors Oski FA, CD DeAngelis, RD Feigin, et al., 667-73. Philadelphia, PA: J.B. Lippincott Company.

Shapiro BK. 1993. Detection and assessment of developmental disabilities. In *Ambulatory Pediatric Care*, Second ed. Editor Dershewitz RA, 145-50. Philadelphia, PA: J.B. Lippincott Company.

Simeonsson RJ, and NE Simeonsson. 1992. Developmental assessment. In *Primary Pediatric Care*, Second ed. Editor Hoekelman RA, 234-9. St. Louis, MO: Mosby-Year Book, Inc.

9. DIABETES MELLITUS[1]
Seven Asch, M.D., M.P.H.

Several recent reviews provided the core references in developing quality indicators for diabetes (Singer et al., in Eddy, 1991; Bergenstal, 1993; Gerich, 1989; Nathan, in Rubenstein and Federman, 1993; Garnick et al., 1994; Plotnick, in Oski, 1994; Golden and Gray, in McAnarney et al., 1992). Where these core references cited studies to support individual indicators, we have included the original references. We also performed narrow searches of the medical literature from 1985 to 1995 to supplement these references for particular indicators. Indicators of quality of care for gestational diabetes are covered in Chapter 16.

IMPORTANCE

Diabetes is a heterogeneous yet often serious and common chronic condition prevalent throughout the world. In 1992, the number of diabetics in the United States alone was estimated to be 7.2 million. The prevalence of insulin-dependent diabetes mellitus (IDDM) among children and adolescents varies somewhat from 1.2 to 1.9 per 1,000 population in the age group (Plotnick, in Oski, 1994). The incidence of diabetes among children reaches its highest rate of onset between 10 and 14 years (Golden and Gray, in McAnarney et al., 1992).

For children and adolescents, the failure to adequately treat (i.e., undertreatment, poor control) diabetes may contribute to delays in growth, skeletal maturation, and sexual maturation. On the other hand, high doses of insulin may result in weight gain, rebound hyperglycemia, ketosis, and growth retardation (Plotnick, in Oski, 1994). Adolescents with IDDM have comorbid hypertension more often than previously believed; treatment can prevent serious complications of cardiovascular disease and diabetic nephropathy. Cigarette smoking,

---

[1]Originally written for the Women's Quality of Care Panel. Some modifications have been made to reflect issues for children and adolescents.

which has been increasing among adolescents, is a risk factor for
macrovascular complications (Golden and Gray, in McAnarney et al.,
1992). Adolescents with IDDM are also at higher risk for other
autoimmune diseases (Golden and Gray, in McAnarney et al., 1992). About
half of insulin-dependent diabetics develop kidney failure (Bergenstal,
1993). All of these complications taken together result in much higher
death rates among diabetics than the remainder of the population
(Palumbo et al., 1976). Much of the benefit of high quality care will
accrue years later from the prevention of morbidity and mortality from
such complications. Death rates from diabetes itself increase with age
ranging from 0.2 per 100,000 for those between 15 and 19 years of age to
14.6/100,000 for those between 50 and 54 years (National Center for
Health Statistics [NCHS], 1994a).

The treatment of diabetes is resource intensive, with total costs
estimated at $30-40 billion annually in 1992 (American Diabetes
Association [ADA], 1993), or $1 of every $7 spent on health care in 1992
(Rubin et al., 1994). Diabetes was the eighth most common reason for a
patient visiting a physician's office in 1992 (NCHS, 1994b).

EFFICACY AND/OR EFFECTIVENESS OF INTERVENTIONS

Screening

Indicators of the quality of screening diabetics for complications
of diabetes are covered under diagnosis below. This section covers
screening patients not known to be diabetic for the disease. Both the
American College of Physicians (Singer et al., in Eddy, 1991) and the
Canadian Task Force on Periodic Health Examination [CTF] (1979)
recommended that asymptomatic patients need not undergo screening for
diabetes. Children who develop IDDM are rarely asymptomatic. These
recommendations turned on the poor evidence that treatment of patients
so identified would prevent complications. Though many persons have
asymptomatic hyperglycemia, most complications of diabetes occur late in
the course of the disease, limiting the benefits of early
identification. Since the publication of those recommendations, the
Diabetes Control and Complications Trial (DCCT) (see below) has added
evidence for the efficacy of tight control in known diabetics in

preventing complications (DCCT, 1993a). However, we have found no subsequent studies either directly evaluating the efficacy of screening asymptomatic patients in reducing morbidity or mortality from diabetes (Singer, 1988; CTF, 1979).

Diagnosis

The initial diagnosis of diabetes depends upon the measurement of a fasting blood sugar greater than 140/mg/dl or a postprandial blood sugar of greater than 200/mg/dl. If a recorded blood sugar meets the above criteria, we recommend looking for notation of the diagnosis of diabetes in the progress notes or problem list. Most experts also recommend a complete history and physical examination, dietary evaluation, urinalysis for protein, measurement of blood creatinine, and a lipid panel at the time of initial diagnosis (ADA, 1989). We do not propose any of these as quality indicators for the initial diagnosis because of the small number of incident cases in our sample and the difficulty of defining the time of initial diagnosis.

We instead concentrate on the routine diagnostic tests that known diabetics should undergo regardless of their clinical status and stage of disease. The first of these is the measurement of glycosylated hemoglobin to monitor glycemic control. Based on a randomized controlled trial of 240 patients, it was found that measuring hemoglobin A_{1c} every three months leads to changes in diabetic treatment and improvement in metabolic control, indicated by a lowering of average hemoglobin A_{1c} values (Larsen et al., 1990). The landmark DCCT followed 1,441 insulin-dependent diabetics (about 14 percent of whom were adolescents) for 9 years and found that tight glycemic control and lower hemoglobin A_{1c} values decreased rates of diabetic complications (DCCT, 1993a). Despite recommendations from a number of specialty and generalist physician societies, there is great variation in the use of this test (ADA, 1993; Bergenstal et al., 1993; Garnick et al., 1994; Goldstein et al., 1994). We suggest looking for a hemoglobin A_{1c} test for all diabetics at 6-month intervals, the longest recommended interval.

Home blood glucose monitoring has been shown to aid glycemic control in diabetics treated with insulin. The DCCT employed home blood glucose monitoring for its population of insulin-dependent diabetics rather than the more easily tolerated urine glucose monitoring to achieve tight control because moderate hyperglycemia (180 mg/dl) may not cause glycosuria. At least one small randomized trial (n=23) has shown home blood glucose monitoring to improve glycemic control in obese insulin-dependent diabetics (Allen et al., 1990). The optimal frequency of monitoring has not yet been determined, though some studies have questioned patients ability to comply with frequent measurement (Bergenstal et al., 1993; Health and Public Policy Committee, 1983; Muchmore et al., 1994; Gordon, 1991). Observational data has failed to find any strong relationship between home blood glucose monitoring and glycemic control in noninsulin-dependent diabetics (Patrick, 1994; Allen et al., 1990). Specialty societies recommend that patients on insulin be offered training and equipment for home glucose monitoring, and we propose this as another indicator of diagnostic quality (ADA, 1993).

Because of the frequency of vision, cardiovascular, and renal complications among diabetics, many of which may be asymptomatic, the ADA (1989) has recommended several screening tests in children: yearly eye exam in children age 12-18 who have had a diagnosis of diabetes for at least 5 years; tests of triglycerides, total cholesterol, and HDL cholesterol every 2 years; routine urinalysis test yearly, and, after 5 years duration of diabetes or after puberty, a test of total urinary protein excretion. An annual eye and vision exam conducted by an ophthalmologist after five years of disease duration has also been recommended by the American College of Physicians (ACP), the ADA, and the American Academy of Ophthalmology (AAO) (ACP, ADA and AAO, 1992). Retinal examination by generalists has been shown to be much less effective in detecting retinopathy at an early treatable stage (Reenders et al., 1992). The routine evaluation of the other screening recommendations has never been tested in controlled trials, but the conditions screened for (hyperlipidemia p.396 and nephropathy p.398-9 ESRD) are both more common in diabetics and amenable to intervention (The Carter Center, 1985). Compliance with ADA screening recommendations has been estimated to vary from 20 to 50 percent (Garnick et al., 1994; Brechner et al., 1993).

Other common treatable complications of diabetes include hypertension, cellulitis, and osteomyelitis. The ADA recommends blood pressure measurement and examination of the feet at every visit to detect these complications early in their course as well as a careful history to elicit signs and symptoms of hypoglycemia and hyperglycemia. No controlled trials have examined the efficacy of a regular history and physical examination.

Treatment

Recent debate in the area of diabetic treatment hinges on the utility of tight glycemic control. The goal of tight control and prevention of long-term complications through aggressive treatment is supported by the DCCT (1993a). The DCCT randomized 1,441 insulin-dependent diabetics into conventional therapy or intensive therapy that included daily adjustments of insulin dosage, frequent home glucose monitoring and nutritional advice. Under the optimal circumstances present in the DCCT trial, 44 percent of the intervention group achieved glycosylated hemoglobin values under the goal of 6.05 mg/dl percent at least once, but only 5 percent maintained average values in that range. The intervention group developed 76 percent less retinopathy, 57 percent less albuminuria, and 60 percent less clinical neuropathy, but this reduction in diabetic complication may come at the expense of quality of life (Nerenz et al., 1992). For example, the tight control group in DCCT experienced a two- to three-fold increase in hypoglycemic episodes. The efficiency of such methods in general practice has not received adequate evaluation. Nonetheless, the ADA recommends that all diabetics over the age of seven be offered similar aggressive therapy.

The DCCT investigators suggest, however, that the risk-benefit ratio for children under 13 may be less favorable. In Type I diabetes (IDDM), emphasis is placed on avoidance of diabetic ketoacidosis and tight control of blood sugar levels through the judicious use of insulin.

Adherence to ADA diet decreases insulin and oral hypoglycemic requirements and serum lipids (Bantle, 1988). The DCCT (1993b) relied on dietitians and revealed that greater adherence to dietary instructions resulted in better control. Exercise improves glucose tolerance and may reduce or eliminate the need for drug therapy (Raz et al., 1994). The ADA and the American Board of Family Practice recommend dietary and exercise counseling at both the initial diagnosis and before starting oral hypoglycemics or insulin (ADA, 1989; Bergenstal et al., 1993). We recommend evaluating the medical record for evidence that all diabetics have received dietary and exercise counseling.

Insulin treatment is essential for Type I diabetics. The literature contains varied recommendations as to the optimal timing and content of insulin injections (Gregerman, 1991, in Barker et al., 1991; Knatterud, 1978), and no one regimen has emerged as superior. It has been suggested that, for children and adolescents, two injections per day of short- and intermediate-acting insulin are generally necessary to achieve reasonable control (Plotkin in Oski, 1994). The ADA recommends that all diabetics taking insulin receive formal instruction in the technique of injection (ADA, 1989; Bergenstal et al., 1993). We recommend evaluating the medical record for evidence that this has taken place.

Though quality indicators for treatment of hypertension are covered elsewhere, the intersection of diabetes and hypertension poses special treatment challenges. Control of hypertension is perhaps the most crucial step in preventing diabetic nephropathy. In particular, ACE inhibitors and possibly calcium channel blockers have been shown to reduce hyperalbuminuria and delay the progression to diabetic nephropathy (Lederle, 1992; Anderson, 1990). Beta blockers on the other hand may block the symptoms of hypoglycemia, and thus may be contraindicated in treated diabetics (Hamilton, 1990).

Follow-up

A study of internists and family practitioners using patient vignettes found wide variation in recommended follow-up intervals for diabetics (Petitti and Grumbach, 1993). The ADA (1989) guidelines recommend that regular visits be scheduled every three months for insulin-dependent diabetics. As a minimum standard of care for patients with diabetes, we suggest a visit every six months.

RECOMMENDED QUALITY INDICATORS FOR DIABETES MELLITUS

The following criteria apply to children with diabetes aged 5-18.

Diagnosis

Indicator	Quality of evidence	Literature	Benefits	Comments
1. Patients with the diagnosis of diabetes should have the following routine monitoring tests:				
a. glycosylated hemoglobin every 6 months	I	Larsen et al., 1990	Prevent diabetic complications.*	Randomized controlled trial of 240 patients indicated a significant decrease in hemoglobin A_{1c} among those whose hemoglobin A_{1c} was monitored. Time interval is that used in most clinical trials.
b. Eye and visual exam if more than 5 years since diagnosis	III	ACP, ADA and AAO, 1992; ADA, 1989	Prevent retinopathy.	Eye and visual exam shown to detect retinopathy at an earlier treatable stage.
c. Triglycerides at least once a year	III	ACP, ADA and AAO, 1992; ADA, 1989	Prevent hyperlipidemia and atherosclorotic complications.	Recommendations based on expert opinion, though studies have shown conditions they screen for to be more common in diabetics and all are susceptible to treatment with improved outcomes resulting from earlier detection.
d. Total cholesterol at least once a year	III	ACP, ADA and AAO, 1992; ADA, 1989	Prevent hyperlipidemia and atherosclorotic complications.	Recommendations based on expert opinion, though studies have shown conditions they screen for to be more common in diabetics and all are susceptible to treatment with improved outcomes resulting from earlier detection.
e. HDL cholesterol at least once a year	III	ACP, ADA and AAO, 1992; ADA, 1989	Prevent hyperlipidemia and atherosclorotic complications.	Recommendations based on expert opinion, though studies have shown conditions they screen for to be more common in diabetics and all are susceptible to treatment with improved outcomes resulting from earlier detection.
f. Urinalysis at least once a year	III	ADA, 1989	Prevent renal disease.	Recommendations based on expert opinion, though studies have shown conditions they screen for to be more common in diabetics and all are susceptible to treatment with improved outcomes resulting from earlier detection.
g. Examination of feet at every visit	III	ADA, 1989	Prevent lower extremity amputation, reduced morbidity from foot infections.	ADA recommendation. Earlier detection of treatable disease reduces probability of developing serious complications. Exam provides an opportunity for patient education.

h. Measurement of blood pressure at every visit	III	ADA, 1989
2. All patients taking insulin should monitor their glucose at home daily.	III	ADA, 1993	Prevent hypoglycemic episodes. Prevent diabetic complications.*	A small RCT found that home glucose monitoring increases glycemic control in insulin dependent diabetics. Another study found no difference in control by frequency of monitoring. Recommended by the ADA.

Treatment

Indicator	Quality of evidence	Literature	Benefits	Comments
3. All diabetics should receive dietary and exercise counseling.	II	Raz et al., 1994; Delahanty and Halford, 1993; ADA, 1989; Bergenstal et al., 1993	Reduce diabetic complications.*	Adherence to ADA diet decreases insulin and oral hypoglycemic requirements and serum lipids. Exercise improves glucose tolerance and may reduce or eliminate need for drug therapy. DCCT used dieticians and found that adherence to diet improved control and the ADA and the ABFP recommend their use. No study has found that dietary counseling reduces diabetic complications.

Follow-up

Indicator	Quality of evidence	Literature	Benefits	Comments
4. All patients with diabetes should have a follow-up visit at least every 6 months.	III	Bergenstal et al., 1993; ADA, 1989	Reduce probability of severe diabetic complications.*	Visits for diabetic patients in control should be every 3-6 months (per ABFP). Routine monitoring facilitates early detection and treatment of complications.

* Diabetic complications include visual loss and dysfunction of the heart, peripheral vasculature, peripheral nerves and kidneys.

Quality of Evidence Codes:

I: RCT
II-1:   Nonrandomized controlled trials
II-2:   Cohort or case analysis
II-3:   Multiple time series
III: Opinions or descriptive studies

REFERENCES - DIABETES MELLITUS

Allen BT, ER DeLong, and JR Feussner. October 1990. Impact of glucose self-monitoring on non-insulin-treated patients with type II diabetes mellitus: Randomized controlled trial comparing blood and urine testing. *Diabetes Care* 13 (10): 1044-50.

American College of Physicians, American Diabetes Association, and American Academy of Ophthalmology. 15 April 1992. Screening guidelines for diabetic retinopathy. *Annals of Internal Medicine* 116 (8): 683-5.

American Diabetes Association. 1993. *Direct and Indirect Costs of Diabetes in the United States in 1992.* Alexandria, VA: American Diabetes Association.

American Diabetes Association. May 1989. Standards of medical care for patients with diabetes mellitus. *Diabetes Care* 12 (5): 365-8.

Anderson S. 1990. Renal effects of converting enzyme inhibitors in hypertension and diabetes. *Journal of Cardiovascular Pharmacology* 15 (Suppl. 3): S11-S15.

Bantle JP. 1988. The dietary treatment of diabetes mellitus. *Medical Clinics of North America* 72 (6): 1285-99.

Bergenstal RM, WE Hall, and JA Haugen. 1993. *Diabetes Mellitus: Reference Guide*, Fourth ed. Lexington, KY: American Board of Family Practice.

Brechner RJ, CC Cowie, LJ Howie, et al. 13 October 1993. Ophthalmic examination among adults with diagnosed diabetes mellitus. *Journal of the American Medical Association* 270 (14): 1714-7.

Canadian Task Force on the Periodic Health Examination. 3 November 1979. The periodic health examination. *Canadian Medical Association Journal* 121: 1193-1254.

The Carter Center. July 1985. Closing the gap: The problem of diabetes mellitus in the United States. *Diabetes Care* 8 (4): 391-406.

Delahanty LM, and BN Halford. November 1993. The role of diet behaviors in achieving improved glycemic control in intensively treated patients in the Diabetes Control and Complications Trial. *Diabetes Care* 16 (11): 1453-8.

The Diabetes Control and Complications Trial Research Group. 30 September 1993. The effect of intensive treatment of diabetes on the development and progression of long-term complications in insulin-dependent diabetes mellitus. *New England Journal of Medicine* 329 (14): 977-86.

The Diabetes Control and Complications Trial Research Group. July 1993. Expanded role of the dietitian in the Diabetes Control and Complications Trial: Implications for clinical practice. *Journal of the American Dietetic Association* 93 (7): 758-67.

Garnick DW, J Fowles, AG Lawthers, et al. 18 February 1994. Focus on quality: Profiling physicians' practice patterns. *In Press, Journal Ambulatory Care Management.*

Gerich JE. 2 November 1989. Oral hypoglycemic agents. *New England Journal of Medicine* 321 (18): 1231-45.

Golden MP, and DL Gray. 1992. Diabetes Mellitus. In *Textbook of Adolescent Medicine.* McAnarney ER, RE Kriepe, DP Orr, et al.,Philadelphia, PA: W. B. Saunders Company.

Goldstein DE, RR Little, H Wiedmeyer, et al. 1994. Is glycohemoglobin testing useful in diabetes mellitus? Lessons from the Diabetes Control and Complications Trial. *Clinical Chemistry* 40 (8): 1637-40.

Gordon D, CG Semple, and KR Paterson. 1991. Do different frequencies of self-monitoring of blood glucose influence control in type 1 diabetic patients. *Diabetic Medicine* 8: 679-82.

Gregerman RI. 1991. Diabetes mellitus. In *Principles of Ambulatory Medicine*, Third ed. Editors Barker LR, JR Burton, and PD Zieve, 913-51. Baltimore, MD: Williams and Wilkins.

Hamilton BP. October 1990. Diabetes mellitus and hypertension. *American Journal of Kidney Diseases* 16 (4-Suppl.1): 20-9.

Health and Public Policy Committee, and American College of Physicians. August 1983. Selected methods for the management of diabetes mellitus. *Annals of Internal Medicine* 99 (2): 272-4.

Knatterud GL, CR Klimt, ME Levin, et al. 7 July 1978. Effects of hypoglycemic agents on vascular complications in patients with adult-onset diabetes. *Journal of the American Medical Association* 240 (1): 37-42.

Larsen ML, M Horder, and EF Mogensen. 11 October 1990. Effect of long-term monitoring of glycosylated hemoglobin levels in insulin-dependent diabetes mellitus. *New England Journal of Medicine* 323 (15): 1021-5.

Lederle RM. 1992. The effect of antihypertensive therapy on the course of renal failure. *Journal of Cardiovascular Pharmacology* 20 (Suppl. 6): S69-S72.

Muchmore DB, J Springer, and M Miller. 1994. Self-monitoring of blood glucose in overweight type 2 diabetic patients. *Acta Diabetologica* 31: 215-9.

Nathan DM. 1993. Diabetes mellitus. In *Scientific American Medicine*. Editor Rubenstein E, and D Federman, New York, NY: Scientific American Illustrated Library.

National Center for Health Statistics. 18 August 1994. *National Ambulatory Medical Care Survey: 1992 summary*. U.S. Department of Health and Human Services, Hyattsville, MD.

National Center for Health Statistics. 1 1994. *Vital statistics of the United States, 1990, vol. II: Mortality-part A*. U.S. Department of Health and Human Services, Hyattsville, MD.

Nerenz DR, DP Repasky, FW Whitehouse, et al. May 1992. Ongoing assessment of health status in patients with diabetes mellitus. *Medical Care Supplement* 30 (5, Supplement): MS112-MS123.

Palumbo PJ, LR Elveback, C Chu, et al. July 1976. Diabetes mellitus: Incidence, prevalence, survivorship, and causes of death in Rochester, Minnesota 1945-1970. *Diabetes* 25 (7): 566-73.

Patrick AW, GV Gill, IA MacFarlane, et al. 1994. Home glucose monitoring in type 2 diabetes: Is it a waste of time? *Diabetic Medicine* 11: 62-5.

Petitti DB, and K Grumbach. September 1993. Variation in physicians' recommendations about revisit interval for three common conditions. *Journal of Family Practice* 37 (3): 235-40.

Plotnick M. 1994. Insulin-dependent diabetes mellitus. *Principles and Practive of Pediatrics*, 2d ed. Editors Oski FA, CD DeAngeles, RD Feigin, et al., 1981-1992. Philadelphia, PA: JB Lippincott Co.

Raz I, E Hauser, and M Bursztyn. 10 October 1994. Moderate exercise improves glucose metabolism in uncontrolled elderly patients with non-insulin-dependent diabetes mellitus. *Israel Journal of Medical Sciences* 30 (10): 766-70.

Reenders K, E De Nobel, H Van Den Hoogen, et al. 1992. Screening for diabetic retinopathy by general practitioners. *Scandinavian Journal of Primary Health Care* 10: 306-9.

Rubin RJ, WM Altman, and DN Mendelson. 1994. Health care expenditures for people with diabetes mellitus, 1992. *Journal of Clinical Endocrinology and Metabolism* 78 (4): 809A-F.

Singer DE, JH Samet, CM Coley, et al. 15 October 1988. Screening for diabetes mellitus. *Annals of Internal Medicine* 109: 639-49.

10. DIARRHEAL DISEASE, ACUTE
Glenn Takata, M.D., M.S.

The recommendations on the evaluation and management of acute diarrheal disease in children were developed by summarizing the guidelines and recommendations of review articles (Hamilton, 1985; DeWitt, 1989; Fitzgerald, 1989; Walker-Smith, 1990; American Academy of Pediatrics [AAP], 1993; Laney and Cohen, 1993; Richards et al., 1993; World Health Organization [WHO], 1993; Northrup and Flanigan, 1994) and the April 1991 supplement to *The Journal of Pediatrics,* found in volume 118, number 4, part 2, which discussed the "Management of Acute Diarrheal Disease." The review articles were selected from a MEDLINE literature search on the key words diarrhea and gastroenteritis, looking for articles in the English language published between the years 1985 and 1995. Focused assessment of the literature with respect to specific areas of importance or disagreement among the reviews were then conducted which relied on reference lists in those review articles.

IMPORTANCE

Acute diarrheal disease is one of the most common presenting conditions in the pediatric population in the United States. Based on longitudinal studies conducted in Charlottesville, Virginia, Washington, D.C., and Winnipeg, Manitoba, done in the period from 1975 to 1980, the incidence of mild diarrheal illness during the first five years of life was estimated to be 6.5 to 11.5 episodes per child, resulting in 21.5 to 38 million episodes per year (Glass et al., 1991). The incidence of diarrheal illness is felt to be highest among children one to three years of age (Glass et al., 1991). The rate of diarrheal illness among children attending daycare centers may be two to three times higher than for other cohorts of children (Cohen, 1991; Northrup and Flanigan, 1994).

The incidence of a diarrheal illness leading to a physician visit was about 0.6 to 1.1 cases per child during the first five years of life based on data from the National Health Interview Survey for 1981 to 1985

and from the 1985 National Ambulatory Care Survey and the National
Ambulatory Care Complement Survey (Glass and Cohen, 1991). Based on the
National Hospital Discharge Survey for 1979 to 1984 and the McAuto data
base of 1982-1985, hospitalization for diarrhea occurred among 1.4
percent of all children up to five years of age; this represented 10.6
percent of all hospitalizations of children in the United States,
constituting 4.2 days per hospitalization (Glass and Cohen, 1991).

Based on the Multiple Cause of Death data files for 1973 to 1983,
one child out of every 15,000 born in the United States died of
complications associated with diarrhea such as dehydration, electrolyte
abnormalities, shock, cardiac arrest, respiratory failure, prematurity,
malnutrition, and bronchopneumonia (Glass et al., 1991). Another
possible cause of death in children with diarrhea is hypoglycemia
(Wapnir and Lebenthal, 1991). Deaths from diarrhea account for ten
percent of preventable postneonatal infant deaths in the United States
(Richards et al., 1993). Most deaths attributable to diarrhea occurred
among infants less than one year of age (Glass et al., 1991). In the
infant less than 36 months of age with diarrhea and fever, the risk of
bacterial enteritis with bacteremia is felt high enough to warrant a
septic work-up. The incidence of diarrheal illnesses is high, and the
morbidity and mortality significant.

Northrup and Flanigan (1994) estimate the typical cost of care for
inpatient parenteral therapy for an episode of acute diarrhea at $2000
and $200 for oral rehydration in an outpatient setting. Listernick et
al. (1986) similarly found that oral rehydration cost about twelve
percent as much as intravenous therapy. Considering the numbers of
cases of acute diarrhea among children, the cost is high.

EFFICACY AND/OR EFFECTIVENESS OF INTERVENTIONS

Screening and Prevention

Though acute diarrheal illness is not a condition or symptom
screened for in the United States health system, the health care
provider in the provision of routine health supervision should inquire
as to factors of high risk for episodes of diarrhea such as attendance
in a child care center, frequent visits to a health care facility (e.g.,

for children with a chronic illness), or the presence of a compromised immune condition. In these high-risk situations, parents, and children who are old enough to understand, should be instructed on the importance of prevention of diarrheal episodes through good sanitation practices such as careful handwashing after toileting (DeWitt, 1989) and care in food preparation (Hamilton, 1985). In the infant, breastfeeding may also afford some degree of protection against infectious diarrheal events (Hamilton, 1985). In addition, various vaccines are presently undergoing development in an effort to prevent diarrhea caused by rotaviruses, typhoid fever, shigella, cholera, enterotoxigenic *E. coli*, and enteropathogenic *E. coli* (Levine, 1991).

Diagnosis

The presence of diarrhea, that is "stools that are abnormally frequent and liquid" (DeWitt, 1989), is established through assessment of the history and the gross examination of a stool sample when available. The health care provider should assess the child's hydration status and the likelihood of sepsis. The health care provider should also determine the etiology of the diarrheal episode, whether viral, bacterial, parasitic, or noninfectious, and the possible need for further intervention, such as the need for antimicrobial agents or public health referral. In most cases in which shock is not present or sepsis is not suspected, however, the episode of diarrhea will be brief and self-limited; the health care provider may reserve more exhaustive etiologic evaluation for the child who does not respond to standard hydration (Richards et al., 1993; Northrup and Flanigan, 1994).

The presence and severity of diarrhea must first be established. The health care provider should inquire as to (1) the date of onset, (2) the consistency and character of the stool, whether voluminous, watery, mucousy, or bloody, and (3) the frequency of stools (DeWitt, 1989). A precise definition of diarrhea is not available; it is assessed in comparison to the individual child's normal frequency, consistency, and volume of stools. The degree of oral intake of fluids is also important to determine, as is the degree of urinary output (DeWitt, 1989; Fitzgerald, 1989). The clinician should also inquire as to the child's affect and the presence of fever, abdominal pain, tenesmus, or vomiting (DeWitt, 1989; Northrup and Flanigan, 1994). Other useful information would include past or present antibiotic use, contact persons with similar symptoms, attendance in a child care setting, recent diet history, recent travel history, recent exposure to livestock or other animals, and history of chronic illness, specifically sickle cell anemia or immunocompromise (DeWitt, 1989; Northrup and Flanigan, 1994). If available, the stool should be examined, especially for presence of gross blood (Northrup and Flanigan, 1994). The physical examination should focus on assessing hydration status as noted below and also on the possibility of sepsis (Baraff et al., 1993), especially in children under three years old. The vital signs should be measured and recorded (DeWitt, 1989). The weight should be recorded (DeWitt, 1989). Information gathering with regard to specific etiology may be postponed until the child's hydration status is stabilized, unless it relates directly to management of fluids and electrolytes or diagnosing sepsis.

Because much of the morbidity and mortality of acute diarrhea are caused by problems of hydration and electrolyte imbalance, the hydration status of the child with diarrhea must be immediately assessed through elements of the history and physical examination. In the World Health Organization Management of the Patient with Diarrhea chart, the assessment of dehydration is based on the factors shown in Table 10.1 (AAP, 1993; WHO, 1993):

Table 10.1

WHO Factors For Assessing Hydration Status

FACTORS	DEGREE OF DEHYDRATION		
	MINIMAL	MILD-TO-MODERATE	SEVERE
General condition	Well, alert	*Restless, irritable	*Lethargic or unconscious; floppy
Eyes	Normal	Sunken	Very sunken and dry
Tears	Present	Absent	Absent
Mouth and tongue	Moist	Dry	Very dry
Thirst	Drinks normally, not thirsty	*Thirsty, drinks eagerly	*Drinks poorly or not able to drink
Skin pinch	Skin goes back quickly	*Skin goes back slowly	*Skin goes back very slowly
<u>DECISION</u>	No signs of dehydration	*≥ 2 of above signs, including at least one "key" sign	*≥ 2 of above signs, including at least one "key" sign

*key signs of dehydration

Based on these five factors the child is assessed as not dehydrated, as having some dehydration (50-100 milliliters per kilogram estimated fluid deficit), or as having severe dehydration (greater than 100 ml/kg fluid deficit (WHO, 1993). Northrup and Flanigan (1994) similarly distinguish between mild (10-40 milliliters/kilogram fluid deficit), moderate (50-90 ml/kg), and severe (100-130 ml/kg) levels of dehydration based on the above and the factors shown in Table 10.2:

Table 10.2

Northrup and Flanigan Factors For Assessing Hydration Status

FACTORS	DEGREE OF DEHYDRATION		
	MILD	MODERATE	SEVERE
Anterior fontanelle	Normal	Depressed	Severely depressed
Radial pulse	Full	Full-weak	Feeble or absent
Pulse rate	Normal	Elevated	Vary rapid
Peripheral blood pressure	Normal	Within normal limits	Low or absent

Fitzgerald (1989) also mentions increased urine specific gravity, decreased urine output, and an increased ratio of blood urea nitrogen to creatinine as signs of dehydration. DeWitt (1989) lists similar criteria but also mentions serum electrolytes with high sodium and low bicarbonate as being consistent with dehydration. DeWitt (1989) also advises a urine culture if excessive white blood cells are seen on the urinalysis.

The possibility of sepsis must also be considered, particularly in infants and in the presence of fever, blood in the stool, and other dysenteric signs and symptoms (Finkelstein et al., 1989; Baraff et al., 1993). If there is any suspicion of sepsis or bacteremia, a sepsis evaluation should be performed (Baraff et al., 1993). (See Chapter 12 for the general approach to the child with possible bacteremia or sepsis.)

Though in most cases of acute diarrhea, determining the specific etiology is unimportant, (Richards et al., 1993; Northrup and Flanigan, 1994) in a few cases, such as when sepsis is suspected or when the clinical course is prolonged, establishing the etiologic agent may be useful in terms of treatment. Initially, the clinician may make a presumptive etiologic determination based on characteristic clinical and epidemiologic patterns (Northrup and Flanigan, 1994). Fitzgerald (1989) and Northrup and Flanigan (1994) recognize two clinical patterns of acute diarrhea. The first is secretory or enterotoxigenic diarrhea characterized by watery diarrhea, sometimes with vomiting and fever but without significant cramping, without blood or leukocytes in the stool. Secretory or enterotoxigenic diarrhea may be caused by enterotoxigenic *Echerichia coli*, *Vibrio cholera*, *Giardia lamblia*, *Cryptosporidium*, Rotavirus, and Norwalk-like virus and organisms associated with food poisoning such as *Staphylococcus aureus*, *Bacillus cereus*, and *Clostridium perfringens* (Northrup and Flanigan, 1994). The second is inflammatory diarrhea characterized by mucous in the stools, fever, cramps, abdominal pain, often myalgias and arthralgias, and blood and leukocytes in the stool; the inflammatory diarrheas include *Shigella*, invasive *E. coli*, *Salmonella*, *Campylobacter*, *C. difficile, and Entameba histolytica* (Northrup and Flanigan, 1994).

Fitzgerald (1989) also lists clinical characteristics for viral diarrheas:

1. low grade temperature elevation
2. vomiting
3. pale, large volume, acidic stools
4. no occult blood
5. rapid development of dehydration.

The factors for bacterial diarrheas are:

1. abrupt onset
2. fever greater than 101°F
3. no vomiting
4. blood in stool
5. dark mucoid stools
6. toxic appearance
7. low serum albumin

Clinical features specific to each of the viral, bacterial, and parasitic diarrheas may be found in the above cited reviews (Hamilton, 1985; DeWitt, 1989; Fitzgerald, 1989; Laney and Cohen, 1993; Northrup and Flanigan, 1994) as well as other sources (Blacklow and Greenberg, 1991; Guerrant and Bobak, 1991; Pickering, 1991).

Epidemiologic data demonstrate that in 50 to 75 percent of stool specimens an enteropathogen is identified (Cohen, 1991). When the etiology of acute diarrhea is established the most common cause is viral, followed by bacterial and then parasitic etiologies (Fitzgerald, 1989; Cohen, 1991; Laney and Cohen, 1993). Rotavirus is the cause of diarrhea in up to 25 percent of children with diarrhea in the outpatient setting and in up to 50 percent of young children requiring hospitalization for diarrhea and dehydration (Cohen, 1991). Blacklow and Greenberg (1991) state that Rotavirus is "responsible for 30 to 60 percent of all cases of severe watery diarrhea in young children." Northrup and Flanigan (1994) cite a median of 34 percent for Rotavirus among children less than 2 years of age requiring hospitalization for diarrhea and dehydration. Rotavirus occurs most commonly in the fall in

the southwest United States and in the late winter and spring in the
northeast United States, especially among children between 3 months and
15 months of age, and may be spread by both fecal-oral and respiratory
routes (Blacklow and Greenberg, 1991; Northrup and Flanigan, 1994).
Norwalk virus tends to occur in outbreaks among children older than 6
years of age and adults (Northrup and Flanigan, 1994). Infection with
Norwalk virus is usually from a common source rather than person-to-
person (Laney and Cohen, 1993). Both Rotavirus and Norwalk virus have
short incubation periods of 1 to 3 days; duration of symptoms is 5 to 7
days for Rotavirus and 1 to 2 days for Norwalk virus (Blacklow and
Greenberg, 1991; Northrup and Flanigan, 1994). Enteric adenoviruses are
another common cause of acute diarrhea, especially in children less than
two years of age (Blacklow and Greenberg, 1991; Laney and Cohen, 1993).
Enteric adenoviruses have been found in 2 to 22 percent of cases of
diarrhea from studies from various parts of the world (Blacklow and
Greenberg, 1991). Enteric adenoviruses have a 8 to 10 day incubation
period and a 5 to 12 day duration (Blacklow and Greenberg, 1991;
Northrup and Flanigan, 1994). Enteric adenovirus infection is usually
passed by the fecal-oral (Laney and Cohen, 1993) or person-to-person
route (Blacklow and Greenberg, 1991). Other viruses that may cause
acute episodes of diarrhea include pestivirus, astrovirus, calicivirus,
parvovirus, and non-group A rotavirus (Cohen, 1991). Despite some
epidemiologic differences noted after the fact, it is difficult to
delineate between viral etiologies of acute diarrhea upon initial
presentation.

Bacterial causes of acute diarrhea are less common. Among the
invasive bacterial enteritides, *Salmonella* is the most common bacterial
cause of diarrhea in the United States (Laney and Cohen, 1993).
Salmonella infections are most common in infants younger than 6 months
(Cohen, 1991) and also among those with acquired immunodeficiency
syndrome, sickle cell anemia, and reticuloendothelial dysfunction and is
acquired through contaminated foods, in particular meat, dairy, and
poultry products (Northrup and Flanigan, 1994). The incubation period
for *Salmonella* is 2 to 3 days, and the duration of illness about 2 to 3
days. *Shigella* is the second most common bacterial cause of diarrhea in

the United States identified among children 6 months to 10 years of age (Cohen, 1991; Laney and Cohen, 1993) and is uncommon in infants less than six months of age (Cohen, 1991). *Shigella* may be transmitted from person to person in child care (Laney and Cohen, 1993; Northrup and Flanigan, 1994) or other group settings (Northrup and Flanigan, 1994). *Shigella* may, in fact, be the most common etiology of bacterial diarrhea in the child care setting (Cohen, 1991). *Campylobacter* is most frequent among children less than 1 year of age and among young adults (Laney and Cohen, 1993). Incubation is for 1 to 7 days; the *campylobacter* is most commonly transmitted by the fecal-oral route (Laney and Cohen, 1993). Aeromonas species, particularly in Australia, and *Plesiomonas shigelloides* are also associated with acute diarrhea (Cohen, 1991). Acute diarrhea caused by *Yersinia enterocolitica,* though common in Europe and Canada, is uncommon in the United States (Cohen, 1991; Northrup and Flanigan, 1994) and is more likely in the child less than 5 years of age (Laney and Cohen, 1993; Northrup and Flanigan, 1994). *Yersinia* outbreaks are usually associated with contaminated foods, particularly milk and milk products (Cohen, 1991). Though not common, enterohemorrhagic *E. coli* has significant epidemiologic association with the hemolytic uremic syndrome which is characterized by microangiopathic hemolytic anemia, uremia, and thrombocytopenia (Laney and Cohen, 1993).

Among those bacteria causing enterotoxigenic diarrhea, some toxins are ingested by the child while others are produced in the infected intestine. Ingestion of toxin in the case of *S. aureus* or *B. cereus* leads to a brief duration of diarrhea after a short incubation period of 1 to 6 hours (Northrup and Flanigan, 1994). *C. perfringens* is found in contaminated foods and leads typically to not more than a three-day bout of severe diarrhea following a 8 to 12 hour incubation period (Northrup and Flanigan, 1994). Enterotoxigenic *E. coli* and *V. cholerae* cause a secretory diarrhea of 3 to 7 day duration (Northrup and Flanigan, 1994). *C. difficile* leading to pseudomembranous colitis is associated with antibiotic use and may spread from patient to patient (Northrup and Flanigan, 1994). Other possible bacterial enteropathogens include *Vibrio parahaemolyticus* and non-O1 Vibrio serogroups (Cohen, 1991).

Parasitic causes of acute diarrhea are even less common. Among parasitic causes, *Giardia lamblia* is the most common (Cohen, 1991). The prevalence of giardiasis is highest among infants and toddlers, with an increased incidence in children attending child care centers (Cohen, 1991). In child care settings, 21 to 26 percent of children may be asymptomatic carriers of Giardia (Laney and Cohen, 1993). Giardia is transmitted via the fecal-oral or person-to-person route (Laney and Cohen, 1993; Northrup and Flanigan, 1994). *Cryptosporidium* is a relatively common parasitic diarrheal illness in developing countries and is passed by the fecal-oral route and via person-to-person transmission (Northrup and Flanigan, 1994). The duration of cryptosporidial diarrhea is about 2 weeks (Northrup and Flanigan, 1994). Cryptosprodium is relatively common in the child care setting (DeWitt, 1989). Both Cryptosporidium and Giardia are more common among children with immune compromise (Northrup and Flanigan, 1994).

Laboratory diagnosis of specific etiologic agents of acute diarrhea is usually not necessary (Richards et al., 1993; Northrup and Flanigan, 1994) except (1) where sepsis is an issue, (2) in those rare cases in which antibiotic therapy is being considered, and (3) in cases that may require public health intervention, as with outbreaks of salmonella. Sepsis may be considered in cases with dysenteric symptoms such as blood in the stool or fever. Microscopic examination of the stool, if positive for erythrocytes and leukocytes and associated with fever, may suggest campylobacter, yersinia, salmonella, or shigella infection (Northrup and Flanigan, 1994). Despite the association with bacterial enteritides, the presence of fecal leukocytes does not necessarily predict a positive stool culture nor the need for antibiotics (Richards et al., 1993). DeWitt (1989) states that the probability of having a positive stool culture given stool leukocytes on microscopic examination is 70 percent; and, given a positive stool culture, the probability of stool leukocytes on examination is 90 percent. DeWitt (1985) indicated that fecal leukocyte determination or stool polymorphonuclear test should be reserved for children with diarrhea of abrupt onset, frequency of greater than four stools a day, and no vomiting before the onset of diarrhea. Positive fecal leukocyte determination, in addition to those three factors, led to a sensitivity in detecting a positive stool culture of 74 percent and a specificity of 94 percent. The sensitivity and specificity of using fecal leukocyte alone was 85 percent and 88 percent, but DeWitt (1985) stated that performing a fecal leukocyte determination on all children with diarrhea was not practical. The presence of erythrocytes without leukocytes suggests entamoeba, and the lack of either erythrocytes or leukocytes suggests noninvasive bacterial or viral causes (Northrup and Flanigan, 1994). Stool cultures, looking for common bacterial etiologies, and rotaviral antigen analysis may be warranted in epidemic situations where public health intervention may be required (Richards et al., 1993). Rotavirus group A and enteric adenoviruses may be detected by enzyme-linked immunosorbant assay techniques (Laney and Cohen, 1993). Stool cultures may be helpful in children who have an inflammatory clinical pattern of acute diarrhea with bloody stools and fever (DeWitt, 1989; Finkelstein et al., 1989; Richards et al., 1993), especially when diarrhea persists more than three days (Northrup and Flanigan, 1994). Finkelstein et al. (1989) found that, for infants less than 12 months old: (1) a history of fever and blood in the stool led to a likelihood ratio (LR) of 13.5 of a positive stool culture; (2) for blood in the stool and more than nine stools in 24 hours a LR or 11.8; and, (3) for fever and more than nine stools in 24 hours, a LR of 3.8. They found that the presence of only one of these factors led to a LR of 1.1. Northrup and Flanigan (1994) note that a simple laboratory evaluation consisting of stool culture, rotavirus determination, and analysis for ova and parasite may cost up to $180 and analysis for *C. difficile* toxin $50. The yield of stool cultures may be as low as two percent and have a cost of greater than $900 per positive result (Richards et al., 1993). Those with persistent symptoms longer than 10 to 14 days may warrant stool examination for ova and parasites (DeWitt, 1989; Northrup and Flanigan, 1994). Diagnosis of Giardia may be made by direct microscopic examination of at least three stool specimens, duodenal fluid sample, or small bowel biopsies or by antigen detection using enzyme-linked immunosorbant assay (Northrup and Flanigan, 1994) or counterimmunoelectrophoresis (Laney and Cohen, 1993). The *C. difficile* toxin may be identified in a stool sample (Northrup and

Flanigan, 1994). It must be noted that the *C. difficile* toxin may be present in children without clinical disease (Northrup and Flanigan, 1994).

The 3 to 5 percent (Santosham and Greenough, 1991) of children whose diarrhea persists for more than ten to fourteen days warrant further evaluation to determine specific etiology.

Treatment

The treatment of acute diarrhea is first directed toward the prevention or correction of fluid and electrolyte imbalance and the prevention or treatment of possible sepsis and then toward pharmacologic or public health intervention for specific etiologic diagnoses. The WHO case management strategy for acute diarrhea includes (Richards et al., 1993):

1. early administration of appropriate fluids at home;
2. treatment of dehydration with WHO oral rehydration solution;
3. treatment of severe dehydration with intravenous electrolyte solution;
4. continued feeding throughout the diarrheal episode;
5. selective use of antibiotics;
6. non-use of antidiarrheal drugs

The WHO approach was associated with a 71 percent decrease in the median diarrhea case-fatality rate in fourteen sites in developing countries and a drop of 28 to 4.6 percent among low birth weight neonates in an Egyptian intensive care unit (Richards et al., 1993), and a decrease in the diarrhea-specific mortality rate during a two-year study in a village in Bangladesh (Santosham and Greenough, 1991). In general, most episodes of acute diarrhea will respond to fluid and electrolyte stabilization and feeding therapy without other intervention (DeWitt, 1989; Northrup and Flanigan, 1994).

Since dehydration is initially the greatest threat to the patient, treatment is directed toward restoration and stabilization of fluid and electrolyte balance. If the child is not yet dehydrated, the health care provider should promote the maintenance of the regular diet and prescribe the early initiation of oral hydration therapy at home with the appropriate carbohydrate-electrolyte solution (20 to 50 milliequivalents of sodium per liter), as well as maintenance of the regular diet (Fitzgerald, 1989; Santosham and Greenough, 1991; Northrup and Flanigan, 1994). Conflicting somewhat with the previous recommendation in terms of the sodium concentration of extra fluids, Richards et al. (1993) state that appropriate home solutions would include WHO oral rehydration solution, soups, unsweetened fruit juices, yogurt-based drinks, and plain water given with starchy foods containing some salt, emphasizing the need to continue the regular diet to the extent possible. According to the 1990 WHO protocol, the child without dehydration should be reevaluated within three days for continuing diarrhea, vomiting, thirst, poor oral intake, fever, or bloody stools.

Northrup and Flanigan (1994) state that the child with mild-to-moderate dehydration should receive oral hydration therapy with an isotonic or hypotonic carbohydrate solution containing electrolytes and that intravenous therapy should be reserved for children with severe dehydration defined by impending cardiovascular collapse or those unable to take oral feedings because of coma, intractable vomiting, or other reasons. Other contraindications to oral rehydration include shock, purging greater than ten milliliters per kilogram per hour, or ileus (Laney and Cohen, 1993) and glucose intolerance causing severe purging with administration of oral rehydration (Santosham and Greenough, 1991). Oral rehydration is effective in both enterotoxigenic or secretory and inflammatory diarrhea (AAP, 1985). Northrup and Flanigan (1994) state that less than 2 percent of cases of acute diarrhea in the community and less than 20 percent of cases presenting for medical care should require intravenous therapy. Bhan et al. (1994) cite two studies with higher oral rehydration treatment failure rates of 7 percent and 24 to 27 percent.

Oral rehydration therapy in the child with mild-to-moderate dehydration consists of replacement of the child's fluid deficit and ongoing losses and provision of maintenance fluid, electrolyte, and nutritional needs. Though the use of the WHO oral rehydration solution, with a glucose-to-sodium molar ratio of 1.2:1 and with supplemental potassium chloride and trisodium citrate dihydrate or sodium bicarbonate, has been shown effective throughout the developing world in treatment of cholera and noncholera diarrheas and in hospital-based and clinic-based studies in the developed countries (Santosham and Greenough, 1991; Richards et al., 1993), solutions varying from the WHO oral rehydration solution have been suggested (Santosham et al., 1985; Walker-Smith, 1990; Northrup and Flanigan, 1994). One major difference in these solutions is their sodium chloride concentration, ranging from 45 milliequivalents per liter in Pedialyte (Ross) to 90 mEq/L in the WHO oral rehydration solution (Santosham and Greenough, 1991). Other modifications to the WHO oral rehydration solution are being tested including the substitution of complex carbohydrates such as rice or other cereals in place of glucose (Greenough and Khin-Maung-U, 1991; Khin-Maung-U and Greenough, 1991; Lebenthal and Lu, 1991) and the addition of amino acids (Ribeiro and Lifshitz, 1991) to facilitate fluid absorption, particularly in patients with excessive purging (Laney and Cohen, 1993; Bhan et al., 1994; Northrup and Flanigan, 1994). These cereal-based and amino acid supplemented oral rehydration solutions may reduce vomiting and diarrheal volume loss and shorten duration of the diarrheal episode (Greenough and Khin-Maung-U, 1991; Khin-Maung-U and Greenough, 1991; Lebenthal and Lu, 1991; Santosham and Greenough, 1991; Bhan et al., 1994). Bhan et al. (1994) in their exhaustive review of this literature come to the following conclusions:

1. Rice-based oral rehydration solutions were superior to the WHO oral rehydration solution for treatment of patients with cholera.

2. Rice-based oral rehydration solutions were as effective as the WHO oral rehydration solution for treatment of children with acute non-cholera diarrhea if feeding was resumed promptly after rehydration. This was also true for young infants, severely malnourished children, and children with increased risk of glucose malabsorption.

3. Maltodextrin-based oral rehydration solutions were as effective as the WHO oral rehydration solution for treatment of children with non-cholera diarrhea.

4. Amino-acid-containing oral rehydration formulas have no clinical advantage over the WHO oral rehydration solution for treatment of children with cholera or non-cholera diarrhea.

In 1985 the AAP endorsed the use of the WHO oral rehydration solution for the rehydration of dehydrated infants, whatever the presenting serum osmolality, and for the maintenance of hydration when given in equal amounts with water, breast milk, or low carbohydrate juices. The AAP recommended that the oral rehydration solution contain 75 to 90 millimoles per liter of sodium, 20 mmol/L potassium, 20 to 30 percent of anions as base and the remainder as chloride, and 2 to 2.5 percent glucose (Santosham and Greenough, 1991). The AAP (1993) also endorsed the basic treatment approach to dehydration due to acute diarrhea advocated by the WHO. Physicians in the developed countries, including Great Britain (Walker-Smith, 1990) and the United States, (Avery and Snyder, 1990; Richards et al., 1993) have been slow to adopt the use of oral rehydration solution despite these recommendations (Santosham and Greenough, 1991). The high cost of oral rehydration solutions in the United States, five-to-six dollars per liter, compared to the ten cents per liter cost borne by the United Nations, may contribute to the lack of adherence by U.S. physicians who fear parental noncompliance due to financial reasons (Richards et al., 1993).

In mild-to-moderate dehydration in the child of any age, oral fluid deficit replacement should occur over the initial 4 to 6 hours of therapy in a health care setting (Fitzgerald, 1989; Santosham and Greenough, 1991; Laney and Cohen, 1993; WHO, 1993; Northrup and Flanigan, 1994). Initially small, frequent feedings may be more appropriate, especially when vomiting is a problem. Vomiting is not an absolute contraindication to oral rehydration (AAP, 1985; Fitzgerald, 1989; Santosham and Greenough, 1991; Laney and Cohen, 1993; Richards et al., 1993). The volume of feedings is increased as tolerated. In certain cases nasogastric feeding may be considered (Fitzgerald, 1989). Ongoing stool losses should be estimated by the health care provider and replaced on a one to one-and-a-half by volume basis with oral carbohydrate-electrolyte solution; maintenance needs must also be met

(Santosham and Greenough, 1991; Northrup and Flanigan, 1994). Richards et al. (1993) believe that the child may continue the WHO oral rehydration solution during the maintenance phase with as much free water allowed as tolerated by the child and resumption of regular feedings as described below. The AAP (1985) also feels the WHO oral rehydration solution is adequate as a maintenance solution as long as it is diluted with equal amounts of low solute fluid. A recent study done in the United States of male infants less than two years of age in mild-to-moderate dehydration seemed to indicate that the a 45-50 mmol/L solution of sodium might be suitable for use in both the rehydration and maintenance phases of intervention; however, these low sodium solutions were not compared to the WHO oral rehydration solution, and the sample size was too small to adequately monitor for adverse effects (Cohen et al., 1995). Once the child has been rehydrated and the maintenance phase established, the child may be discharged home. The AAP (1985) recommends that the daily volume of maintenance solution not be greater than 150 milliliters per kilogram per day and that the excess needs be provided with a low-solute fluid. The child's hydration status must be monitored by the health care provider (Richards et al., 1993; Northrup and Flanigan, 1994), perhaps the day following discharge from the health care setting. Richards et al. (1993) note that the non-breast-fed infant less than six months of age should be given 100 to 200 milliliters of additional water during the rehydration phase while the breast-fed infant should continue breast-feeding as noted below. The use of oral rehydration solution in an urban American hospital resulted in a decrease in treatment time, eleven hours compared to 103 hours for intravenous therapy, and a decrease in cost, $273 versus $2300 (Richards et al., 1993).

In severe dehydration or where oral replacement is not possible, intravenous fluids administered in the health care setting may be needed. In contrast to intravenous infusion rates typical in the United States in which rehydration occurs over the initial 24-48 hours of treatment (DeWitt, 1989; Kallen, 1990), Richards et al. (1993) and Northrup and Flanigan (1994), echoing the WHO recommendations, stress the need for much more rapid rates of intravenous resuscitation.

Northrup and Flanigan (1994) advocate replacing the initial fluid deficit in addition to ongoing losses in no more than six hours with 30 milliliters per kilogram in infants and 40 milliliters per kilogram in older children being infused in the first 30 minutes and the remainder in the next five hours for infants and two-and-a-half hours for the older child. Isotonic solutions such as Ringer lactate or normal saline are required for resuscitation in these cases (Santosham and Greenough, 1991; Northrup and Flanigan, 1994). Though such rapid rates might be a problem in cases of hypernatremic dehydration if a hypotonic solution was infused (Kallen, 1990), with isotonic solutions this might not be a problem. According to the 1990 WHO guidelines, the child's hydration status should be reassessed every one to two hours by the health care provider. Oral hydration is begun as soon as the child is stable, as assessed by the pulse, blood pressure, and state of consciousness (Santosham and Greenough, 1991), or as soon as tolerated (Richards et al., 1993; Northrup and Flanigan, 1994). Once intravenous resuscitation has been successful, the child may be treated as for mild-to-moderate dehydration with complete rehydration being accomplished within four to six hours (Santosham and Greenough, 1991).

In addition to fluid and electrolyte resuscitation, the issue of refeeding in children of all ages, particularly infants, has been a controversial one (Brown, 1991). In Great Britain and the United States it has been the practice to cease breast milk, formula or milk, and solids until after at least the initial twenty-four hours of glucose-electrolyte solution therapy and then to slowly reintroduce regular feeds (Darrow et al., 1949; Hamilton, 1985; Walker-Smith, 1990). Northrup and Flanigan (1994) advocate "the basic principle of giving more food and giving it earlier than previously recommended." The AAP (1995) has recommended that feeding resume within twenty-four hours of the onset of diarrhea. The majority of U.S. pediatricians do not follow the WHO or AAP recommendations regarding refeeding much less for oral rehydration (Snyder, 1991; Bezerra, 1992; Richards et al., 1993). Benefits of refeeding include an increase in intestinal disaccharidases and pancreatic secretion leading to induction of mucosal cell growth and proliferation, preventing natriuria and decreasing the incidence of malnutrition (Laney and Cohen. 1993). Fitzgerald (1989) mentions increased protein production in intestinal epithelial cells. Some studies have shown improved weight gain and shorter duration of diarrhea when full nutrition is restored soon after rehydration (Brown, 1991; Northrup and Flanigan, 1994). Other studies show improved nutritional status and no increase in duration of diarrhea (Richards et al., 1993). On balance, many studies show no difference in the duration of diarrhea with early refeeding (Ransome and Roode, 1984; Isolauri et al., 1986; Brown et al., 1988; Gazala et al., 1988; Margolis et al., 1990; Santosham et al., 1990; Chew et al., 1993) though a few show a slight decrease (Isolauri and Vesikari, 1985; Santosham et al., 1985; Santosham et al., 1991). Breastfeeding should continue through the diarrheal episode (Hamilton, 1985; Walker-Smith, 1990; Santosham and Greenough, 1991; Laney and Cohen, 1993; Richards et al., 1993; Northrup and Flanigan, 1994). Those continued on breast milk had lower stool output in one study (Khin-Maung-U et al., 1985) and shorter illness duration in rotaviral diarrhea (Brown, 1991).

Differences of opinion exist with regard to the use of nonhuman milk formulas in refeeding of children with acute diarrhea (Brown et al., 1994). Northrup and Flanigan (1994) state that children on milk-based formulas may continue these formulas in smaller, more frequent feedings or diluted with cereals and other foods. The AAP (1985), Hamilton (1985), Fitzgerald (1989), Walker-Smith (1990), Richards et al. (1993), and Northrup and Flanigan (1994) acknowledge that some clinicians advocate lactose-free formulas for children with acute diarrhea, though they feel it is not routinely required. DeWitt (1989) and Laney and Cohen (1993) still advocate lactose-free formula for the first 48 hours of refeeding. Brown et al. (1994) in a meta-analytic review of studies addressing this question concluded that the routine use of lactose-free milk formula was not warranted since the increased duration of diarrhea with lactose-containing formula was not clinically significant. Brown et al. (1994) felt that lactose-free formula might be justified in children with severe dehydration on presentation, previous treatment failure, underlying severe malnutrition, or worsening diarrhea upon consumption of lactose-containing formula.

Another point of contention has been the need for dilution of formula during the period of refeeding (Brown et al., 1994). Santosham and Greenough (1991) state that lactose-free formula may be given without dilution while other formulas should be diluted one-to-one. Richards et al. (1993) assert that dilution is not necessary though they find dilution acceptable if diarrhea worsens when milk is given. The AAP (1985) and Hamilton (1985), in contrast, recommend the reintroduction of formula or milk in dilute mixtures. Brown et al. (1994) in their meta-analytic review concluded that routine dilution of formula was not necessary as a small increased risk of treatment failure with undiluted formula was balanced by a poorer weight gain with diluted formula.

Richards et al. (1993) state that children normally on a semisolid or solid diet should continue on a "balanced, energy-rich and easily digestible diet" such as "lentils, meat or fish, eggs and dairy products, mashed cooked vegetables and bananas" and "starches such as cooked cereals" rather than sugar. Brown (1991) summarizes the studies with regard to refeeding of mixed diets as indicating "that mixtures of accessible staple foods are safe to use during diarrheal illness and yield purging rates during early therapy that are generally similar to, or in some cases possibly less than, those observed with milk- or soy-based formula diets. Of particular interest was the consistent finding that the duration of diarrhea was markedly reduced among the groups that received the staple foods." Brown (1991) also goes on to warn that "it is somewhat worrisome that the children tended to consume more dietary energy and to gain slightly more weight when they received the formula diets." Laney and Cohen (1993) and Northrup and Flanigan (1994) agree in general with these recommendations regarding reintroduction of solids.

Concomitant to fluid and electrolyte stabilization, concerns about possible sepsis must be addressed during the initial phase of treatment. (See review of Chapter 12 for the general approach to the child with possible bacteremia or sepsis.)

Though treatment of acute diarrhea is primarily concerned with issues of hydration, in a few cases knowledge of specific etiology may aid to eradicate infection, shorten the duration of disease, reduce shedding of infectious material through the use of antimicrobial agents, and promote necessary public health intervention. In viral diarrheas, hydration is the mainstay of treatment whether it be oral or parenteral, and specific pharmacologic therapy is not available.

Of the bacterial diarrheas, very few are aided by pharmacologic therapy. Fitzgerald (1989) states that "(E)mpirical antibiotic treatment is unwarranted in the management of the nontoxic infant with acute diarrhea." In Salmonella diarrhea, though amoxicillin, trimethoprim-sulfamethoxasole, or the new quinolones are thought to be effective, treatment guided by susceptibility testing is usually considered only for patients with sickle cell anemia, lymphoma, leukemia, and immunocompromise to prevent or treat possible bacteremia (Northrup and Flanigan 1994) or metastatic pyogenic infection (Pickering, 1991). Laney and Cohen (1993) also recommend that any child less than one year of age with a positive blood culture with Salmonella or any infant less than three months of age with a positive stool culture with Salmonella be treated with parenteral antibiotics. Antibiotic treatment of salmonella diarrhea, however, may prolong the period of fecal shedding of the organism (Richards et al., 1993) and increase the risk of the asymptomatic carrier state (Laney and Cohen, 1993). Northrup and Flanigan (1994) recommend amoxicillin, trimethoprim-sulfamethoxasole, or the new quinolones for treatment of Salmonella; and, Pickering (1991) also recommends consideration of ampicillin, chloramphenical, ceftriaxone, and cefotaxime. Treatment of shigellosis is generally felt to be effective in decreasing the duration of symptoms and decreasing the length of excretion (Laney and Cohen, 1993). Treatment of Shigella should be directed by susceptibility testing, though trimethoprim-sulfamethoxazole is the initial antibiotic of choice (Pickering, 1991; Northrup and Flanigan, 1994) and nalidixic acid or pivmecillinam may be alternatives (Richards et al., 1993). Pickering (1991) and Laney and Cohen (1993) mention ampicillin as a choice in treating Shigella; however, ampicillin resistance has become a problem. Tetracylcine (Laney and Cohen, 1993) and ciprofloxacin and norfloxacin (Pickering, 1991; Laney and Cohen, 1993) are other alternatives for treating Shigella in the older patient. Antibiotic therapy, specifically erythromycin, for campylobacter diarrhea may only be effective when given early in the course of the illness (Richards et al., 1993), within four days of onset of symptoms (Pickering, 1991) or in epidemic situations, such as in child care centers, or for illness associated with severe fever or bloody diarrhea (Northrup and Flanigan, 1994). Campylobacter is also susceptible to furazolidone, the quinolones, aminoglycosides, tetracycline, chloramphenicol, and clindamycin (Pickering, 1991). Antibiotic therapy is not useful for the treatment of *Y. enterocolitica* diarrhea though it may be used in those with severe diarrhea or underlying illness (Pickering, 1991; Laney and Cohen, 1993). In cases of suspected cholera with severe dehydration, trimethoprim-sulfamethoxazole or the alternatives of tetracycline, furazolidone, erythromycin, or chloramphenicol may be helpful in shortening the duration of illness and the period of excretion (Pickering, 1991; Richards et al., 1993). Ampicillin may also be an alternative treatment for cholera (Pickering, 1991). Cessation of antibiotic usage is the primary treatment of *C. difficile* pseudomembranous colitis, though in some cases metronidazole or vancomycin may be necessary (Pickering, 1991; Northrup and Flanigan, 1994). Treatment of hemolytic uremic syndrome associated with *E. coli* enteritis, requires mainly supportive treatment.

Giardia may be treated with furazolidone, which has fewer side effects, or with metronidazole or quinacrine hydrochloride (Northrup and Flanigan, 1994). Richards et al. (1993) note that giardiasis should only be treated if symptoms persist for at least fourteen days and if cysts or trophozoites are found in stool or small bowel fluid samples and lists tinidazole and ornidazole as alternative antimicrobials. Paromomycin, a nonadsorbable aminoglycoside, may be an effective agent against cryptosporidium (Northrup and Flanigan, 1994). Pickering (1991) states that antimicrobial therapy is usually not needed in cryptosporidial diarrhea. Richards et al. (1993) state that amoebiasis may be treated with metronidazole though only if fresh stool samples reveal trophozoites with ingested erythrocytes. Pickering (1991) recommends iodoquinol, paromomycin, or diloxanide furoate for the asymptomatic cyst excretor and reserves metronidazole for mild-to-moderate or severe intestinal disease or liver abscess or other extraintestinal amebic disease. When metronidazole is ineffective, Pickering (1991) mentions various alternatives for the antimicrobial treatment of recalcitrant amebiasis.

All articles reviewed agreed that antimotility medications and nonabsorbable antibiotics or adsorbents should not be used in the treatment of acute diarrhea in children (Hamilton, 1985; DeWitt, 1989; Fitzgerald, 1989; Avery and Snyder, 1990; WHO, 1990; Richards et al., 1993; Northrup and Flanigan, 1994). Most of these so-called antidiarrheal compounds are not approved for use in children less than two or three years of age (Pickering, 1991). Apparently none have been shown effective in well-controlled studies in decreasing stool volume or duration of symptoms (Richards et al., 1993). In particular, adsorbents and lactobacillus compounds have not been shown effective in well-controlled studies (Pickering, 1991). Fitzgerald (1989) postulates that prolonging the transit time of the intestine increases the time "injurious agents" remain in contact with the intestinal epithelium. Pickering (1991) notes that side effects may occur due to salicylate or bismuth absorption from bismuth-subsalicylate preparations, impairment of absorption of needed medications or nutrients, and interference with identification of enteropathogens. Antimotility medications have been shown to worsen the clinical course in shigellosis and in antimicrobial-associated colitis and have the risks attendant with overdose (Pickering, 1991). Others mention the possibility of dangerous side effects (Richards et al., 1993), including toxic megacolon and colonic hemorrhage (Northrup and Flanigan, 1994) and ileus (Avery and Snyder, 1990) with the use of antimotility or antidiarrheal medications.

Follow-up

Follow-up may be necessary in certain cases. The health care provider should check the child with acute diarrhea without dehydration for continued diarrhea, vomiting, thirst, poor oral intake, fever, or bloody stools three days after initiation of therapy and the child with mild-to-moderate or severe diarrhea one week after discharge from therapy in the health care setting. Persistent diarrhea may be more likely in younger children, malnourished children, or immunocompromised children, such as those with acquired immunodeficiency syndrome (Northrup and Flanigan, 1994). Young infants and those with severe diarrhea are more likely to be treatment failures (Brown and Lifshitz, 1991) Children who have parasitic diarrheas or those with more severe, invasive bouts of acute diarrhea leading to enterocyte brush border damage and decreased disaccharidase levels may also be more prone to persistent diarrhea (Northrup and Flanigan, 1994). Children with diarrheal illness of greater than 14 day duration should be evaluated for persistent or chronic diarrhea (Walker-Smith, 1990; Northrup and Flanigan, 1994).

RECOMMENDED QUALITY INDICATORS FOR ACUTE DIARRHEA

The following clinical indicators apply to children up to age 3-5 years.

Diagnosis

Indicator	Quality of evidence	Literature	Benefits	Comments
1. In all children presenting with acute diarrhea, history should be obtained regarding:	III	DeWitt, 1989; Richards et al., 1993; Northrup and Flanigan, 1994	Prevent or correct dehydration.	This information is useful in assessing the hydration status. An accurate assessment of hydration status is essential for appropriate treatment. If the duration has been greater than 2 weeks the child should be evaluated for chronic diarrhea rather than acute diarrhea.
a. the date of onset or duration of diarrheal stools;	III	DeWitt, 1989; Richards et al., 1993; Northrup and Flanigan, 1994		
b. stool consistency, frequency (e.g., number per day), and volume;	III	DeWitt, 1989; Northrup and Flanigan, 1994	Prevent or correct dehydration.	This information is useful in establishing the presence of diarrhea. One must admit, however, that the definition of diarrhea is not well established and dependent on a relative departure from the child's normal bowel pattern in terms of increased frequency and decreased consistency.
c. presence or absence of blood in the stool;	III	DeWitt, 1989; Baraff et al., 1993; Richards et al., 1993; Northrup and Flanigan, 1994	Decrease morbidity from untreated diarrhea.* Prevent sepsis and its complications.**	This information is useful in establishing the presence of inflammatory or bacterial diarrhea and the possibility of sepsis. The possibility of a bacterial etiology for diarrhea in a child will lead the health care provider to consider diagnostic procedures such as fecal leukocyte examination and stool culture, to consider an evaluation to rule-out sepsis or bacteremia, and to consider the possible need for antibiotic therapy.
d. presence or absence of fever, as reported by the parent;	III	DeWitt, 1989; Baraff et al., 1993; Northrup and Flanigan, 1994	Decrease morbidity from untreated diarrhea.* Prevent sepsis and its complications.**	This information is useful in establishing the presence of inflammatory or bacterial diarrhea and the possibility of sepsis. The possibility of a bacterial etiology for diarrhea in a child will lead the health care provider to consider diagnostic procedures such as fecal leukocyte examination and stool culture, to consider an evaluation to rule-out sepsis or bacteremia, and to consider the possible need for antibiotic therapy.

e. presence or absence of vomiting;	III	DeWitt, 1989; Northrup and Flanigan, 1994	Prevent or correct dehydration.	This information is useful in determining the hydration status and the possible course of treatment. If the child has intractable vomiting, oral rehydration therapy may fail. Intractable vomiting is a relative contraindication for oral rehydration therapy; but, it is felt that less than 2 percent of all children with diarrhea in the community will not respond well to oral rehydration therapy for any reason.
f. frequency and volume of fluid intake;	III	DeWitt, 1989; Northrup and Flanigan, 1994	Prevent or correct dehydration.	This information is useful in determining the hydration status and the possible course of treatment. The child who is comatose and unable to take fluids orally will require intravenous rehydration.
2. History should be obtained regarding the frequency and volume of urinary output.	III	DeWitt, 1989; Fitzgerald, 1989; Northrup and Flanigan, 1994	Prevent or correct dehydration.	This information is useful in assessing the hydration status.
3. The weight should be recorded and, if available, compared to a recent weight obtained prior to the onset of diarrhea.	III	DeWitt, 1989; AAP, 1993	Prevent or correct dehydration.	This information is useful in assessing the hydration status and monitoring the progress of therapy. Weight measurement is the gold standard of hydration status. Progress in treatment of dehydration is most easily assessed by comparative weights from the start to the end of therapy.
4. Documentation should also include: a. heart rate b. respiratory rate c. blood pressure d. temperature	III	DeWitt, 1989	Prevent or correct dehydration.	This information is useful in assessing the hydration status and monitoring the progress of therapy.
5. All of the following findings regarding hydration status should be recorded:	III	DeWitt, 1989; AAP, 1993; WHO, 1993; Northrup and Flanigan, 1994	Prevent or correct dehydration. Decrease morbidity from untreated diarrhea.* Prevent sepsis and its complications.**	These factors represent the World Health Organization's criteria for assessing the degree of dehydration of the child with diarrhea. Also, if shock or fever is present, the health care provider should consider the possibility of sepsis. The possibility of a bacterial etiology for diarrhea in a child will lead the health care provider to consider diagnostic procedures such as fecal leukocyte examination and stool culture, to consider an evaluation to rule-out sepsis or bacteremia, and to consider the possible need for antibiotic therapy.

a. general condition;	III	DeWitt, 1989; AAP, 1993; WHO, 1993; Northrup and Flanigan, 1994		General condition characterized by: well, alert; restless, irritable; or lethargic or unconscious, floppy.
b. appearance of eyes;	III	DeWitt, 1989; AAP, 1993; WHO, 1993; Northrup and Flanigan, 1994		Appearance of eyes characterized by: normal; sunken; or very sunken and dry.
c. presence or absence of tears;	III	DeWitt, 1989; AAP, 1993; WHO, 1993; Northrup and Flanigan, 1994		
d. degree of oral moisture;	III	DeWitt, 1989; AAP, 1993; WHO, 1993; Northrup and Flanigan, 1994		Degree of oral moisture characterized by: moist; dry; or very dry.
e. degree of thirst;	III	DeWitt, 1989; AAP, 1993; WHO, 1993; Northrup and Flanigan, 1994		Degree of thirst characterized by: drinks normally, not thirsty; thirsty, drinks eagerly; or drinks poorly or not able to drink.
f. degree of skin turgor; and	III	DeWitt, 1989; AAP, 1993; WHO, 1993; Northrup and Flanigan, 1994		Degree of skin turgor characterized by: skin goes back quickly; skin goes back slowly; or skin goes back very slowly.
g. condition of anterior fontanelle.	III	DeWitt, 1989; AAP, 1993; WHO, 1993; Northrup and Flanigan, 1994		Condition of anterior fontanelle characterized by: normal/flat; slightly sunken; or severely sunken.
6. The exam should note the presence or absence of blood in the stools, either by visual inspection or by chemical means.	III	DeWitt, 1989; Northrup and Flanigan, 1994	Prevent or correct dehydration. Decrease morbidity from untreated diarrhea.* Prevent sepsis and its complications.**	This information is useful in establishing the presence of inflammatory or bacterial diarrhea and the possibility of sepsis. The possibility of a bacterial etiology for diarrhea in a child will lead the health care provider to consider diagnostic procedures such as fecal leukocyte examination and stool culture, to consider an evaluation to rule-out sepsis or bacteremia, and to consider the possible need for antibiotic therapy.

#	Recommendation		References		
7.	The assessment of hydration status should be recorded in terms of percent dehydration or fluid deficit in milliliters per kilogram or as: • not dehydrated (less than 50 milliliters per kilogram fluid deficit), • mild-moderate dehydration (50-100 milliliters per kilogram fluid deficit), or • severe dehydration (greater than 100 milliliters per kilogram fluid deficit).	III	AAP, 1993; WHO, 1993; Northrup and Flanigan, 1994	Prevent or correct dehydration.	This information is useful in determining the possible course of treatment.
8.	Serum electrolytes should have been obtained if the child's dehydration was severe or if the pulse rate was elevated and the blood pressure was low.	III	DeWitt, 1989; Kallen, 1990; Northrup and Flanigan, 1994	Avoid complications of cerebral edema and seizures.	A child in severe dehydration may have severe electrolyte imbalances requiring correction and requiring modification of intravenous therapy. For example, with severe hypernatremia, the health care provider may opt to correct the sodium concentration excess over a period of 48 hours rather than 24 hours or less. Blood pressure and pulse changes will be specified based on the age of the child.
9.	Urinalysis should have been obtained if the child's dehydration was severe or if the pulse rate was elevated and the blood pressure was low.	III	DeWitt, 1989; Fitzgerald, 1989; Kallen, 1990; Northrup and Flanigan, 1994	Prevent or correct dehydration.	Urine specific gravity, as part of the urinalysis, would provide a useful monitor as to the success or failure of hydration therapy and may be particularly useful in the case of severe dehydration.
10.	Fecal leukocytes should have been obtained if the child with diarrhea is less than 36 months of age and had fever or blood in the stool.	II-2	DeWitt et al., 1985; Finkelstein et al., 1989;	Prevent morbidity/mortality due to bacterial infection.	The reviews on acute diarrhea indicate fecal leukocyte determination might not be needed until diarrhea has persisted despite three days of hydration therapy. In their guideline on workup of fever, Baraff et al. (1993) indicate that fecal leukocytes should be obtained in the child less than 36 months of age with fever and diarrhea. Though not well documented, this recommendation seems to be based on the findings of DeWitt et al. (1985) and Finkelstein et al. (1989). The appropriate use of the fecal leukocyte determination would lead to appropriate treatment of bacterial diarrhea and reduced costs of evaluation since not all children would require fecal leukocyte determination.

209

	Indicator	Quality of evidence	Literature	Benefits	Comments
11.	Stool culture should be obtained if the child with diarrhea is less than 36 months of age and had fever or blood in the stool or > 5 fecal leukocytes per high power field.	II-2	DeWitt et al., 1985; Finkelstein, 1989;	Prevent morbidity/mortality due to bacterial infection.	See above discussion of the use of fecal leukocyte examination. In their guideline on workup of fever, Baraff et al. (1993) indicate that a stool culture should be obtained in the child less than 36 months of age with fever and diarrhea with blood and mucous or with > 5 fecal leukocytes per high power field. The appropriate use of the stool culture would lead to appropriate treatment of bacterial diarrhea and reduced costs of evaluation since not all children would require stool culture determination.
12.	A stool examination for ova and parasites should be obtained if the child had a history of recent travel to a developing country, acquired or congenital immunocompromise, or exposure to a potential carrier of parasitic diarrhea.	III	DeWitt, 1989; Laney and Cohen, 1993; Northrup and Flanigan, 1994	Decrease morbidity from untreated diarrhea.*	Parasites are the least common cause of diarrhea in children. Evaluation for possible parasitic causes of diarrhea should, therefore, be limited to children at high risk for parasitic infection. Such focused evaluation will reduce the overall costs of evaluation of diarrhea among children. Conversely, even with a history of recent travel, residence in a child care setting, immunocompromise or exposure to a potential carrier of parasitic diarrhea, stool examination for ova and parasite might not be needed unless diarrhea has persisted greater than 10-14 days or a public health concern existed.
13.	If stool was obtained for ova and parasite examination, three stool samples, obtained on three consecutive days, should have been ordered.	III	Northrup and Flanigan, 1994	Decrease morbidity from untreated diarrhea.*	The false negative rate may be high with a single stool specimen. Though the incidence of parasitic diarrhea is low, when present appropriate treatment will be enhanced by identifying the parasite on stool examination. Although these should ideally be obtained on 3 consecutive days, extension of that period to 5-7 days may be appropriate.

Treatment

	Indicator	Quality of evidence	Literature	Benefits	Comments
14.	If the child had diarrhea but was not dehydrated, the practitioner should recommend additional fluid intake beyond what is normal for the child.	III	AAP, 1993; Richards et al., 1993; Northrup and Flanigan, 1994	Prevent dehydration.	The extra fluid should have a sodium concentration of about 20-50 milliequivalents per liter of fluid.

#	Recommendation	Grade	Objective	References	Comments
15.	If the child had mild-moderate dehydration, is not comatose, and is without intractable vomiting, has evidence of ileus, and moderate or severe purging upon administration of oral electrolyte-sugar solution, oral rehydration therapy should be prescribed and consist of: a. electrolyte, sugar solution as specified by the American Academy of Pediatrics (1993) or the World Health Organization (Richards et al., 1993); b. correction of the initial fluid deficit in the first 6 hours of treatment; and c. be monitored in the office or emergency room setting during entire period of rehydration.	I	Prevent or correct dehydration.	Santosham et al., 1982; Santosham et al., 1985; Tamer et al., 1985; Listernick et al., 1986; Herzog et al., 1987; AAP, 1993; WHO, 1993	Oral rehydration therapy has been shown to be an effective treatment for the child with mild-moderate dehydration and avoids the need for intravenous therapy and its possible morbidity. It is felt that less than 2 percent of all children with diarrhea in the community will not respond well to oral rehydration therapy. In some cases, nasogastric feedings may be an alternative rather than intravenous intervention. References AAP (1993) and Richards et al. (1993) review the American Academy of Pediatrics and World Health Organization guidelines.
16.	If the child had severe dehydration, intravenous rehydration should be prescribed and consist of: a. replacement of the fluid deficit with either isotonic fluid, such as normal-saline or Ringer's Lactate solution as specified by the World Health Organization, or electrolyte solution based on serum electrolyte deficits; b. the pulse and blood pressure should be stabilized within normal limits for age within 6 hours of initiation of treatment; c. replacement of the fluid deficit within 48 hours of initiation of treatment; d. monitoring of input and output; and e. completion of all rehydration in the inpatient setting or observation unit.	III	Reverse the complications of severe dehydration and prevent end-organ damage and death.	DeWitt, 1989; Kallen, 1990; AAP, 1993; WHO, 1993; Northrup and Flanigan, 1994	Complications of severe dehydration include death, cardiovascular collapse, seizure, and coma.
17.	If while healthy the child was being breast fed, the health care provider should advise the parent to continue breast feeding if the child is able to feed orally.	I	Prevent or correct dehydration.	Khin-Maung-U et al., 1985; AAP, 1993; WHO, 1993	In children 6 to 24 months of age with moderate or severe dehydration due to diarrhea, the continued provision of breast feeding in addition to oral rehydration solution resulted in decreased number of bowel movements, while in the hospital 12.1 versus 17.4, and stool output, 89.2 milliliters/kilogram/patient versus 115.8 ml/kg/patient, while requiring less total volume of oral rehydration solution. AAP (1993) and Richards et al. (1993) review the American Academy of Pediatrics and World Health Organization guidelines.

18.	If while healthy the child was formula fed or weaned, the health care provider should have instituted refeeding within twenty-four hours of the onset of hydration therapy.	I	Rees and Brook, 1979; Placzek and Walker-Smith, 1984; Ransome et al., 1984; Isolauri and Vesikari, 1985; Santosham et al., 1985; Isolauri et al., 1986; Brown et al., 1988; Gazala et al., 1988; Conway and Ireson, 1989; Fox et al., 1990; Margolis et al., 1990; Santosham et al., 1990; Lifshitz et al., 1991; Santosham et al., 1991; AAP, 1993; Chew et al., 1993	Prevent malnutrition and associated complications of poor nutrition.	On balance the randomized controlled studies show at best a small decrease in duration of diarrhea; but, the theoretical positive effect on nutritional status would warrant early refeeding, especially in the young infant or child with underlying malnutrition.
19.	Antimicrobial agents should be used in a child with: a. suspected or culture-proven cholera with severe dehydration; or b. salmonella in patients with sickle cell anemia, lymphoma, leukemia, other immune compromise (acquired or congenital), positive stool culture for bacterial pathogen and less than 3 months of age, or bacteremia with salmonella and less than 6 months of age; or c. giardia with symptoms of greater than 10-14 days duration and with positive stool ova and parasite examination; or d. amoeba with positive stool ova and parasite examination.	III	WHO, 1990; Pickering, 1991; Laney and Cohen, 1993; Northrup and Flanigan, 1994	Decrease morbidity from untreated diarrhea.* Prevent sepsis and its complications.**	If antimicrobials are to be used, in order to enhance the probability of eradicating the intended target, the choice of antimicrobial agent should be based on the most likely organism. Conversely, even when a bacterial or parasitic etiology of diarrhea is identified, the health care provider need not automatically treat with an antimicrobial. Antibiotics may be useful in diarrhea caused by shigella as well as the listed indications.

212

Indicator	Quality of evidence	Literature	Benefits	Comments
20. Antidiarrheal or antimotility medications should never be used in treatment of diarrhea in a child.	III	Hamilton, 1985; DeWitt, 1989; Fitzgerald, 1989; Avery and Snyder, 1990; WHO, 1990; Pickering, 1991; Northrup and Flanigan, 1994	Prevent side effects of antidiarrheal and antimotility medications.	No evidence is cited by any of the reviews that antidiarrheal or antimotility medications are effective in the treatment of diarrhea in children. The reviews cited on the contrary all indicate that the use of these medications have been associated with serious side effects, such as toxic megacolon, colonic hemorrhage, and ileus.

Follow-up

Indicator	Quality of evidence	Literature	Benefits	Comments
21. The young infant less than three months of age with acute diarrhea should have follow-up by the health care provider within: a. three days of intervention for diarrhea without dehydration; b. one week after rehydration (either inpatient or outpatient) of mild-moderate or severe diarrhea.	III	Brown and Lifshitz, 1991; AAP, 1993; Northrup and Flanigan, 1994	Prevent dehydration.	The cited reviews do not define young infant. The choice of three months is based on clinical opinion. The young infant is at greater risk of failing therapy. Since diarrhea may continue for several days as noted in the text, the health care provider needs to monitor the hydration status of the child over the natural course of the disease process. Maintenance of normal hydration status depends on the continuation of appropriate treatment outside of the medical setting by the child's guardians. Through close followup, the health care provider can increase the likelihood that the child will maintain normal hydration status until the end of the diarrhea process. Children whose hydration status has been corrected through medical intervention are more likely to be close to the end of their illness. The choice of three days and one week for follow-up is partly based on clinical opinion and partly on the natural course of the majority of acute diarrheal episodes.

213

#	Statement		Reference		Explanation
22.	The child with growth delay or malnutrition should have follow-up by the health care provider within: a. three days of intervention for diarrhea without dehydration; b. one week after rehydration (either inpatient or outpatient) of mild-moderate or severe diarrhea.	III	Northrup and Flanigan, 1994	Prevent dehydration.	The child with growth delay or malnutrition is at greater risk than the child without these conditions to fail therapy. Since diarrhea may continue for several days as noted in the text, the health care provider needs to monitor the hydration status of the child over the natural course of the disease process. Maintenance of normal hydration status depends on the continuation of appropriate treatment outside of the medical setting by the child's guardians. Through close followup, the health care provider can increase the likelihood that the child will maintain normal hydration status until the end of the diarrhea process. The choice of three days and one week for follow-up is partly based on clinical opinion and partly on the natural course of the majority of acute diarrheal episodes.
23.	The child with immunocompromise should have follow-up by the health care provider within: a. three days of intervention for diarrhea without dehydration; b. one week after rehydration (either inpatient or outpatient) of mild-moderate or severe diarrhea.	III	Northrup and Flanigan, 1994	Prevent dehydration.	The child with immunocompromise is at greater risk than the child without these conditions to fail therapy. The choice of three days and one week for follow-up is partly based on clinical opinion and partly on the natural course of the majority of acute diarrheal episodes.
24.	Any child with severe dehydration should have follow-up by the health care provider within one week after discharge for intervention.	III	Brown and Lifshitz, 1991	Prevent dehydration.	Maintenance of normal hydration status depends on the continuation of appropriate treatment outside of the medical setting by the child's guardians. The choice of one week for follow-up is partly based on clinical opinion and partly on the natural course of the majority of acute diarrheal episodes.
25.	Any child with inflammatory or invasive diarrhea should have follow-up by the health care provider within: a. three days of intervention for diarrhea without dehydration; b. one week after discharge for intervention of mild-moderate or severe diarrhea.	III	Northrup and Flanigan, 1994	Prevent dehydration.	Through close follow-up, the health care provider can increase the likelihood that the child will maintain normal hydration status until the end of the diarrhea process. The choice of three days and one week for follow-up is partly based on clinical opinion and partly on the natural course of the majority of acute diarrheal episodes.

214

| 26. | Any child with diarrhea and culture positive for parasites should have follow-up by the health care provider within:
a. three days of intervention for diarrhea without dehydration;
b. one week after discharge for intervention of mild-moderate or severe diarrhea. | III | Northrup and Flanigan, 1994 | Prevent dehydration. | Parasitic diarrhea may be quite persistent and may require follow-up stool examinations to document its eradication. The choice of three days and one week for follow-up is partly based on clinical opinion and partly on the natural course of the majority of acute diarrheal episodes. |
| 27. | If there is no improvement in diarrhea after 3 days of hydration therapy, the following work-up should be performed:
a. serum electrolytes
b. urinalysis
c. fecal leukocyte examination
d. stool culture | III | DeWitt et al., 1985; DeWitt, 1989; Fitzgerald, 1989; Kallen, 1990; Richards et al., 1993; Northrup and Flanigan, 1994 | Prevent dehydration. | The child with diarrhea persisting greater than three days while on treatment is at risk of advancing degrees of dehydration. |

*Morbidity may include severe hydration, abdominal and rectal pain, weight loss, lost school days, and lost work days for the parent.

**Complications of sepsis include multi-organ failure and death.

Quality of Evidence Codes:

I: RCT
II-1:   Nonrandomized controlled trials
II-2:   Cohort or case analysis
II-3:   Multiple time series
III: Opinions or descriptive studies

215

REFERENCES - ACUTE DIARRHEAL DISEASE

American Academy of Pediatrics, Committee on Nutrition, and LA Barness. 1993. *Pediatric Nutrition Handbook*, Third ed.Elk Grove Village, Illinois: American Academy of Pediatrics.

American Academy of Pediatrics, Committee on Nutrition. 1985. Use of oral fluid therapy and post-treatment feeding following enteritis in children in a developed country. *Pediatrics* 76 (2): 358-61.

Avery ME, and JD Snyder. 1990. Oral therapy for acute diarrhea. *New England Journal of Medicine* 323 (13): 891-4.

Baraff LJ, JW Bass, GR Fleisher, et al. 1993. Practice guideline for the management of infants and children 0 to 36 months of age with fever without source. *Pediatrics* 92 (1): 1-12.

Bezerra JA, TH Stathos, B Duncan, et al. 1992. Treatment of infants with acute diarrhea: What's recommended and what's practiced. *Pediatrics* 90 (1): 1-4.

Bhan MK, D Mahalanabis, O Fontaine, et al. 1994. Clinical trials of improved oral rehydration salt formulations: a review. *Bulletin of the World Health Organization* 72 (6): 945-55.

Blacklow NR, and HB Greenberg. 1991. Viral gastroenteritis. *New England Journal of Medicine* 325 (4): 252-64.

Brown KH. 1991. Dietary management of acute childhood diarrhea: Optimal timing of feeding and appropriate use of milks and mixed diets. *Journal of Pediatrics* 118 (4, Part 2): S92-S98.

Brown KH, AS Gastanaduy, JM Saavedra, et al. 1988. Effect of continued oral feeding on clinical and nutritional outcomes of acute diarrhea in children. *Journal of Pediatrics* 112 (2): 191-200.

Brown KH, and F Lifshitz. 1991. Management of acute diarrheal disease: Discussion V. *Journal of Pediatrics* 118 (4, Part 2): S109-S110.

Brown KH, and WC MacLean. 1984. Nutritional management of acute diarrhea: An appraisal of the alternatives. *Pediatrics* 73 (2): 119-25.

Brown KH, JM Peerson, and O Fontaine. 1994. Use of nonhuman milks in the dietary management of young children with acute diarrhea: A meta-analysis of clinical trials. *Pediatrics* 93 (1): 17-27.

Chew F, FJ Penna, LAP Filho, et al. 1993. Is dilution of cows' milk formula necessary for dietary management of acute diarrhoea in infants aged less than 6 months? *Lancet* 341: 194-7.

Cohen MB. 1991. Etiology and mechanisms of acute infectious diarrhea in infants in the United States. *Journal of Pediatrics* 118 (4, Part 2): S34-S39.

Cohen MB, AG Mezoff, DW Laney, et al. 1995. Use of a single solution for oral rehydration and maintenance therapy of infants with diarrhea and mild to moderate dehydration. *Pediatrics* 95 (5): 639-45.

Conway SP, and A Ireson. 1989. Acute gastroenteritis in well nourished infants: comparison of four feeding regimens. *Archives of Disease in Childhood* 64: 87-91.

Darrow DC, EL Pratt, J Flett, et al. 1949. Disturbances of water and electrolytes in infantile diarrhea. *Pediatrics* 3 (2): 129-56.

DeWitt TG. 1989. Acute diarrhea in children. *Pediatrics in Review* 11 (1): 6-13.

DeWitt TG, KF Humphrey, and P McCarthy. 1985. Clinical predictors of acute bacterial diarrhea in young children. *Pediatrics* 76 (4): 551-6.

Finkelstein JA, JS Schwartz, S Torrey, et al. 1989. Common clinical features as predictors of bacterial diarrhea in infants. *American Journal of Emergency Medicine* 7 (5): 469-73.

Fitzgerald JF. 1989. Management of acute diarrhea. *Pediatric Infectious Disease Journal* 8 (8): 564-9.

Fox R, CLS Leen, EM Dunbar, et al. 1990. Acute gastroenteritis in infants under 6 months old. *Archives of Disease in Childhood* 65: 936-8.

Gazala EY, S Weitzman, Z Weizman, et al. 1988. Early vs. late refeeding in acute infantile diarrhea. *Israel Journal of Medical Sciences* 24: 175-9.

Ghishan FK. 1988. The transport of electrolytes in the gut and the use of oral rehydration solutions. *Pediatric Clinics of North America* 35 (1): 35-51.

Glass RI, and MB Cohen. 1991. Management of acute diarrheal disease: Discussion I. *Journal of Pediatrics* 118 (4, Part 2): S40-S43.

Glass RI, JF Lew, RE Gangarosa, et al. 1991. Estimates of morbidity and mortality rates for diarrheal diseases in American children. *Journal of Pediatrics* 118 (4, Part 2): S27-S33.

Greenough WB, and Khin-Maung-U. 1991. Cereal-based oral rehydration therapy. II. Strategic issues for its implementation in national diarrheal disease control programs. *Journal of Pediatrics* 118 (4, Part 2): S80-S85.

Guerrant RL, and DA Bobak. 1991. Bacterial and protozoal gastroenteritis. *New England Journal of Medicine* 325 (5): 327-40.

Hamilton JR. 1985. Treatment of acute diarrhea. *Pediatric Clinics of North America* 32 (2): 419-27.

Herzog LW, WG Bithoney, and RJ Grand. 1987. High sodium rehydration solutions in well-nourished outpatients. *Acta Paediatrica Scandinavica* 76: 306-10.

Isolauri E, T Vesikari, P Saha, et al. 1986. Milk versus no milk in rapid refeeding after acute gastroenteritis. *Journal of Pediatric Gastroenterology and Nutrition* 5 (2): 254-61.

Isolauri E, and T Vesikari. 1985. Oral rehydration, rapid feeding, and cholestyramine for treatment of acute diarrhea. *Journal of Pediatric Gastroenterology and Nutrition* 4: 366-74.

Kallen RJ. 1990. The management of diarrheal dehydration in infants using parenteral fluids. *Pediatric Clinics of North America* 37 (2): 265-86.

Khin-Maung-U, and WB Greenough III. 1991. Cereal-based oral rehydration therapy. I. Clinical studies. *Journal of Pediatrics* 118 (4, Part 2): S72-S79.

Khin-Maung-U, Nyunt-Nyunt-Wai, Myo-Khin, et al. 1985. Effect on clinical outcome of breast feeding during acute diarrhoea. *British Medical Journal* 290: 587-9.

Laney DW, and MB Cohen. 1993. Approach to the pediatric patient with diarrhea. *Gastroenterology Clinics of North America* 22 (3): 499-516.

Lebenthal E, and R Lu. 1991. Glucose polymers as an alternative to glucose in oral rehydration solutions. *Journal of Pediatrics* 118 (4, Part 2): S62-S69.

Levine MM. 1986. Antimicrobial therapy for infectious diarrhea. *Reviews of Infectious Diseases* 8 (Suppl. 2): S207-S216.

Levine MM. 1991. Vaccines and milk immunoglobulin concentrates for prevention of infectious diarrhea. *Journal of Pediatrics* 118 (4, Part 2): S129-S136.

Lifshitz F, UF Neto, CAG Olivo, et al. 1991. Refeeding of infants with acute diarrheal disease. *Journal of Pediatrics* 118 (4, Part 2): S99-S108.

Listernick R, E Zieserl, and AT Davis. 1986. Outpatient oral rehydration in the United States. *American Journal of Diseases in Children* 140: 211-5.

Margolis PA, T Litteer, N Hare, et al. 1990. Effects of unrestricted diet on mild infantile diarrhea. *American Journal of Diseases of Children* 144 (2): 162-4.

Northrup RS, and TP Flanigan. 1994. Gastroenteritis. *Pediatrics in Review* 15 (12): 461-72.

Pickering LK. 1991. Therapy for acute infectious diarrhea in children. *Journal of Pediatrics* 118 (4, Part 2): S118-S128.

Pickering L, and MM Levine. 1991. Management of acute diarrheal disease: Discussion VII. *Journal of Pediatrics* 118 (4, Part 2): S137-S138.

Placzek M, and JA Walker-Smith. 1984. Comparison of two feeding regimens following acute gastroenteritis in infancy. *Journal of Pediatric Gastroenterology and Nutrition* 3 (2): 245-8.

Ransome OJ, and H Roode. 1984. Early introduction of milk feeds in acute infantile gastro-enteritis. *South African Medical Journal* 65 (127-8):

Rees L, and CGD Brook. 7 April 1979. Gradual reintroduction of full-strength milk after acute gastroenteritis in children. *Lancet* 770-1:

Ribeiro HDC, and F Lifshitz. 1991. Alanine-based oral rehydration therapy for infants with acute diarrhea. *Journal of Pediatrics* 118 (4, Part 2): S86-S90.

Richards L, M Claeson, and NF Pierce. 1993. Management of acute diarrhea in children: Lessons learned. *Pediatric Infectious Disease Journal* 12 (1): 5-9.

Santosham M, B Burns, V Nadkarni, et al. 1985. Oral rehydration therapy for acute diarrhea in ambulatory children in the United States: A double-blind comparison of four different solutions. *Pediatrics* 76 (2): 159-66.

Santosham M, RS Daum, L Dillman, et al. 1982. Oral rehydration therapy of infantile diarrhea: A controlled study of well-nourished children hospitalized in the United States and Panama. *New England Journal of Medicine* 306 (18): 1070-6.

Santosham M, IM Fayad, M Hashem, et al. 1990. A comparison of rice-based oral rehydration solution and "early feeding" for the treatment of acute diarrhea in infants. *Journal of Pediatrics* 116: 868-75.

Santosham M, S Foster, R Reid, et al. 1985. Role of soy-based, lactose-free formula during treatment of acute diarrhea. *Pediatrics* 76 (2): 292-8.

Santosham M, J Goepp, B Burns, et al. 1991. Role of a soy-based lactose-free formula in the outpatient management of diarrhea. *Pediatrics* 87 (5): 619-22.

Santosham M, and WB Greenough. 1991. Oral rehydration therapy: A global perspective. *Journal of Pediatrics* 118 (4, Part 2): S44-S51.

Snyder JD. 1991. Use and misuse of oral therapy for diarrhea: Comparison of US practices with American Academy of Pediatrics recommendations. *Pediatrics* 87 (1): 28-33.

Tamer AM, LB Friedman, SRW Maxwell, et al. 1985. Oral rehydration of infants in a large urban U. S. medical center. *Journal of Pediatrics* 107 (1): 14-9.

Walker-Smith JA. 1990. Management of infantile gastroenteritis. *Archives of Disease in Childhood* 65: 917-8.

Wapnir RA, and E Lebenthal. 1991. Management of acute diarrheal disease: Discussion III. *Journal of Pediatrics* 118 (4, Part 2): S70-S71.

World Health Organization. 1993. *The Management and Prevention of Diarrhoea: Practice Guidelines*, Third ed.Geneva, Switzerland: World Health Organization.

World Health Organization (WHO). 1990. *The Rational Use of Drugs in the Management of Acute Diarrhoea in Children*.Geneva, Switzerland: World Health Organization.

11. FAMILY PLANNING/CONTRACEPTION[1]
Deidre Gifford, M.D.

The USPSTF (1989) review of "Counseling to Prevent Unintended Pregnancy," as well as the background papers in *Preventing Disease, Beyond the Rhetoric* (Goldbloom and Lawrence, 1990) were used for the sections describing the importance of and recommendations for screening and counseling. For specific indicators regarding contraceptive methods, the relevant American College of Obstetricians and Gynecologists (ACOG) Committee Opinions and Technical Bulletins were consulted. In addition, *Contraceptive Technology* (Hatcher et al., 1989, pp. 233-284) and the textbook, *Infertility, Contraception and Reproductive Endocrinology* (Mishell, 1991, in Mishell et al., 1991) were used.

IMPORTANCE

Unintended and unwanted pregnancies are common in the United States. It has been estimated that about 37 percent of births among women aged 15-44 are unintended, and just over one-quarter of those (10 percent of births) are thought to be unwanted. Unwanted pregnancy is a risk factor for late entry into prenatal care, which has been associated with low birthweight and other poor pregnancy outcomes (USPSTF, 1989). Children born as a result of unwanted pregnancies are at increased risk for child abuse and neglect, and for behavioral and educational problems later in life. Unwanted pregnancies among adolescents are common, with as many as 10 percent of girls in the United States aged 15-19 becoming pregnant each year. Sixty-six percent of unmarried teenage girls are sexually active by the age of 19 (USPSTF, 1989).

---

[1]Originally written for the Women's Quality of Care Panel.

EFFICACY OF INTERVENTION

Screening for Risk of Unintended Pregnancy

While there is no direct evidence available that taking a sexual history and offering contraception when appropriate will lower the rate of unintended pregnancy, counseling to prevent unintended pregnancy is widely recommended (USPSTF, 1989; Fielding and Williams, 1990, in Goldbloom and Lawrence, 1990). Except for abstinence, the most highly effective methods of contraception (hormonal methods, sterilization, and IUD) all require a visit to a health professional. There is evidence that teens who use hormonal methods of contraception are less likely to have an unwanted pregnancy than those using nonprescription contraceptives. Physicians, and others providing primary care to women, who do not ask about sexual activity and contraceptive practices may miss the opportunity to offer an intervention (contraception) which is known to be effective in preventing a serious adverse health outcome (unintended pregnancy). One study of Canadian teens revealed that although 85 percent had seen their doctor in the preceding year, only one third of sexually active girls had ever discussed contraception with their doctors (Feldman, 1990, in Goldbloom and Lawrence, 1990). According to a report by the World Health Organization, if all sexually active couples had routinely used effective contraception in 1980, there would have been almost 1 million fewer abortions, 340,000 fewer unintended births, 5,000 fewer infant deaths, and a reduction in the infant mortality rate of 10 percent (IOM, 1995). Furthermore, if the proportion of unintended pregnancies were reduced by 30 percent in the U.S., there would be 200,000 fewer unwanted births, and 800,000 fewer abortions each year (IOM, 1995).

Once it has been determined that an individual is at risk for unintended pregnancy (i.e., is sexually active without contraception or with ineffective contraception and does not desire pregnancy at that time), it is appropriate to discuss the risks and benefits of the various methods, and to offer the most acceptable contraceptive method (USPSTF, 1989; Fielding and Williams, 1990, in Goldbloom and Lawrence, 1990). In a recent report on prevention of unintended pregnancy, the

IOM (1995) concluded that "...too few providers of health care...use all available opportunities to discuss contraception and the importance of intended pregnancy to the health and well-being of women and men, children and families." The appropriate interval for screening for risk of unintended pregnancy has not been determined.

Treatment

Highly effective methods exist for preventing unintended pregnancy. These include abstinence, sterilization, hormonal contraceptives (oral, injectable, and implants), intra-uterine devices and barrier methods. Other methods, such as periodic abstinence, coitus interruptus and spermicides are less effective. Oral contraceptives (OCs) are the most commonly used non-permanent form of contraception in the United States. Approximately 10 million women in the U.S. currently use this method (USPSTF, 1989). OCs generally contain both an estrogen and progestin component ("combination" OCs), although a progestin only pill is also available. Combination OCs are highly effective in preventing pregnancy, with failure rates of 0.1 to 3.0 percent. In actual use, they may be less effective in teen-aged girls because of a lack of compliance (Hatcher et al., 1989; ACOG Technical Bulletin, 1994). In their original formulation, combination pills contained 50 mcg of synthetic estrogen, while the majority of OCs prescribed today contain 35 mcg or less.

While OCs have many non-contraceptive benefits (e.g., reduction in menstrual flow, decreased dysmenorrhea, decreased anemia, lower risk of ovarian and endometrial cancer) (ACOG Technical Bulletin, 1994), they are also associated with health risks which may exceed their contraceptive benefit in some groups of women. Specifically, women who smoke and take oral contraceptives are at increased risk of cardiovascular disease when compared to non-smoking OC users. The Royal College of General Practitioners' OC study (Croft and Hannaford, 1989) recruited 1400 OC users and 1400 non-users in 1968 and has followed this cohort to study the health effects of OC use. A nested case-control study using these data showed that neither current nor past OC use was a risk factor for myocardial infarction (MI) when other risk factors were controlled for. However, OC users who smoked were at increased risk of MI compared to non-smoking OC users. Those who smoked fewer than 15 cigarettes per day had a relative risk of MI of 3.5 (95 percent CI 1.3-9.5), and those who smoked more than 15 cigarettes per day had a relative risk of MI of 20.8 (5.2-83.1). (These relative risks are not adjusted for age, hypertension or other risk factors for MI.) Although data on OC formulation were not reported, many of the pill users in this study were likely to have been using a 50 mcg OC at the time of recruitment. Data regarding the risk of smoking and low-dose OC use, stratified by age, are not available.

RECOMMENDED QUALITY INDICATORS FOR FAMILY PLANNING/CONTRACEPTION

The following criteria apply to all post-menarchal girls up to age 18 for whom the medical record documents a history of vaginal intercourse; selected indicators also apply to adolescent boys (ages 13-18).

Screening

	Indicator	Quality of evidence	Literature	Benefits	Comments
1.	A history to determine risk for unintended pregnancy should be taken yearly on all women. In order to establish risk, the following elements of the history need to be documented: a. Menstrual status (e.g., pre- or post-menopausal, history of hysterectomy, etc.), last menstrual period, or pregnancy test; b. Sexual history (presence or absence of current sexual intercourse); c. Current contraceptive practices; d. Desire for pregnancy.	III	USPSTF, 1989	Prevent unwanted pregnancies and births. Prevent abortions.	The USPSTF does not make a recommendation for screening interval. As many as 37% of births among women aged 15-44 are unintended and over one quarter are unwanted. The goal of these recommendations is to identify women at risk for unintended pregnancies and counsel appropriately those who are interested in contraception.

Treatment

	Indicator	Quality of evidence	Literature	Benefits	Comments
2.	All adolescent girls and boys at risk for unintended pregnancy (i.e., sexually active) should receive counseling about effective contraceptive methods.	III	USPSTF, 1989	Prevent unwanted pregnancies and births. Prevent abortions.	Women at risk for unintended pregnancy are those who are sexually active without effective contraception and who do not desire pregnancy. Effective contraception is defined as: 1) Hormonal contraception (OC, injectable prostaglandins or implants) 2) IUD 3) Barrier + spermicide 4) Sterilization 5) Complete abstinence
3.	The smoking status of all women prescribed combination OCs should be documented in the medical record.	II	ACOG Technical Bulletin, 1994	Prevent myocardial infarction and other thromboembolic complications.*	Women who smoke and use combination oral contraceptives (containing both estrogen and progestin component) are at risk for myocardial infarction (relative risk is 20 times greater than in women who do not smoke). Therefore, if prescribing oral contraceptives, the smoking status should be documented.

| 4. | All women who smoke and are prescribed oral contraceptives should be counseled and encouraged to quit smoking. | II-2 | Croft and Hannaford, 1989; Kottke et al., 1988 | Prevent myocardial infarction and other thromboembolic complications.* | Because smoking increases risk of MI among women using oral contraception, and also has other long term toxicities (lung cancer, chronic lung disease, etc.), women should be counseled to quit. Counseling by physicians has been shown to be effective. |

*Thromboembolic complications include myocardial infarction, cerebrovascular accident, thrombophlebitis, and pulmonary emboli.

Quality of Evidence Codes:

I:	RCT
II-1:	Nonrandomized controlled trials
II-2:	Cohort or case analysis
II-3:	Multiple time series
III:	Opinions or descriptive studies

REFERENCES - FAMILY PLANNING/CONTRACEPTION

American College of Obstetricians and Gynecologists. October 1994. Hormonal contraception. *ACOG Technical Bulletin* 198: 1-12.

Croft P, and PC Hannaford. 21 January 1989. Risk factors for acute myocardial infarction in women: Evidence from the Royal College of General Practitioners' oral contraception study. *British Medical Journal* 298: 165-8.

Feldman W. 1990. Unwanted teenage pregnancy: A Canadian perspective. In *Preventing Disease: Beyond the Rhetoric*. Editors Goldbloom RB, and RS Lawrence, 92-3. New York, NY: Springer-Verlag.

Fielding JE, and CA Williams. 1990. Unwanted teenage pregnancy: A US perspective. In *Preventing Disease: Beyond the Rhetoric*. Editors Goldbloom RB, and RS Lawrence, 94-100. New York, NY: Springe-Verlag.

Hatcher RA, J Trussell, F Stewart, et al. 1994. The pill: Combined oral contraceptives. In *Contraceptive Technology*, 16th revised ed. 223-84. New York, NY: Irvington Publishers, Inc.

Institute of Medicine, Committee on Unintended Pregnancy. 1995. *The Best Intentions: Unintended Pregnancy and the Well-Being of Children and Families*. Washington, DC: National Academy Press.

Kottke TE, RN Battista, GH DeFriese, et al. 20 May 1988. Attributes of successful smoking cessation interventions in medical practice: A meta-analysis of 39 controlled trials. *Journal of the American Medical Association* 259 (19): 2883-9.

Mishell DR. 1991. Oral steroid contraceptives. In *Infertility, Contraception and Reproductive Endocrinology*, Third ed. Editors Mishell DR, V Davajan, and RA Lobo, 839-71. Boston, MA: Blackwell Scientific Publications.

U.S. Preventive Services Task Force. 1989. *Guide to Clinical Preventive Services: An Assessment of the Effectiveness of 169 Interventions*. Baltimore, MD: Williams and Wilkins.

12. FEVER WITHOUT SOURCE OF INFECTION IN CHILDREN UNDER 3 YEARS OF AGE
Glenn Takata, M.D., M.S.

The recommendations on the evaluation of fever without obvious source of infection in children less than 3 years old were developed by summarizing the guidelines and recommendations of review articles (Downs et al., 1991; Lieu et al., 1991; Baraff et al., 1993; Harper and Fleisher, 1993). The review articles were selected from this reviewer's personal library and a MEDLINE literature search on the key words fever and sepsis, looking for English-language articles related to infants and children published between 1985 and 1995. Focused assessment of the literature with respect to specific areas of importance or disagreement among the reviews were then conducted which relied on reference lists in the review articles.

IMPORTANCE

In children under 3 years old, fever is a common presenting symptom to the physician. Fever may be an indication of a mild infectious process such as a viral upper respiratory infection or a more serious infectious process such as bacteremia, meningitis, bone and joint infections, urinary tract infection, pneumonia, soft tissue infection, or a bacterial enteritis. The source of fever may not be readily apparent on initial assessment. The evaluation of fever in this age group has great clinical importance, as any of the serious bacterial infections whose presence it may signal may have grave morbidity if not treated.

The summary of the 1991 National Ambulatory Medical Care Survey estimated that 9.1 percent of all office visits to pediatric specialists was for fever. Fever was a much more common presenting complaint among those less than 15 years of age than for older age groups (National Center for Health Statistics [NCHS], 1994c). For children less than 15 years of age, fever was the principal reason for a visit among 7.1 percent of that population (NCHS, 1994c). Non-population-based studies have described the prevalence of fever in various ways. Pantell et al.

(1980), looked at all infants under 6 months old at a family practice center in Charleston County, South Carolina. An increasing proportion with fever were found with increasing age, 1.2 percent of neonates versus 13.2 percent of infants 5 to 6 months age (Pantell et al., 1980). Baraff et al. (1993), cited a study that estimated that 65 percent of all children between birth and 2 years of age visit a physician for the complaint of fever. Two studies done at academic medical centers indicated that about 1 percent of all emergency department (ED) visits were for fever, which would extrapolate to about 220,000 ED visits by infants less than 3 years of age per year in the United States (Baskin, 1993). Harper and Fleischer (1993) estimated that fever was the chief complaint for 15 to 25 percent of ED visits of children ages 3 to 36 months.

The costs of the work-up and treatment of fever in children under 3 years old include the costs of blood, urine, cerebrospinal, and stool studies, radiographic or nuclear medicine studies, hospitalization, antibiotics, and complications of medical management, such as allergic reactions to antibiotics (Lieu et al., 1991). Lieu et al. (1991) estimated the following costs for services provided to febrile children at the Children's Hospital of Philadelphia in 1989: blood culture $60, leukocyte count $3, oral amoxicillin $5, outpatient visit $40, extended emergency room visit $210, hospitalization for meningitis $5,247, for pneumococcal bacteremia $1,096, for Hemophilus influenza bacteremia $3,029, and for anaphylaxis to antibiotic $3,020 (Lieu et al., 1991). Although the figures are dated, DeAngelis et al. (1983) reported that the average cost of medical care for an infant less than 60 days of age with a fever of greater than or equal to 38°C admitted to The Johns Hopkins Hospital in Baltimore in 1979-80 was $2,130. The costs ranged from $1,480 for infants with aseptic meningitis to $6,345 for those with meningitis.

Lieu et al. (1991) concluded in their decision analysis of options available for the management of the febrile child without obvious focus of infection that the average cost per major infection prevented of the optimal alternative in their analysis was about $50,503 while that for the least effective alternative examined was $66,758. Downs et al.

(1991) found in their decision analysis that the optimal strategy
resulted in 69.99 quality-adjusted life-years and prevented 60 events of
death or permanent disability as compared to the least effective
strategy, which resulted in 69.96 additional quality-adjusted life-
years. The appropriate management of the many children under 3 years
old who present to health care providers with fever without obvious
source of infection may result in improved health outcomes.

EFFICACY AND/OR EFFECTIVENESS OF INTERVENTIONS

Screening

Screening for fever is not a routine aspect of health care for
children less than 36 months old. Prevention of the sequelae of
possible bacteremia or sepsis include instructing parents to monitor the
acutely ill child for signs and symptoms of bacteremia or sepsis,
including the proper measurement of temperature, as detailed below.

Diagnosis

The goal of diagnosis is initially to confirm the presence of
fever. The determination of the source of the fever, when it is not
initially apparent, is reserved until the presence of fever is
established. If the child is without fever upon evaluation of the
health care provider, further evaluation may be undertaken based on
other signs or symptoms, including a temperature measured by the parent
at home, especially if by rectal thermometry. One cannot rely on a
report of tactile temperature. In one study, axillary glass thermometry
in a group of children younger than six years of age had a sensitivity
of 33.3 percent in detecting fever with a specificity of 97.3 percent
compared to rectal thermometry (Kresch, 1984). A similar finding was
made with electronic thermometry comparing axillary temperatures to oral
and rectal temperatures (Ogren, 1990). Oral or rectal thermometry are
thought to be the most accurate methods, with rectal temperatures being
about 1 degree Fahrenheit higher than oral temperatures (Bonadio, 1993).
Devices measuring skin temperature with temperature-sensitive liquid
crystals are inaccurate because they underestimate core body
temperature, and problems also exist with infrared ear thermometry

(Bonadio, 1993). Temperatures may also be affected by overbundling with blankets and clothing and the administration of acetaminophen and other antipyretics (Bonadio, 1993). The degree of reduction in temperature with administration of acetaminophen is not related to the probability of a serious bacterial illness, nor is the improvement in clinical appearance with defervescence (Baker et al., 1989). Baker et al. (1989) also concluded that administration of acetaminophen prior to evaluation may interfere with the health care provider's assessment of the child.

Though the range of normal body temperatures is thought to be 36.2 to 37.8 degrees centigrade, fever itself is not well-defined (Bonadio, 1993). For infants less than 3 months of age, fever is usually defined as a body temperature greater than or equal to 38 degrees centigrade; for children older than 3 months, the threshold temperature for fever is between 37.7 and 38.3 degrees centigrade (Bonadio, 1993). In one study, the median value defined as fever was 38.0°C by pediatric residency directors and 38.1°C by emergency department residency directors (Baraff, 1991). An expert panel reviewed that study and, based on the clinical opinion of its individual members, defined the threshold temperature as 38.0°C taken rectally (Baraff et al., 1993).

Treatment

Once the presence of fever is established, the physician must decide which febrile infants require further evaluation and treatment. In that sense, the treatment of fever or its therapeutic intervention is the diagnosis of the need for further work-up and treatment of potentially serious bacterial infections. Much effort has been spent trying to identify clinical indicators of bacteremia or serious bacterial infections in the febrile child without obvious source of infection that would indicate the need for further work-up and then specific treatment; however, the results have not been conclusive. Clinical judgments for identifying high risk among febrile infants have been shown to be inadequate (McCarthy et al., 1980; Lieu et al., 1991; Baraff et al., 1993; Harper and Fleisher, 1993). Early studies by McCarthy and colleagues (1985, 1987) indicated that an Acute Illness Observation Scale, which attempted to quantify the quality of cry, reaction to parent stimulation, state variation, color, hydration, and response to social overtures, might have utility in identifying febrile infants at high risk. In a study of 4- to 8-week-old infants, however, the Acute Illness Observation Scale had a sensitivity of only 46 percent in identifying serious illness and 33 percent in identifying bacterial disease (Baker et al., 1990). Baraff et al. (1993), in their Bayesian review of the literature, concluded that the Observation Scale was inadequate to discriminate between febrile infants with and without bacteremia. Despite their reservations, Baraff and his colleagues still recommended that the clinician make a gestalt assessment of the young febrile infant as toxic-appearing or not--that is, meeting the "clinical picture consistent with the sepsis syndrome (lethargy, signs of poor perfusion, or marked hypoventilation, hyperventilation, or cyanosis)" (Baraff et al., 1993).

Other clinical indicators of risk for bacteremia and serious bacterial infection among febrile children have been evaluated. Harper and Fleischer (1993) noted that a higher temperature was associated with a higher risk of bacteremia; however, they concluded that response to antipyretics was not a useful indicator. The leukocyte count may be a useful indicator of risk; Harper and Fleisher (1993) and Lieu et al. (1991) both cited a study that estimated the sensitivity in identifying bacteremia in a febrile child with a leukocyte count above 10,000/microliter at 92 percent. An increased band cell count, an increased erythrocyte sedimentation rate, and an increased C-reactive protein did not add utility to the leukocyte count (Harper and Fleisher, 1993). Blood culture, cerebrospinal fluid studies and culture, urinalysis, urine gram stain, and urine culture are helpful in identifying specific bacterial infections. The blood culture has been estimated to have a sensitivity of 70 percent in identifying bacteremia (Lieu et al., 1991). The chest radiograph may be helpful in identifying pneumonia in the infant or child with signs of lower respiratory infection. The stool smear and stool culture assists with the identification of bacterial enteritis in the infant or child with diarrhea (Baraff et al., 1993).

The Rochester Criteria, developed at the University of Rochester, combine history, physical examination, and laboratory findings to identify febrile children, particularly infants less than one year old who are at risk of bacteremia or a serious bacterial infection (Jaskiewicz et al., 1994). The child is considered to be at low risk for bacteremia or a serious bacterial infection if all the following criteria are met:

1. Infant appears generally well.

2. Infant has been previously healthy

    a. born at term ($\geq$37 weeks gestation)

    b. did not receive perinatal antimicrobial therapy

    c. was not treated for unexplained hyperbilirubinemia

    d. had not received and was not receiving antimicrobial agents

    e. had not been previously hospitalized

    f. had no chronic underlying illness

    g. was not hospitalized longer than mother

3. No evidence of skin, soft tissue, bone, joint, or ear infection

4. Laboratory values:

    a. peripheral blood white blood count 5.0 to 15.0 x 10^9 cells/L

    b. absolute band form count $\leq$1.5 x 10^9 cells/L

    c. $\leq$10 WBC per high power field (x40) on microscopic examination of a spun urine sediment

    d. $\leq$5 WBC per high power field (x40) on microscopic examination of a stool smear (only for infants with diarrhea)

In a recent study, the negative predictive value of the Rochester Criteria was estimated at 98.9 percent in ruling out serious bacterial infection and 99.5 percent in ruling out bacteremia (Jaskiewicz et al., 1994). A previous meta-analytic study had found that the probability of a serious bacterial infection declined from a baseline of 7 percent to 0.2 percent if the Rochester criteria for low risk were met (Klassen and Rowe, 1992). McCarthy (1994), in commenting on the Jaskiewicz et al. (1994) study, which advocates applying the Rochester criteria to infants less than 28 days of age, notes that another study evaluating the Rochester Criteria found a much lower negative predictive value of 95.1

percent for serious bacterial illnesses with a sensitivity of 67.5 percent. A sensitivity of 52 percent was estimated in a study done at a pediatric emergency room at an academic center (Baskin et al., 1992). In another commentary, he recommends that, because of the low sensitivity of the Rochester Criteria, the initial evaluation and therapeutic intervention be based on clinical examination and a full, rather than the partial, septic work-up of the Rochester criteria (McCarthy, 1993). Baraff et al. (1993), using Bayesian meta-analysis, estimated the probability of a serious bacterial infection at 0.2 percent in a febrile infant less than or equal to 90 days of age who is also at low risk based on the Rochester Criteria.

Several recent literature reviews contain recommendations regarding the intervention in an infant or child with fever. Lieu et al. (1991), performed a decision analysis using information from the literature, comparing six strategies for treating the child with fever aged 3 to 36 months old:

1. no intervention
2. treatment alone with oral amoxicillin
3. blood culture alone
4. blood culture and oral amoxicillin
5. blood culture with the decision to use oral amoxicillin based on a leukocyte count threshold of 10,000
6. blood culture and oral amoxicillin based on clinical judgment alone

Management of positive blood cultures was dependent on the organism. Other management issues and outcomes considered were hospitalization, intravenous antibiotics, repeat blood culture, and reactions to antibiotic therapy. Lieu et al. (1991) concluded that the lowest base cost per adverse outcome (i.e., any serious bacterial infection) prevented was options 4 or 5. The decision analysis was sensitive to the specificity of the blood culture, the leukocyte count threshold value, the sensitivity of clinical judgment, the effectiveness of the initial treatment, the cost of the initial treatment, the cost of the leukocyte count, and the cost of hospitalization for pneumococcal bacteremia (Lieu et al., 1991).

Downs et al. (1991), performed a decision analysis looking at the child 2 to 24 months of age with fever greater than or equal to 39°C and compared the following strategies:

1. obtaining a blood culture and empiric treatment with antibiotics;

2. obtaining a blood culture and treating based on a leukocyte count; or

3. watchful waiting.

Based on quality-adjusted life-years, the authors found that empiric treatment with antibiotics and blood culture was the optimal treatment alternative. This finding remained true as long as the probability of bacteremia was above 1.4 percent and the efficacy of treatment was above 21 percent (Downs et al., 1991). A multicenter prospective, randomized study also found that children at high risk of occult bacteremia, as defined by fever greater than or equal to 39.5°C, a high white blood cell count greater than or equal to 15 x 10^9 per liter, and no focus of infection, benefited from intramuscular ceftriaxone treatment as compared to treatment with amoxicillin/potassium clavulanate (Bass et al., 1993).

Baraff et al. (1993) made recommendations based on a Bayesian meta-analytic review of the literature and the final determination of an expert panel. The meta-analysis estimated that the negative predictive probability of a serious bacterial infection was 99.3 percent among nontoxic, low-risk infants less than 28 days of age, with a 95 percent confidence interval ranging from 98.0 percent to 99.9 percent. Though the rationale was not explicitly stated in the article,[1] the expert panel recommended that all febrile infants less than 28 days of age be hospitalized for sepsis evaluation, including complete blood count, urinalysis, cerebrospinal fluid glucose, protein, and cell count, and cultures of blood, urine, and cerebrospinal fluid. While they thought intravenous antibiotics should most likely be administered, they left that decision to the discretion of the physician.

---

[1]This is probably because the estimate was based on a single study.

For infants 28 to 90 days old at low risk for bacteremia or serious bacterial infection determined using the Rochester Criteria, Baraff et al. (1993) felt outpatient evaluation was appropriate if the parents or caretakers were reliable and close follow-up was possible. In infants meeting these criteria, a blood culture and urine culture were recommended as well as a lumbar puncture and a stool culture in infants with bloody diarrhea or with >5 white blood cells per high power field in the stool. In a previous publication, lumbar puncture was recommended for infants less than 8 weeks of age (Baraff et al., 1992). In the most recent guidelines, Baraff, et al. (1993) recommend intramuscular ceftriaxone, which would warrant a prior lumbar puncture in any case. Though by the Rochester Criteria infants with otitis media would be considered at high risk for bacteremia or serious bacterial infection, Baraff et al. (1993) decided that infants with otitis media could be considered at low risk though they do not cite evidence to support this recommendation.

Follow-up of these 28- to 90-day-old infants would occur in 18 to 24 hours with a second dose of intramuscular ceftriaxone given. If the infant had otitis media, oral antibiotics would be prescribed if the initial cultures were negative. If the initial blood or cerebrospinal fluid culture was positive, the infant was to be admitted for parenteral antibiotics. An exception was made for pneumococcal bacteremia in the afebrile, normal appearing infant who could be treated as an outpatient on oral amoxicillin and with close follow-up. If the initial urine culture was positive and the infant was afebrile, nontoxic in appearance, with a negative blood culture, that infant could be treated as an outpatient on oral antibiotics with outpatient radiologic work-up. An alternative approach for the low risk febrile infant 28 to 90 days old is to obtain a urine culture and to withhold antibiotics (Baraff et al., 1993). In this case, the blood and cerebrospinal fluid cultures are optional, and follow-up again occurs at 24 hours. Parental preferences for these treatment options were elicited (Oppenheim et al., 1994). Though knowing the possible risks of serious bacterial infections, 78.8 percent of parents preferred the option without lumbar puncture and without antibiotics because it entailed less pain, less time, and less medication, yet included the follow-up visit (Oppenheim et al., 1994). The febrile infant aged 28 to 90 days who is not low risk as determined by the Rochester Criteria, with the exception of infants with otitis media as noted above, should be hospitalized for sepsis evaluation and parenteral antibiotics (Baraff et al., 1993).

In the case of the child aged 3 to 36 months old with fever without obvious source of infection, Baraff et al. (1993) recommended the following treatment. If the child does not appear toxic and the temperature is less than 39°C, no further work-up or intervention is recommended unless the fever persists for greater than 48 hours or the clinical condition deteriorates. If the child does not appear toxic but has a temperature greater than or equal to 39°C, various decisions with regard to evaluation and treatment are made. A urine culture is obtained for males less than six months of age and females less than two years of age. Stool culture is obtained for patients with blood and mucus in the stool or with greater than 5 white blood cells per high power field in the stool. A chest radiograph is obtained for children with lower respiratory symptoms. A blood culture may be obtained and empiric antibiotic therapy administered based on temperature alone or on temperature and the leukocyte count. Parental preferences were elicited for the options of obtaining a blood culture and empiric antibiotic treatment versus blood culture and antibiotics based on a white blood count (Oppenheim et al., 1994); 67.1 percent of parents preferred to base the need for blood culture and antibiotics on a white blood count (Oppenheim et al., 1994). In any case, a follow-up evaluation must be done by the clinician (i.e., interval history, examination, and review of laboratory results, specifically cultures) within 24 to 48 hours of the initial evaluation. If the blood culture is positive for pneumococcus and the patient has a persistent fever, the child should be admitted to the hospital for sepsis evaluation and parenteral antibiotics. For bacteremia with other bacteria, hospital admission is automatic for sepsis evaluation and parenteral antibiotics. If the urine culture is positive, the child is admitted if febrile or ill-appearing. If the febrile child aged 3 to 36 months appears toxic, then the child is admitted to the hospital from the outset for sepsis evaluation and parenteral antibiotics. Much of the decision making is thus based on the subjective assessment of the clinician (Baraff et al., 1993).

A recent study surveyed primary-care pediatricians in Utah as to their adherence to these guidelines (Young, 1995). Based on case scenarios, these pediatricians managed febrile infants with fewer laboratory tests and hospitalizations than recommended by the Baraff guidelines (Young, 1995). Young (1995) concludes that until immunization programs are successful against all serious bacterial pathogens or a test is developed that effectively identifies bacteremic children that "clinicians will find the [Baraff] practice guidelines a helpful standard against which to compare their management of nontoxic febrile infants."

Follow-up

Required follow-up care is described under treatment.

RECOMMENDED QUALITY INDICATORS FOR FEVER IN CHILDREN UNDER 3 YEARS OF AGE

The following clinical indicators apply to children less than 36 months of age.

Diagnosis

	Indicator	Quality of evidence	Literature	Benefits	Comments
1.	The diagnosis of fever should be based on a temperature measurement of 38 degrees centigrade or greater taken at home or in the medical setting.	III	Bonadio, 1990; Baraff et al., 1993; Bonadio, 1993	Prevent morbidity or mortality due to untreated serious bacterial infection.*	The presence of fever when based on parental report is more likely if based on an actual measurement rather than just a feel of the child's skin surface. Though the method and site of thermometry may also affect the temperature reading, more errors would be in a falsely low temperature than a falsely high temperature.
2.	The health care provider should document if the child had received an antipyretic and, if so, the time and the dose.	II-2	Baker et al., 1989	Prevent morbidity or mortality due to untreated serious bacterial infection.*	The health care provider may avoid a false negative confirmation of the presence of fever or of clinical appearance of serious illness if assessment is tempered with knowledge of recent acetaminophen administration to the child with fever. Temperature was reduced in children with occult bacteremia given acetaminophen; the clinical appearance of serious illness was greater prior to acetaminophen administration in children with occult bacteremia compared to following acetaminophen administration.
3.	The health care provider should document a temperature measured by oral or rectal thermometry in the medical setting.	III	Bonadio, 1993	Prevent morbidity or mortality due to untreated serious bacterial infection.*	The method and site of thermometry may also affect the temperature reading. More errors would be in a falsely low temperature than a falsely high temperature if only measuring skin surface temperatures or tympanic membrane temperatures.
	Treatment regardless of age				
4.	In all children presenting with fever, the child's age should be recorded.	III	Baraff et al., 1993	Reduce risk of serious bacterial infection with fever and the attendant risks of morbidity and mortality.	Treatment is modified based on the child's age. Baraff et al. (1993) presents a guideline based on meta-analytic review and expert panel opinion.
5.	In all children presenting with fever, the following should be documented: a. heart rate; b. respiratory rate; and c. blood pressure.	III		Reduce risk of cardiovascular compromise.	A review of the vital signs should aid the health care provider in assessing for the presence of sepsis.

240

Treatment for the infant less than 28 days of age presenting with fever (T>38.0)

#	Recommendation	Grade	References	Objective	Comments
6.	If the infant has fever, the infant should be hospitalized.	III	Baraff et al., 1993; McCarthy, 1994	Prevent mortality and morbidity due to untreated infection.*	The infant less than 28 days of age is felt to be functionally immunocompromised compared to the older child and at particular risk of serious bacterial infection with the presence of fever and at risk of significant mortality and morbidity. Aggressive treatment (e.g., hospitalization and full septic work-up) are required. Baraff et al. (1993) presents a guideline based on meta-analytic review and expert panel opinion.
7.	The assessment should include: a. a complete blood count, b. urinalysis, c. cerebrospinal fluid analysis of glucose and protein, d. gram stain, e. cell count, f. blood culture, g. urine culture, and h. cerebrospinal fluid culture.	III	Baraff et al., 1993	Prevent mortality and morbidity due to untreated infection.*	The most likely sites of bacterial infection in the child under 28 days old with fever would include the blood, the urine, and the cerebrospinal fluid; so, work-up should concentrate in these areas to avoid missing treatment of these serious bacterial infections.
8.	If the infant has lower respiratory symptoms, a chest radiograph should be obtained.	II-2	Patterson, 1990; Crain et al., 1991; Baraff et al., 1993	Reduce morbidity from pulmonary disease.	The yield of chest radiographs in detecting lower respiratory infections is quite low (estimates range from 0-3%) if specific respiratory signs are absent in the infant. Obtaining a chest radiograph only in the presence of one of these symptoms decreases unnecessary use of resources. Though 30% reduction in use is possible. A respiratory rate of 60 was chosen by Crain et al. (1991) in their study of infants less than 8 weeks old, one could make an argument for a threshold of 40. Baraff et al. (1993) present a guideline based on meta-analytic review and expert opinion. Lower respiratory symptoms are defined as tachypnea, grunting, flaring, retractions, decreased breath sounds, rales, or rhonchi. Tachypnea is defined as a respiratory rate above 60.
9.	If the infant has bloody diarrhea or a fecal leukocyte count >= 5 leukocytes per high power field, a stool culture should be obtained.	II-2,	DeWitt et al., 1985; Finkelstein et al., 1989; Baraff et al., 1993	Reduce morbidity/mortality from bacterial infection.*	The likelihood of bacterial diarrhea increases with the presence of bloody diarrhea (likelihood ratio 13.5) or the presence of leukocytes in the stool smear thus increasing the yield of a stool culture. Baraff et al. (1993) present a guideline based on meta-analytic review and expert opinion.

#	Recommendation	Level	Citation	Outcome	Comments
10.	If the infant is nontoxic and at low risk,** then the infant should be treated with empiric antibiotics.	III	Baraff et al., 1993	Reduce morbidity/mortality from serious bacterial infection.*	
11.	If the infant is toxic in appearance (e.g., lethargic; poor perfusion; or marked hypoventilation, hyperventilation, or cyanosis), or at high risk,** then the infant should be treated with empiric parenteral antibiotics pending the culture results.	III	Baraff et al., 1993	Reduce morbidity/mortality from serious bacterial infection.*	
12.	If: • any culture is positive, or • the cerebrospinal fluid studies are abnormal, or • the chest radiograph demonstrates an infiltrate or effusion, or • skin, soft tissue, bone, joint, or ear infection are present, then the infant should be treated with parenteral antimicrobials.	III	Baraff et al., 1993; Baraff et al., 1992	Decrease morbidity/mortality from serious bacterial infection.*	This review does not deal with the specific management issues for specific diagnoses. If the health care provider strongly feels the infant is bacteremic or septic, even with negative laboratory assessment, the health care provider would treat empirically with a full course of antibiotics. A meta-analytic review found that parenteral antibiotic treatment of occult bacteremia decreased the subsequent mean probability of meningitis from 9.8 to 0.3 percent.

Treatment for the infant 28 to 90 days of age with fever (>38°C)

#	Recommendation	Level	Citation	Outcome	Comments
13.	The assessment should document whether or not the infant appears toxic, i.e., if the infant has signs of sepsis based on: • lethargy, • poor perfusion, or • hypoventilation, hyperventilation, or cyanosis.	II-2	Baraff et al., 1993; Jaskiewicz et al., 1994	Reduce morbidity/mortality from serious bacterial infection.*	These are based in part on the Rochester criteria for determining which febrile infants, without obvious focus of infection, are at low risk for bacteremia or other serious bacterial infection. Infants who meet all criteria are deemed nontoxic and at low risk and those who are toxic are automatically at high risk.
14.	The assessment should include whether or not the infant had been healthy up to the point of this illness.†	II-2	Baraff et al., 1993; Jaskiewicz et al., 1994	Reduce morbidity/mortality from serious bacterial infection.*	These are based in part on the Rochester criteria for determining which febrile infants, without obvious focus of infection, are at low risk for bacteremia or other serious bacterial infection. Infants who meet all criteria are deemed nontoxic and at low risk and those who are toxic are automatically at high risk.
15.	All children who present with fever > 39°C should receive: a) CBC b) UA.	III	Baraff et al., 1993	Prevent mortality and morbidity due to untreated infection.*	
16.	If the child has fever and diarrhea, a fecal leucocyte evaluation should be done.	II-2	Baraff et al., 1993	Prevent mortality and morbidity due to untreated infection.*	

#	Recommendation		Citation		Comments
17.	If the infant is at high risk, the infant should be hospitalized.	III	Baraff et al., 1993	Avoid morbidity/mortality from serious bacterial infections.*	The infant 28-90 days of age at high risk based on the above criteria which are based on the Rochester criteria will have a higher probability of a serious bacterial infection and will require a complete work-up consisting of hospitalization and full septic work-up.
18.	If the infant is toxic or at high risk, the assessment should also include: a. cerebrospinal fluid analysis of glucose and protein, b. gram stain, c. cell count, d. blood culture, e. urine culture, and f. cerebrospinal fluid culture.	III	Baraff et al., 1993	Avoid morbidity/mortality from serious bacterial infections.*	The most likely sites of bacterial infection in the infant 28 to 90 days of age who are at high risk include the blood, the urine, and the cerebrospinal fluid; so, work-up should concentrate in these areas.
19.	If the infant is not toxic and is at low risk, the infant may be managed as an outpatient. One of the following courses should be followed: a. Obtain cerebrospinal fluid for glucose, protein, gram stain, and cell count determination; obtain blood, urine, and cerebrospinal fluid cultures; and, administer intramuscular ceftriaxone; or b. Obtain at least a urine culture and withhold antimicrobial treatment.	III	Baraff et al., 1993	Prevent morbidity due to untreated serious bacterial infection.*	The probability of a serious bacterial infection in an infant at low risk is 0.2 percent. This estimate was based on two studies. Close follow-up is warranted in these cases.
20.	If the infant with fever is at low risk and is being managed as an outpatient, the infant's condition should be reassessed in 18-24 hours in the medical care setting.	III	Baraff et al., 1993	Prevent morbidity due to untreated serious bacterial infection.*	
21.	If the infant who was initially nontoxic and at low risk is still nontoxic at follow-up in the outpatient setting, then: a. under the first course: - a second dose of ceftriaxone is administered, and - the culture results are reviewed; and b. under the second course - the culture result(s) are reviewed.	III	Baraff et al., 1993	Prevent morbidity due to untreated serious bacterial infection.*	
22.	The infant who was nontoxic and initially at low risk and was still nontoxic and at low risk on first follow-up in the outpatient setting should receive another follow-up in the medical care setting within 24 hours.	III		Prevent morbidity due to untreated serious bacterial infection.*	In many laboratories, the final reading of cerebrospinal fluid and urine cultures does not occur until two days after collection of the specimen.

#	Recommendation	Level	Reference	Objective	Rationale
23.	If the infant with fever has lower respiratory symptoms, a chest radiograph should be obtained.	II-2, III	Patterson, 1990; Crain et al., 1991; Baraff et al., 1993	Reduce morbidity from pulmonary infection.	The yield of chest radiographs in detecting lower respiratory infections is quite low (0-3%) if specific respiratory signs are absent in the infant. Obtaining a chest radiograph only in the presence of one of these symptoms decreases unnecessary use of resources. Though a respiratory rate of 60 was chosen by Crain et al. (1991) in their study of infants less than 8 weeks of age, one could make an argument for a threshold of 40. Baraff et al. (1993) presents a guideline based on meta-analytic review and expert panel opinion. Lower respiratory symptoms are defined as tachypnea, grunting, flaring, retractions, decreased breath sounds, rales, or rhonchi. Tachypnea is defined as a respiratory rate greater than 60 breaths per minute.
24.	If the infant with fever has bloody diarrhea or a fecal leukocyte count greater than 5 leukocytes per high power field, a stool culture should be obtained.	II-2	DeWitt et al., 1985; Finkelstein et al., 1989; Baraff et al., 1993	Reduce risk of morbidity and mortality from serious bacterial infection.*	The likelihood of bacterial diarrhea increases with the presence of bloody diarrhea or the presence of leukocytes in the stool smear thus increasing the yield of a stool culture. Baraff et al. (1993) presents a guideline based on meta-analytic review and expert panel opinion.
25.	If at any point the blood culture is positive, the infant should be hospitalized for parenteral antibiotic treatment appropriate to the specific diagnosis except in the case of bacteremia due to *Streptococcus pneumonia*.	III	Baraff et al., 1993	Reduce risk of morbidity and mortality from serious bacterial infection.*	Any serious bacterial infection warrants inpatient parenteral antibiotic therapy for successful treatment. Oral amoxicillin or penicillin is appropriate in the afebrile, well-appearing infant with bacteremia due to pneumococcus.
26.	If at any point the urine culture is positive, the infant should be hospitalized for parenteral antibiotic treatment appropriate to the specific diagnosis except in the case of an afebrile and nontoxic infant.	III	Baraff et al., 1993	Reduce risk of morbidity and mortality from serious bacterial infection.*	Any serious bacterial infection warrants inpatient parenteral antibiotic therapy for successful treatment. Outpatient oral antibiotic therapy is appropriate in the afebrile, well-appearing infant with a positive urine culture, as long as close follow-up and radiologic work-up is done.
27.	If at any point the cerebrospinal fluid results are abnormal or the cerebrospinal fluid culture is positive, the infant should be hospitalized for parenteral antimicrobial treatment appropriate to the specific diagnosis.	III	Baraff et al., 1993	Reduce risk of morbidity and mortality from serious bacterial infection.*	Any serious bacterial infection warrants inpatient parenteral antibiotic therapy for successful treatment.
28.	If at any point pneumonia is diagnosed, the infant should be hospitalized for parenteral antimicrobial treatment appropriate to the specific diagnosis.	III	Baraff et al., 1993	Reduce risk of morbidity and mortality from serious bacterial infection.*	Any serious bacterial infection warrants inpatient parenteral antibiotic therapy for successful treatment.

No.	Recommendation		Reference	Objective	Comments
29.	If at any point a skin, soft tissue, bone, or joint infection is diagnosed, the infant should be hospitalized for parenteral antimicrobial treatment appropriate to the specific diagnosis.	III	Baraff et al., 1993	Reduce risk of morbidity and mortality from serious bacterial infection.*	Any serious bacterial infection warrants inpatient parenteral antibiotic therapy for successful treatment.
	Treatment for the child 3 to 36 months of age				
30.	The assessment should document: a. the level of consciousness, b. the temperature, c. the heart rate, d. the respiratory rate, e. the blood pressure, f. the perfusion, g. the degree of cyanosis.	III	Baraff et al., 1993	Reduce risk of cardiovascular compromise. Reduce risk of morbidity and mortality from serious bacterial infection.*	A review of the vital signs, level of consciousness, perfusion, and skin color should aid the health care provider in assessing for the presence of sepsis, a possible complication of any serious bacterial infection. Baraff et al. (1993) presents a guideline based on meta-analytic review and expert panel opinion.
31.	If the infant/child is at high risk for sepsis,** the infant should be hospitalized.	III	Baraff et al., 1993	Reduce risk of morbidity and mortality from serious bacterial infection.*	The child 3 to 36 months of age at high risk based on criteria for sepsis will have a higher probability of a serious bacterial infection and will require a complete work-up consisting of hospitalization and full septic work-up. The risk status of the child will affect which treatment options the health care provider will undertake. The older febrile child with toxic appearance has a 10-90% chance of a serious bacterial infection.
32.	If the infant/child is at high risk for sepsis,** the assessment should include a complete blood count; urinalysis; cerebrospinal fluid analysis of glucose, protein, gram stain, and cell count; and, blood, urine, and cerebrospinal fluid cultures.	III	Baraff et al., 1993	Reduce risk of morbidity and mortality from serious bacterial infection.*	The most likely sites of bacterial infection in the child 3 to 36 months of age at high risk include the blood, the urine, and the cerebrospinal fluid; so, work-up should concentrate in these areas to avoid missing treatment of these serious bacterial infections.
33.	If the infant/child is at low risk for sepsis** and the temperature is greater than or equal to 39°C and there is no obvious source of infection, a urine culture should be obtained if the child is a female less than two years of age or a male less than six months of age.	III	Baraff et al., 1993	Reduce risk of morbidity and mortality from serious bacterial infection.*	Male children are at greater risk for urinary tract infections under the age of six months, and female children are at greater risk for urinary tract infections under the age of two years. If the infant/child has a urinary tract infection, appropriate treatment and further evaluation of the urinary tract, e.g., renal ultrasound and vesicoureterogram, will be required.
34.	If the infant/child is at low risk for sepsis** and the temperature is greater than or equal to 39°C and diarrhea is present, a stool culture should be obtained if there is blood and mucus in the stool or if there are ≥5 leukocytes per high power field in the stool.	II-2	DeWitt et al., 1985; Finkelstein et al., 1989; Baraff et al., 1993	Reduce risk of morbidity and mortality from serious bacterial infection.*	The likelihood of bacterial diarrhea increases with the presence of bloody diarrhea or the presence of leukocytes in the stool smear thus increasing the yield of a stool culture. Baraff et al. (1993) presents a guideline based on meta-analytic review and expert panel opinion.

245

#	Recommendation	Rating	Citation	Objective	Comments
35.	If the infant/child is at low risk for sepsis** and the temperature is greater than or equal to 39°C, a chest radiograph should be obtained in a child with dyspnea, tachypnea, rales, or decreased breath sounds.	III, II-2	Patterson, 1990; Crain et al., 1991; Baraff et al., 1993	Reduce morbidity from pulmonary disease.	The yield of chest radiographs in detecting lower respiratory infections is quite low (0-3%) if specific respiratory signs are absent in the infant. Obtaining a chest radiograph only in the presence of one of these symptoms decreases unfruitful use of resources. These references do not define tachypnea except for a respiratory rate greater than 60 in the infant less than 8 weeks old in Crain et al. (1991). Baraff et al. (1993) presents a guideline based on meta-analytic review and expert panel opinion. Tachypnea is defined as a respiratory rate (breaths per minute) above: • 40 for infants/children age 3 months to one year, and • 30 for children 1-3 years old.
36.	If the infant/child is at low risk for sepsis** and the temperature is greater than or equal to 39°C, then: a. a blood culture should be obtained, and b. the child should be treated empirically with parenteral antibiotics.	III	Baraff et al., 1993	Prevent morbidity due to untreated serious bacterial infection.*	The risk of occult bacteremia in the febrile 3 to 36 month old infant/child is 4.3 percent with a 95 percent confidence interval of 2.6 percent to 6.5 percent.
37.	If the infant/child is at low risk for sepsis** and the temperature is greater than or equal to 39°C, then: a. a blood culture should be obtained, and b. a CBC should be obtained, and c. the child should be treated with antibiotics only if the WBC is ≥15,000.	III	Baraff et al., 1993	Prevent morbidity due to untreated serious bacterial infection.*	The risk of occult bacteremia in the febrile 3 to 36 month old infant/child is 4.3 percent with a 95 percent confidence interval of 2.6 percent to 6.5 percent.
38.	If the infant/child is at low risk for sepsis** and the temperature is greater than or equal to 39°C, then the infant/child should be reassessed in 24-48 hours in the medical setting.	III	Baraff et al., 1993	Prevent morbidity due to untreated serious bacterial infection.*	
39.	If the infant/child at low risk for sepsis** with an initial temperature greater than or equal to 39°C is well-appearing at outpatient follow-up, no further intervention is required; but, the parent should be advised to return if the fever persists greater than 48 hours.	III	Baraff et al., 1993	Prevent morbidity/mortality from serious bacterial infection.*	
40.	If at any point the blood culture is positive, the infant/child should be hospitalized for parenteral antibiotic treatment appropriate to the specific diagnosis except in the case of bacteremia due to Streptococcus pneumonia.	III	Baraff et al., 1993	Reduce risk of morbidity and mortality from serious bacterial infection.*	Any serious bacterial infection warrants inpatient parenteral antibiotic therapy for successful treatment. Oral amoxicillin or penicillin is appropriate in the afebrile, well-appearing infant/child with bacteremia due to pneumococcus.

#		Level	Source	Objective	
41.	If at any point the urine culture is positive, the infant/child should be hospitalized for parenteral antibiotic treatment appropriate to the specific diagnosis except in the case of an afebrile, nontoxic infant/child.	III	Baraff et al., 1993	Reduce risk of morbidity and mortality from serious bacterial infection.*	Any serious bacterial infection warrants inpatient parenteral antibiotic therapy for successful treatment. Outpatient oral antibiotic therapy is approrpiate in the afebrile, well-appearing infant/child with a positive urine culture.
42.	If at any point the cerebrospinal fluid results are abnormal or the cerebrospinal fluid culture is positive, the infant/child should be hospitalized for parenteral antimicrobial treatment appropriate to the specific diagnosis.	III	Baraff et al., 1993	Reduce risk of morbidity and mortality from serious bacterial infection.*	Any serious bacterial infection warrants inpatient parenteral antibiotic therapy for successful treatment.
43.	If at any point pneumonia is diagnosed, the infant/child should be hospitalized for parenteral antimicrobial treatment appropriate to the specific diagnosis.	III	Baraff et al., 1993	Reduce risk of morbidity and mortality from serious bacterial infection.*	Any serious bacterial infection warrants inpatient parenteral antibiotic therapy for successful treatment.
44.	If at any point a skin, soft tissue, bone, or joint infection is diagnosed, the infant/child should be hospitalized for parenteral antimicrobial treatment appropriate to the specific diagnosis.	III	Baraff et al., 1993	Reduce risk of morbidity and mortality from serious bacterial infection.*	Any serious bacterial infection warrants inpatient parenteral antibiotic therapy for successful treatment.

Follow-up is included in the treatment indicators.

*Morbidity of serious bacterial (and sometimes viral) infection includes cardiovascular collapse, anoxia, multiorgan failure, and cerebral ischemia.

An infant is considered to be at high risk if any two of the criteria listed below are **not met:
- appears generally well,
- previously healthy,†
- no evidence of skin, soft tissue, bone, joint, or ear infection found, and
- laboratory values negative
  - peripheral blood white blood count 5.0 to 15.0 x 10^9 cells/L,
  - absolute band from count ≤ 1.5 x 10^9 cells/L,
  - ≤ 10 WBC per high-power field (x 40) on microscopic examination of a spun urine sediment, and
  - < 5 WBC per high-power filed (x 40) on microscopic examination of a stool smear (only for infants with diarrhea).
  If all criteria are met, the infant is considered to be at low risk.

High risk in a child 3-36 months of age would be indicated by: lethargy; poor perfusion; hyperventilation, hyperventilation, or cyanosis. An infant meeting none of these criteria is considered to be at low risk.

†An infant is considered to have been previously healthy if all the following apply:
- born at term (≥ 37 weeks' gestation)
- did not receive perinatal, antimicrobial therapy
- was not treated for unexplained hyperbilirubinemia,
- had not received and was not receiving antimicrobial agents,
- had not been previously hospitalized,
- had no chronic underlying illness, and
- was not hospitalized longer than the mother.

247

Quality of Evidence Codes:

I: RCT
II-1:   Nonrandomized controlled trials
II-2:   Cohort or case analysis
II-3:   Multiple time series
III: Opinions or descriptive studies

REFERENCES - FEVER IN CHILDREN UNDER 3 YEARS OF AGE

Baker MD, JR Avner, and LM Bell. 1990. Failure of infant observation scales in detecting serious illness in febrile, 4- to 8-week-old infants. *Pediatrics* 85 (6): 1040-3.

Baker RC, T Tiller, JC Bausher, et al. 1989. Severity of disease correlated with fever reduction in febrile infants. *Pediatrics* 83 (6): 1016-9.

Baraff LJ. 1991. Management of the febrile child: A survey of pediatric and emergency medicine residency directors. *Pediatric Infectious Disease Journal* 10 (11): 795-800.

Baraff LJ, JW Bass, GR Fleisher, et al. 1993. Practice guideline for the management of infants and children 0 to 36 months of age with fever without source. *Pediatrics* 92 (1): 1-12.

Baraff LJ, and SI Lee. 1992. Fever without source: Management of children 3 to 36 months of age. *Pediatric Infectious Disease Journal* 11 (2): 146-51.

Baraff LJ, SI Lee, and DL Schriger. 1993. Outcomes of bacterial meningitis in children: A meta-analysis. *Pediatric Infectious Disease Journal* 12 (5): 389-94.

Baraff LJ, S Oslund, and M Prather. 1993. Effect of antibiotic therapy and etiologic microorganism on the risk of bacterial meningitis in children with occult bacteremia. *Pediatrics* 92 (1): 140-3.

Baraff LJ, SA Oslund, DL Schriger, et al. 1992. Probability of bacterial infections in febrile infants less than three months of age: A meta-analysis. *Pediatric Infectious Disease Journal* 11 (4): 257-64.

Baskin MN. 1993. The prevalence of serious bacterial infections by age in febrile infants during the first 3 months of life. *Pediatric Annals* 22 (8): 462-466.

Baskin MN, EJ O'Rourke, and GR Fleisher. 1992. Outpatient treatment of febrile infants 28 to 89 days of age with intramuscular administration of ceftriaxone. *Journal of Pediatrics* 120 (1): 22-27.

Bass JW, RW Steele, RR Wittler, et al. 1993. Antimicrobial treatment of occult bacteremia: A multicenter cooperative study. *Pediatric Infectious Disease Journal* 12 (6): 466-73.

Bonadio WA. 1993. Defining fever and other aspects of body temperature in infants and children. *Pediatric Annals* 22 (8): 467-73.

Bonadio WA. 1990. Evaluation and management of serious bacterial infections in the febrile young infant. *Pediatric Infectious Disease Journal* 9 (12): 905-12.

Crain EF, D Bulas, PE Bijur, et al. 1991. Is a chest radiograph necessary in the evaluation of every febrile infant less than 8 weeks of age? *Pediatrics* 88 (4): 821-4.

DeAngelis C, A Joffe, M Wilson, et al. 1983. Iatrogenic risks and financial costs of hospitalizing febrile infants. *American Journal Disease of Children* 137: 1146-9.

DeWitt TG, KF Humphrey, and P McCarthy. 1985. Clinical predictors of acute bacterial diarrhea in young children. *Pediatrics* 76 (4): 551-6.

Downs SM, RA McNutt, and PA Margolis. 1991. Management of infants at risk for occult bacteremia: A decision analysis. *Journal of Pediatrics* 118 (1): 11-20.

Finkelstein JA, JS Schwartz, S Torrey, et al. 1989. Common clinical features as predictors of bacterial diarrhea in infants. *American Journal of Emergency Medicine* 7 (5): 469-73.

Harper MB, and GR Fleisher. 1993. Occult bacteremia in the 3-month-old to 3-year-old age group. *Pediatric Annals* 22 (8): 484-93.

Jaskiewicz JA, CA McCarthy, AC Richardson, et al. 1994. Febrile infants at low risk for serious bacterial infection--an appraisal of the Rochester criteria and implications for management. *Pediatrics* 94 (3): 390-96.

Klassen TP, and PC Rowe. 1992. Selecting diagnostic tests to identify febrile infants less than 3 months of age as being at low risk for serious bacterial infection: A scientific review. *Journal of Pediatrics* 121 (5): 671-6.

Kresch MJ. 1984. Axillary temperature as a screening test for fever in children. *Journal of Pediatrics* 104 (4): 596-99.

Lieu TA, S Schwartz, DM Jaffe, et al. 1991. Strategies for diagnosis and treatment of children at risk for occult bacteremia: Clinical effectiveness and cost-effectiveness. *Journal of Pediatrics* 118 (1): 21-9.

McCarthy PL. 1994. The febrile infant (commentary). *Pediatrics* 94 (3): 397-9.

McCarthy PL. 1993. Infants with fever (editorial). *New England Journal of Medicine* 329 (20): 1493-4.

McCarthy PL, JF Jekel, CA Stashwick, et al. 1980. History and observation variables in assessing febrile children. *Pediatrics* 65 (6): 1090-5.

McCarthy PL, RM Lembo, HD Fink, et al. 1987. Observation, history, and physical examination in diagnosis of serious illnesses in febrile children <= 24 months. *Journal of Pediatrics* 110 (1): 26-30.

McCarthy PL, RM Lembo, MA Baron, et al. 1985. Predictive value of abnormal physical examination findings in ill-appearing and well-appearing febrile children. *Pediatrics* 76 (2): 167-171.

National Center for Health Statistics. 1994. *National Ambulatory Medical Care Survey: 1991 summary*. U.S. Department of Health and Human Services, Hyattsville, MD.

Ogren JM. 1990. The inaccuracy of axillary temperatures measured with an electronic thermometer. *American Journal of Diseases of Children* 144: 109-11.

Oppenheim PI, G Sotiropoulos, and LJ Baraff. 1994. Incorporating patient preferences into practice guidelines: Management of children with fever without source. *Annals of Emergency Medicine* 24 (5): 836-41.

Pantell RH, M Naber, R Lamar, et al. 1980. Fever in the first six months of life. *Clinical Pediatrics* 19 (2): 77-82.

Patterson RJ, GS Bisset, DR Kirks, et al. 1990. Chest radiographs in the evaluation of the febrile infant. *American Journal of Radiology* 155: 833-5.

Young PC. 1995. The management of febrile infants by primary-care pediatricians in Utah: Comparisons with published practice guidelines. *Pediatrics* 95 (5): 623-7.

13. HEADACHE[1]

Pablo Lapuerta, M.D., and Steven Asch, M.D., M.P.H.

We identified articles on the evaluation and management of headache
by conducting a MEDLINE search of English language articles between 1990
and 1995 (keywords headache, diagnosis, treatment) and by reviewing two
textbooks on primary care (Pruitt, in Goroll et al., 1995; Bleeker and
Meyd, in Barker et al., 1991) and one for children and adolescents
(Prensky in Oski, 1994). Of the fourteen relevant articles that were
retrieved, nine were review articles and five were observational
studies. Several of these articles addressed the selection of
diagnostic tests and principles of pharmacological management, with a
focus on tension headache and migraine. We did not find controlled
trials that analyzed elements of an appropriate history or physical
examination, and for these topics expert opinion was the primary source
of information.

IMPORTANCE

The prevalence of frequent headaches among children has been
estimated to be 2.5 percent for 7-year-olds and 15.7 among 15-year-olds
(Prensky, in Oski, 1994). Among children presenting to a physician with
headache, about half are experiencing migraines.

EFFICACY AND/OR EFFECTIVENESS OF INTERVENTIONS

Diagnosis

The International Headache Society (IHS) has developed a thorough
and comprehensive etiologic classification system for headaches
(Dalessio, 1994). Common categories include: tension, migraine,
cluster, noncephalic infection (e.g., influenza), head trauma,
intracranial vascular disorders (e.g., hemorrhage), intracranial
nonvascular disorders (e.g., meningitis, neoplasm), substance
withdrawal, and neuralgias. Much of the initial diagnostic work-up for

---

[1]This review was originally prepared for the Women's Quality of
Care Panel.

headaches focuses on distinguishing benign etiologies like tension headaches from the more serious causes like meningitis, hemorrhage, or neoplasm. Once that distinction is made, clinicians should distinguish among the more common benign etiologies in order to prescribe the most efficacious treatment.

All sources recommended a detailed history as the first step in making these distinctions. Essential elements include: temporal profile (chronology, onset, frequency), associated symptoms (nausea, aura, lacrimation, fever), location (unilateral, bilateral, frontal, temporal), severity, and family history (Dalessio, 1994; Bleeker and Meyd, in Barker et al., 1991). There is less confusion about the essential elements of the neurologic examination, though most sources recommend at least an evaluation of the cranial nerves, a fundoscopic examination to rule out papilledema, and examination of reflexes (Dalessio, 1994; Larson et al., 1980; Frishberg, 1994).

One of the most difficult diagnostic decisions in the evaluation of new onset headache is the indications for computerized tomography (CT) and magnetic resonance imaging (MRI) of the head to find structural lesions like arteriovascular malformations, subdural hematomas, and tumors. Several observational studies suggest that a head CT scan is a low-yield evaluation tool in patients with normal neurological examinations (Larson et al., 1980; Masters et al., 1987; Becker et al., 1988; Nelson et al., 1992; Becker et al., 1993; Frishberg, 1994), though even in such patients severe headaches may indicate subarachnoid hemorrhage and constant headaches may indicate intracranial tumors. As a consequence, guidelines from a 1981 National Institutes of Health (NIH) Consensus Panel on the use of CT recommended imaging only when the patient has an abnormal neurological examination or a severe or constant headache (NIH Consensus Statement, 1981). Others have expressed reservations that using severity alone as criteria for head imaging may lead to extensive overuse (Becker et al., 1988). The American Academy of Neurology (1993) previously reviewed 17 case series to define the yield of pathology when CT or MRI scanning is used to evaluate headache patients. In 897 migraine patients, they found only 4 abnormalities, none of which were clinically unsuspected. Of the 1825 patients with headaches and normal neurologic examinations, 2.4 percent had intracranial pathology. Based on these data, the Academy recommended against scanning migraine patients, but concluded there was insufficient evidence to recommend for or against scanning other headache patients with normal neurologic examinations.

Head trauma is another strong indication for imaging. In a study of 3658 head trauma patients, the Skull X-Ray Referral Criteria Panel identified focal neurologic signs, decreasing level of consciousness and penetrating skull injury as indications for CT scanning (Masters et al., 1987). In a separate study of 374 blunt trauma patients there were 7 abnormal head CT results in patients without abnormal neurological findings, but the best initial treatment for these cases was observation alone (Nelson et al., 1992).

While there is still some debate as to the proper indications for CT or MRI in headache patients, there is little controversy surrounding the use of skull radiographs in such patients. Clinical trials have shown skull radiographs to be poor predictors of adverse outcomes in patients with head trauma or others presenting for evaluation of headache (Masters et al., 1987).

Treatment

Our quality indicators address the two most common etiologies for headaches in children and adolescents: migraine and tension headaches. Unlike adults, migraines are more commonly found among males (66 percent vs. 33 percent among adults) (Prensky in Oski, 1994).

The treatment of migraine headache depends on the frequency and severity of symptoms. Placebo-controlled trials support the use of aspirin, acetaminophen, and nonsteroidal anti-inflammatory medications in mild cases. In children under age 5, the usual dose is 1 grain per year of age; for those aged 5-10, the dose is 5 grains; and for those over age 10, the dose is 10 grains (Prensky in Oski, 1994). For more severe pain, clinicians often rely on ergot preparations, antiemetics, opioids, and sumatriptan. Children under 12 should not take more than 3 mg of ergot per headache; older children should not take more than 6 mg (Prensky in Oski, 1994). Though clinical trials have found intravenous dihydroergotamine to be effective in reducing both pain and emergency room use, three clinical trials failed to find any effect of oral ergotamines on migraine pain. Metoclopramide and chlorpromazine also have clinical trial support in the treatment of acute migraine headaches. The newest agent in the migraine pharmacopoeia is sumatriptan, a 5-hydroxytryptamine 1D agonist, available only in injectable form in the United States. Sumatriptan reduced the pain and associated symptoms of migraine headaches in 70 to 90 percent of subjects in several clinical trials (Kumar and Cooney, 1995). However, sumatriptan should not be used concurrently with ergotamine due to an interactive vasoconstrictive effect (Raskin, 1994; Kumar and Cooney, 1995). At the time this was written, the safety and effectiveness of sumatriptan in children had not been established (Physicians' Desk Reference, 1995).

A consensus exists that if a patient has more than two migraine headaches per month then prophylactic treatment is indicated, and this concept has been endorsed by the International Headache Society. The use of beta blockers, valproic acid, calcium channel blockers, tricyclic antidepressants, naproxen, aspirin, cyrohepatadine and valproate are supported by controlled clinical trials. No clinical trials have compared any of these agents with another in preventing migraines (Raskin, 1993; Sheftell, 1993; Raskin, 1994; Rapoport, 1994; Kumar and Cooney, 1995).

Treatment options for tension headaches include aspirin, acetaminophen, and nonsteroidal anti-inflammatory agents. At least one clinical trial found prophylaxis with tricyclic antidepressants to be beneficial. Tension headache and migraine have been considered to be part of a continuum of the same process and as a result clear distinctions between appropriate treatments for the two diagnoses are not always present. While clinical trials support the effectiveness of oral opioid agonists and barbiturates in these two conditions, most sources recommend against initial therapy with these agents due to the risk of dependence. Butorphanal nasal spray has been encouraged as an outpatient opioid agent because it is less addictive and has been shown to reduce emergency room visits for severe migraine headache (Markley, 1994; Kumar, 1994).

Follow-up Care

The need for physician visits depends on the frequency and severity of headache and cannot be precisely defined. Indeed, in the United States, most people who experience headaches do not seek evaluation or treatment from physicians (Kumar and Cooney, 1995). Accepted guidelines for specialist referral are not present in the literature, and most cases of migraine and tension headache can be handled adequately by a primary care physician.

RECOMMENDED QUALITY INDICATORS FOR HEADACHE

These indicators apply to children ages 2 to 18.

Diagnosis

	Indicator	Quality of evidence	Literature	Benefits	Comments
1.	All patients with new onset headache should be asked about: a. Location of the pain (e.g., frontal, bilateral) b. Associated symptoms (e.g., aura) c. Temporal profile (e.g., new onset, constant) d. Severity e. Family history	III	Dalessio, 1994; Larson et al., 1980; Frishberg, 1994	Decrease symptoms of sinusitis (e.g., post nasal drip, fever) and prevent potential complications of mastoiditis, periosteal and epidural abcess. Decrease neurologic symptoms from migraines. Reduce tension headache symptoms and side effects of unwarranted therapy. Preserve neurologic function.	Location can distinguish sinus, tension, and cluster. Associated symptoms can distinguish migraine and cluster headaches. Temporal profile can distinguish cluster, tension, and tumors. Severity can distinguish hemorrhage. Family history can distinguish migraine. Accurate diagnosis of sinusitis can prompt antibiotic or decongestant treatment. Accurate diagnosis of migraine and cluster can prompt treatment (see below). Accurate diagnosis of tension headaches can prompt treatment (see below). Accurate diagnosis of tumors can prompt lifesaving radiation or surgery.
2.	All patients with new onset headache should have a neurological examination evaluating the: a. Cranial nerves b. Fundi c. Deep tendon reflexes	III	Dalessio, 1994; Larson et al., 1980; Frishberg, 1994	Preserve neurologic function.	Abnormal neurologic examination is an indication for CT or MRI scanning. Increased detection of tumors, cerebrovascular accidents and intracranial hemmorhage can lead to lifesaving radiation or surgery.
3.	CT or MRI scanning is indicated in patients with new onset headache and any of the following circumstances: a. Abnormal neurological examination b. Constant headache c. Severe headache	III	NIH Consensus Statement, 1981	Preserve neurologic function.	Recommendations of NIH Consensus Panel on Computed Tomographic Scanning of the Brain.
4.	Skull X-rays should not be part of an evaluation for headache.	II	Masters et al., 1987	Averts side effects (e.g., radiation) of skull X-ray. Averts delays in CT or MRI scanning where indicated.	Four observational trials found a combined incidence of pathology of 0.7% in patients who would not otherwise receive a CT or MRI scan.

258

Treatment

	Indicator	Quality of evidence	Literature	Benefits	Comments
5.	If the patient has an acute mild migraine or tension headache, he or she should receive aspirin, tylenol, or other nonsteroidal anti-inflammatory agents before being prescribed any other medication.	I	Kumar and Cooney, 1995	Reduced migraine symptoms* with fewest side effects from other potential agents.*	More effective than placebo in reducing headaches, nausea and photophobia, but no effect on vomiting.
6.	If the patient has an acute moderate or severe migraine headache, he or she should receive one of the following before being prescribed any other agent: a. Intramuscular ketorolac b. Intravenous dihydroergotamine c. Intravenous chlorpromazine d. Intravenous metaclopramide	I	Kumar and Cooney, 1995; Raskin, 1993; Raskin, 1994; Sheftell, 1993; Rapoport, 1994	Reduced migraine symptoms.*	All listed agents have clinical trial support, but none have been compared against one another. Clinical trials did not find an effect for oral ergot preparations alone, though they have not been evaluated in their usual combination with caffeine or barbiturates. Sumatriptan has not been approved for use in children.
7.	Recurrent moderate or severe tension headaches should be treated with a trial of tricyclic antidepressant agents.	I	Kumar and Cooney, 1995	Reduced rate of tension headache recurrence. Improve quality of life and functioning.	Clinical trials show reduction in pain scores.
8.	If a patient has more than 2 migraine headaches each month, then prophylactic treatment is indicated with one of the following agents: a. Beta blockers b. Calcium channel blockers c. Tricyclic antidepressants d. Naproxen e. Fluoxitene f. Valproate g. Cyproheptadine	I	Kumar and Cooney, 1995; Sheftell, 1993; Markley, 1994	Reduced rate of recurrent migraine symptoms.*	All listed agents have clinical trial support, but none have been compared against one another.
9.	Sumatriptan and ergotamine should not be concurrently administered.	III	Kumar and Cooney, 1995	Averts adverse effects of vasoconstriction: exacerbation of chest pain in ischemic disease, hypertension, painful extremties.	Synergistic effect may cause prolonged vasoconstriction.
10.	Opioid agonists and barbiturates should not be first-line therapy for migraine or tension headaches.	III	Markley, 1994; Kumar, 1994	Averts adverse effects of opiate therapy.*	Other less habit-forming alternative treatment should be tried first. If patient has already tried other medications at home, administration of opioid agonists is not considered first-line.

* Side effects of migraine therapeutic agents include:
Ergotamines: vasoconstriction, exacerbation of coronary artery disease, nausea, abdominal pain, somnolence
Opiates: dependence, somnolence, withdrawal
Phenothiazines: dystonic reactions, anticholinergic reactions, insomnia

Migraine symptoms include: headache, nausea, photophobia, vomiting, phonophobia, scotomota, other focal neurologic symptoms

Quality of Evidence Codes:

I: RCT
II-1:   Nonrandomized controlled trials
II-2:   Cohort or case analysis
II-3:   Multiple time series
III: Opinions or descriptive studies

REFERENCES - HEADACHE

American Academy of Neurology. 1993. *Summary statement: The Utility of Neuroimaging in the Evaluation of Headache in Patients With Normal Neurological Examinations.* American Academy of Neurology, Minneapolis, MN.

Becker LA, LA Green, D Beaufait, et al. 1993. Use of CT scans for the investigation of headache: A report from ASPN, Part 1. *Journal of Family Practice* 37 (2): 129-34.

Becker L, DC Iverson, FM Reed, et al. 1988. Patients with new headache in primary care: A report from ASPN. *Journal of Family Practice* 27 (1): 41-7.

Bleecker ML, and CJ Meyd. 1991. Headaches and facial pain. In *Principles of Ambulatory Medicine*, Third ed. Editors Barker LR, JR Burton, and PD Zieve, 1082-96. Baltimore, MD: Williams and Wilkins.

Dalessio DJ. May 1994. Diagnosing the severe headache. *Neurology* 44 (Suppl. 3): S6-S12.

Frishberg BM. July 1994. The utility of neuroimaging in the evaluation of headache in patients with normal neurologic examinations. *Neurology* 44: 1191-7.

Kumar KL. 1994. Recent advances in the acute management of migraine and cluster headaches. *Journal of General Internal Medicine* 9 (June): 339-48.

Kumar KL, and TG Cooney. 1995. Headaches. *Medical Clinics of North America* 79 (2): 261-86.

Larson EB, GS Omenn, and H Lewis. 25 January 1980. Diagnostic evaluation of headache: Impact of computerized tomography and cost-effectiveness. *Journal of the American Medical Association* 243 (4): 359-62.

Markley HG. May 1994. Chronic headache: Appropriate use of opiate analgesics. *Neurology* 44 (Suppl. 3): S18-S24.

Masters SJ, PM McClean, JS Arcarese, et al. 8 January 1987. Skull x-ray examinations after head trauma: Recommendations by a multidisciplinary panel and validation study. *New England Journal of Medicine* 316 (2): 84-91.

National Institutes of Health. 1981. Computed tomographic scanning of the brain. *NIH consensus statement (online), November 4-6* 4 (2): 1-7.

Nelson JB, MA Bresticker, and DL Nahrwold. November 1992. Computed tomography in the initial evaluation of patients with blunt trauma. *The Journal of Trauma* 33 (5): 722-7.

Physicians' desk reference : PDR : 1995. 49th ed. Montvale, N.J. : Medical Economics Company, 1995.

Prensky AL. 1994. Headache. In *Principles and Practice of Pediatrics*, Second ed. Editors Oski FA, CD DeAngelis, RD Feigin, et al., 2135-2140. Philadelphia, PA: J. B. Lippincott Company.

Pruitt AA. 1995. Approach to the patient with headache. In *Primary Care Medicine: Office Evaluation and Management of the Adult Patient*, Third ed. Editors Goroll AH, LA May, and AG Mulley Jr., 821-9. Philadelphia, PA: J.B. Lippincott Company.

Rapoport AM. May 1994. Recurrent migraine: Cost-effective care. *Neurology* 44 (Suppl. 3): S25-S28.

Raskin NH. 1993. Acute and prophylactic treatment of migraine: Practical approaches and pharmacologic rationale. *Neurology* 43 (Suppl. 3): S39-S42.

Raskin NH. 1994. Headache. In: Neurology-from basics to bedside [Special Issue]. *Western Journal of Medicine* 161 (3): 299-302.

Sheftell FD. August 1993. Pharmacologic therapy, nondrug therapy, and counseling are keys to effective migraine management. *Archives of Family Medicine* 2: 874-9.

14. IMMUNIZATIONS
Mark Schuster, M.D., Ph.D.

The United States Public Health Service Immunization Practice Advisory Committee (ACIP) and the American Academy of Pediatrics (AAP) Committee on Infectious Diseases traditionally provide recommendations for immunization schedules and procedures in the United States (Centers for Disease Control [CDC], 1995). These organizations publish their recommendations primarily in the *Morbidity and Mortality Weekly Report (MMWR)* and the *Red Book*, respectively; their recommendations usually agree (Dennehy et al., in Feigin and Cherry, 1992). This review draws heavily on these recommendations.

In January 1995, the ACIP and the AAP, along with the American Academy of Family Physicians (AAFP), released a joint set of recommendations (CDC, 1995).[1] These organizations developed this immunization schedule in collaboration with representatives from the Food and Drug Administration and the National Institutes of Health. State immunization programs, the Maternal and Child Health Bureau; vaccine manufacturers also provided advice (Hall, 1995).

Additional sources include textbooks on pediatrics (Wilson in Oski et al., 1994), primary care pediatrics (Rennels in Dershewitz, 1993), and pediatric infectious disease (Dennehy et al., in Feigin and Cherry, 1992). Several articles were also identified from the bibliographies of the previously described sources and from a MEDLINE search of English-language articles on missed opportunities (the common term for episodes of clinical interaction in which children who could have been immunized were not) published between January 1990 and March 1995.

IMPORTANCE

Immunizations are the primary method of preventing many communicable diseases. They work both by inducing immunity in the

---

[1]Clinicians who have not adapted to the new immunization schedule from the ACIP's prior schedule (released in the fall, 1993) will not be placed at a disadvantage because the new one only lengthens the time period during which several immunizations are recommended.

recipient and by creating herd immunity in a community that is well-immunized (if more than a threshold percentage of a community is immunized, the disease cannot get enough of a foothold to spread). Thus, there are personal and public health reasons for children to be immunized.

Most (if not all) public school districts require children to have received the full immunization schedule to start school, so the United States has high immunization rates for school-aged children. For example, in the early 1980s, more than 95 percent of school-aged children were completely immunized (Cutts et al., 1992). By contrast, the United States has a poor record for two-year olds, who should have received the primary series for all childhood immunizations. A median of 46 percent of children among various studied populations had completed immunizations by their second birthday (Cutts et al., 1992).[1]

All diseases for which immunizations are routinely recommended can cause serious illness. Hepatitis B is the only disease that is not traditionally associated with childhood. Immunization of children for hepatitis B is recommended primarily because targeted immunization of high-risk adolescents and adults has failed; therefore, the AAP decided to recommend immunization of all infants as well (AAP, 1992).

GENERAL ISSUES PERTINENT TO ALL IMMUNIZATIONS

Contraindications to Immunization

Contraindications specific to individual vaccines are described in the discussions of those vaccines. The following list covers contraindications that apply to all vaccines:

1. Anaphylactic reaction to a vaccine (AAP in Peter, 1994; CDC, 1993b). Clinicians should ask about prior reactions to vaccines.

2. Anaphylactic reaction to a vaccine constituent (AAP in Peter, 1994; CDC, 1993b). Known allergies to specific vaccine

---

[1]These data exclude immunizations for *Haemophilus influenzae* type b (Hib), which were not yet included in most states' school entry requirements.

constituents are rare, so it would be difficult to incorporate clinician inquiries about them into quality indicators.

3. Moderate or severe illnesses with or without a fever (AAP in Peter, 1994; CDC, 1993b). The ACIP/AAP recommendations do not define the distinction between mild vs. moderate/severe illnesses. Even when the ACIP provides an example of a mild illness--a mild upper respiratory infection (URI) with or without low-grade fever (CDC, 1989)--it does not specify what temperature and what thermometer site constitute the cut off for a fever that is higher than low grade. Clinicians are given wide discretion in deciding when to delay immunizations. Researchers conducting studies of missed opportunities (which uniformly show that physicians frequently delay immunizations for mild illnesses) have developed their own criteria for symptoms that warrant immunization delay (Farizo et al., 1992; Szilagyi et al., 1993; McConnochie and Roghmann, 1992), but their protocols have not been widely disseminated and have not become standards for the profession. Thus, there are no published guidelines or professional standards to incorporate into quality indicators for immunization delay. One solution to this problem is to select quality indicators that allow a sufficient grace period so that most children who miss an immunization because of a moderate/severe illness would have had enough time to catch up. The number who do not catch-up because of prolonged or chronic illnesses would be small and so should have little impact on the overall quality score. More comprehensive approaches to measuring quality could be added in the future.

4. Guardian refusal. Guardian refusal (for religious or other reasons) should be documented for legal reasons and so that other clinicians will know the context in which they are offering immunizations at future visits.

Documentation

One component of quality is the quality of documentation. It is important to document specific details such as lot number in case a vaccine lot is recalled later. Documentation standards are set by federal law in the United States. The National Childhood Vaccine Injury Act of 1986, which went into effect in 1988, requires that health care providers record in the child's permanent medical record the date of administration of all childhood-mandated vaccines, the manufacturer, the lot number, and the name of the health care provider administering the vaccine (Dennehy et al., in Feigin and Cherry, 1992).[1]

POLIO

The standard vaccine is oral polio vaccine (OPV), which is a live virus vaccine. An alternative is the inactivated polio vaccine (IPV).

Recommendations

The recommendation is to give OPV at 2 months, 4 months, 6 to 18 months, and 4 to 6 years (CDC, 1995). The first dose can be administered as early as 6 weeks (CDC, 1994).

Children with HIV infection or a known altered immunodeficiency (hematologic and solid tumors, congenital immunodeficiency, and long-term immunosuppressive therapy) (AAP in Peter, 1994; CDC, 1993b) should not receive OPV; instead, they should receive IPV (AAP in Peter, 1994; CDC, 1993b). Elsewhere, the CDC (1993a) provides a more expansive list of immunosuppressive conditions, including congenital immunodeficiency, leukemia, lymphoma, generalized malignancy or therapy with alkylating agents, antimetabolites, radiation, or large amounts of corticosteroids. Pregnancy is a questionable contraindication (AAP in Peter, 1994; CDC, 1993b) but is unlikely to turn up for this population (since most pregnant adolescents would have received the complete polio series in order to attend school). If a pregnant adolescent is at high risk for

---

[1]While Hib (Haemophilus influenza type b) and HBV (Hepatitis b vaccination) were not mandated at the time of this Act, it is safe to assume that they are covered by it now or that it would be viewed as reasonable for a quality indicator to apply the same standards to them that it applies to vaccines that were mandated at the time.

exposure to the against polio virus, OPV rather than IPV should be given (AAP in Peter, 1994; CDC, 1993b). Corticosteroid therapy does not contraindicate live virus vaccination when it is less than two weeks duration, low to moderate dose, long-term alternative day treatment with short-acting preparations, maintenance physiologic doses (replacement therapy), or administered topically (skin or eyes), by aerosol, or by intra-articular, bursal, or tendon injection.

IPV should be given to anyone with a household contact who is immunosuppressed (AAP in Peter, 1994; CDC, 1993b; see list of conditions qualifying as immunosuppression in preceding paragraph). Therefore, an inquiry must be made at each visit about possible immunosuppressed contacts. Some families may not want the household contact's immunosuppression listed in the child's chart for privacy reasons, so administration of IPV should be interpreted as presumptive evidence of an immunosuppressed child or contact.

Contraindications to IPV include anaphylactic reaction to neomycin or streptomycin (AAP in Peter, 1994; CDC, 1993b).

DIPHTHERIA-TETANUS-PERTUSSIS

The standard formulation is a combination of diphtheria and tetanus toxoids and pertussis vaccine (DTP). A formulation with acellular pertussis vaccine is also available (DTaP). Other formulations include Td (with a smaller amount of diphtheria toxoid) and DT.

DTP should be given at 2 months, 4 months, 6 months, 12-18 months, and 4-6 years. If the child is at least 15 months old, the fourth (and fifth) dose can be given as either DTaP or DTP (CDC, 1995). The first dose can be administered as early as 6 weeks (CDC, 1994). There must be at least 6 months between the third and fourth doses (CDC, 1995). As of the seventh birthday, a child should only receive formulations that do not contain the pertussis vaccine.

Td should be given between 11 and 16 years of age (CDC, 1995). However, the CDC used to recommend and the Guidelines for Adolescent Preventive Services (Elster and Kuznets, 1994) recommend that adolescents receive Td 10 years after the last DTP (due, but not necessarily given, between 4 and 6 years). Therefore, an indicator should reflect that a person who received a DTP between 7 and 10 years old would not need to be revaccinated until 10 years later when he or she would be 17 to 20 years old.

DTP should not be given if the patient has had encephalopathy within seven days of administration of a previous dose of DTP (AAP in Peter, 1994; CDC, 1993b). It is also acceptable (but not necessary) to withhold DTP/DTaP when, within 48 hours of receiving a prior DTP vaccine, the patient has experienced fever greater than or equal to 40.5°C (105°F), collapse or shock-like state (hypotonic-hyporesponsive episode), persistent, inconsolable crying lasting at least three hours; within 72 hours of receiving a prior DTP vaccine, the child has a seizure; and if the child has a proven or suspected underlying neurologic disorder (AAP in Peter, 1994; CDC, 1993).

HAEMOPHILUS INFLUENZAE TYPE B

There are two schedules for Haemophilus influenzae type b vaccine (Hib), depending on which vaccine formulation is used (CDC, 1995):

- HbOC (HibTITER[R]), PRP-T (ActHib[TM] and OmniHIB[TM]), or DTP/HbOC (TETRAMUNE[TM]) are due at 2, 4, 6, and 12-15 months.
- PRP-OMP (PedvaxHIB[R]) are due at 2,4, and 12-15 months. The guidelines imply but do not directly state that if either of the first two are not PRP-OMP, then there should be a 6-month vaccine. This formulation is also known as the Meningococcal Protein Conjugate.

Either type can be given at 12-15 months, regardless of which were used for the first year. The first Hib can be given as early as the sixth week (CDC, 1994a).

A recent study comparing various sequences and substitutions of the different Hib formulations suggests that the immune response to using PRP-OMP alone during the first year is inferior to the response when at least one HbOC is given and also inferior to a sequence of three HbOC shots (Anderson et al., 1995). While the study's authors draw the conclusion that changing vaccines during the primary sequences is acceptable, they recommend further study rather than advise against using only PRP-OMP.

MEASLES-MUMPS-RUBELLA

Measles, mumps, and rubella (German measles) vaccines are generally combined (MMR).

The first MMR is due at 12 to 15 months. The second shot is due at 4 to 6 years or 11 to 12 years (CDC, 1995), and is generally dictated by the requirements of local school districts. Though the recommendations specify either time period for the second shot, but not the time in between, it seems most reasonable for an indicator to allow the second vaccine to be given during the full range of time between these two time periods. For example, if an eight-year-old child not yet immunized with a second MMR moved to a school district that requires the second MMR, he or she would need to be immunized and would have no reason to get a repeat MMR at 11 to 12 years old.

The second shot should not be given within a month of the first. This would probably only come up as an issue if a child of at least 4 years old has had no MMRs and is presently catching up.

During measles outbreaks in preschool children, vaccination may be recommended for children as young as 6 months old; these children should still have a vaccination after they reach 12 months.

Reasons not to be vaccinated specific to MMR (AAP in Peter, 1994; CDC, 1993b) include anaphylactic reaction to neomycin, pregnancy (for theoretical reasons (CDC, 1994)), and known altered immunodeficiency other than HIV (hematologic and solid tumors, congenital immunodeficiency, and long term immunosuppressive therapy). Anaphylactic reaction to egg ingestion is also an acceptable contraindication, though protocols exist for immunizing people with such histories (Greenberg and Birx, 1988; Herman et al., 1983). If a child has had immunoglobulin administered within the prior three months, it is acceptable to delay MMR if one has done a risk-benefit analysis for the individual patient.

HEPATITIS B VACCINE

The Hepatitis B vaccine is referred to as HBV. Though not a vaccine, Hepatitis B Immune Globulin (HBIG) will also be discussed below because it is sometimes used in tandem with HBV.

In the United States, 200,000 to 300,000 acute Hepatitis B infections occur each year. More than one million people in the U.S. have chronic Hepatitis B infection, and about 4,000 to 5,000 people die each year from chronic liver disease and hepatocellular carcinoma resulting from Hepatitis B. Depending on region, gender, and race, between 3.3 percent and 25 percent of the population have had Hepatitis B. The likelihood of becoming chronically infected with Hepatitis B varies inversely with the age at which infection occurs. Newborns who become infected from Hepatitis B surface antigen (HBsAg)-positive mothers have a 90 percent probability of becoming chronic carriers. It is estimated that more than 25 percent of infants who are chronic carriers will die from primary hepatocellular carcinoma or cirrhosis of the liver, generally while adults (AAP, 1992).

All pregnant women should be screened for HBsAg during an early prenatal visit (CDC, 1995) (See Chapter 16).

If the mother is HBsAg-negative, the child should receive HBV at birth to 2 months, 1 to 4 months, and 6 to 18 months with at least one month between the first two doses (CDC, 1995; AAP, 1992; AAP in Peter, 1994).

If the mother is HBsAg-positive, a newborn should receive HBIG within 12 hours of birth, and the initial dose of HBV should be given concurrently at a different site. (Because of differences in different manufacturer's formulations, this initial dose should be either Merck Sharpe & Dohme's Recombivax HB[R] or SmithKline Beecham's Engerix-B[R].) The second and third HBV doses should be given at 1 and 6 months of age (CDC, 1995; AAP, 1992; AAP in Green, 1994).

If the mother's HBsAg status is not known, a newborn should receive HBV within 12 hours of birth in the dose recommended for children whose mothers are HBsAg-positive. The mother should be tested immediately. Though not specifically recommended, it seems clear that a mother who was not screened prenatally should be screened soon enough to allow administration of HBIG to the child before he/she is one week old. If the mother is found to be HBsAg-positive, the child should receive HBIG as soon as possible and within seven days of birth. The recommendations for the second and third dose of HBV follow the guidelines according to whether the mother is positive or negative (AAP, 1992; AAP in Peter, 1994). Although the recommendations do not address what should occur if the mother's status remains unknown, one might argue that the child should be treated as if the mother were positive.

The AAP recommends vaccinating adolescents who have sexually transmitted infections, have had more than one sexual partner in the previous six months, are injection drug users, are males who are sexually active with other males, have sexual contacts with individuals at high risk, or have tasks as employees, volunteers, or trainees that involve contact with blood or blood-contaminated body fluids (AAP in Peter, 1994). Some of this information would not necessarily be recorded in the chart because of privacy concerns and the last risk factor would not be asked routinely, but when such risk factors appear in the chart, delivery (or an offer) of the vaccine should be noted as well.

Children or adolescents who are Alaskan Natives or Pacific Islanders or whose parents are immigrants from countries with high rates of HBV infection should be vaccinated as well (AAP in Peter, 1994). It would be difficult to incorporate countries with high rates of HBV into an indicator, but the list would be available from the CDC if desired.

CATCHING UP FOR LATE IMMUNIZATIONS

Patients who are behind on immunizations are supposed to follow an accelerated schedule to catch-up. The general approach is not to delay age-appropriate immunizations while catching up on missed immunizations (e.g., a thirteen-month-old can receive the first MMR while catching up on missed DTPs). If the child is at least 4 months old but less than 7 years old and has not begun any of the initial series, the interval between the first, second, and third DTPs and Hibs should be reduced to one month. Except in special circumstances, Hib should not be given after the fifth birthday. Additional Hib recommendations vary with the particular manufacturer and are detailed in CDC (1994b). The second OPV is given 2 months after the first, and the third 6 weeks after the second. The second HBV is given 1 month after the first, and the third is given 6 months after the second. The fourth DTP/DTaP is given at least 6 months after the third one; likewise for the fourth Hib. If the child reaches his/her 7th birthday during this catch-up sequence, remaining DTPs should be given as Td (CDC, 1994b).

A child who is at least 7 years but less than 18 years of age and has never been vaccinated should receive on the first visit, Td, OPV, MMR; 6-8 weeks after the first visit, the same set should be given again. Six months after the second visit, Td and OPV are given. DTP/DTaP is not given to people who are 7 or older. OPV is not given to people who are 18 or older. Hepatitis B vaccination generally depends on risk factors (CDC 1994b). Additional details appear in CDC (1994b).

UNKNOWN PRIOR IMMUNIZATION RECORD

There are no guidelines for how quickly a physician should track down a new patient's immunization history from other clinicians if the guardian does not know it. However, given that there are no adverse reactions to being reimmunized with MMR, OPV/IPV, Hib, HBV, a child whose immunization record cannot be obtained should be reimmunized (CDC 1994b).

RECOMMENDED QUALITY INDICATORS FOR CHILDHOOD IMMUNIZATIONS

The following criteria apply to routine immunizations for infants, children, and adolescents.

	Indicator	Quality of Evidence	Literature	Benefits	Comments
	Polio				
1.	All children should have had two OPV/IPV between six weeks and the first birthday.*	I, III	CDC, 1995; CDC, 1994a; Cherry in Feigin and Cherry, 1992; CDC, 1991	Prevent polio.[a]	OPV and IPV both help prevent individuals from contracting polio and help decrease the chances of polio spreading through a community.
2.	All children should have had three OPV/IPV between six weeks and the second birthday.*	I, III	CDC, 1995; CDC, 1994a; Cherry in Feigin and Cherry, 1992; CDC, 1991	Prevent polio.[a]	OPV and IPV both help prevent individuals from contracting polio and help decrease the chances of polio spreading through a community.
3.	All children should have had four OPV/IPV between six weeks and the seventh birthday.*	I, III	CDC, 1995; CDC, 1994a; Cherry in Feigin and Cherry, 1992; CDC, 1991	Prevent polio.[a]	OPV and IPV both help prevent individuals from contracting polio and help decrease the chances of polio spreading through a community.
4.	Children with immunocompromise (hematologic and solid tumors, congenital immunodeficiency, and long-term immunosuppressive therapy) or HIV infection should receive IPV rather than OPV (at the same ages as OPV).	III	AAP in Peter, 1994; CDC, 1993b	Prevent polio.[a] Prevent polio transmission from the vaccine.	OPV can cause polio in an immunocompromised person.
5.	Before each OPV, guardians should be questioned about the presence of an immunocompromised contact in the household.	III	Inferred from AAP in Peter, 1994; CDC, 1993b	Prevent sprreading polio to an immunocompromised contact of a recipient of OPV.[a]	OPV can cause polio in an immunodeficient contact of the recipient. Many people probably do not document this; however, it is quite important to ask. An expectation of documentation increases the likelihood that it is really done, allows for quality review, and provides some legal protection. One might argue that if the parent signs a consent that says to tell the clinician about immunosuppressed household contacts, that is adequate. Such consents should be in the chart for documentation. A physician who takes care of the whole household might argue that he or she knows everyone's immune status and doesn't need to ask again or to document in the child's chart that no one is immunosuppressed.
6.	If there is a household contact with immunocompromise, children should receive IPV instead of OPV.	III	AAP in Peter, 1994; CDC, 1993b	Prevent polio.[a]	The live virus presents a risk for infection among immunocompromised persons.
	Diphtheria/Tetanus/Pertussis				

273

#	Recommendation	Quality	Citations	Objective	Explanation
7.	All children should have had three DTP between six weeks and the first birthday.*	I, III	CDC, 1995; CDC, 1994a; Dennehy et al., in Feigin and Cherry, 1992; CDC, 1991	Prevent diphtheria.[b] Prevent tetanus.[c] Prevent pertussis.[d]	DTP helps prevent individuals from contracting diphtheria, tetanus, and pertussis.
8.	All children should have had four DTP between six weeks and the second birthday, with at least six months between the third and fourth dose (the fourth may be DTaP if given after 15 months old).*	I, III	CDC, 1995; CDC, 1994a; Dennehy et al., in Feigin and Cherry, 1992; CDC, 1991	Prevent diphtheria.[b] Prevent tetanus.[c] Prevent pertussis.[d]	DTP/DTaP helps prevent individuals from contracting diphtheria, tetanus, and pertussis.
9.	All children should have had five DTP/DTaP between six weeks and the seventh birthday, with at least six weeks between the third and fourth doses (the fourth and fifth may be DTaP if given after 15 months old).*	I, III	CDC, 1995; CDC, 1994a; Dennehy et al., in Feigin and Cherry, 1992; CDC, 1991	Prevent diphtheria.[b] Prevent tetanus.[c] Prevent pertussis.[d]	DTP/DTaP helps prevent individuals from contracting diphtheria, tetanus, and pertussis.
10.	By age 17, all children should have had one Td between age 7 and 17. A formulation that includes pertussis is acceptable.	I, III	CDC, 1995; Dennehy et al., in Feigin and Cherry, 1992; CDC, 1991	Prevent diphtheria.[b] Prevent tetanus.[c]	Booster vaccines for tetanus are indicated every 10 years. Though the pertussis vaccine has generally not been given to patients over 7 years old because of concerns about increased side effects, there is growing concern that adults are spreading the disease to children. Though official recommendations have not emerged, an infectious disease expert has indicated that some clinicians are now giving the pertussis vaccine to persons older than 7.
11.	Children who have had encephalopathy within 7 days of a prior dose of DTP should not receive any further vaccination with DTP.	III	AAP in Peter, 1994; CDC, 1993b	Prevent recurrent encephalopathy. Prevent neurologic deficits.	Risk of encephalopathy due to DTP is higher in people with a prior episode of encephalopathy associated with DTP.

Haemophilus influenzae type B

#	Recommendation	Quality	Citations	Objective	Explanation
12.	All children should have had two PRP-OMP Hib or three Hib (any combination of formulations) between six weeks and the first birthday.*	I, III	CDC, 1995; CDC, 1994a; Dennehy et al., in Feigin and Cherry, 1991b	Prevent infection with Haemophilus influenzae type B.[e]	Hib helps prevent individuals from contracting Haemophilus influenzae type B and helps decrease the chances of it spreading through a community.
13.	Between the ages of six weeks and 2 years, all children should have had either: – four Hib vaccinations, or – three Hib vaccinations if the first two were PRP-OMB Hib.*	I, III	CDC, 1995; CDC, 1994a; Dennehy et al., in Feigin and Cherry, 1991b	Prevent infection with Haemophilus influenzae type B.[e]	Hib helps prevent individuals from contracting Haemophilus influenzae type B and helps decrease the chances of it spreading through a community.

Measles/Mumps/Rubella

#	Recommendation	Quality	Citations	Objective	Explanation
14.	All children should have had one MMR between their first and second birthdays.*	I, III	CDC, 1995; Dennehy et al., in Feigin and Cherry, 1992; Cherry in Feigin and Cherry, 1992a, 1992b; Brunell in Feigin and Cherry, 1992; CDC, 1990a; CDC, 1989a	Prevent measles.[f] Prevent mumps.[g] Prevent rubella.[h]	MMR helps prevent individuals from contracting measles, mumps, and rubella and helps decrease the chances of it spreading through a community.

#	Recommendation	Category	References	Purpose	Explanation
15.	All children should have had an MMR between their fourth and thirteenth birthdays.*	I, III	CDC, 1995; Dennehy et al., in Feigin and Cherry, 1992; Cherry in Feigin and Cherry, 1992; Brunell in Feigin and Cherry, 1992; CDC, 1990; CDC, 1989a	Prevent measles.f Prevent mumps.g Prevent rubella.h	MMR helps prevent individuals from contracting measles, mumps, and rubella and helps decrease the chances of it spreading through a community. The recommendation is to give the second MMR between 4-6 years or 11-12 years, with local school requirements having a major impact on the choice. For our purposes, it will be easiest to make sure a second has been given between 4-12 years. Thus the acceptable range ends on the thirteenth birthday.
16.	Children who are immunocompromised (with the exception of children with HIV infection) (hematologic and solid tumors, congenital immunodeficiency, and long-term immunosuppressive therapy) should not receive MMR.	III	AAP in Peter, 1994; CDC, 1993b	Prevent contraction of measles from the vaccine.f	
Hepatitis B					
17.	The mother's HBsAg status should be documented in the child's chart within one week of birth.	III	Inferred from AAP, 1992	Prevent perinatal transmission of Hepatitis B. Prevent liver disease from Hepatitis B.	If a mother is HBsAg positive, the infant should receive immune globulin within 12 hours to prevent development of Hepatitis B.
18.	All children whose mothers are known to be HBsAg-Negative should have had at least two HBV by the first birthday with at least one month between the first two doses.*	I, III	CDC, 1995; Dennehy et al., in Feigin and Cherry, 1992; CDC, 1990a	Prevent Hepatitis B infection and subsequent liver disease.	HBV helps prevent individuals from contracting Hepatitis B and helps decrease the chances of it spreading through a community.
19.	All children whose mothers are known to be HBsAg-Negative should have had three HBV by the second birthday with at least one month between the first two doses.*	I, III	CDC, 1995; Dennehy et al., in Feigin and Cherry, 1992; CDC, 1990a	Prevent Hepatitis B infection and subsequent liver disease.	HBV helps prevent individuals from contracting Hepatitis B and helps decrease the chances of it spreading through a community.
20.	All children whose mothers are known to be HBsAg-Positive at birth should receive HBIG and HBV by the beginning of the twelfth hour of life.	I, III	CDC, 1995; AAP, 1992 and 1994; Dennehy et al., in Feigin and Cherry, 1992; CDC, 1990a	Prevent perinatal or subsequent transmission of Hepatitis B from the mother. Prevent liver disease from Hepatitis B.	HBV helps prevent individuals from contracting Hepatitis B and helps decrease the chances of it spreading through a community. HBIG helps prevent the child from contracting Hepatitis B over the short run.
21.	All children whose mothers are known to be HBsAg-Positive should have had three HBV by the beginning of the ninth month of life.*	I, III	CDC, 1995; AAP, 1992 and 1994; Dennehy et al., in Feigin and Cherry, 1992; CDC, 1990a	Prevent perinatal or subsequent transmission of Hepatitis B from the mother. Prevent liver disease from Hepatitis B.	HBV helps prevent individuals from contracting Hepatitis B and helps decrease the chances of it spreading through a community. Given that the child has a known risk of becoming infected with Hepatitis B, it seems reasonable to provide a narrower grace period for vaccination.
22.	All children whose mother's HBsAg status is not known should receive HBV by the beginning of the twelfth hour of life.	I, III	CDC, 1995; AAP, 1992; AAP in Peter, 1994; Dennehy et al., in Feigin and Cherry, 1992; CDC, 1990a	Prevent perinatal or subsequent transmission of Hepatitis B from the mother. Prevent liver disease from Hepatitis B.	HBV helps prevent individuals from contracting Hepatitis B and helps decrease the chances of it spreading through a community.

275

Influenza

No.	Recommendation	Rating	Citation	Objective	Comments
23.	All children whose mother's HBsAg status is not known by the end of the first week of life should receive HBIG.	I, III	Inferred from CDC, 1995; AAP, 1992; AAP in Peter, 1994; Dennehy et al., in Feigin and Cherry, 1992; CDC, 1990a	Prevent perinatal or subsequent transmission of Hepatitis B from the mother. Prevent liver disease from Hepatitis B.	While this is not specifically recommended, it seems to flow logically from the recommendation that mothers of unknown Hepatitis B status be checked in time for the child to receive HBIG by the end of the first week of life. HBIG helps prevent the child from contracting Hepatitis B over the short run.
24.	Adolescents with any of the following risk factors should recieve the full three-part HBV series within one year of the clinician becoming aware of the risk factor: – have a history of sexually transmitted infection; – have had more than one sexual partner in the previous six months; – use injection drugs; – are males who are sexually active with other males; – are sexual contacts of high-risk individuals; or – have tasks as employees, volunteers, or trainees that involve contact with blood or blood-contaminated body fluids.	I, III	AAP in Peter, 1994; Dennehy et al., in Feigin and Cherry, 1992; CDC, 1990a	Prevent infection with Hepatitis B. Prevent liver disease from Hepatitis B.	The AAP does not make this recommendation in as strong a manner as it makes other vaccine recommendations. There appears to be concern about the increased cost of the vaccine in adolescents compared to children (because of a larger dose). However, in an environment in which there is a risk of underuse, particularly of expensive therapies, Hepatitis B vaccine may be susceptible to omission. HBV helps prevent individuals from contracting Hepatitis B and helps decrease the chances of it spreading through a community.

Influenza

No.	Recommendation	Rating	Citation	Objective	Comments
25.	Children with asthma and other chronic pulmonary diseases, hemodynamically significant cardiac disease, hemoglobinopathies (e.g., sickle cell disease) or undergoing immunosuppresssive therapy should receive a yearly influenza vaccine. Other children at high risk may also benefit from an annual influenza vaccine, including those with: HIV infection, diabetes mellitus, chronic renal disease, and chronic metabolic diseases.	I-III	CDC, 1994a; AAP, 1994; Dennehy et al., in Feigin and Cherry, 1991a	Prevent pneumonia. Prevent mortality from influenza.	The influenza vaccine has been shown to prevent influenza. Patients at risk for developing complications from influenza should be vaccinated.

General Indicators

No.	Recommendation	Rating	Citation	Objective	Comments
26.	An inquiry should be made before each new set of immunizations (or after each prior set) about reactions to prior vaccines.	III	Inferred from AAP in Peter, 1994; CDC, 1993b	Prevent potentially life-threatening immunization reactions.	If consent forms that mention prior reactions are used, these may substitute for a specific notation in the chart.
27.	Children who have had an anaphylactic reaction to a prior vaccine should not receive that vaccine again.	III	AAP in Peter, 1994; CDC, 1993b	Prevent potentially life-threatening immunization reactions.	It will usually be unclear which vaccine caused the reaction, so presumably all given just prior to the reaction will be discontinued.
28.	Each immunization given at that institution should be documented with the date of administration, manufacturer, lot number, and name of health care provider administering the vaccine.	III	Dennehy et al., in Feigin and Cherry, 1992	Prevent infectious diseases covered by vaccines.	Proper documentation enables reimmunization if a batch is subsequently found to be bad.

Catch-Up Immunizations

276

#	Indicator		Source	Goal	Comments
29.	Children at least 8 months old but less than 5 years old who are behind on their immunizations should receive three OPV/IPV, four DTP/DTaP/Td, three Hib, three HBV, and one MMR within one year of the first visit with the managed care provider.	III	CDC, 1994	Prevent infectious diseases covered by each vaccine.	The guidelines start at 4 months old, but most children less than 8 months should be able to catch up easily by one year. Depending on the type of Hib, either three or four would be required; therefore, the indicator requires three so that the brand of Hib does not need to be specified.
30.	Children at least 5 years old but less than 7 years old who are behind on their immunizations should receive three OPV/IPV, four DTP/DTaP/Td, three HBV, and one MMR within one year of the first visit with the managed care provider.	III	CDC, 1994	Prevent infectious diseases covered by each vaccine.	This guideline is separated from the prior one because children should not receive Hib after their fifth birthday.
31.	Children who are at least 7 years old but less than 18 years old and who are behind on their immunizations should have had three OPV/IPV, three Td, and two MMR within one year of the first visit with the managed care provider.	III	CDC, 1994	Prevent infectious diseases covered by each vaccine.	Though the pertussis vaccine is not usually given after the seventh birthday, a tetanus formulation that includes pertussis will be considered acceptable.

Prior Immunization Record

#	Indicator		Source	Goal	Comments
32.	For children less than five years old who are new to the practice, there should be a notation of prior immunization history or a notation of an effort to obtain such information (e.g., parent will call in or bring it to next visit, letter will be sent to prior provider) at the first visit.	III		Prevent infectious diseases covered by vaccines.	This indicator does not come directly from recommendations in standard immunization guidelines, but it follows from them. It would be reasonable to omit the age cap. It is included because almost all children become up-to-date on their immunizations shortly after starting school, so it seems reasonable for a physician to take school attendance as a proxy for a complete immunization record, particularly if the parent says it is complete.
33.	If a prior immunization record for a child less than five years old has not been obtained within six months of the first visit, the child should be given catch-up immunizations.	III	Inferred from CDC, 1994	Prevent infectious diseases covered by vaccines.	This indicator does not come directly from recommendations in standard immunization guidelines, but it seems reasonable. It would be reasonable to omit the age cap. It is included because almost all children become up-to-date on their immunizations shortly after starting school, so it seems reasonable for a physician to take school attendance as a proxy for a complete immunization record, particularly if the parent says it is complete.

* Any of the following (if documented in the chart) can serve as adequate justification for not having given the particular immunization: Refusal by guardian or persistent contraindication to immunization (for all immunizations), anaphylaxis; for IPV, anaphylactic reaction to streptomycin or neomycin; for DTP, encephalopathy within 7 days of prior DTP, fever at least 40.5 C (105 F) within 48 hours of prior DTP, collapse or shocklike state within 48 hours of prior DTP, seizures within 3 days of prior DTP, at least three hours of persistent inconsolable crying within 48 hours of prior DTP, proven or suspected underlying neurologic disorders; for MMR, anaphylactic reaction to egg ingestion or neomycin, altered immune status other than HIV infection, immunoglobulin administration in the prior 3 months.)

a Polio can be asymptomatic or cause a minor illness, aseptic meningitis, asymmetric acute flaccid paralysis with areflexia of the involved limb, residual paralytic disease, bulbar paralysis, or respiratory muscle paralysis. A child who has recently received OPV can spread polio to an immunocompromised contact or become infected with polio if he/she is immunocompromised.

[b]Diphtheria can cause membranous nasopharyngitis, obstructive laryngotracheitis, subcutaneous infection, vaginal infection, conjunctival infection, otic infection, thrombocytopenia, myocarditis, or neurologic problems such as vocal cord paralysis or ascending paralysis.

[c]Tetanus can cause neurologic disease with severe muscle spasms, which generally last more than one week, and subside over 6 weeks if the person recovers.

[d]Pertussis can cause mild upper respiratory symptoms, severe paroxysms of coughing, and vomiting. Symptoms can last 6-10 weeks. It can cause apnea in children less than 6 months old. Complications include seizures, pneumonia, encephalopathy, and death.

[e]Haemophilus influenzae type B can cause meningitis, epiglottitis, septic arthritis, etc.

[f]Complications of measles include otitis media, bronchopneumonia, laryngotracheobronchitis, croup, diarrhea, encephalitis (which can cause permanent brain damage), death, and subacute sclerosing panencephalitis (SSPE; causes behavioral and intellectual deterioration and convulsions).

[g]Mumps causes swelling of salivary glands, meningeal signs, encephalitis, orchitis in post-pubescent males (which can cause sterility), other rare complications, and death.

[h]Rubella can cause mild disease with rare complications. The major concern is that it can be spread to pregnant women (not previously infected) and cause serious congenital anomalies.

Quality of Evidence Codes:

I: RCT
II-1:   Nonrandomized controlled trials
II-2:   Cohort or case analysis
II-3:   Multiple time series
III: Opinions or descriptive studies

Note: There are multiple legitimate reasons why a child might not have received immunizations for which he/she was due at a particular visit. However, these reasons should not vary by location and should be infrequent enough so that they should not have a major impact on quality indicators. The time period over which these indicators expect immunizations to have been given is broad enough that most children who had a high fever or other transient illness at any particular visit should have had ample opportunity to catch up.

Note: We will try to collect the exact date of immunization so that we can do a sensitivity analysis on the impact of having shorter or longer grace periods for giving immunizations after the recommended age and on the impact of creating a graded scale for the length of delay (e.g., one point off for a one month delay, ten points off for a one year delay).

278

REFERENCES - CHILDHOOD IMMUNIZATION

American Academy of Pediatrics. 1994. Section 1: Active and passive immunization. *1994 Red Book: Report of the Committee on Infectious Diseases*. Editor Peter G. American Academy of Pediatrics, Elk Grove Village, IL.

American Academy of Pediatrics, and Committee on Infectious Diseases. April 1992. Universal hepatitis B immunization. *Pediatrics* 89 (4): 795-9.

Anderson EL, MD Decker, JA Englund, et al. 15 March 1995. Interchangeability of conjugated haemophilus influenzae type b vaccines in infants. *Journal of the American Medical Association* 273 (11): 849-53.

Brunell PA. 1992. Mumps. In *Textbook of Pediatric Infectious Diseases*, Third ed. Editors Feigin RD, and JD Cherry, 1610-1613. Philadelphia, PA: W.B. Saunders Company.

Centers for Disease Control. 8 August 1991. Diphtheria, tetanus, and pertussis: Recommendations for vaccine use and other preventive measures: Recommendations of the Immunization Practices Advisory Committee (ACIP). *Morbidity and Mortality Weekly Report* 40 (RR-10): 1-28.

Centers for Disease Control. 7 April 1989. Recommendations of the Immunization Practices Advisory Committee: General recommendations on immunization. *Morbidity and Mortality Weekly Report* 38 (13): 205-27.

Centers for Disease Control. 9 June 1989. Recommendations of the Immunization Practices Advisory Committee (ACIP): Mumps Prevention. *Morbidity and Mortality Weekly Report* 38 (22): 388-400.

Centers for Disease Control. 9 February 1990. Recommendations of the Immunization Practices Advisory Committee (ACIP): protection against viral hepatitis. *Morbidity and Mortality Weekly Report* 39 (RR-2): 1-26.

Centers for Disease Control. 23 November 1990. Recommendations of the Immunization Practices Advisory Committee: Rubella Prevention. *Morbidity and Mortality Weekly Report* 39 (RR-15): 1-18.

Centers for Disease Control. 11 January 1991. Recommendations of the Advisory Committee on Immunization Practices (ACIP): *Haemophilus b* conjugate vaccines for prevention of *haemophilus influenzae* type b disease among infants and children two months of age and older. *Morbidity and Mortality Weekly Report* 40 (RR-1): 1-7.

Centers for Disease Control. 24 May 1991. Recommendations of the Immunization Practices Advisory Committee: Prevention and Control of Influenza. *Morbidity and Mortality Weekly Report* 40 (RR-6): 1-15.

Centers for Disease Control. 9 April 1993. Recommendations of the Advisory Committee on Immunization Practices (ACIP): Use of vaccines and immune globulins for persons with altered immunocompetence. *Morbidity and Mortality Weekly Report* 42 (RR-4): 1-18.

Centers for Disease Control. 28 January 1994. Recommendations of the Advisory Committee on Immunization Practices (ACIP). *Morbidity and Mortality Weekly Report* 43 (RR-1): 1-38.

Centers for Disease Control. 6 January 1995. Recommended childhood immunization schedule--United States, January 1995. *Morbidity and Mortality Weekly Report* 43 (51 & 52): 959-61.

Centers for Disease Control. 23 April 1993. Standards for pediatric immunization practices. *Morbidity and Mortality Weekly Report* 42 (RR-5): 1-13.

Cherry JD. 1992. Enteroviruses. In *Textbook of Pediatric Infectious Diseases*, Third ed. Editors Feigin RD, and JD Cherry, 1737-1753. Philadelphia, PA: W.B. Saunders Company.

Cherry JD. 1 1992. Measles. In *Textbook of Pediatric Infectious Diseases*, Third ed. Editors Feigin RD, and JD Cherry, 1591-1609. Philadelphia, PA: W.B. Saunders Company.

Cherry JD. 2 1992. Rubella. In *Textbook of Pediatric Infectious Diseases*, Third ed. Editors Feigin RD, and JD Cherry, 1792-1817. Philadelphia, PA: W.B. Saunders Company.

Cutts FT, ER Zell, D Mason, et al. 8 April 1992. Monitoring progress toward US preschool immunization goals. *Journal of the American Medical Association* 267 (14): 1952-5.

Dennehy PH, EE Jost, and G Peter. 1992. Active immunizing agents. In *Textbook of Pediatric Infectious Diseases*, Third ed. Editors Feigin RD, and JD Cherry, 2231-61. Philadelphia, PA: W.B. Saunders Company.

Elster, AB, and NJ Kuznets. 1994. *AMA Guidelines for Adolescent Preventive Services (GAPS): Recommendations and rationale.* Chicago, IL: American Medical Association.

Farizo KM, PA Stehr-Green, LE Markowitz, et al. April 1992. Vaccination levels and missed opportunities for measles vaccination: A record audit in a public pediatric clinic. *Pediatrics* 89 (4): 589-92.

Greenberg MA, and DL Birx. September 1988. Safe administration of mumps-measles-rubella vaccine in egg-allergic children. *Journal of Pediatrics* 113 (3): 504-6.

Hall CB. 1995. The recommended childhood immunization schedule of the United States. *Pediatrics* 95 (1): 135-7.

Herman JJ, R Radin, and R Schneiderman. 1983. Allergic reactions to measles (rubeola) vaccine in patients hypersensitive to egg protein. *Journal of Pediatrics* 102 (2): 196-9.

McConnochie KM, and KJ Roghmann. June 1992. Immunization opportunities missed among urban poor children. *Pediatrics* 89 (6):

Rennels MB. 1993. Childhood immunizations. In *Ambulatory Pediatric Care*, Second ed. Editor Dershewitz RA, 55-66. Philadelphia, PA: J.B. Lippincott Company.

Szilagyi PG, LE Rodewald, SG Humiston, et al. 1993. Missed opportunities for childhood vaccinations in office practices and the effect on vaccination status. *Pediatrics* 91 (1): 1-7.

Wilson MH. 1994. Immunization. In *Principles and Practice of Pediatrics*, Second ed. Editors Oski FA, CD DeAngelis, RD Feigin, et al., 612-33. Philadelphia, PA: J.B. Lippincott Company.

15. OTITIS MEDIA
Lee Hilborne, M.D., and Cheryl Damberg, Ph.D.

OTITIS MEDIA WITH EFFUSION (SEROUS OTITIS MEDIA)

Quality indicators for otitis media were derived based on a review of the following sources: (1) a MEDLINE search of the English language medical literature from 1990 to 1995;[1] (2) *The AHCPR Clinical Practice Guideline on Otitis Media with Effusion in Young Children* (Stool et al., 1994); (3) relevant references in articles identified by the medical literature search; and (4) a general pediatrics textbook (Williams, in Hoekelman et al., 1992). The review pertains to children 1 to 3 years of age.

IMPORTANCE

Second to respiratory tract infections, otitis media is the most common childhood disease. Williams (in Hoekelman et al., 1992) reports that approximately 75 percent of children will develop at least one episode of otitis media before the age of 10. The term otitis media refers to a broad range of clinical conditions, including acute middle ear infections (acute otitis media, purulent otitis media, suppurative otitis media), the accumulation of fluid in the middle ear (otitis media with effusion, serous otitis media), or both (Kemp, 1990). Table 15.1 defines the different otitis conditions.

---

[1]This search yielded 70 references specifically addressing management of otitis media and the effectiveness of that management.

Table 15.1

Classification of Otitis Media

Clinical Terms	Synonyms and Definitions
Otitis media without effusion	Synonym: myringitis Presence of erythema and opacificaiton of the tympanic membrane without the presence of an effusion. May be seen in the early states of acute otitis media or as otitis media resolves.
Acute otitis media (AOM)	Synonyms: Acute suppurative, purulent or bacterial otitis media Clinically identifiable infection of the middle ear. Recent, rapid onset of signs and symptoms associated with middle ear inflammation.
Otitis media with effusion (OME)	Synonyms: Secretory, nonsuppurative, serous or mucoid otitis media Otitis media without signs or symptoms of acute disease, but with the presence of a middle ear effusion. May be subdivided into acute, subacute, and chronic based on duration of effusion.
Chronic otitis media (COM)	Synonym: Chronic suppurative, purulent, or intractable otitis media Presence of pronounced intractable middle ear pathology with or without suppurative otorrhea. Suppurative refers to an active infection while otorrhea refers to a discharge through a perforated tympanic membrane.

Source: Sagraves et al., 1992.

This review focuses on otitis media with effusion, a process that frequently follows acute otitis media. Stool et al. (1994) estimate otitis media with effusion represents 25 to 35 percent of all otitis media cases.

In 1990, there were 24.5 million physician visits with the diagnosis of otitis media. Of the total number of visits, children under age 15 accounted for 19.7 million visits (Schappert, 1992). For children younger than age 15, otitis media represented the most frequent diagnosis for physician visits (Schappert, 1992). According to Williams (in Hoekelman et al., 1992), young children are more prone to otitis media, especially those between 6 and 24 months of age. Although specific incidence rates vary, the Greater Boston Study found that more than 60 percent of children had at least one episode of acute otitis media by age one; 80 percent had one episode by three years of age, and more than 40 percent had at least three episodes (Teele et al., 1989). The prevalence of otitis media by age group is shown in Table 15.2.

Table 15.2

Prevalence of Otitis Media by Age

Age	Prevalence
Neonate	0-12%
1 year	12%
2 years	7-12%
3-4 years	12-18%
5 years	4-17%
6-8 years	3-9%
9 years	0-6%

Source: Sagraves et al., 1992.

With respect to pediatric visits, otitis media was second only to well-child care as a reason for a physician visit (Schappert, 1992). Children under age two have the highest rate of visits to physician offices for otitis media (Stool et al., 1994; Schappert, 1992). Visits for otitis media are roughly the same for males and females. Approximately 25 percent of all prescriptions for children under age 10 are for oral antibiotics to treat otitis media (Bluestone, 1986). Berman (1995) notes that inappropriate antibiotic treatment of otitis media facilitates multidrug-resistant strains of bacterial pathogens. The estimated annual costs of medical and surgical treatment of otitis media range between $3 and $4 billion (Stool et al., 1994; Schappert, 1992).

Hearing loss is the most prevalent functional impairment resulting from otitis media. If hearing loss persists, evidence, although not entirely conclusive, suggests that patients may have impaired speech, hearing, and language development (Lous et al., 1988; Callahan and Lazoritz, 1988). These problems are most common when otitis media affects younger children.

EFFICACY AND/OR EFFECTIVENESS OF INTERVENTIONS

Screening

Although an ear examination is part of the recommended general pediatric history and physical examination, controversy remains regarding explicit screening for otitis media. Gates et al. (1989) recommend a screening battery when children enter school to guard against learning problems secondary to hearing loss. An abnormal screen exists when the middle ear pressure is more negative than -200 mm H_2O and there is low compliance on tympanometry. Screen failure also exists when audiometric testing reveals inability to detect a 25 dB tone at 4,000 Hz. However, when otitis media with effusion is suspected, certain diagnostic tests are warranted. Furthermore, because otitis media with effusion frequently follows an episode of acute otitis media, diagnostic tests are recommended for these patients.

Diagnosis

Otitis media with effusion may be asymptomatic or patients may experience ear discomfort, hearing loss, tinnitus, possibly vertigo, or a feeling of ear fullness. Diagnostic tests include otoscopy (viewing the tympanic membrane with illumination) and pneumatic otoscopy (otoscopy viewing the tympanic membrane with small amounts of positive and negative air pressure). The AHCPR Guideline panel strongly recommended the use of pneumatic otoscopy as the diagnostic evaluation tool for suspected otitis media with effusion, because pneumatic otoscopy can suggest the presence of effusion, even when visual inspection of the eardrum (i.e., otoscopy alone) gives no indication of middle ear pathology (Stool et al., 1994). Based on limited scientific evidence and expert opinion, tympanometry may be useful to confirm the diagnosis of otitis media with effusion, with the inference that this technique is more reliable than audiometry alone (Gates et al., 1989; Kemp, 1990).

Hearing loss evaluation may be beneficial early in the disease process (i.e., in the first 3 months of disease) and, based on expert opinion and limited scientific evidence, is recommended for a child who has bilateral otitis media with effusion for a total of three months

(Stool et al., 1994). Tympanometry is neither an appropriate nor reliable predictor of hearing impairment (Stool et al., 1994), given that its positive predictive value for hearing loss can be as low as 49 percent.

Treatment

The antibiotic treatment of otitis media with effusion remains controversial because most cases of otitis media resolve without any intervention within 3 months (Zielhuis et al., 1990; Stool et al., 1994). Furthermore, there is a lack of consensus in the literature with respect to the efficacy of antibiotics for otitis media with effusion. (Mandel et al., 1987; Cantekin et al., 1991). Most studies conclude that antibiotics have a small but significantly positive effect on the resolution of otitis media with effusion.

Williams et al. (1993) completed a meta-analysis of the literature and demonstrated that antibiotics provided benefit in the short-term treatment of otitis media with effusion (relative difference = 0.16; 95 percent confidence interval = 0.03 to 0.29). However, long-term benefit was not found when comparing the use of antibiotics to placebo (relative difference = 0.06; confidence interval = -0.03 to 0.14). Rosenfeld and Post (1992), also by meta-analysis, found that antibiotics favor more rapid resolution of serous otitis media and recommend their use in otitis media with effusion patients. AHCPR's meta-analysis showed a 14 percent increase in the probability that otitis would resolve when antibiotic therapy was given versus no treatment (Stool et al., 1994).

During the initial management period (up to 12 weeks), observation of the otherwise healthy child with a unilateral effusion is the treatment of choice (Berman et al., 1994). Myringotomy, with or without insertion of tympanostomy tubes, is not recommended for initial management of otitis media with effusion in an otherwise healthy child (Stool et al., 1994). Early antibiotic therapy is also an option and should be more strongly considered in the following situations:

- bilateral serous otitis media, particularly when accompanied by a hearing loss;
- very young infants unable to verbalize complaints;

- in association with a purulent upper respiratory infection;
- when the tympanic membrane or middle ear appear possibly damaged;
- when episodes frequently recur (i.e., three or more times); or
- in the presence of associated vertigo.

The choice of antibiotics is the same as those recommended for acute otitis media given that similar organisms are isolated from both disease processes. Recommended antibiotics include, among others:

1) Amoxicillin (Pukander et al., 1993; Mandel et al., 1991)

2) Amoxicillin-clavulanate (McCarty et al., 1993);

3) Cefaclor (Mandel et al., 1991);

4) Cefuroxime axetil (McLinn et al., 1994);

5) Cefixime (Asmar et al., 1994);

6) Erythromycin-sulfisoxazole (Mandel et al., 1991);

7) Trimethoprim-sulfamethoxazole (Daly et al., 1991); and

8) Clarithromycin (Pukander et al., 1993; Mandel et al., 1991).

Evidence from cohort studies suggests that second hand smoke (i.e., passive smoke) may increase the likelihood of otitis media with effusion, although, at present, the data are not conclusive (Maw and Bawden, 1994; Maw et al., 1992). Nevertheless, given the overall health benefits to smoking cessation for both parents and children, parents who smoke should be advised to stop and referred to a smoking cessation program.

When considering treatment options for patients with uncomplicated otitis media with effusion, antihistamines, decongestants, and steroid therapy are contraindicated because they have not been shown to offer benefit, particularly given their associated risks such as central nervous system depression and steroid dependence (Estelle and Simons, 1994). The AHCPR clinical guideline also recommends against adenoidectomy and/or tonsillectomy for the treatment of otitis media with effusion (Stool et al., 1994).

Patients identified as having otitis media with effusion, whether treated or not, should be evaluated every 4-6 weeks to determine whether there is persistence or resolution of the process (Stool et al., 1994).

Patients who have persistent bilateral otitis media with effusion ($\geq$ 3 months in duration) should be evaluated for hearing loss. If hearing loss is not severe (less than 20 db in the best ear) and the disease is unilateral, continued observation or continuation/introduction of antibiotics is appropriate (Mandel et al., 1991). In the presence of a bilateral hearing deficit (defined as 20 decibels hearing threshold level or worse in the better-hearing ear), antibiotics or myringotomy with tympanostomy tube placement is recommended (Bluestone et al., 1986). However, 10 percent of children with otitis media with effusion will have persistent disease at three months and many of these cases will resolve without intervention (Stool et al., 1994). Some argue that tympanostomy tube placement is never appropriate treatment for otitis media with effusion in the absence of a significant hearing loss (Kleinman et al., 1994). In any case, placement of tympanostomy tubes as a first line of treatment is considered inappropriate (Kleinman et al., 1994).

At subsequent follow-up (about 4-6 months), if antibiotics have failed to resolve the effusion in patients with significant bilateral hearing loss (as defined above), placement of tympanostomy tubes is recommended (Stool et al., 1994). Patients with persistent otitis media with effusion should be evaluated for possible hearing loss (Stool et al., 1994).

RECOMMENDED QUALITY INDICATORS FOR OTITIS MEDIA WITH EFFUSION

These indicators apply to children ages 1-3 years.

Diagnosis

	Indicator	Quality of evidence	Literature	Benefits	Comments
1.	All patients with the diagnosis of suspected otitis media with effusion should be evaluated with pneumatic otoscopy.	III	Stool et al., 1994	Prevent allergic reactions from antibiotics. Avoid unnecessary placement of tubes. Prevent antimicrobial drug resisitance.	Achieves better precision in making diagnosis. Reduces false positives and false negatives. Otoscopy alone is not recommended since visual inspection of the eardrum may give no indication of middle ear pathology. Inappropriate antibiotic treatment can lead to drug resistance.
2.	Patients with persistent (≥3 months duration) bilateral otitis media with effusion should have a hearing evaluation.	II/III	Lous, 1988; Stool et al., 1994; Daly, 1982; Callahan & Lazoritz, 1988	Prevent delayed language development and hearing loss.	Recommendation based on limited scientific evidence and expert opinion.

Treatment

	Indicator	Quality of evidence	Literature	Benefits	Comments
3.	All patients with the diagnosis of otitis media with effusion should receive either: – antibiotics, or – trial of observation.	I, II/III	Stool et al., 1994; Mandel, 1987; Cantenkin, 1991; Williams, 1992; Behrman, 1992	Prevent hearing and language development problems. Minimize discomfort and behavior changes.	Most effusions spontaneously resolve by 3 months. Antibiotics are considered for treatment because studies show that in 27 to 50 percent of cases, aspirates contain bacteria or provide a medium for bacteria to grow. Meta-analysis showed a 14-percent increase in the probability that otitis would resolve when antibiotic therapy was given versus no treatment. Use of antibiotics must be weighed against the side effects and costs of treatment.
4.	For all paitents with a diagnosis of otitis media with effusion, during the initial management period (up to 12 weeks), myringotomy with or without insertion of tympanostomy tubes should not be performed in an otherwise healthy child (no other complications).	II	Stool et al., 1994	Prevent complications of surgery.* Prevent complications of anesthesia.** Prevent tympanosclerosis and persistent perforation.	Myringotomy at this stage has not been shown to be of benefit and may cause morbidity, such as external auditory canal wall laceration, persistent otorrhea, granuloma formation of the myringotomy site, cholesteatoma, and permanent membrane perforation.

290

	Indicator	Quality of evidence	Literature	Benefits	Comments
5.	All patients with the diagnosis of otitis media with effusion who have tympanostomy tubes should have a bilateral hearing loss (defined as 20 decibels hearing threshold level or worse in both ears) documented in the record.	III	Stool et al., 1994	Restoration of hearing. Prevent language delay.	Because of risks associated with insertion of tympanostomy tubes and the lack of controlled studies documenting benefits, this procedure should be limited to children with more severe symptoms.
6.	Patients with persistent otitis media with effusion (>= 3 months duration) and hearing loss (bilateral hearing deficits of 20 decibels hearing threshold or worse) should receive: a. oral antibiotic therapy if child has not been on antibiotics, or b. a change in antibiotics, or c. bilateral myringotomy with tube placement; and d. environmental risk factor control counseling.	III	Stool et al., 1994	Prevent hearing loss and problems with language development.	Scientific evidence is limited to support recommendation of tube replacement; however, strong panel consensus exists. Exposure to cigarette smoke has been shown to increase risk of otitis media with effusion. The panel also noted that parents may wish to remove children from a child care facility.
7.	Management of patients with otitis media with effusion for 4-6 months and a history of significant bilateral hearing loss (at least 20 decibels) and a failure of adequate antibiotic therapy should include: a. bilateral myringotomy with tube placement, and b. environmental risk factor counseling.	III	Stool et al., 1994	Prevent hearing loss and problems with language development.	Severity and duration of disease suggest intervention is warrranted. Assumes failure of antibiotic therapy.

Follow-up

	Indicator	Quality of evidence	Literature	Benefits	Comments
8.	All patients identified as having otitis media with effusion must either have a recommendation for follow-up visit or have been seen for reevaluation within 8 weeks of diagnosis.	II/III	Lous, 1988; Stool et al., 1994; Daly, 1982	Prevent hearing loss and problems with language development.	The AHCPR Guideline recommends a six-week follow-up period. Eight weeks allows plans addition time to have accomplished follow-up.

*Complications of surgery include: external auditory canal wall laceration, persistent otorrhea, granuloma formation at the myringotomy site, cholesteatoma, and permanent tympanic membrane perforation. Structural changes in the tympanic membrane are also possible, especially with repeated tube insertions. The risk of repeated tube insertions has been estimated to be as high as 30 percent within 5 years of initial surgery.

**Complications of anesthesia include mortality, cardiac arrest, and allergic reactions.

Quality of Evidence Codes:

I: RCT
II-1:   Nonrandomized controlled trials
II-2:   Cohort or case analysis
II-3:   Multiple time series
III: Opinions or descriptive studies

ACUTE OTITIS MEDIA

IMPORTANCE

This review focuses on acute otitis media (AOM), a process that frequently precedes otitis media with effusion (Fliss, et al., 1994). Recurrent acute otitis media is defined as repeated episodes of acute otitis, conventionally defined as three episodes of acute otitis media (Teele et al., 1989). The propensity for recurrent acute otitis media is associated with onset of disease before one year of age (Fliss et al., 1994). Persistent acute otitis media is defined as symptoms beyond six days of initiating therapy or recurrence within a few days of completing at least a 10 day course of antibiotics (Fliss et al., 1994). These children should be watched closely.

EFFICACY AND/OR EFFECTIVENESS OF INTERVENTIONS

Screening

Because acute otitis media is an acute episodic illness, screening for this process is not appropriate.

Diagnosis

Patients with acute otitis media usually experience some or all of the following symptoms often following an acute upper respiratory illness: ear pain (otalgia), fever (23 percent of patients) (Schwartz et al., 1981), and hearing loss. A suggestion of these symptoms by history or nondescript findings (Baker, 1991) provided by the parents or patient, such as irritability, lethargy, decreased appetite, vomiting, or diarrhea should result in an otoscopic examination to observe for redness and opacity, possibly with bulging of the tympanic membrane. In acute disease, the membrane will usually be less compliant and therefore less mobile on pneumatic otoscopy. The presence of a mucopurulent drainage (otorrhea) may occur should the tympanic membrane be ruptured or compromised by tympanostomy tubes.

Treatment

Initial treatment of acute otitis media is with antibiotics, although studies do suggest that there is a spontaneous cure rate, in some studies up to 80 percent (Haddad, 1994; Pichichero, 1994). The choice of antibiotics is the same as those recommended for otitis media with effusion because similar organisms are isolated from both disease processes. Recommended antibiotics include, among others:

1) Amoxicillin (Pukander et al., 1993; Mandel et al., 1991; Berman, 1995);

2) Amoxicillin-clavulanate potassium (McCarty et al., 1993);

3) Cefaclor (Mandel et al., 1991);

4) Cefuroxime axetil (McLinn et al., 1994);

5) Cefixime (Asmar et al., 1994);

6) Erythromycin-sulfisoxazole (Mandel et al., 1991);

7) Trimethoprim-sulfamethoxazole (Daly et al., 1991; Berman, 1995);

8) Clarithromycin (Pukander et al., 1993; Mandel et al., 1991);

9) Erythromycin (Berman, 1995) and;

10) Sulfisoxazole.

Most general discussions of the antimicrobial treatment of acute otitis media favor the use of amoxicillin in the child without allergy to penicillin drugs (Pichichero, 1994).

For patients who do not respond within the first two days of treatment (i.e., 48 hours), aspiration, both for diagnosis and therapy, should be considered; at the very least, the patient's antibiotic coverage should be expanded to achieve broader coverage. The pediatrician should inform the parents to watch the child closely for either lack of resolution or progressive clinical signs (e.g., increasing lethargy) that may suggest extension of the disease. However, Berman (1995) notes that the effectiveness of antibiotics for acute otitis media is controversial, since in two-thirds of treated children the clinical signs and symptoms resolve without eradication of the middle-ear pathogen.

Follow-up Care

Once resolved, the child should be seen again to ensure that serous otitis media is not present. This evaluation should occur after the course of antibiotics is completed.

RECOMMENDED QUALITY INDICATORS FOR ACUTE OTITIS MEDIA

These indicators apply to children ages 1-3 years.

Diagnosis

	Indicator	Quality of evidence	Literature	Benefits	Comments
1.	All children presenting to the clinician with fever, nonspecific behavioral changes (e.g., irritability, lethargy, decreased appetite, vomiting, diarrhea), or ear pain should receive an ear examination using a pneumatic otoscope.	III	Fliss et al., 1994; Howie et al., 1993	Prevent hearing loss and problems with language development from untreated infections.	In young children, fever and/or nonspecific complaints may be the only symptoms of ear infection. Pneumatic otoscopy is more informative than otoscopy alone as a diagnostic tool.

Treatment

	Indicator	Quality of evidence	Literature	Benefits	Comments
2.	For all patients with the diagnosis of acute otitis media, at least 10 days of antibiotics should be prescribed.	III	Pichichero, 1994	Prevent hearing loss and problems with language development.	Treatment failure may be greater of the course of antibiotic therapy is less than 10 days.

Follow-up

	Indicator	Quality of evidence	Literature	Benefits	Comments
3.	Once a diagnosis of acute otitis media is made, follow-up chart review should document a return visit after the course of antibiotics within 8 weeks of diagnosis.	III	Berman, 1995	Prevent hearing loss and problems with language development.	Follow-up visit is necessary to determine whether inflammation of the tympanic membrane has resolved; persistent infection may not be symptomatic.

Quality of Evidence Codes:

I: RCT
II-1:   Nonrandomized controlled trials
II-2:   Cohort or case analysis
II-3:   Multiple time series
III: Opinions or descriptive studies

REFERENCES - OTITIS MEDIA

Asmar BI, AS Dajani, MA Del Beccaro, et al. December 1994. Comparison of cefpodoxime proxetil and cefixime in the treatment of acute otitis media in infants and children. *Pediatrics* 94 (6): 847-52.

Baker RC. November 1991. Pitfalls in diagnosing acute otitis media. *Pediatric Annals* 20 (11): 591-8.

Berman S. 8 June 1995. Otitis media in children. *New England Journal of Medicine* 332 (23): 1560-5.

Berman S, R Roark, and D Luckey. 1994. Theoretical cost effectiveness of management options for children with persisting middle ear effusions. *Pediatrics* 93 (3): 353-63.

Bluestone CD. 1986. Otitis media and sinusitis in children. *Drugs* 31 supp (3): 132-41.

Bluestone CD, TJ Fria, SK Arjona, et al. January 1986. Controversies in screening for middle ear disease and hearing loss in children. *Pediatrics* 77 (1): 57-70.

Callahan CW, and S Lazoritz. May 1988. Otitis media and language development. *American Family Physician* 37 (5): 186-90.

Cantekin EI, TW McGuire, and TL Griffith. 18 December 1991. Antimicrobial therapy for otitis media with effusion ('secretory' otitis media). *Journal of the American Medical Association* 266 (23): 3309-17.

Daly KA. August 1991. Epidemiology of otitis media. *Otolaryngologic Clinics of North America* 24 (4): 775-86.

Estelle F, and R Simons. 1994. H1-receptor antagonists: Comparative tolerability and safety. *Drug Experience* 10 (5): 350-80.

Fliss DM, A Leiberman, and R Dagan. 1994. Medical sequelae and complications of acute otitis media. *Pediatric Infectious Disease Journal* 13 (1): S34-40.

Gates GA, JL Northern, HP Ferrer, et al. April 1989. Diagnosis and screening. In: *Recent Advances in Otitis Media: Report of the Fourth Research Conference (Suppl 139)*. *Annals of Otology, Rhinology and Laryngology* 98 (Number 4, Part 2): 39-41.

Haddad Jr. J. June 1994. Treatment of acute otitis media and its complications. *Pediatric Otology* 27 (3): 431-41.

Kemp ED. June 1990. Otitis media. *Primary Care* 17 (2): 267-87.

Kleinman LC, J Kosecoff, RW Dubois, et al. 27 April 1994. The medical appropriateness of tympanostomy tubes proposed for children younger than 16 years in the United States. *Journal of the American Medical Association* 271 (16): 1250-5.

Lous J, M Fiellau-Nikolajsen, and AL Jeppesen. 1988. Secretory otitis media and language development: A six-year follow-up study with case-control. *International Journal of Pediatric Otorhinolaryngology* 15: 185-203.

Mandel EM, D Kardatzke, CD Bluestone, et al. 1993. A comparative evaluation of cefaclor and amoxicillin in the treatment of acute otitis media. *Pediatric Infectious Disease Journal* 12 (9): 726-32.

Mandel EM, HE Rockette, JL Paradise, et al. 1991. Comparative efficacy of erythromycin-sulfisoxazole, cefaclor, amoxicillin or placebo for otitis media with effusion in children. *Pediatric Infectious Disease Journal* 10 (12): 899-906.

Mandel EM, HE Rockette, CD Bluestone, et al. 19 February 1987. Efficacy of amoxicillin with and without decongestant-antihistamine for otitis media with effusion in children. *New England Journal of Medicine* 316 (8): 432-7.

Maw AR, and R Bawden. 1994. Factors affecting resolution of otitis media with effusion in children. *Clinical Otolaryngology* 19: 125-30.

Maw AR, AJ Parker, GN Lance, et al. 1992. The effect of parental smoking on outcome after treatment for glue ear in children. *Clinical Otolaryngology* 17: 411-4.

McCarty JM, A Phillips, and R Wiisanen. 1993. Comparative safety and efficacy of clarithromycin and amoxicillin/clavulanate in the treatment of acute otitis media in children. *Pediatric Infectious Disease Journal* 12 (12): S122-S127.

McLinn SE, M Moskal, J Goldfarb, et al. February 1994. Comparison of cefuroxime axetil and amoxicillin-clavulanate suspensions in treatment of acute otitis media with effusion in children. *Antimicrobial Agents and Chemotherapy* 38 (2): 315-8.

Pichichero ME. 1994. Assessing the treatment alternatives for acute otitis media. *Pediatric Infectious Disease Journal* 13 (1): S27-34.

Pukander JS, JP Jero, EA Kaprio, et al. 1993. Clarithromycin vs amoxicillin suspensions in the treatment of pediatric patients with acute otitis media. *Pediatric Infectious Disease Journal* 12 (12): S118-21.

Rosenfeld RM, and JC Post. April 1992. Meta-analysis of antibiotics for the treatment of otitis media with effusion. *Otolaryngology-Head and Neck Surgery* 106 (4): 378-86.

Sagraves R, W Maish, and A Kameshka. December 1992. Update on otitis media: Part 1. Epidemiology and pathophysiology. *American Pharmacy* NS32 (12): 27-31.

Schappert, SM. 8 September 1992. *Office Visits for Otitis Media: United States, 1975-90*. U.S. Department of Health and Human Services, Hyattsville, MD.

Schwartz RH, WJ Rodriguez, I Brook, et al. 22 May 1981. The febrile response in acute otitis media. *Journal of the American Medical Association* 245 (20): 2057-8.

Stool, SE, AO Berg, S Berman, et al. July 1994. *Otitis Media with Effusion in Young Children: Clinical Practice Guideline*. Agency for Health Care Policy and Research, Public Health Service, U.S. Department of Health and Human Services, No. 12. Rockville, MD.

Teele DW, JO Klein, B Rosner, et al. July 1989. Epidemiology of otitis media during the first seven years of life in children in greater Boston: A prospective, cohort study. *The Journal of Infectious Diseases* 160 (1): 83-94.

van Buchem FL, JHM Dunk, and MA van't Hof. 24 October 1981. Therapy of acute otitis media: Myringotomy, antibiotics, or neither? A double-blind study in children. *Lancet* 2 (8252): 883-7.

Williams RL. Otitis media and otitis externa. 1992. In *Primary Pediatric Care*, Second ed. Editor Hoekelman RA, 1417-20. St. Louis, MO: Mosby-Year Book, Inc.

Williams RL, TC Chalmers, KC Stange, et al. 15 September 1993. Use of antibiotics in preventing recurrent acute otitis media and in treating otitis media with effusion. *Journal of the American Medical Association* 270 (11): 1344-51.

Zielhuis GA, GH Rach, and P van den Broek. 1990. The natural course of otitis media with effusion in preschool children. *European Archives of Oto-Rhino-Laryngology* 247: 215-21.

16. PRENATAL CARE

The pediatric expert panel agreed to defer scoring and modification of the pediatric prenatal care indicators to the women's expert panel. In doing so, the pediatric expert panel agreed to accept any changes (modifications, deletions, additions) the women's expert panel made to the prenatal care indicators.

The literature review and proposed adult women's prenatal care indicators can be found in Chapter 14, "Prenatal Care," in the RAND document *Quality of Care for Women: A Review of Selected Clinical Conditions and Quality Indicators,* DRU-1720-HCFA. The final set of pediatric prenatal care indicators can be found in the indicator crosswalk table in Appendix C of this document. The only difference between the two sets of indicators is that the pediatric indicators exclude any women's indicators that exceed the pediatric age range.

17. SICKLE CELL SCREENING AND SELECT TOPICS IN PREVENTION OF COMPLICATIONS
Mark Schuster, M.D., Ph.D.

We used the following sources to construct indicators for sickle cell disease screening for newborns and selected topics in prevention of complications for infants and children: appropriate chapters from textbooks on pediatrics (Martin and Pearson in Oski et al., 1994) and pediatric primary care (Platt in Dershewitz, 1993; Whitten in Hoekelman et al., 1992) and the Agency for Health Care Policy and Research (AHCPR) clinical practice guideline *Sickle Cell Disease: Screening, Diagnosis, Management, and Counseling in Newborns and Infants* (Sickle Cell Disease Guideline Panel, 1993).

IMPORTANCE

There are several types of sickle cell diseases, among them sickle cell anemia (Hb SS), hemoglobin SC disease (Hb SC), and sickle beta-thalassemia. In the United States, these diseases are most commonly found in people of African ancestry, but they also affect people of Mediterranean, Caribbean, South and Central American, Arabian, and East Indian ancestry. In the United States, sickle cell anemia affects more than 50,000 people and occurs in about 1 in 375 African-American live births. Estimated prevalence of hemoglobin SC disease is 1 in 835 African-American live births; for sickle beta-thalassemia, it is 1 in 1,667 African-American live births (Sickle Cell Disease Guideline Panel, 1993).

EFFICACY/EFFECTIVENESS OF INTERVENTIONS

Screening

The AHCPR practice guideline recommends screening of all newborns for sickle cell disease regardless of racial or ethnic background. The rationale is (1) there is a benefit to screening (prophylaxis, which is discussed below), (2) it is not possible to identify accurately a person's heritage by appearance or surname, and (3) much screening is conducted by state-sponsored programs supported at least in part by public funds. More than 40 states, the District of Columbia, Puerto Rico, and the Virgin Islands conduct universal newborn hemoglobinopathy screening (Sickle Cell Disease Guideline Panel, 1993).

The Sickle Cell Disease Guideline Panel (1993) states that screening of populations with a low prevalence of sickle cell disease is cost-effective when the screening is integrated into a laboratory that is also testing samples from a population with a high prevalence. In states that provide universal screening, all managed care plans should conduct the screening and obtain the results. However, low prevalence states that do not have universal screening programs may not provide access to laboratories in high prevalence areas. Therefore, managed care plans that serve low prevalence populations in these states might decide that it is not cost-effective to screen all newborns. However, there would probably be little disagreement that they should be screening all African-American newborns.

Platt (in Dershewitz, 1993), Whitten (in Hoekelman et al., 1992), and Martin and Pearson (in Oski et al., 1994) all recommend hemoglobin electrophoresis for definitive diagnosis. The Sickle Cell Disease Guideline Panel (1993) lists three methods that can be used to make a definitive diagnosis: electrophoresis, immunologic testing, or DNA analysis. The panel also says that testing both parents' blood can assist in diagnosis. Some types of sickle cell disease do not need confirmation (e.g., Hb SE, Hb SD, or Hb SO$_{Arab}$), but these forms of the disease are quite rare (Sickle Cell Disease Guideline Panel, 1993). Whitten (in Hoekelman et al., 1992) says that parents generally do not need to be tested when a child is found to have sickle cell disease since the diagnosis is usually clear.

If a child has a positive screen at birth, it should be repeated after the child is at least one month old (unless both parents have sickle trait) since the initial test could also have detected hereditary persistence of fetal hemoglobin or sickle cell-beta thalassemia (Whitten in Hoekelman et al., 1992). While Platt (in Dershewitz, 1993) does not give a specific timetable for screening, she states that diagnosis should be made in the newborn period.

Prophylaxis

Infections with *Streptococcus pneumoniae* are one of the major causes of death in infants with sickle cell anemia. Without prophylaxis, about 30 percent will become infected during the first three years of life, and about one-third of them will die from infection (Gaston and Verter, 1990). This occurs because of functional asplenia that develops over the first two years of life (Sickle Cell Disease Guideline Panel, 1993). A randomized, controlled clinical trial showed that twice-daily oral penicillin reduces the morbidity and mortality from Streptococcus pneumoniae infections in children with sickle cell disease (Gaston et al., 1986).

The Sickle Cell Disease Guideline Panel (1993) recommends beginning penicillin prophylaxis by 2 months of age for infants with suspected sickle cell anemia and sickle beta-thalessemia, whether or not definitive diagnosis has been made yet. Martin and Pearson (in Oski et al., 1994), however, say that prophylaxis should begin by 6 months of age (Martin and Pearson in Oski et al., 1994), and the American Academy of Pediatrics (AAP) (in Peter, 1994) says it should begin before 4 months. Platt (in Dershewitz, 1993) says that it should begin as soon as possible.

While there is general support for the use of penicillin prophylaxis, there is some disagreement on the age at which it can be discontinued. Some state that prophylaxis should continue twice a day for the first five years of life (Platt in Dershewitz, 1993; Whitten in Hoekelman et al., 1992), while at least one other states that it should continue until at least 6 years of age (Martin and Pearson in Oski et al., 1994). The AAP (in Peter, 1994) says that prophylaxis should be strongly considered in children younger than 5 years old and considered for older children. Research to determine the age at which to discontinue prophylaxis is currently being conducted (AAP in Peter, 1994).

Children with sickle cell disease should receive the pneumococcal vaccine when they are at least two years old (AAP in Peter, 1994; Platt, in Dershewitz, 1993).

Monitoring

Children of all ages with sickle cell disease should be seen every few months to monitor baseline laboratory data such as complete blood cell count and reticulocyte count and to monitor intercurrent events (Platt, in Dershewitz, 1993).

RECOMMENDED QUALITY INDICATORS FOR SICKLE CELL SCREENING FOR NEWBORNS AND PREVENTION OF COMPLICATIONS

The following criteria apply to sickle cell screening for newborns and select topics in prevention of complications for infants and children.

Screening

	Indicator	Quality of evidence	Literature	Benefits	Comments
1.	All children in states with mandatory newborn sickle cell testing should be screened before hospital discharge or within 48 hours of birth, whichever comes later.	III	Inferred from Sickle Cell Disease Guideline Panel, 1993	Prevent pneumococcal infection. Decrease heart failure from splenic sequestration.	Screening allows for early diagnosis and prophylactic therapy (e.g., penicillin) before the patient develops the first pneumococcal infection. It also enables monitoring (which helps treatment of sickle crises) to begin. It allows time to teach the family about symptoms to watch for in children with sickle cell.
2.	African-American children should be tested for sickle cell disease by the end of the third month of life.	III	Whitten, in Hoekelman et al., 1992	Prevent pneumococcal infection. Decrease heart failure from splenic sequestration.	Though the AHCPR guideline recommends testing for all newborns regardless of race or ethnicity, it also says that universal testing has only been shown to be cost-effective when low prevalence regions. However, individual managed care organizations located in states that do not offer universal screening may not consider it cost-effective to test all newborns and may not have the ability to coordinate with high prevalence states. Testing through a state newborn screening program is adequate if results are noted in the chart. This indicator will be difficult to operationalize if racial background is not typically recorded in the chart.
3.	Children with a positive sickle screen at less than or equal to one month of age should have a repeat screen after one month of age and prior to the end of six months of age.	III	Sickle Cell Disease Guideline Panel, 1993; Whitten, in Hoekelman et al., 1992	Prevent allergic reactions from antibiotics. Prevent antibiotic resistance. Improve quality of life.	Confirmatory tests are necessary because of the possibility of false positive diagnoses. False positive diagnoses lead to unnecessary prophylaxis and vigilance for symptoms. Prophylactic antibiotics can have side effects, increase resistance in the community, and are disruptive to take on a daily basis. The purpose is to confirm the diagnosis.

305

Prevention of Complications

	Indicator	Quality of evidence	Literature	Benefits	Comments
4.	Children with a positive sickle screen or children suspected of being positive for sickle cell disease should be placed on daily penicillin prophylaxis from at least six months of age until at least five years of age.	I	Gaston et al., 1986; AAP, in Peter, 1994; Martin & Pearson, in Oski et al., 1994; Platt, in Dershewitz, 1993; Sickle Cell Disease Guideline Panel, 1993	Prevent pneumococcal infections.	Pneumococcal infections are prevalent and are often fatal in persons with sickle cell disease. The references recommend different age ranges for prophylaxis. The one specified here is the narrowest found in the reviewed literature.
5.	Children with sickle cell disease should have a hematocrit or hemoglobin, and reticulocyte count performed at least every four months.	III	Platt, in Dershewitz, 1993	Prevent worsening anemia and death. Improve quality of life. Decrease heart failure from splenic sequestration.	This information provides baseline values for comparison during periods of acute illness. It also allows determination of when the patient is more anemic than baseline so that he/she can receive potentially life-saving transfusions, and it avoids inappropriate transfusion by clinicians who do not recognize that the patient is at a stable level of anemia.
6.	Children with sickle cell disease should have received the pneumococcal vaccine between 2 years and 3 years of age.	III	Inferred from AAP in Peter, 1994; Platt, in Dershewitz, 1993	Prevent penumococcal infections.	The literature does not say how soon after the second birthday one should receive this vaccine, but it seems clear that the sooner the better to prevent possible infection.
7.	A child older than 2 years with sickle cell disease who joins a new managed care organization should have documented at the first visit whether or not he/she has ever had a pneumococcal vaccine or that efforts are being made to determine the vaccine history.	I, III		Prevent penumococcal infections.	This is not specifically recommended, but the importance of this vaccine suggests that it should be addressed immediately by new providers.
8.	The patient should receive the vaccination within one month of this visit if the patient or the patient's caregiver does not know if the vaccine has been given and it has not been confirmed by other means. If the patient or patient's caregiver does not believe the vaccine had been given before, the vaccine should be given at that visit.	I, III	Hales and Barriere, 1979; Ammann et al., 1977	Prevent penumococcal infections.	This is not specifically recommended, but the importance of this vaccine suggests that it should be addressed immediately by new providers.

Quality of Evidence Codes:

I: RCT
II-1: Nonrandomized controlled trials
II-2: Cohort or case analysis
II-3: Multiple time series
III: Opinions or descriptive studies

REFERENCES - SICKLE CELL SCREENING FOR NEWBORNS

American Academy of Pediatrics. 1994. Asplenic children. *1994 Red Book: Report of the Committee on Infectious Diseases.* Editor Peter G. American Academy of Pediatrics. 57-9, Elk Grove Village, IL.

Ammann AJ, J Addiego, DW Wara, et al. 1977. Polyvalent pneumococcal-polysaccharide immunization of patients with sickle-cell anemia and patients with splenectomy. *New England Journal of Medicine* 297: 897-900.

Gaston MH, JI Verter, G Woods, et al. 19 June 1986. Prophylaxis with oral penicillin in children with sickle cell anemia: A randomized trial. *New England Journal of Medicine* 314 (25): 1593-9.

Gaston MH, and J Verter. 1990. Sickle cell anemia trial. *Statistics in Medicine* 9: 45-51.

Hales K, and SL Barriere. 1979. Polyvalent pneumococcal vaccines: A review. *American Journal of Hospital Pharmacy* 36: 773-777.

Martin PL, and HA Pearson. 1994. The hemoglobinopathies and thalassemias. In *Principles and Practice of Pediatrics*, Second ed. Editors Oski FA, CD DeAngelis, RD Feigin, et al., 1660-3. Philadelphia, PA: J.B. Lippincott Company.

Platt OS. 1993. Sickle cell anemia. In *Ambulatory Pediatric Care*, Second ed. Editor Dershewitz RA, 479-81. Philadelphia, PA: J.B. Lippincott Company.

Sickle Cell Disease Guideline Panel. April 1993. *Sickle Cell Disease: Screening, Diagnosis, Management, and Counseling in Newborns and Infants. Clinical Practice Guideline No. 6.* Agency for Health Care Policy and Research, Public Health Service, U.S. Department of Health and Human Services, Rockville, MD.

Whitten CF. 1992. Sickle cell conditions. In *Primary Pediatric Care*, Second ed. Editors Hoekelman RA, SB Friedman, NM Nelson, et al., 240-2. St. Louis, MO: Mosby-Year Book, Inc.

18. TUBERCULOSIS SCREENING
Mark Schuster, M.D., Ph.D.

The American Thoracic Society (ATS) and the Centers for Disease Control and Prevention (CDC) traditionally provide guidance on the diagnosis, treatment, prevention, and control of tuberculosis (ATS, 1990; CDC, 1990). In addition, the American Academy of Pediatrics (AAP) makes specific recommendations regarding children. This review therefore draws heavily on the published recommendations of these three organizations. Additional sources include the U.S. Preventive Services Task Force's (USPSTF) Guide to Clinical Preventive Services (1989) and textbooks on pediatrics (Starke et al. in Oski et al., 1994), general pediatrics (Niederman in Dershewitz, 1993), and pediatric infectious disease (Smith et al., in Feigin and Cherry, 1992). Several articles were also identified from the bibliographies of the previously described sources and from a MEDLINE search of English-language articles on tuberculosis screening in pediatric and adolescent age groups published between January 1990 and March 1995.

IMPORTANCE

Epidemiology

Mycobacterium tuberculosis is the bacterium responsible for tuberculosis (TB). It can cause significant pulmonary and extrapulmonary disease, but in most otherwise healthy people, untreated infection becomes dormant and never progresses to clinical disease. The risk for developing disease is highest in the first two years after initial infection, but disease may develop months or years later (AAP, 1994a).

Newly-infected children are more likely to progress to disease than newly-infected adults. Without treatment, disease eventually develops in 5 to 10 percent of immunologically normal adults with TB infection. By comparison, disease develops in up to 43 percent of untreated children less than 1 year old, 24 percent of 1-5 year olds, and 15 percent of 11-15 year olds (Starke et al. in Oski et al., 1992). In addition to age, risk factors for progression of infection to disease include recent close contact with an infected person, recent skin test conversion (see below), intravenous drug use, and medical conditions and treatments that adversely affect the cellular immune system (e.g., HIV infection, Hodgkin's disease, lymphoma, diabetes mellitus, chronic renal failure, malnutrition, and daily corticosteroid therapy) (AAP, 1994a; Starke et al. in Oski et al., 1992).

Transmission is usually by inhalation of droplet nuclei produced by an adult or adolescent with infectious pulmonary TB, though transmission through or across skin, gastrointestinal tract, mucous membranes, placenta, or amniotic fluid has been reported. Children with primary pulmonary TB are usually not contagious (AAP, 1994a).

After decades of consistently declining incidence of TB, the United States has been experiencing a resurgence (Starke et al. in Oski et al., 1992). In 1992, over 26,000 cases of TB were reported, a 13 percent increase per 100,000 population over 1985 (the year with the lowest number of reported TB cases since reporting began). The increase was 25 percent for children 0-4 years old and 21 percent for children 5-14 years old (CDC, 1993). In 1990, the CDC (1990) estimated that there were 10 to 15 million people in the U.S. with latent TB infection.

Case rates of TB for all ages are highest in urban, low-income areas. More than two-thirds of cases are reported in nonwhite racial and ethnic groups (Asians and Pacific Islanders, African Americans, Native Americans and Alaskan Natives, and Latinos) and more than one quarter are reported in people born outside the United States. Rates are also high among the homeless and residents of correctional facilities (AAP, 1994a).

Screening Methods

The purpose of TB screening is to identify asymptomatic infected people so that they can take chemoprophylaxis to prevent the development of TB disease and so their potentially infected contacts can be identified. A tuberculin skin test is used for screening. The incubation period from infection to development of a positive reaction

to a tuberculin skin test is about two to ten weeks. Tuberculin
reactivity usually lasts throughout a person's lifetime (AAP, 1994a).

There are two techniques for applying the tuberculin test:

1) The Mantoux technique consists of intracutaneous administration
   of 5 Tuberculin Units (5-TU) of purified protein derivative
   (PPD) into the forearm. Two other concentrations of PPD, 1-TU
   and 250-TU, are not appropriate for routine screening (ATS,
   1990). A positive test consists of an indurated area of
   adequate size (discussed below). This method is generally
   necessary to make a diagnosis of TB infection, and it is the
   method recommended by the AAP (1994a), the ATS (1990), and the
   USPSTF (1989) for screening people with risk factors for TB.

2) The multiple-puncture test (MPT) punctures the skin with a
   pointed applicator that is either coated with dried tuberculin
   or passes through a film of liquid tuberculin. MPTs use either
   PPD or Old Tuberculin (OT). The quantity of tuberculin
   introduced into the skin cannot be precisely controlled so they
   are not as reliable as the Mantoux and must be interpreted with
   caution. Though a negative MPT is a good indication that the
   Mantoux would be negative, an MPT reaction is not adequate
   evidence that a Mantoux would be positive. An exception is a
   vesicular MPT reaction, which can be read as positive.
   Therefore, nonvesicular MPT reactions must be confirmed by a
   Mantoux (ATS, 1990).

Because of the inferiority of the MPT, the AAP (1994a), the ATS
(1990), and the USPSTF (1989) all recommend the Mantoux for screening
people with TB risk factors. MPTs are not recommended for screening
high-risk populations or for diagnosis (AAP, 1994a; ATS, 1990). The AAP
strongly recommends that "MPTs are not appropriate for diagnosis, and
their use should be severely restricted if not eliminated" (AAP, 1994b).
Because detection of newly infected persons requires accurate testing
and reading, multiple-puncture devices should not be used in tuberculin
testing surveillance programs designed to detect newly infected persons
(ATS, 1990). However, MPTs may be used for surveys or screening among

groups of asymptomatic unexposed persons in whom only a small proportion
are expected to have TB infection (ATS, 1990).

Interpretation of Mantoux Results (AAP, 1994a)

The definition of a positive Mantoux skin test (5TU-PPD) varies
somewhat among the guidelines of different organizations, but there is
much overlap. The CDC, ATS, and AAP all interpret an indurated area of
at least 15 mm as positive in any person. Interpretation of smaller
areas as positive depends on epidemiologic and clinical factors, and
recommendations are not uniform. We will base our indicators on the
AAP's guidelines (AAP, 1994a) since they are the only ones targeted
specifically at the pediatric and adolescent age groups. (The ATS
(1990) recommendations are quite similar but are slightly less expansive
in the list of reasons for calling a reaction positive when smaller than
15 mm.)

A positive Mantoux includes induration that is (AAP, 1994a):

1) at least 15 mm in anyone;

2) at least 10 mm in a child who:

   a. is less than 4 years old, or

   b. has other medical risk factors putting him/her at increased
      risk of developing TB disease (e.g., Hodgkin's disease,
      lymphoma, diabetes mellitus, chronic renal failure, and
      malnutrition), or

   c. who was born, or whose parents were born, in regions of the
      world where TB is highly prevalent, or

   d. who is frequently exposed to adults who are HIV-infected,
      homeless, users of intravenous and other street drugs, poor
      and medically indigent city dwellers, residents of nursing
      homes, incarcerated or institutionalized persons, and
      migrant farm workers.

3) at least 5 mm in a child who:

   a. is in close contact with someone with a known or suspected
      infectious case of TB (households with active or previously
      active cases) if: (1) treatment cannot be verified as
      adequate before exposure, (2) treatment was initiated after

the period of the child's contact began, or (3) reactivation is suspected), or

b. is suspected of having TB disease clinically or by chest x-ray, or

c. has an immunosuppressive condition or HIV infection or is receiving an immunosuppressive treatment.

Tuberculin skin tests should be read 48-72 hours after they are placed (ATS, 1990; USPSTF, 1989; AAP, 1994a). Delayed hypersensitivity reactions to tuberculin (i.e., a positive test) begin at 5 to 6 hours, are maximal at 48-72 hours, and subside over a period of days. In a few persons (who are elderly or have not been tested previously), reactions may develop slowly and may not peak until after 72 hours. Immediate hypersensitivity reactions begin shortly after injection, but disappear by 24 hours and should not be confused with positive tests (ATS, 1990). The AAP (1994a) recommends that qualified medical personnel read positive and negative tuberculin skin tests 48 to 72 hours after placement. In practice, it may be quite difficult to get parents to bring their children back in two or three days to have the test read. This may be even more difficult when the test is negative, and parents believe they can adequately read them. Recent studies have shown that parents often misread positive skin tests (Cheng et al., 1995b) and that parents often do not bring their children back to have the test read even with incentives and reminder phone calls (Cheng et al., 1995a). Studies show that 28-82 percent of skin tests in pediatric patients are not read in the requisite 48-72 hour period (USPSTF, 1989). If tests are read late, positive responses may have subsided enough to be read as negative.

For each tuberculin test, a record should be made of the technique of administration (Mantoux or multiple-puncture), the kind and dose of tuberculin, and the size of reaction in millimeters of induration (ATS, 1990). In a clinic in which only one type of tuberculin is used, it would be unnecessary to document these in each chart. However, the size of reaction would be important.

The frequency of false-positive and false-negative tests depends on a number of variables, including immunologic status, the size of the hypersensitivity reaction, and the prevalence of atypical mycobacteria (nontuberculosis mycobacteria that cross-react with the tuberculin skin test) (USPSTF, 1989). Vaccination with BCG (a TB vaccine rarely given in the U.S. but common among immigrants from some parts of the world) can produce a false positive. Guidelines for interpreting skin tests take this into account (ATS, 1990). Anergy testing can help distinguish true from false negatives in HIV-infected and immunosuppressed people (ATS, 1992; CDC, 1991).

Populations To Be Screened

The AAP and ATS recommend a strategy of identifying high-risk populations for annual Mantoux skin-testing rather than routinely testing all persons, many of whom would be at low risk (AAP, 1994b; ATS, 1990).

Specifically, the AAP (1994a) defines as high risk children or adolescents who:

- are contacts of adults [or adolescents][1] with infectious tuberculosis, or
- are from or have parents [or household contacts] from regions of the world with high prevalence of tuberculosis, or
- have abnormalities on chest X-ray suggestive of tuberculosis, or
- have clinical evidence of tuberculosis, or
- are HIV-infected, or
- have immunosuppressive conditions, or
- have other medical risk factors, e.g., Hodgkin's disease, lymphoma, diabetes mellitus, chronic renal failure, malnutrition, or
- are incarcerated, or
- are frequently exposed to adults [or adolescents] who are HIV-infected, homeless, users of intravenous and other street

---

[1]Material that seems consistent with the AAP list has been added in brackets.

drugs, poor and medically-indigent city dwellers, residents of nursing homes, migrant farm workers.

If no household contacts have current TB disease but one or more contacts have a positive tuberculin skin test, an infant should be tested with a Mantoux skin test at 3 to 4 months of age (AAP, 1994a). The AAP (1994a) provides guidelines for what to do if a contact does have current disease or if all contacts cannot be promptly tested. These detailed guidelines will not be incorporated into the indicators because they will not apply to many patients in the current study and because they fit better in a review of management of adult TB rather than a review of routine screening.

The ATS (1990), the CDC (1990), and the USPSTF (1989) do not define high-risk specifically for children and adolescents, but their general recommendations are essentially the same as the AAP's.

The CDC and ATS do not recommend routine skin testing in low-risk groups in communities with a low prevalence of tuberculosis except for one-time testing during childhood for epidemiologic assessment of tuberculosis infection in the area. Positive skin tests in such populations would be more likely to be false than true positives (AAP, 1994a). The AAP (1994a) makes an additional recommendation for children with no risk factors living in high-prevalence regions and for children whose risk factor history is incomplete or unreliable: periodic Mantoux tests (e.g., 1, 4, 6, and 11-16 years) may be performed depending on local epidemiology. These recommendations will not be incorporated into an indicator because of the variability of local epidemiology and because the timing of testing for this recommendation is left to the discretion of the clinician.

Many people who should receive skin-testing do not. In one study, three-quarters of TB patients had had contact with a health-care provider within the 5 year period prior to diagnosis, but less than one-third had been skin-tested, even though many had risk factors for TB (ATS, 1992). The CDC estimates that more than 90 percent of persons reported to have clinical TB disease have been infected for at least a year (CDC, 1990).

Chemoprophylaxis

Screening is important because chemoprophylaxis can be given to asymptomatic people to prevent progression from TB infection to disease and to prevent spread to others.

Isoniazid (INH) is the primary drug used for prophylaxis. When taken as prescribed, preventive therapy with INH is highly effective. In controlled trials conducted by the U.S. Public Health Service, 12 months of INH preventive therapy reduced the incidence of disease by 54-88 percent. The main reason for variation appears to have been the amount of medication actually taken. In a large trial in eastern Europe among infected adults with abnormal chest x-rays, a 12-month course of INH was 75 percent effective among all persons assigned to the regimen and 93 percent effective among those who were compliant with therapy. A six month course was 69 percent effective among those who were compliant (ATS, 1992). The AAP (1994a) reports that efficacy of chemoprophylaxis is almost 100 percent when the medication is taken properly. The current recommendation for children without HIV is 9 months and with HIV is at least 12 months (AAP, 1994a). INH is not without risks, primarily a risk of hepatotoxicity that increases with age, but the benefits are generally considered to outweigh the risks until a person is at least 35 years old. Other prophylaxis regimens may be necessary when there is reason to believe the organisms are resistant to INH (ATS, 1992). If INH-resistance is suspected, Rifampin should be given along with INH until the suspected source of infection can be tested for susceptibilities. If the index case is susceptible to INH, Rifampin would be discontinued; if the index case is susceptible only to Rifampin, the INH should be discontinued. If the index case is susceptible to neither, an (infectious disease) expert should be consulted (AAP, 1994a).

Children receiving chemoprophylaxis should have a visit with medical personnel at least monthly during therapy so they can be checked for symptoms of side effects. Because of possible visual impairment, children who are old enough should have a baseline visual acuity test done. Follow-up tests are only necessary if indicated by symptoms of changing vision (ATS, 1986). Children should receive a chest x-ray when chemoprophylaxis is begun. If it is normal and the child remains asymptomatic, it does not need to be repeated (AAP, 1994a).

Hepatotoxic reactions to INH are rare in children and adolescents, so routine monitoring of lower enzymes is not necessary. Pyrodaxine helps prevent peripheral neuritis and should be given daily (Niederman in Dershewitz, 1993).

RECOMMENDED QUALITY INDICATORS FOR TUBERCULOSIS SCREENING AND TREATMENT

The following criteria apply to tuberculosis screening for infants, children, and adolescents.

Indicator	Quality of evidence	Literature	Benefits	Comments
1. By the time a child is four months old, there should be documentation of whether or not the child has tuberculosis risk factors* or documentation that the child has had a Mantoux test.	III	Inferred from AAP, 1994a; ATS, 1990	Prevent development of TB disease and its complications.** Prevent spread of TB.	Though guidelines call for annual screening in people at risk for TB, they do not say how often or at what interval a clinician should ask about TB risk factors. Setting the time at one year old should provide ample opportunity to have asked about risk factors at least once. By asking about risk factors, the clinician can determine the need for testing, prophylaxis to prevent infection from developing into disease, and treatment. Clinicians would often know that a child's parents were not from regions of the world with high prevalence of TB and therefore would not typically ask about this risk factor. However, they would not necessarily know whether there was another relative, boarder, household employee, or other contact from another part of the world. Therefore, it seems appropriate to ask about household contacts and to document it. TB risk factors include: - whether the child has had contact with an adult/adolescent with infectious TB; - whether the child or household contacts are from a region of the world with high TB prevalence; and - whether the child is frequently exposed to adults or adolescents who are HIV-infected, homeless, users of injection and other street drugs, poor and medically-indigent city dwellers, residents of nursing homes, or migrant farm workers.
2. If no contacts have evidence of current TB disease but at least one has a positive tuberculin skin test, newborns should be Mantoux tested by the end of the fourth month of life.	III	AAP, 1994a	Prevent development of TB disease and its complications.** Prevent spread of TB.	

318

#	Recommendation	Grade	Source	Objective	Comments
3.	If a child has any of the TB risk factors listed below, he/she should receive an annual Mantoux skin test during the duration of the risk factor: a. has abnormalities on chest X-ray suggestive of TB; or b. has clinical evidence of TB; or c. has HIV-infection, Hodgkin's disease, lymphoma, diabetes mellitus, chronic renal failure, malnutrition, or another immunosuppressive condition; or d. has had contact with an adult/adolescent with infectious TB; or e. is from, or household contacts are from, a region of the world with high TB prevalence; or f. is frequently exposed to adults or adolescents who are HIV-infected, homeless, users of injection and other street drugs, poor and medically-indigent city dwellers, residents of nursing homes, or migrant farm workers.	III	AAP, 1994a; ATS, 1990	Prevent development of TB disease and its complications. Prevent spread of TB.	Regular screening facilitates early detection of infection so that prophylaxis or treatment can be given in a timely fashion.
4.	Children with immunodeficiency or HIV-infection should have anergy testing (e.g., Candida or Mumps antigen) at the same time as TB testing.	III	ATS, 1992; CDC, 1991	Prevent development of TB disease and its complications.** Prevent spread of TB.	Immunocompromised persons may have a negative TB skin test but still have exposure to or infection with TB.
5.	Mantoux skin tests in children with risk factors should be read by a health professional or other trained personnel within 48-72 hours.	III	AAP, 1994a	Prevent development of TB disease and its complications.** Prevent spread of TB.	This may be clinically difficult to implement, given the effort it takes for parents to bring their children back in 2-3 days later. However, it is the recommendation of organized medicine, and there are good reasons for the recommendation. Many clinicians will have the family report if the skin test was positive, but parental assessments in at least some populations are not reliable.
6.	Results of tuberculin skin tests in children with risk factors should be documented within 96 hours of placing the test.	III	ATS, 1990	Prevent development of TB disease and its complications.** Prevent spread of TB.	Even if the clinician trusts the parent's ability to read a positive or negative test properly, the parent may forget to check if there is not an incentive for the clinician to get a response in the proper time period.
7.	All Mantoux skin tests read as positive should document that there was induration and should document the diameter of the induration in millimeters.	III	ATS, 1990	Prevent development of TB disease and its complications.** Prevent spread of TB. Prevent toxicities of anti-TB medications.	Though a positive test requires induration, people often mistake erythema without induration for a positive. The diameter in millimeters is used to determine whether the test is positive.
8.	A Mantoux skin test with ≥15 mm should be read as positive.	III	AAP, 1994a	Prevent development of TB disease and its complications.** Prevent spread of TB. Prevent toxicities of anti-TB medications.	The definition of a positive test depends on both the diameter of induration and characteristics of the patient.

319

#	Recommendation		Source	Purpose	Comment
9.	A Mantoux skin test should be read as positive if there is induration that is at least 10 mm in a child who: - is less than 4 years old; - has other medical risk factors for developing TB disease (Hodgkin's disease, lymphoma, diabetes mellitus, chronic renal failure, malnutrition); - who was born, or whose parents were born, in regions of the world where TB is highly prevalent; or - who is frequently exposed to adults who are HIV-infected, homeless, users of intravenous and other street drugs, poor and medically indigent city dwellers, residents of nursing homes, incarcerated or institutionalized persons, and migrant farm workers.	III	AAP, 1994a	Prevent development of TB disease and its complications.** Prevent spread of TB. Prevent toxicities of anti-TB medications.	The definition of a positive test depends on both the diameter of induration and characteristics of the patient.
10.	A Mantoux skin test should be read as positive if there is induration that is at least 5 mm in a child who: - is in close contact with someone with a known or suspected infectious case of TB (households with active or previously active cases) if (a) treatment cannot be verified as adequate before exposure, (b) treatment was initiated after the period of the child's contact began, or (c) reactivation is suspected; - is suspected of having TB disease clinically or by chest X-ray; or - has an immunosuppressive condition or HIV infection or is receiving immunosuppressive treatment	III	AAP, 1994a	Prevent development of TB disease and its complications.** Prevent spread of TB. Prevent toxicities of anti-TB medications.	The definition of a positive test depends on both the diameter of induration and characteristics of the patient.
11.	All children with positive Mantoux skin tests should have a chest x-ray within two weeks.	III	AAP, 1994a	Prevent development of TB disease and its complications.**	The AAP does not specify how quickly the chest x-ray should be done, but this time period seems reasonable so that active TB can be diagnosed and addressed expeditiously for a condition that should be addressed quickly.
12.	Children with a positive Mantoux test and negative chest x-ray and no other symptoms of TB should receive prophylaxis with INH and/or Rifampin.	I, III	Comstock et al., 1974; Smith et al., in Feigin and Cherry, 1992; AAP, 1994a	Prevent development of TB disease and its complications.**	Prophylaxis greatly reduces the risk of developing TB disease.
13.	Children with a positive Mantoux test and negative chest x-ray and no other symptoms of TB, whose presumed index case (source of infection) has TB resistant to INH and Rifampin, should have a referral made to an infectious disease specialist.	III	AAP, 1994a	Prevent development of TB disease and its complications.**	TB that is resistant to standard medications is becoming more common.

320

14.	Prophylaxis with INH should be given for 9 months to asymptomatic children without HIV and 12 months to asymptomatic children with HIV.	III	AAP, 1994a	Prevent development of TB disease and its complications.**	
15.	Children receiving TB chemoprophylaxis should have contact with a clinician at least once every 5 weeks during therapy.	III	ATS, 1986; Niederman in Dershewitz, 1993	Prevent development of TB disease and its complications.** Prevent toxicities from medications.	Periodic visits ensure patients are taking medications and check for side effects. Side effects are rare in children and include hepatitis and peripheral neuritis or convulsions (due to inhibition of pyridoxine metabolism). The ATS recommendation is for once a month. This indicator allows a grace period.
16.	All children three years and older who are receiving TB chemoprophylaxis with INH should have a baseline visual acuity test performed or attempted.	III	ATS, 1986	Prevent vision loss.	Vision loss is an uncommon side effect of INH. Three-year olds will not always participate in a visual acuity test, but they are young enough to try. Most four-year olds will participate.

*TB risk factors include:
- whether the child has had contact with an adult/adolescent with infectious TB;
- whether the child or household contacts are from a region of the world with high TB prevalence; and
- whether the child is frequently exposed to adults or adolescents who are HIV-infected, homeless, users of injection and other street drugs, poor and medically-indigent city dwellers, residents of nursing homes, or migrant farm workers.

**Disease can cause serious and disabling illness affecting lungs and most other parts of the body.

Quality of Evidence Codes:

I: RCT
II-1:   Nonrandomized controlled trials
II-2:   Cohort or case analysis
II-3:   Multiple time series
III: Opinions or descriptive studies

REFERENCES - TUBERCULOSIS SCREENING AND TREATMENT

American Academy of Pediatrics, and Committee on Infectious Diseases. January 1994. Screening for tuberculosis in infants and children. *Pediatrics* 93 (1): 131-4.

American Academy of Pediatrics. 1994. Tuberculosis. *1994 Red Book: Report of the Committee on Infectious Diseases*. Editor Peter G. American Academy of Pediatrics, Elk Grove Village, IL.

American Thoracic Society. 1992. Control of tuberculosis in the United States. *American Review of Respiratory Disease* 146: 1623-33.

American Thoracic Society. 1990. Diagnostic standards and classification of tuberculosis. *American Review of Respiratory Disease* 142: 725-35.

American Thoracic Society. 1986. Treatment of tuberculosis and tuberculosis infection in adults and children. *American Review of Respiratory Disease* 134: 355-63.

Centers for Disease Control. 17 September 1993. Emerging infectious diseases: Tuberculosis morbidity--United States, 1992. *Morbidity and Mortality Weekly Report* 42 (36): 696-704.

Centers for Disease Control. 26 April 1991. Purified protein derivative (PPD)-tuberculin anergy and HIV infection: Guidelines for anergy testing and management of anergic persons at risk of tuberculosis. *Morbidity and Mortality Weekly Report* 40 (RR-5): 27-33.

Centers for Disease Control. 18 May 1990. Screening for tuberculosis and tuberculous infection in high-risk populations: Recommendations of the Advisory Committee for Elimination of Tuberculosis. *Morbidity and Mortality Weekly Report* 39 (RR-8): 1-7.

Cheng TL, MC Ottolini, K Baumhaft, et al. April 1995. Effectiveness of strategies to increase adherence with tuberculosis test reading in a high risk population. From *Archives of Pediatrics and Adolescent Medicine. Program and Abstracts from the Ambulatory Pediatric Association's 35th Annual Meeting: May 7-11, 1995 in San Diego, California,* 149(4):P72.

Cheng TL, MC Ottolini, P Getson, et al. April 1995. Poor validity of parent reading of skin test induration in a high risk population. From *Archives of Pediatrics and Adolescent Medicine. Program and Abstracts from the Ambulatory Pediatric Association's 35th Annual Meeting: May 7-11, 1995 in San Diego, California,*

Comstock GW, VT Livesay, and SF Woolpert. 1974. Prognosis of a positive tuberculin reaction in childhood and adolescence. *American Journal of Epidemiology* 99: 131-138.

Niederman LG. 1993. Tuberculosis: Screening and prophylaxis. In *Ambulatory Pediatric Care*, Second ed. Editor Dershewitz RA, 624-6. Philadelphia, PA: J.B. Lippincott Company.

Smith MHD, JR Starke, and JR Marquis. 1992. Tuberculosis and opportunistic mycobacterial infections. In *Textbook of Pediatric Infectious Diseases*, Third ed. Editors Feigin RD, and JD Cherry, 1321-61. Philadelphia, PA: W.B. Saunders Company.

Starke JR. 1994. Tuberculosis. In *Principles and Practice of Pediatrics*, Second ed. Editors Oski FA, CD DeAngelis, RD Feigin, et al., 1244-56. Philadelphia, PA: J.B. Lippincott Company.

Starke JR, RF Jacobs, and J Jereb. June 1992. Medical progress: Resurgence of tuberculosis in children. *Journal of Pediatrics* 120 (6): 839-55.

U.S. Preventive Services Task Force. 1989. *Guide to Clinical Preventive Services: An Assessment of the Effectiveness of 169 Interventions*. Baltimore, MD: Williams and Wilkins.

19. UPPER RESPIRATORY INFECTIONS[1]

Eve Kerr, M.D., M.P.H., and Mark Schuster, M.D., Ph.D.

We conducted a MEDLINE search of the medical literature for all English-language review articles published between 1990 and 1995 for the following topics: pharyngitis, common cold, influenza, rhinovirus, bronchitis- acute, cough, and rhinitis. We selected articles from the MEDLINE results and references from the review articles were obtained in areas of controversy. In addition, we consulted two medical texts (Panzer et al., 1991; Barker et al., 1991) for general clinical approaches to respiratory infections.

Respiratory tract infections account for more than 10 percent of all office visits to the primary care physician (Perlman and Ginn, 1990). According to the 1993 National Health Interview Survey (NHIS), over 250 million cases of respiratory infections occur in the U.S. yearly (NCHS, 1994b). Respiratory infections include the common cold, influenza, pharyngitis, sinusitis, bronchitis, and pneumonia. Influenza and the common cold account for the majority of cases. Children under 5 years had 424.7 restricted activity days per 100 persons per year due to acute respiratory conditions; this represents 49 percent of all restricted activity days for acute conditions for children in this age category (NCHS, 1994b). Children age 5 to 17 had 295.2 restricted activity days per 100 persons per year for acute respiratory conditions, or 47 percent of all restricted activity days due to acute conditions for this age group (NCHS, 1994b).

---

[1]Portions of this chapter (the sections on acute bronchitis, influenza, nasal congestion and rhinorrhea, acute sinusitis, and chronic sinusitis) were originally prepared for the Women's Quality of Care Panel.

PHARYNGITIS IN CHILDREN AND ADOLESCENTS
Mark Schuster, M.D., Ph.D.

This review is based primarily on textbooks of pediatrics (El-Said in Oski et al., 1994; Hammerschlag in Oski et al., 1994), pediatric primary care (Niederman and Marcinak in Dershewitz, 1993; Widome in Hoekelman et al., 1992), pediatric infectious disease (Cherry in Feigin and Cherry, 1992), and adolescent medicine (Krilov in Friedman et al., 1992; Biro in McAnarney et al., 1992). We have also used the American Academy of Pediatrics' (AAP's) book of infectious disease recommendations (AAP in Peter, 1994). This review covers people up to 18 years old.

IMPORTANCE

Acute pharyngitis is the third most common diagnosis made by office-based pediatricians after otitis media and undifferentiated upper respiratory tract infections (Widome in Hoekelman et al., 1992). It peaks during ages 5-8 years (Niederman and Marcinak in Dershewitz, 1993).

Pharyngitis can be caused by bacteria, viruses, or fungi (Hammerschlag in Oski et al., 1994), though bacteria and viruses account for most cases (Widome in Hoekelman et al., 1992). In normal, healthy children, over 90 percent of cases are caused by (in order of decreasing frequency): Group A beta-hemolytic Streptococcus (GABHS); adenoviruses; influenza viruses A and B; parainfluenza viruses 1, 2, and 3; Epstein-Barr virus; enteroviruses; *Mycoplasma pneumoniae*; and *Chlamydia pneumoniae* (Hammerschlag in Oski et al., 1994).

EFFICACY/EFFECTIVENESS OF INTERVENTIONS

Diagnosis

History and Physical Examination

Since many causes of pharyngitis are not susceptible to treatment, the diagnostic challenge is to determine which cases are due to a treatable cause, primarily GABHS. Because GABHS can have significant

complications, it must be considered in all cases of acute pharyngitis
(Cherry in Feigin and Cherry, 1992; Hammerschlag in Oski et al., 1994).
The major complication of GABHS is acute rheumatic fever (ARF), which
can cause serious long-term heart disease. About 1 to 5 percent of
untreated GABHS throat infections are followed by ARF (El-Said in Oski
et al., 1994).

Age is a major factor in the epidemiology of and thus diagnosis of
pharyngitis. GABHS accounts for about 25-50 percent of cases of acute
pharyngitis in primary school-aged children (Widome in Hoekelman et al.,
1992). It is uncommon in children less than 3 years old, though
outbreaks have been reported in child care settings (AAP in Peter,
1994). Only 3 to 4 percent of cases of pharyngitis in children younger
than 2 years old are due to GABHS (Widome in Hoekelman et al., 1992).

In one study, viruses were responsible for 42 percent of all cases
of pharyngitis in children aged 6 months to 17.9 years (Hammerschlag in
Oski et al., 1994). Viral etiologies (e.g., influenza and
parainfluenza) predominate in pre-school children (Widome in Hoekelman
et al., 1992).

Pharyngitis can be divided into two categories: with nasal symptoms
(nasopharyngitis) and without (pharyngitis or tonsillopharyngitis).
Nasopharyngitis is almost always caused by a virus, most typically
adenovirus, influenza, or parainfluenza (Cherry in Feigin and Cherry,
1992; Hammerschlag in Oski et al., 1994). Nasopharyngitis will not be
addressed further in this review.

Pharyngitis is an inflammatory illness of the mucous membranes and
underlying structures of the throat. Diagnosis requires objective
evidence of inflammation (i.e., erythema, exudate, or ulceration)
(Cherry in Feigin and Cherry, 1992). While sore throat is always
present with pharyngitis, it does not guarantee that pharyngitis is
present. Children with colds without evidence of pharyngeal
inflammation may report sore throats (Cherry in Feigin and Cherry, 1992;
Hammerschlag in Oski et al., 1994). In addition to sore throat,
pharyngitis is often accompanied by fever, headache, nausea, vomiting,
anorexia, some degree of lessened activity, and sometimes abdominal

pain. Cervical lymph nodes may be enlarged and tender (Cherry in Feigin and Cherry, 1992).

Pharyngitis in children is almost always acute and self-limited. Cases with viral etiology generally last 4-10 days, while those caused by GABHS last slightly longer when untreated (Cherry in Feigin and Cherry, 1992).

In one study of children with acute febrile exudative tonsillitis, the only clinical clues to the nature of the infecting agent were cough and rhinitis, both of which were observed in 45 percent of patients with viral disease and in only 10 percent of children with GABHS (Hammerschlag in Oski et al., 1994).

GABHS usually has an acute onset and is characterized by a sore throat (often with dysphagia), fever (often above 101 F), pharyngeal and tonsillar erythema, and tonsillar exudate. Anterior cervical lymph nodes are enlarged and tender. Erythema of the soft palate and an enanthem of doughnut lesions on the soft palate suggest GABHS. Headache, abdominal pain, and vomiting are common. Upper respiratory tract symptoms such as cough, rhinorrhea, and conjunctivitis reduce the possibility of GABHS (Niederman and Marcinak in Dershewitz, 1993). Evidence of lower respiratory tract disease suggests parainfluenza and mycoplasma (Widome in Hoekelman et al., 1992).

Other etiologies of pharyngitis can cause similar symptoms. Nonetheless, given the possible complications of GABHS, the diagnosis should be considered in a child older than the appropriate cutoff age who has pharyngitis with or without exudate in the absence of a cold (Widome in Hoekelman et al., 1992).

There is some disagreement about the age below which it is not necessary to diagnose or treat GABHS. Widome (in Hoekelman et al., 1992) says the diagnosis should be considered in children older than 2 years who have appropriate signs and symptoms, while the AAP (in Peter, 1994) and Hammerschlag (in Oski et al., 1994) put the cutoff at 3 years old. The AAP (in Peter, 1994) specifies that diagnosis and treatment are not important under 3 years old because ARF is not of concern in this age group.

Scarlet fever has a characteristic sandpaper-like rash, which is caused by one or more of the several erythrogenic exotoxins produced by GABHS strains. With the exception of rare cases of severe scarlet fever with systemic toxicity, the epidemiology, symptoms, sequelae, and treatment of scarlet fever are the same as for GABHS pharyngitis (AAP in Peter, 1994).

Gonococcal pharyngitis may present as an acute inflammatory, exudative tonsillopharyngitis or as a chronic sore throat (Niederman and Marcinak in Dershewitz, 1993). However, in adolescents with *N. gonorrhoeae* infection, the pharynx is the sole site in only 1-4 percent of cases, and over 90 percent of pharyngeal infections are asymptomatic. *C. trachomatis* also appears to be an uncommon cause of pharyngitis. Only 2 percent of adolescents presenting with pharyngitis had *C. trachomatis* on culture, and none in an asymptomatic group did (Biro in McAnarney, 1992). While *N. gonorrhoeae* should be considered in sexually active adolescents, most abused children with *N. gonorrhoeae* isolated from the nasopharynx are asymptomatic (Hammerschlag in Oski et al., 1994).

Infectious mononucleosis (due to Epstein-Barr virus) may present as pharyngitis, with or without exudative tonsillitis. Fever is common, although children rarely appear very ill. Cervical or more general lymphadenopathy, palatal petechiae, splenomegaly, and edema of the eyelids support this diagnosis. Signs of upper respiratory tract infection, including rhinitis and cough, are more common in children younger than 4 years old. The child may also have a macular erythematous rash (Niederman and Marcinak in Dershewitz, 1993).

Laboratory Tests

Throat culture is the standard method of diagnosing GABHS. Throat cultures have up to 10 percent false-negatives (usually due to improper collection or transport) (Niederman and Marcinak in Dershewitz, 1993) and up to 50 percent false positives, which are not associated with an antibody rise, suggesting the presence of a different etiologic agent with coincident carriage of GABHS (Widome in Hoekelman et al., 1992).

If the child has obvious viral infection (e.g., pharyngocon-junctival fever consistent with adenovirus, herpangina), antibiotics would not be needed so culture is not necessary (Hammerschlag in Oski et al., 1994).

Rapid Streptococcal identification tests can permit identification of infection during the visit. Though it is generally agreed that these tests have high specificity (AAP in Peter, 1994; Cherry in Feigin and Cherry, 1992; Hammerschlag in Oski et al., 1994; Krilov in Friedman et al., 1992; Niederman and Marcinak in Dershewitz, 1993; Widome in Hoekelman et al., 1992). Reports of sensitivities range from 85-90 percent (Widome in Hoekelman et al., 1992) to lower than 50-70 percent (AAP in Peter, 1994), with Hammerschlag (in Oski et al., 1994) reporting that sensitivities are not always as high as reported because some researchers use as a reference culture methods with lower than desired sensitivities. Many patients with negative rapid tests have true infection (indicated by a rise in convalescent antibody titers) (Hammerschlag in Oski et al., 1994; Widome in Hoekelman et al., 1992). Hammerschlag (in Oski et al., 1994) reports that false-negative rates average around 15 percent. Therefore, a culture should be sent if results of a rapid screen are negative (AAP in Peter, 1994; Hammerschlag in Oski et al., 1994; Niederman and Marcinak in Dershewitz, 1993; Widome in Hoekelman et al., 1992).

Gram stain examination is not an accurate way to identify GABHS, *N. gonorrhoeae*, or *C. haemolyticum* (Hammerschlag in Oski et al., 1994). However, a gram-stained smear from an exudative area may be useful if anaerobic agents are suspected (Cherry in Feigin and Cherry, 1992).

Cultures for organisms other than GABHS should be reserved for unusual situations, such as persistent symptomatology, indicative epidemiology, or other pertinent historical data (Cherry in Feigin and Cherry, 1992). In the sexually active adolescent, gonococcal pharyngitis with appropriate culture methods should be considered (Krilov in Friedman et al., 1992).

The heterophil antibody test should be used when infectious mononucleosis is suspected (Hammerschlag in Oski et al., 1994; Niederman and Marcinak in Dershewitz, 1993; Widome in Hoekelman et al., 1992). However, it may be negative in children younger than 4 years and also early in the course of illness. The mono spot test can remain positive

for several months (Niederman and Marcinak in Dershewitz, 1993).
Differentiation of infectious mononucleosis from streptococcal
pharyngitis by looking for atypical lymphocytes in a Wright-Giemsa-
stained smear of pharyngeal exudate is an inferior method (Hammerschlag
in Oski et al., 1994).

Blood counts have little diagnostic value in distinguishing among
the causes of pharyngitis unless infectious mononucleosis is suspected.
Patients with infectious mononucleosis have a relative and absolute
lymphocytosis, with 10-20 percent Downey cells (basophylic, vacuolated,
and foamy cytoplasm) (Widome in Hoekelman et al., 1992). A peripheral
lymphocytosis greater than 50-60 percent or atypical lymphocytosis
greater than 10 percent is suggestive of mononucleosis (Niederman and
Marcinak in Dershewitz, 1993).

If a retropharyngeal abscess is suspected, a lateral x-ray of the
neck may reveal a posterior pharyngeal mass, sometimes with gas
(Niederman and Marcinak in Dershewitz, 1993).

Treatment for GABHS

The primary purpose of treatment for GABHS pharyngitis is
prevention of subsequent development of ARF (Widome in Hoekelman et al.,
1992). In recent outbreaks of ARF in the United States, many of the
patients had had an illness suggestive of pharyngitis within one month
of onset of ARF symptoms, but had received either no antibiotics or less
than a 10-day course (Hammerschlag in Oski et al., 1994). During
epidemics, as many as 3 percent of untreated patients with acute GABHS
pharyngitis may develop ARF. With endemic infections, the attack rates
are lower but still constitute a risk. The risk of ARF can be virtually
eliminated with adequate treatment of the antecedent infection (AAP in
Peter, 1994).

In addition to preventing ARF, antibiotic treatment can shorten the
duration and severity of symptoms (Niederman and Marcinak in Dershewitz,
1993; Widome in Hoekelman et al., 1992). It also prevents suppurative
complications (e.g., otitis media, lymphadenitis, peritonsillar abscess
(Niederman & Marcinak in Dershewitz, 1993)) and prevents spread of
illness to contacts. It also eliminates the streptococci from the

pharynx and prevents a rise in titers of the streptococcal antibodies. It has not been proven that treatment affects the incidence or severity of acute glomerulonephritis (Widome in Hoekelman et al., 1992).

If the rapid screen is positive, the person should be treated. Otherwise, treatment can generally await culture results since rheumatic fever can be prevented if treatment is started as late as the ninth day of symptoms. However, a physician might choose to treat immediately if the clinical evidence strongly suggested streptococcal infection and there was concern that the family would not follow through for subsequent treatment (Widome in Hoekelman et al., 1992). While Cherry (in Feigin and Cherry, 1992) agrees that there may be clinical situations in which one may treat immediately because one cannot be certain of follow-up, he warns that early treatment may also result in a decreased desirable antibody response allowing reinfection with type-specific organisms. However, Krilov (in Friedman et al., 1992) reports that other studies have not borne out the theory that early therapy might abort host antibody response, making the individual more susceptible to recurrent infection.

Treatment options include intramuscular benzathine penicillin G or procaine penicillin, oral potassium penicillin V for 10 days, or if the patient is allergic to penicillin, erythromycin for 10 days (Hammerschlag in Oski et al., 1994; Niederman and Marcinak in Dershewitz, 1993; Widome in Hoekelman et al., 1992). These treatments will be about 90 percent effective (Hammerschlag in Oski et al., 1994). First generation cephalosporins are acceptable for individuals allergic to penicillin. However, tetracyclines and sulfonamides should not be used for treating GABHS pharyngitis because many strains are resistant to the former and because the latter does not eradicate the organism (AAP in Peter, 1994).

Follow-up

Routine follow-up cultures after treatment for GABHS are generally unnecessary (Widome in Hoekelman et al., 1992).

Persistent or Recurrent GABHS Infection

Bacteriologic treatment failures with or without clinical relapse occur in up to 25 percent of patients. This is due to either failure to take medication, reinfection from close contacts, antimicrobial tolerance and the coexistence in the pharynx of beta-lactamase-producing bacteria (e.g., *Bacteroides fragilis, Bacteroides melaninogenicus* (Hammerschlag in Oski et al., 1994)), or carrier state (Widome in Hoekelman et al., 1992).

Carriers are people who have colonization but not infection. They have neither an antibody response nor a risk of rheumatic fever. They are not very contagious (Widome in Hoekelman et al., 1992). Up to 50 percent of children symptomatic with sore throats and positive GABHS cultures do not have serologic evidence of streptococcal infection. The failure rate for penicillin is high for asymptomatic carriers. Penicillin and rifampin are more efficacious in eradicating carriage (Niederman and Marcinak in Dershewitz, 1993).

With clinical relapse, a second course of treatment should be given, and cultures of family members may be appropriate. With repeated relapse or persistent failure to eradicate streptococci from the throat, a beta-lactamase-resistant antibiotic may be effective (Widome in Hoekelman et al., 1992). Beta-lactamase-resistant and antistaphylococcal medications (e.g., amoxicillin-clavulanate, narrow-spectrum cephalosporins, dicloxacillin, and clindamycin) can be useful in retreatment of people who have failed penicillin treatment (AAP in Peter, 1994; Hammerschlag in Oski et al., 1994).

Treatment for Gonorrhea

Pharyngitis caused by *N. gonorrhoeae* can be treated by intramuscular ceftriaxone or oral amoxicillin plus probenicid. Contacts must be checked, and in children, sexual abuse must be considered (Widome in Hoekelman et al., 1992). See Chapter 21 for indicators on treatment of gonorrhea.

Treatment for Viral Pharyngitis

In viral pharyngitis, antibiotics do not affect the course of disease and have not been shown to prevent secondary bacterial infection (Widome in Hoekelman et al., 1992).

Aspirin should not be used in children and teenagers with pharyngitis because of its etiologic role in influenza-associated Reye's syndrome and because it can be difficult to differentiate influenza viral infections from other respiratory viral infections (Cherry in Feigin and Cherry, 1992; Widome in Hoekelman et al., 1992).

Household contacts of a patient with streptococcal pharyngitis who have recent or current symptoms suggestive of streptococcal infection should be cultured. Culturing asymptomatic household contacts is not recommended except during outbreaks or in other unique epidemiologic situations, such as presence of a person in the family with rheumatic heart disease or streptococcal toxic shock syndrome (AAP in Peter, 1994).

BRONCHITIS, ACUTE
Eve Kerr, M.D., M.P.H.

IMPORTANCE

Acute bronchitis is an inflammatory disorder of the tracheobronchial tree that results in acute cough without signs of pneumonia (Billas, 1990). Preschool children had an estimated 22 million episodes of acute bronchitis in 1992, while school-aged children and adolescents had 1.9 million episodes of acute bronchitis in 1992 (NCHS, 1994b).

EFFICACY AND/OR EFFECTIVENESS OF INTERVENTIONS

Diagnosis

The causative organism of acute bronchitis is usually viral, but a variety of bacterial organisms may cause or contribute to bronchitis (e.g., *Mycoplasma pneumoniae*, *Chlamydia pneumoniae*, *B. catarrhalis*, and

Bordetella pertussis) (Billas, 1990; Barker et al., 1991). Cough may be nonproductive initially but generally becomes mucopurulent. The duration of cough is two weeks or less. Sputum characteristics are not helpful in distinguishing etiology of cough (Barker et al., 1991). Pharyngitis, fatigue and headache often precede onset of cough. Examination of the chest is usually normal, but may reveal rhonchi or rales without any evidence of consolidation. A detailed history must be obtained to rule in or out other possible causes for acute cough. Acute cough is defined as lasting less than three weeks (Pratter et al., 1993). Bronchitis, sinusitis, and the common cold are probably the most common causes of acute cough. Cough secondary to irritants (e.g., tobacco smoke) and allergies (e.g., from allergic rhinitis) are the next most common causes of cough (Zervanos and Shute, 1994).

Treatment

Most authorities agree that treatment with antibiotics in patients who are otherwise healthy and free of systemic symptoms is not useful (Barker et al., 1991; Billas, 1990). Orr et al. (1993) conducted a review of all randomized placebo-controlled trials of antibiotics for acute bronchitis published in the English language between 1980 and 1992. Four studies showed no significant benefit of using antibiotics, while two studies (one using erythromycin and the other using trimethoprim sulfa) did show benefit in decrease of subjective symptoms.

INFLUENZA
Eve Kerr, M.D., M.P.H.

IMPORTANCE

Children under 5 had 11 million episodes of influenza and children from 5-17 had 28 million episodes in 1992 (NCHS, 1994b). Most influenza symptoms are caused by the influenza A virus, which is dispersed by sneezing, coughing, or talking. Among school-aged children and adolescents, the clinical presentation of influenza is similar to that

found in adults.   In younger children and infants, the illness is an
undifferentiated febrile upper respiratory illness (Cherry in Oski,
1994).   While generally a self-limited disease, pandemics of influenza
have caused heavy death tolls (Wiselka, 1994).   Influenza causes between
10,000 and 20,000 deaths in the United States annually, especially among
infants, the elderly, and those with chronic medical conditions (Fiebach
and Beckett, 1994).   In addition, influenza can cause complications such
as pneumonitis, secondary pneumonia, Reye's syndrome, myositis and
myoglobinuria, myocarditis, and neurologic sequelae (Wiselka, 1994;
Barker et al., 1991).   Influenza takes its toll in restricted activity
days, amounting to 158 million restricted activity days per 100 persons
per year for children under 5 and 143 million restricted activity days
per 100 persons per year for those age 5-17 (NCHS, 1994c).

EFFICACY AND/OR EFFECTIVENESS OF INTERVENTIONS

Diagnosis

Uncomplicated influenza has an abrupt onset of systemic symptoms
including fever, chills, headache and myalgias.   The fever generally
persists 3-4 days, but may persist up to 7 days.   Respiratory symptoms
(e.g., cough, hoarseness, nasal discharge, pharyngitis) begin when
systemic symptoms begin to resolve.   Physical findings include toxic
appearance, cervical lymphadenopathy, hot skin watery eyes and rarely,
localized chest findings (e.g., rales).

Treatment

Treatment for uncomplicated influenza is generally symptomatic,
with rest, fluid intake, and aspirin (in adults only) or acetaminophen.
Dyspnea, hemoptysis, wheezing, purulent sputum, fever persisting more
than 7 days, severe muscle pain, and dark urine, may indicate onset of
influenza complications (Barker et al., 1991).   Amantadine has been
shown to decrease virus shedding and shorten duration of influenza
symptoms if treatment was started within 48 hours of symptom onset.
Common side-effects include headache, light headedness, dizziness and
insomnia.   Amantadine should be considered for use in children who are

severely ill or hospitalized if the illness is likely to be caused by
the influenza A virus (Cherry in Oski, 1994).

Prevention

Yearly influenza vaccination is recommended for children who are at
high risk for complications, including those who:

- have chronic bronchopulmonary disease (e.g., TB, cystic
  fibrosis, asthma, bronchiectasis); or
- have cardiovascular disorders (e.g., rheumatic, congenital, or
  hypertensive heart disease); or
- have chronic metabolic diseases (e.g., diabetes mellitus,
  chronic glomerulonephritis, and chronic neurologic disorders
  that affect the respiratory muscles (Cherry in Oski, 1994).

NASAL CONGESTION AND RHINORRHEA
Eve Kerr, M.D., M.P.H.

IMPORTANCE

Over 8 million visits for nasal congestion as the principal reason
for patient visit occurred in 1991 across all age groups in the United
States (NCHS, 1994c). More than half of those visits (4.5 million) were
for children under age 15. Nasal congestion may be due to a variety of
causes, the principal of these being acute viral infection (i.e., common
cold), allergic rhinitis and infectious sinusitis (acute or chronic)
(Canadian Rhinitis Symposium, 1994). Other common causes include
vasomotor rhinitis and rhinitis medicomentosa. Appropriate treatment
rests in making distinctions among these causes. Other less common
reasons for rhinitis include atrophic rhinitis and hormonal rhinitis and
mechanical/obstructive rhinitis. For a more detailed discussion of
allergic rhinitis, see Chapter 3.

The Canadian Rhinitis Symposium convened in January of 1994 to
develop a guide for assessing and treating rhinitis (Canadian Rhinitis

Symposium, 1994). While the guidebook is extensive, essential elements for diagnosis and treatment are discussed below.

EFFICACY AND/OR EFFECTIVENESS OF INTERVENTIONS

Diagnosis and Treatment

The following may serve to differentiate between (1) allergic rhinitis, (2) infectious viral rhinitis (common cold) and (3) sinusitis.

Allergic rhinitis

Symptoms: Nasal congestion, sneezing, palatal itching, rhinorrhea with or without allergic conjunctivitis. Symptoms are seasonal or perennial and may be triggered by allergens such as pollens, mites, molds, and animal danders.

Physical exam: nasal mucosa is pale or hyperemic; edema with or without watery secretions are frequently present.

Treatment: Treatment of allergic rhinitis should include antihistamines, nasal cromolyn and/or nasal glucocorticoid sprays. Oral decongestants may be used for symptomatic relief. If prescribed, topical nasal decongestants are indicated for short term use only.

Infectious viral rhinitis

Symptoms: Nasal congestion and rhinorrhea. Other symptoms of viral infectious rhinitis include mild malaise, sneezing, scratchy throat, and variable loss of taste and smell. Colds due to rhinoviruses typically last one week, and rarely as long as two weeks (Barker et al., 1991). Symptoms are generally of acute onset, unless chronic sinusitis is present (see Section F of this chapter). Symptoms of coexisting acute sinusitis may also be present (see Section E of this chapter).

Physical exam: Mucosa hyperemic and edematous with or without purulent secretions; physical exam should include nasal cavity and sinuses (for presence of sinusitis) and ears (for presence of otitis media) (Barker et al., 1991). Sinus tenderness and fever may be present with sinusitis

Treatment: Treatment of infectious viral rhinitis without sinusitis is symptomatic. Use of oral decongestants or short term nasal decongestants is appropriate but not necessary. For coexisting sinusitis, treatment should be with antibiotics in addition to decongestants (see Section F of this chapter).

Sinusitis

Symptoms/Physical Exam/Treatment: See discussions below on acute and chronic sinusitis (Sections E and F, respectively).

SINUSITIS, ACUTE
Eve Kerr, M.D., M.P.H.

IMPORTANCE—ACUTE AND CHRONIC SINUSITIS

According to the 1991 National Ambulatory Medical Care Survey, chronic sinusitis was the eighth most common diagnosis rendered by physicians for office visits in 1991. This translates to 1.7 percent of all visits among children and adults. Patients frequently mentioned symptoms which could be attributable to sinusitis--headache in 1.5 percent of visits and nasal congestion in 1.3 percent of visits. In children under 15 years of age, sinusitis accounted for 2.5 percent of visits; for persons age 15 to 24 years, allergic rhinitis accounted for 1.9 percent (NCHS, 1994c). While little data exists on the incidence of acute sinusitis, chronic sinusitis was reported by over 37 million persons (about 5 million of whom were under age 18) in the 1992 NHIS (NCHS, 1994b).

EFFICACY AND/OR EFFECTIVENESS OF INTERVENTIONS

Diagnosis

Acute sinusitis is a complication in about 1 to 5 percent of upper respiratory tract infections (Wald in Oski, 1994). By definition, acute sinusitis has a duration of less than 4 to 6 weeks (Wald in Oski, 1994).

Symptoms that may increase the likelihood of acute sinusitis being present in children include persistence of rhinorrhea, cough lasting more than 10 days, mild periorbital swelling, and malodorous breath. Headache is a less common symptom among children as compared to adults and is most often seen in children over age 5. Transillumination may improve the accuracy of diagnosis for maxillary sinusitis, but its usefulness is operator sensitive (Williams and Simel, 1993).

Treatment

Treatment is based on controlling infection and reducing tissue edema. Ten to fourteen days of antibiotics should be instituted for treatment of acute sinusitis; if full recovery has not occurred, antibiotics may be continued for another week (Wald in Oski, 1994). The use of oral or topical decongestants in children has not been adequately studied and is not generally recommended (Wald in Oski, 1994). Antihistamines, because of their drying action on the nasal mucosa, have no role in the treatment of most patients with acute sinusitis, except when patients also manifest symptoms of allergic rhinitis (thin, watery rhinorrhea, and sneezing) (Stafford, 1992).

Follow-up

If symptoms fail to improve after 48 hours, clinical re-evaluation of the patient is recommended and an alternate antibiotic may be required (Wald in Oski, 1994). If symptoms persist after 2 courses of antibiotics, referral to an otolaryngologist and/or more definitive diagnostic studies (e.g., x-ray, sinus CT, nasal endoscopy) is indicated (Stafford, 1992).

SINUSITIS, CHRONIC
Eve Kerr, M.D., M.P.H.

EFFICACY AND/OR EFFECTIVENESS OF INTERVENTIONS

Diagnosis

Chronic sinusitis is common among children with asthma or allergic rhinitis and is sometimes missed (Simons in Oski, 1994). Chronic sinusitis generally presents with nasal discharge, post-nasal drip, nasal obstruction, chronic cough, and loss of taste or smell (Simons in Oski, 1994).

Conditions that commonly predispose to chronic sinusitis include nasal foreign body, previous acute sinusitis, allergic rhinitis, environmental irritants, nasal polyposis, and viral infection (Godley, 1992).

Diagnosis rests on history, evaluation by nasal endoscopy, and CT scanning (Bolger and Kennedy, 1992). In general, if the history is strongly suggestive of chronic sinusitis, one should treat first with antibiotics (see below). If medical therapy is unsuccessful or if disease recurs repeatedly, referral to an otolaryngologist for endoscopic examination is indicated (Bolger and Kennedy, 1992). Endoscopic examination is more specific for chronic sinusitis than is CT scanning. If endoscopic findings are equivocal, a CT scan may demonstrate underlying sinus disease. However, a CT is best performed four to six weeks after optimal medical therapy is instituted to optimize specificity (Bolger and Kennedy, 1992).

Treatment

Medical treatment should be attempted first. First-line therapy for chronic disease is amoxicillin or trimethoprim-sulfamethoxazole three times daily for 21 to 28 days (Simons in Oski, 1994). Amoxicillin/clavulanate or a second- or third-generation cephlasporin is recommended if ß-lactamase-producing *H. influenzae* or *M. catarrhalis* is suspected (Simons in Oski, 1994). Other medications that may be used include topical oral decongestants, nasal steroids, and antihistamines for patients with an allergic component.

Surgical treatment is reserved for cases when medical therapy fails. Currently, endoscopic surgery is the method of choice (Bolger and Kennedy, 1992). Endoscopic examination and debridement of the operative cavity are required once or twice weekly for four to six weeks to promote healing and prevent stenosis of the sinus ostia. Complications of surgery include CSF rhinorrhea, diplopia, blindness and meningitis. However, the rates of complications are very low among experienced surgeons. In studies reporting success rates of surgery in consecutive patients, up to 93 percent of patients reported substantial symptomatic improvement in two-year follow-up, and subsequent revision surgery is reported in 7-10 percent (Bolger and Kennedy, 1992). It should be noted that no randomized controlled trials or case-controlled studies for endoscopic surgery have been performed.

RECOMMENDED QUALITY INDICATORS FOR UPPER RESPIRATORY INFECTIONS

These indicators apply to all children aged 2-18.

Diagnosis

	Indicator	Quality of evidence	Literature	Benefits	Comments
	Pharyngitis				
1.	All patients with sore throat should be asked about presence or absence of fever.	III	Inferred from Niederman & Marcinak in Dershewitz, 1993	Prevent ARF. Prevent suppurative complications of strep throat.* Reduce symptoms. Prevent spread of GABHS.	Presence of fever increases the probability of GABHS.
2.	All patients with sore throat should be asked about nasal symptoms.	III	Inferred from Cherry in Feigin and Cherry, 1992	Prevent ARF. Prevent suppurative complications of strep throat.* Reduce symptoms. Prevent spread of GABHS.	Nasal symptoms decrease the probability of GABHS.
3.	If a rapid streptococcal test is negative, a culture should be sent within 24 hours.	III	AAP in Peter, 1994; Hammerschlag in Oski et al., 1994; Niederman & Marcinak in Dershewitz, 1993; Widome in Hoekelman, 1992	Prevent ARF. Prevent suppurative complications of strep throat.* Reduce symptoms. Prevent spread of GABHS.	Follow-up culture decreases false-negative results. In practice, it should generally be sent immediately, since the most efficient way to perform the sequence is to send two throat swabs at the same time, one for the rapid test and one for culture if the rapid test is negative.
4.	Diagnosis of GABHS, *N. gonorrhoeae*, or *C. haemolyticum* by gram stain in the absense of culture or rapid test is not appropriate.	III	Hammerschlag in Oski et al., 1994	Prevent allergic reactions from antibiotics. Prevent resistance. Prevent ARF. Prevent suppurative complications.* Prevent spread of GABHS, gonorrhea, and chlamydia.	Gram stain is not sufficiently sensitive or specific for making these diagnoses, though it is useful if anaerobic agents are suspected. Use of antibiotics involves allergy risk, contributes to community resistance, and has associated expense and inconvenience.
	Bronchitis/Cough				
5.	The history of patients presenting with cough of less than 3 weeks' duration should document presence or absence of preceding viral infection (e.g., common cold, influenza).	III	Zervanos and Shute, 1994	Decrease cough. Prevent allergic reactions from antibiotics.	If preceding viral infection were present and the patient has no other complications (e.g., fever, shortness of breath), a diagnosis of viral bronchitis is likely. This diagnosis is self-limited and antibiotics are not necessary. No preceding viral infection would lead one to search for non-viral causes of bronchitis.

343

#	Recommendation		Reference	Objective	Rationale
6.	The history of patients presenting with cough of less than 3 weeks' duration should document presence or absence of fever and shortness of breath (dyspnea).	III	Barker et al., 1991	Decrease cough. Decrease shortness of breath. Prevent development of empyema. Prevent development of sepsis.	These symptoms are consistent with possible pneumonia, which would require antibiotic treatment. If the cause is viral, then antibiotics are not required.
7.	Patients presenting with acute cough should receive a physical examination of the chest for evidence of pneumonia.	III	Barker et al., 1991	Decrease cough. Decrease shortness of breath. Prevent development of empyema. Prevent development of sepsis.	Signs of consolidation would lead one on a different diagnostic and treatment path.
8.	Patients presenting with acute cough and with evidence of consolidation on physical exam of the chest (dullness to percussion, egophony, etc.) should receive a chest x-ray to look for evidence of pneumonia.	III	Barker et al., 1991	Decrease cough. Decrease shortness of breath. Prevent development of empyema. Prevent development of sepsis.	Presence of pneumonia would necessitate different treatment and follow-up plans.

Nasal Congestion

#	Recommendation		Reference	Objective	Rationale
9.	If a patient presents with the complaint of nasal congestion and/or rhinorrhea not attributed to the common cold, the history should include: seasonality of symptoms, presence or absence of sneezing, facial pain, fever, specific irritants, use of topical nasal decongestants.	III	Canadian Rhinitis Symposium, 1994	Decrease nasal congestion. Decrease rhinorrhea.	Nasal congestion can result from multiple causes in addition to the common cold. The most important of these, because of availability of treatment, are allergic rhinitis, sinusitis, and topical nasal decongestant abuse (rhinitis medicamentosa). If the practitioner does not attribute symptoms to the common cold, symptoms specific to these alternate diagnoses should be elicited.

Acute Sinusitis

#	Recommendation		Reference	Objective	Rationale
10.	If the diagnosis of acute sinusitis is made, symptoms should be present for a duration of less than 3 weeks (e.g., fever, malaise, cough, nasal congestion, purulent nasal discharge, ear pain or blockage, post-nasal drip, dental pain, headache, or facial pain).	III	Barker et al., 1991; Williams & Simel, 1993	Decrease nasal congestions, fever, post-nasal drip, headache and facial pain.	Acute sinusitis is defined as lasting less than 3 weeks. If symptoms last longer, the patient may have chronic sinusitis, which is more difficult to treat and requires longer duration of antibiotic therapy.

Indicator	Quality of evidence	Literature	Benefits	Comments
Pharyngitis				
11. Patients with documented or presumed streptococcal infection should be treated with intramuscular benzathine penicillin G or procaine penicillin, oral potassium penicillin V for 10 days, or (if the patient is allergic to penicillin) erythromycin for 10 days. First generation cephalosporins are acceptable for individuals allergic to penicillin.	III	AAP in Peter, 1994; Hammerschlag in Oski et al., 1994; Widome in Hoekelman et al., 1992	Prevent ARF. Prevent suppurative complications of strep throat.* Reduce symptoms. Prevent spread of GABHS.	Penicillin is the standard treatment for GABHS; erythromycin is the preferred alternative for patients allergic to penicillin.
12. Tetracyclines and sulfonamides should not be used for treating GABHS pharyngitis.	III	AAP in Peter, 1994	Prevent ARF. Prevent suppurative complications of strep throat.* Prevent spread of GABHS.	Many strains are resistant to the former, and the latter does not eradicate the organism.
13. No antibiotics should be used for a patient with a diagnosis of viral pharyngitis (unless antibiotics were prescribed before culture results were obtained).	III	Widome in Hoekelman et al., 1992	Prevent allergic reactions. Prevent resistance.	Given that antibiotics will sometimes be prescribed at the time of culture because the clinician is not confident the patient will return or be reachable if culture results are positive, it may be difficult to notify the patient that continuation of the full course of antibiotics is unnecessary.
14. Antibiotics should only be prescribed in a patient with conjunctivitis and pharyngitis if a rapid streptococcal test or throat culture is obtained.	III	Hammerschlag in Oski et al., 1994	Prevent allergic reactions. Prevent resistance.	While this is not specified by any particular source, strong evidence of adenovirus (i.e., the combination of sore throat and conjunctivitis) should strongly reduce suspicion of GABHS. If the clinician is nonetheless concerned enough about the possibility of GABHS to treat, he/she should investigate this with a culture. Use of antibiotics involves allergy risk, contributes to community resistance, and has associated expense and inconvenience.
15. Beta-lactamase-resistant and antistaphylococcal medications (e.g., amoxicillin-clavulanate, narrow-spectrum cephalosporins, dicloxacillin, and clindamycin) should be prescribed in patients who have had four episodes of documented or presumed and treated Strep throat in a one-year period.	III	AAP in Peter, 1994; Hammerschlag in Oski et al., 1994	Prevent future GABHS infections. Reduce disability/school loss days. Prevent ARF.	Some persons with frequent episodes of Strep throat despite therapy with penicillin have resistant strains. Children < 2 years old do not require treatment for GABHS because ARF is not observed in this age group.
16. Aspirin should not be used in children and teenagers with pharyngitis.	III	Cherry in Feigin and Cherry, 1992; Widome in Hoekelman et al., 1992; PDR, 1995	Prevent death from Reye's syndrome. Prevent neurologic deficits from Reye's syndrome.	Aspirin has been associated with Reye's syndrome.

#	Indicator		Objective	Reference	Comments
17.	If a diagnosis of infectious mononucleosis is made, it should be on the basis of a positive heterophil antibody test or other EBV antibody tests.	III	Prevent delayed diagnosis of hematologic malignancy. Prevent rupture of spleen.	Hammerschlag in Oski et al., 1994; Widome in Hoekelman et al., 1992	Use of the heterophil test decreases false positive diagnosis, in which case more serious illness might be missed, and false negative diagnosis, in which case a patient might not get proper symptomatic care and might not avoid activities that could lead to serious consequences (e.g., rupture of spleen because athletic activities were not avoided).
Bronchitis/Cough					
18.	If an antibiotic is prescribed for acute cough, documentation of drug allergies should be in the chart.	III	Avoid allergic reactions.	———	Allergy to antibiotics is relatively common. Approximately 2% of persons treated with penicillin derivatives develop an allergic reaction. Since alternative antibiotic regimens usually exist, it is wise to be aware of patients' allergy status before prescribing antibiotic.
19.	If the history documents cigarette smoking in a patient with acute cough, encouragement to stop smoking should be documented.	III	Prevent future bronchitic episodes. Prevent smoking-related morbidity and mortality.	Barker et al., 1991	Smokers are predisposed to bronchitis. Symptomatic patients present a window of opportunity to counsel regarding smoking cessation.
Nasal Congestion					
20.	If nasal decongestants are prescribed, duration of treatment should be for no longer than 4 days.	II	Prevent rhinitis medicamentosa.	Stafford et al., 1992; Barker et al., 1991	Long-term treatment with topical decongestants can cause rebound congestion (rhinitis medicamentosa).
Acute Sinusitis					
21.	Treatment for acute sinusitis should be with antibiotics for 10-14 days.	I-III	Decrease nasal congestion. Decrease fever. Prevent development of chronic sinusitis.	Williams et al., 1995	Antibiotics have proven benefit but the length of treatment is somewhat controversial.
22.	If an antibiotic is prescribed for acute sinusitis, documentation of presence or absence of drug allergies should be in the chart.	III	Avoid allergic reactions.	———	Allergy to antibiotics is relatively common. Approximately 2% of persons treated with penicillin derivatives develop an allergic reaction. Since alternative antibiotic regimens usually exist, it is wise to be aware of patients' allergy status before prescribing antibiotic.
23.	In the absence of symptoms of allergic rhinitis (thin, watery rhinorrhea, and sneezing), antihistamines should not be prescribed for acute sinusitis.	III	Prevent antihistamine side effects.	Stafford et al., 1992	Therefore, they should only be used if allergic symptoms are present. No RCTs have been done in this area.
24.	If symptoms fail to improve after 48 hours of antibiotic treatment, clinical re-evaluation and therapy with another antibiotic should be instituted.	III	Decrease nasal congestion. Decrease fever. Prevent development of chronic sinusitis.	Simons in Oski, 1994	Response should be within 48 hours; if not, alternative diagnosis and therapy should be considered.
25.	If the patient does not improve after two courses of antibiotics, referal to an otolaryngologist for a diagnostic test (CT, x-ray, ultrasound of the sinuses) is indicated.	III	Decrease nasal congestion. Prevent development of chronic sinusitis.	Stafford et al., 1992	Reevaluation of diagnosis and/or surgical treatment may be indicated.

346

Chronic Sinusitis

26.	If a diagnosis of chronic sinusitis is made, the patient should be treated with at least 3 weeks of antibiotics.	III	Decrease nasal congestion and other symptoms of chronic sinusitis.** Prevent recurrence of sinusitis.	Stafford et al., 1992	It is generally agreed that a longer duration of treatment for chronic sinusitis is necessary than for acute sinusitis. However, the exact number of days has not been defined in RCTs. The literature cites 3 weeks as standard of care.
27.	If patient has repeated symptoms after 2 separate 3 week trials of antibiotics, a referral to an otolaryngologist should be ordered.	III	Decrease nasal congestion and other symptoms of chronic sinusitis.** Prevent recurrence of sinusitis.	Bolger and Kennedy, 1992	While medical treatment is still first-line therapy, surgical treatment may be indicated if two course of antibiotics fail to relieve symptoms.
28.	If topical or oral decongestants are prescribed, duration of treatment should be for no longer than 4 days.	II	Prevent rhinitis medicamentosa.	Stafford et al., 1992; Barker et al., 1991	Long-term treatment with topical decongestants can cause rebound congestions (rhinitis medicamentosa).
29.	In the absence of symptoms of allergic rhinitis (thin, watery rhinorrhea, and sneezing), antihistamines should not be prescribed.	III	Prevent antihistamine side effects.	Stafford et al., 1992	Antihistamines may be detrimental to treatment secondary to drying properties. Therefore, they should only be used if allergic symptoms are present. No RCTs have been done in this area.

*Suppurative complications include otitis media, sinusitis, peritonsillar abscess, and suppurative cervical adentis.

**Symptoms of chronic sinusitis include nasal congestions, fever, headache, facial pain, toothache, rhinorrhea, and purulent nasal discharge.

Quality of Evidence Codes:

I:	RCT
II-1:	Nonrandomized controlled trials
II-2:	Cohort or case analysis
II-3:	Multiple time series
III:	Opinions or descriptive studies

REFERENCES - UPPER RESPIRATORY INFECTIONS

American Academy of Pediatrics. 1994. Streptococcal infections. In *1994 Red Book: Report of the Committee on Infectious Diseases*, Twenty-third ed. Editor Peter G, 439-43. Elk Grove Village, IL: American Academy of Pediatrics.

Barker LR, JR Burton, and PD Zieve, Editors. 1991. *Principles of Ambulatory Medicine*, Third ed. Baltimore, MD: Williams and Wilkins.

Billas A. December 1990. Lower respiratory tract infections. *Primary Care* 17 (4): 811-24.

Biro FM. 1992. Disorders of eyes, ears, nose, and mouth. In *Textbook of Adolescent Medicine*. Editors McAnarney ER, RE Kreipe, DP Orr, et al., 283-8. Philadelphia, PA: W.B. Saunders Company.

Bolger WE, and DW Kennedy. 30 September 1992. Changing concepts in chronic sinusitis. *Hospital Practice* 27 (9A): 20-2, 26-8.

Canadian Rhinitis Symposium. 1994. Assessing and treating rhinitis: A practical guide for Canadian physicians. Proceedings of the Canadian Rhinitis Symposium; Toronto, Ontario; January 14-15, 1994. *Canadian Medical Journal* 15 (Suppl. 4): 1-27.

Cherry JD. 1994. Influenza viruses. In *Principles and Practice of Pediatrics*, Second ed. Editors Oski FA, CD DeAngelis, RD Feigin, et al., 1294-1296. Philadelphia: J.B. Lippincott Company.

Cherry JD. 1992. Pharyngitis (pharyngitis, tonsillitis, tonsillopharyngitis, and nasopharyngitis). In *Textbook of Pediatric Infectious Diseases*, Third ed. Editors Feigin RD, and JD Cherry, 159-66. Philadelphia, PA: W.B. Saunders Company.

El-Said GM. 1994. Rheumatic fever. In *Principles and Practice of Pediatrics*, Second ed. Editors Oski FA, CD DeAngelis, RD Feigin, et al., 1626-31. Philadelphia, PA: J.B. Lippincott Company.

Fiebach N, and W Beckett. 28 November 1994. Prevention of respiratory infections in adults: Influenza and pneumococcal vaccines. *Archives of Internal Medicine* 154: 2545-57.

Godley FA. May 1992. Chronic Sinusitis: An Update. *American Family Physician* 45 (5): 2190-9.

Hammerschlag MR. 1994. Pharyngitis. In *Principles and Practice of Pediatrics*, Second ed. Editors Oski FA, CD DeAngelis, RD Feigin, et al., 969-70. Philadelphia, PA: J.B. Lippincott Company.

Krilov LR. 1992. Respiratory tract infections. In *Comprehensive Adolescent Health Care*. Editors Friedman SB, M Fisher, and SK Schonberg, 280-4. St. Louis, MO: Quality Medical Publishing, Inc.

National Center for Health Statistics. December 1994. *Current estimates from the National Health Interview Survey, 1993*. U.S. Department of Health and Human Services, Hyattsville, MD.

National Center for Health Statistics. 1994. *National Ambulatory Medical Care Survey: 1991 summary*. U.S. Department of Health and Human Services, Hyattsville, MD.

Niederman LG, and JF Marcinak. 1993. Sore throat. In *Ambulatory Pediatric Care*, Second ed. Editor Dershewitz RA, 315-9. Philadelphia, PA: J.B. Lippincott Company.

Orr PH, K Scherer, A Macdonald, et al. 1993. Randomized placebo-controlled trials of antibiotics for acute bronchitis: A critical review of the literature. *Journal of Family Practice* 36 (5): 507-12.

Panzer RJ, ER Black, and PF Griner, Editors. 1991. *Diagnostic Strategies for Common Medical Problems*.Philadelphia, PA: American College of Physicians.

Physician's Desk Reference. 1995. *PDR 49th Edition*. Montvale, NJ: Medical Economics Data Production Company.

Pratter MR, T Bartter, S Akers, et al. 15 November 1993. An algorithmic approach to chronic cough. *Annals of Internal Medicine* 119 (10): 977-83.

Simons FE. 1994. Allergic rhinitis. In *Principles and Practice of Pediatrics*, Second ed. Editors Oski FA, CD DeAngelis, RD Feigin, et al., 236-240. Philadelphia: J.B. Lippincott Company.

Stafford CT. November 1990. The clinician's view of sinusitis. *Otolaryngology-Head and Neck Surgery* 103 (Volume 5, Part 2): 870-5.

Wald ER. 1994. Paranasal sinusitis. In *Principles and Practice of Pediatrics*, Second ed. Editors Oski FA, CD DeAngelis, RD Feigin, et al., 951-957. Philadelphia: J.B. Lippincott Company.

Widome MD. 1992. Pharyngitis and tonsillitis. In *Primary Pediatric Care*, Second ed. Editors Hoekelman RA, SB Friedman, NM Nelson, et al., 1448-52. St. Louis, MO: Mosby-Year Book, Inc.

Williams JW, DR Holleman Jr., GP Samsa, et al. 5 April 1995. Randomized controlled trial of 3 vs 10 days of trimethoprim/sulfamethoxazole for acute maxillary sinusitis. *Journal of the American Medical Association* 273 (13): 1015-21.

Williams JW, and DL Simel. 8 September 1993. Does this patient have sinusitis? Diagnosing acute sinusitis by history and physical examination. *Journal of the American Medical Association* 270 (10): 1242-6.

Wiselka M. 21 May 1994. Influenza: Diagnosis, management, and prophylaxis. *British Medical Journal* 308: 1341-5.

Zervanos NJ, and KM Shute. March 1994. Acute, disruptive cough: Symptomatic therapy for a nagging problem. *Postgraduate Medicine* 95 (4): 153-68.

20. URINARY TRACT INFECTIONS
Mark Schuster, M.D., Ph.D.

This review is based on textbooks of pediatrics (Roth and Gonzales in Oski et al., 1994), pediatric primary care (Woodhead in Dershewitz, 1993), and pediatric infectious disease (Marks and Arrieta in Feigin and Cherry, 1992). Several articles were also identified from the textbook bibliographies and from a MEDLINE search of English-language review articles on urinary tract infections (UTIs) and pyelonephritis in pediatric age groups published between January 1990 and March 1995.

IMPORTANCE

The urinary tract ranks second only to the upper respiratory tract as a source of morbidity from bacterial infection in children (Roth and Gonzales in Oski et al., 1994). About one percent of boys and three percent of girls will have had a symptomatic UTI by their eleventh birthday (Stull and LiPuma, 1991).

Most UTIs are successfully treated without significant sequelae (Zelikovic et al., 1992). However, vesicoureteral reflux (VUR) of infected urine into the renal parenchyma (also known as reflux nephropathy) can cause renal scarring. Reflux-associated scarring is the most common single cause of renal hypertension and chronic renal failure in children (White, 1990); it can also cause growth failure. Once renal scarring has occurred, no remedial or preventive measures can be taken (Treves, 1994).

Up to 50 percent of children younger than five years old who have UTI and fever (which is common with UTI) also have VUR, and over 80 percent of children younger than five years old who have recurrent UTI and persistent VUR develop renal scarring (Woodhead in Dershewitz, 1993). Most renal scars seem to appear before five years old, though new scar formation and progression of scarring have been shown in older children (Andrich and Majd, 1992). Timely identification of acute infection, appropriate treatment, detection of patients at risk for renal scarring, and prevention of recurrent infection can greatly reduce the risk of an adverse outcome (Woodhead in Dershewitz, 1993). UTI management thus has two primary aims: the relief of symptoms and the prevention of renal damage (White, 1990).

EFFICACY AND/OR EFFECTIVENESS OF INTERVENTIONS

Screening

There is no consensus on whether asymptomatic children should be screened routinely for bacteriuria (bacteria in the urine). Kemper and Avner (1992) make the case that because of high costs and false positive rates, routine screening of asymptomatic preschool children with urinalysis (UA) should not be done.

Diagnosis

Infants with a UTI may have nonspecific symptoms such as fever, irritability, and other signs of systemic illness, including failure to thrive, vomiting, and diarrhea. Signs of bladder obstruction such as abdominal distention, weak or threadlike urinary stream, infrequent voiding, and discolored or malodorous urine may be present (Woodhead in Dershewitz, 1993). Decreased feeding, lethargy, jaundice, hepatomegaly, and splenomegaly may also be present. A child with UTI may also be asymptomatic (Lebel in Oski et al., 1994). Febrile infants without an apparent source of fever should be evaluated for UTI (Stull and LiPuma, 1991). UTIs are diagnosed in 7.5 percent of infants less than two months who have fever (Lebel in Oski et al., 1994). Infants with UTI should be evaluated for other potential sources of infection with examination of blood and cerebrospinal fluid (Sherbotie and Cornfeld, 1991; Lebel in Oski et al., 1994).

Preschool children may complain of voiding discomfort, or they may develop recurrent (secondary) enuresis, in addition to fever and abdominal or flank pain. School-age children typically have "classic" signs and symptoms of UTI, including dysuria, frequency, urgency, abdominal or flank pain, and fever (Woodhead in Dershewitz, 1993). Hematuria may occur with UTI (Marks and Arrieta in Feigin and Cherry, 1992a). An association between sexual abuse and UTIs has been proposed but has not been demonstrated (Stull and LiPuma, 1991).

Diagnosis is made by urine culture. A midstream clean-catch urine specimen may be used if the child is toilet-trained. If not, urine may be obtained by percutaneous bladder tap or urethral catheterization. In addition, a urine bag collection is adequate if the culture is negative; however, a positive culture could result from a contaminant from the rectum, skin, or prepuce, so it must be confirmed by one of the other two methods (Roth and Gonzales in Oski et al., 1994; Woodhead in Dershewitz, 1993). Urine cultures from bags may sometimes be so suggestive of UTI that some physicians might believe it is unnecessary to collect a more reliable culture, particularly since antibiotic therapy does not present much risk. However, the radiologic work-up (discussed below) is quite invasive and so treatment based on bag urine cultures should be the exception rather than the rule. The culture must be obtained before antibiotics are given because a single dose prior to urine collection can lead to a false-negative result (Roth and Gonzales in Oski et al., 1994).

Bacterial colony counts greater than 100,000 colonies/ml urine for a single organism should be interpreted as diagnostic of a UTI. Colony counts of 10,000 to 100,000 colonies/ml urine associated with clinical signs and symptoms are suggestive of a UTI, but a repeat culture should be done (this may not always be possible if the patient has already started antibiotics). Colony counts less than 10,000/ml may be considered positive if the organism is staphylococcus or a fungus or if the patient has an indwelling catheter. Any bacterial growth from a suprapubic aspirate should be considered positive (Marks and Arrieta in Feigin and Cherry, 1992a).

Though urinalysis may be used to screen for possible UTI (Woodhead in Dershewitz, 1993), a positive urinalysis must be confirmed with a culture in order to make the diagnosis.

UTIs can be subdivided into two categories based on anatomical location: lower tract infection (cystitis) and upper tract infection (pyelonephritis) (Zelikovic et al., 1992). It can be difficult to distinguish between the two in children. Dysuria, frequency, urgency, enuresis, suprapubic pain, and a low-grade fever are more common in cystitis, whereas high fever, nausea, vomiting, flank pain, and lethargy are usually associated with acute pyelonephritis. Overlap in symptoms occurs often (Roth and Gonzales in Oski et al., 1994) and can make specific diagnosis difficult.

Andrich and Majd (1992) say that clinical and laboratory findings are not adequate to diagnose pyelonephritis, and therefore argue for performing renal cortical scintigraphy (RCS) with DMSA (dimercaptosuccinic acid) or GHA (glucoheptonate) in all patients with a febrile UTI, especially young children who are particularly susceptible to scarring. RCS is recommended during the first 2-3 days if the child is hospitalized and within the first 2-3 weeks if the child is treated as an outpatient. However, this is not a typical recommendation of pediatric textbooks, and we have found no analysis weighing the costs and benefits of performing RCS on all children with a UTI. Standard clinical practice remains presumptive treatment of all young children with a UTI for pyelonephritis.

Treatment

Infants with UTI are at risk of developing serious sequelae, including sepsis, electrolyte abnormalities, and shock. They should be treated with parenteral antibiotics. A repeat urine culture should be obtained after 48 hours to assure that urine has been sterilized (Sherbotie and Cornfeld, 1991; Lebel in Oski et al., 1994). Parenteral antibiotic therapy should be continued in infants for 5-7 days. If the baby has improved clinically after 3-5 afebrile days and has sterile urine, antibiotics may be given orally to complete a 10-14 day course. For ill-appearing patients and those with genitourinary abnormalities and pyelonephritis, at least 7 days of parenteral antibiotics are recommended, followed by prolonged oral antimicrobial therapy (e.g., 2-3 weeks) once clinical improvement and microbiologic cure are documented (Sherbotie and Cornfeld, 1991). If the child is not afebrile within 1-2 days or if the repeat urine culture is positive, the child needs an immediate evaluation for urologic obstruction or abscess (in addition to reconfirming bacterial antibiotic susceptibilities) (see radiologic work-up below) (Lebel in Oski et al., 1994).

A repeat culture should be obtained 2-3 days after the start of standard 10-day therapy or 3-4 days after completion of short-course therapy. Sterile urine demonstrates antibiotic effectiveness. If urine is not sterile or the patient remains symptomatic, another urine specimen should be sent for bacterial identification and susceptibility testing and a broad-spectrum antibiotic should be prescribed. Urine should be recultured 3 days later to confirm effectiveness (Woodhead in Dershewitz, 1993).

Any child with symptomatic pyelonephritis should be managed in hospital with parenteral antibiotics (Woodhead in Dershewitz, 1993). Other children can be treated adequately on an outpatient basis with a 7-10 day course. A higher recurrence rate occurs with shorter courses of antibiotics (Roth and Gonzales in Oski et al., 1994). A broad-spectrum antibiotic is used initially (Roth and Gonzales in Oski et al., 1994; Woodhead in Dershewitz, 1993). It must be changed if the organism is not sensitive to it. Treatment for 10 days is adequate (Woodhead in Dershewitz, 1993).

Some clinicians believe that bacterial identification and determination of antibiotic susceptibilities are not necessary in most uncomplicated UTIs. Because most UTIs are caused by *E. coli* (a type of bacteria) sensitive to commonly used antibiotics, rapid clinical response to treatment and a negative culture 2-4 days after initiation of treatment serve the same ends as sensitivity testing. However, the patient with systemic toxicity at initial presentation or who fails to respond promptly to treatment should have these done (Woodhead in Dershewitz, 1993).

Follow-up Care

Recommendations for follow-up culture (to document eradication of infection) are quite variable, ranging from one week after completion of therapy (Roth and Gonzales in Oski et al., 1994) to one month afterwards or just before radiologic evaluation (Woodhead in Dershewitz, 1993). Woodhead (in Dershewitz, 1993) recommends further follow-up every three months for one year and then annually for 2-3 years. However, others do not mention such persistent follow-up.

Prophylaxis

Children with at least four UTIs per year should receive daily prophylactic low-dose antibiotics for 9-12 months (Roth and Gonzales in Oski et al., 1994). Woodhead (in Dershewitz, 1993) recommends prophylaxis for 6 months. Lebel (in Oski et al., 1994) also recommends prophylaxis for recurrent UTIs. Because the length of prophylaxis is open to debate, the shorter time period (6 months) will be used for an indicator.

Any child who needs a radiologic study for VUR should receive low dose prophylactic antibiotics until the voiding cystourethrogram (VCUG) has been done (Woodhead in Dershewitz, 1993).

Radiologic Studies

There is consensus that some children with UTIs need to have a radiologic work-up, but there is disagreement over the particulars of which ages and which genders need what type of work up. Work-up is recommended for all boys (Roth and Gonzales in Oski et al., 1994; Woodhead in Dershewitz, 1993; Sherbotie and Cornfeld, 1991; Gillenwater, 1991). Andrich and Majd (1992) specify that it is necessary only for boys less than 10 years old. There is less consensus for girls, with recommendations including: girls less than 3 years old or girls older than 3 with systemic toxicity, recurrent UTIs, or failure of infection to respond promptly to therapy (Woodhead in Dershewitz, 1993); girls less than 5 years old, girls with evidence of genitourinary abnormalities, and girls older than 5 with recurrent symptomatic bacteriuria (Sherbotie and Cornfeld, 1991); girls less than 10 years old, girls who fail to respond to antibiotic therapy, and girls with recurrent UTIs (Andrich and Majd, 1992); all girls (Gillenwater, 1991). Given these disagreements, our indicators for radiologic work-ups cover all boys less than 10 years old, all girls less than 3 years old, and any other children who require hospitalization (as a proxy for systemic toxicity).

There are several radiographic studies that can be done to evaluate urinary tract anatomy and function. Recommendations for which studies to use vary. Roth and Gonzales (in Oski et al., 1994) recommend (1)

VCUG and (2) renal ultrasound (RUS), intravenous pyelogram (IVP), or nuclear medicine renal scan, though they say the VCUG is not necessary for the older girl with simple cystitis. Woodhead (in Dershewitz, 1993) recommends (1) VCUG or radionuclide cystogram and (2) IVP or RUS. Gillenwater (1991) recommends (1) radionuclide or contrast cystograms and (2) RUS or intravenous urograms. Andrich and Majd (1992) recommend (1) VCUG in boys and isotope cystogram (IC) or VCUG in girls and (2) RUS for afebrile, nontoxic-appearing children. If the cystogram is positive, RCS should be done to see if there is evidence of previous unsuspected renal parenchymal infection. If RUS shows hydronephrosis, diuretic renography (with DTPA or MAG3) must be done to determine if it is obstructive or nonobstructive (Andrich and Majd, 1992).

Our indicators accept any of several options for radiologic work-up: (1) VCUG for boys and IC or VCUG in girls, and (2) RUS, IVP, or nuclear medicine renal scan. A key concern is the amount of radiation exposure from these various methods. IC may be preferred for girls under 5 because of the lower radiation exposure as compared to VCUG and concerns about effect on the ovaries. Similarly, IVP has higher levels of radiation exposure than the other tests and may not provide enough additional information to justify the increased risk. This review does not address recommendations for further work-up and treatment following these radiologic studies.

There are variable recommendations for how long after diagnosis the VCUG (or IC) should be done, ranging from a few days or as soon as the patient is asymptomatic (Andrich and Majd, 1992) to 4-6 weeks after the infection has been treated (Woodhead in Dershewitz, 1993). Our indicator accepts any time within the first three months after diagnosis, as long as the patient has been on prophylactic antibiotics from completion of the treatment regimen until the time of the VCUG or IC.

If the symptoms with each recurrence remain consistent with cystitis, there is no need for repeated invasive evaluations. However, for the child with a persistent problem with UTIs, it seems prudent to repeat a renal ultrasound every 2-3 years to document normal renal growth (Roth and Gonzales in Oski et al., 1994).

Reflux and Other Abnormalities

There is consensus that children with VUR need prophylactic
antibiotics until the reflux resolves (Woodhead in Dershewitz, 1993;
Andrich and Majd; Gillenwater, 1991). Lebel (in Oski et al., 1994)
specifies that children with Grade II or higher reflux need prophylaxis.

In addition, Andrich and Majd raise the idea that any child whose
RCS shows renal parenchymal involvement should be considered for
prophylaxis as well (Andrich and Majd, 1992). However, neither doing
RCS nor prophylaxing all children with a positive RCS has become a
standard of practice.

When VUR is diagnosed, it must be evaluated yearly with VCUG or
radionuclide cystogram. There should be monitoring of renal growth with
US or IVP as long as VUR persists. Low-grade VUR resolves spontaneously
in almost 80 percent of cases and urologic evaluation is unnecessary
unless VUR is complicated by poor growth, hypertension, or reduced renal
function (Woodhead in Dershewitz, 1993). Andrich and Majd prefer IC to
minimize radiation exposure. Infants with reflux should have RUS and
VCUG or radionuclide scan repeated in 6-12 months (Lebel in Oski et al.,
1994).

Higher grades of reflux do not spontaneously resolve and indicate
more severe urinary tract damage. Patients with high grade VUR should
have urologic evaluation and almost always require urethral
reimplantation (Woodhead in Dershewitz, 1993; Gillenwater, 1991),
although exact management is controversial (White, 1990; O'Donnell,
1990). Optimal treatment for moderate degrees of reflux has not been
established (Gillenwater, 1991).

Infants with obstructive signs (e.g., midline lower abdominal
distention; flank mass; infrequent or prolonged voiding; weak,
dribbling, or threadlike urinary stream; or ballooning of the penile
urethra) must be evaluated by a pediatric urologist. Children with any
degree of VUR with hypertension, growth retardation, reduced renal
function, anemia, or other structural renal abnormalities should also
have urologic evaluation (Woodhead in Dershewitz, 1993).

Asymptomatic siblings of children with VUR require screening
because up to 45 percent will also have VUR compared to less than one

percent of the general population (Andrich and Majd, 1992). Andrich and Majd (1992) prefer IC to limit radiation but acknowledge that some radiologists will find the VCUG more reliable because they perform it more often.

RECOMMENDED QUALITY INDICATORS FOR URINARY TRACT INFECTION

The following criteria apply to urinary tract infections for infants and children.

Diagnosis

	Indicator	Quality of evidence	Literature	Benefits	Comments
1.	If an infant or child presents with any of the following symptoms/signs,* either a urine culture should be performed or a urinalysis should be performed; if urinalysis is positive, a urine culture should be performed: a. malodorous urine, abnormal urinary stream, or change in urinary stream in an infant or child; b. failure to thrive in an infant or child; c. vomiting associated with fever in an infant; d. jaundice associated with fever in a neonate; e. pain/discomfort with urination (dysuria), frequency, urgency, flank pain (unrelated to trauma) in a child; f. hematuria unrelated to trauma in infant or child; or g. secondary enuresis in a child.	III	Marks and Arietta in Feigin and Cherry, 1992a; Woodhead in Dershewitz, 1993; Lebel in Oski et al., 1994	Prevent chronic renal failure. Prevent scarring and renal hypertension.	Without proper diagnosis, an untreated UTI in children can cause complications, including vesicoureteral reflux of infected urine (which can lead to renal scarring, which can cause renal hypertension and chronic renal failure). Of note, the sources used in this review sometimes distinguish between infants and children without specifying the age cut-off between them. We will define infants as children who have not reached their first birthday.
2.	In order to diagnose UTI, a positive culture from one of the following methods of urine collection is necessary: – bladder tap, or – catheterization, or – clean catch.	III	Roth and Gonzales in Oski et al., 1994; Woodhead in Dershewitz, 1993	Prevent allergic reactions from antibiotics. Prevent complications of invasive procedures.	Bag urine collection has a high false positive rate. False positives are not trivial, not only because of inappropriate antibiotic usage but also because of potential complications of radiologic procedures discussed below.
3.	In order to rule out UTI, a negative UA or culture from one of the following methods of urine collection is necessary: – bladder tap, or – catheterization, or – clean catch, or – urine bag.	III	Roth and Gonzales in Oski et al., 1994; Woodhead in Dershewitz, 1993	Prevent allergic reactions from antibiotics. Prevent complications of invasive procedures.	Bag urine collection has a high false positive rate. False positives are not trivial, not only because of inappropriate antibiotic usage but also because of potential complications of radiologic procedures discussed below.
4.	If the culture shows greater than 100,000 colonies/ml urine of a single organism, then the patient should be diagnosed and treated for UTI.	III	Marks and Arrieta in Feigin and Cherry, 1992a	Prevent allergic reactions from antibiotics. Prevent complications of invasive radiologic procedures. Prevent chronic renal failure. Prevent renal scarring and hypertension.	

360

#	Recommendation	Level	Reference	Benefits	Comments
5.	If there is bacterial growth of a single organism with at least 10,000 colonies/ml urine from a catherized specimen, then UTI should be diagnosed and treated.	III	Marks and Arrieta in Feigin and Cherry, 1992a	Prevent allergic reactions from antibiotics. Prevent complications of invasive radiologic procedures. Prevent chronic renal failure. Prevent renal scarring and hypertension.	Specimens from clean catch and catheter collection are less likely to have contaminants.
6.	Growth of 10,000 to 100,000 colonies/ml urine from clean catch should be followed up with a repeat urine culture if the patient has not already been treated.	III	Marks and Arrieta in Feigin and Cherry, 1992a	Prevent allergic reactions from antibiotics. Prevent complications of invasive radiologic procedures. Prevent chronic renal failure. Prevent renal scarring and hypertension.	This is a borderline result that may be due to contamination or infection. Repeat culture helps determine whether there is true infection.
7.	If there is any bacterial growth from a specimen obtained from a bladder tap then a UTI should be diagnosed and treated.	III	Marks and Arrieta in Feigin and Cherry, 1992a	Prevent pyelonephritis.	A bladder tap specimen is unlikely to have a contaminant.
8.	Urine culture must be obtained by clean catch, catheterization, or bladder tap before antibiotics are given.	III	Roth and Gonzales in Oski et al., 1994	Prevent allergic reactions from antibiotics. Prevent pyelonephritis. Prevent chronic renal failure. Prevent renal hypertension. Avoid invasive radiologic work-up.	Pre-antibiotic culture allows determination of whether the patient actually has a UTI. It also allows determination of antibiotic sensitivities, which enables switching to proper treatment if necessary. There may be extenuating circumstances where antibiotics cannot wait for culture. For example, a child may have strong evidence of meningococcal sepsis but clinicians may be unsuccessful in obtaining a urine sample. This child will need antibiotics immediately. However, such situations should be uncommon and distributed randomly among sites, so that they will not need to be accounted for at present.

Treatment

	Indicator	Quality of evidence	Literature	Benefits	Comments
9.	All infants with a diagnosis of UTI must initially receive intravenous antibiotics.	III	Sherbotie and Cornfeld, 1991	Prevent sepsis. Prevent renal scarring, renal hypertension, and chronic renal failure.	IV antibiotics are more likely than oral antibiotics to be effective in infants.
10.	IV antibiotics may be switched to oral antibiotics if the infant has had at least 3 days without fever, a negative repeat urine culture, and negative blood and CSF culture.	III	Sherbotie and Cornfeld, 1991	Prevent sepsis. Prevent renal scarring, renal hypertension, and chronic renal failure.	Once it is clear the infection is under control, it is safe to switch to oral antibiotics.
11.	Infants with UTI should receive a total of at least 10 days of antibiotics (IV and oral).	III	Sherbotie and Cornfeld, 1991	Prevent sepsis. Prevent renal scarring, renal hypertension, and chronic renal failure.	Once it is clear the infection is under control, it is safe to switch to oral antibiotics.
12.	Infants with UTI should have a repeat urine culture between 48 hours and the end of the fifth day of IV therapy.	III	Sherbotie and Cornfeld, 1991	Prevent sepsis. Prevent renal hypertension, and chronic renal failure.	Sherbotie and Cornfeld recommend the repeat culture after 48 hours, but do not give a deadline for the culture. Repeat culture assures that treatment is effective. If a UTI is untreated, a child with vesicoureteral reflux of infected urine can develop renal scarring, which can cause renal hypertension and chronic renal failure.
13.	Children with UTI and systemic symptoms such as hypotension, poor perfusion, anorexia, or emesis, should be treated initially with IV antibiotics.	III	Woodhead in Dershewitz, 1993	Prevent sepsis. Prevent renal hypertension, and chronic renal failure.	IV antibiotics assure adequate treatment so that complications (see benefits) are less likely to occur, but oral antibiotics allow for less invasive treatment (and decreased hospitalization) when that is acceptable.
14.	If the child is being treated with oral antibiotics, by the fourth day, either (1) antibiotic sensitivities must be determined, or (2) a repeat culture must be sent.	III	Woodhead in Dershewitz, 1993	Prevent sepsis. Prevent renal hypertension, and chronic renal failure.	If sensitivities are not available to show that the antibiotic is appropriate, a repeat culture will show whether the antibiotic is working.
15.	When antibiotic sensitivities are checked, if the organism is not sensitive to the antibiotic, the antibiotic should be switched to one to which the organism is sensitive within 1 day.	III	Inferred from Woodhead in Dershewitz, 1993	Prevent sepsis. Prevent renal hypertension, and chronic renal failure.	If the child is being treated with an inappropriate antibiotic, one would want to correct the treatment immediately.
16.	All children with the diagnosis of UTI should receive at least 7 days of antibiotics.	III	Roth and Gonzales in Oski et al., 1994	Prevent sepsis. Prevent renal hypertension, and chronic renal failure.	Antibiotics must be taken long enough to ensure adequate treatment.
17.	All children with the diagnosis of pyelonephritis should be treated initially with IV antibiotics.	III	Woodhead in Dershewitz, 1993	Prevent sepsis. Prevent renal hypertension, and chronic renal failure.	Oral antibiotics are not considered adequate for pyelonephritis, which is more serious than simple UTI.
18.	A child with four UTIs in a single year should receive prophylactic antibiotics for at least six months.	III	Woodhead in Dershewitz, 1993	Prevent sepsis. Prevent renal hypertension, and chronic renal failure.	Prophylaxis prevents future UTIs and therefore damage to kidneys and urologic system.

Radiologic Work-up

#	Indicator		References		
19.	Any boy less than 10 years old with a first UTI or with systemic symptoms** (and/or who has not had the following study before) should have a VCUG and one of the following within three months of diagnosis: – RUS, or – IVP, or – nuclear medicine renal scan.	III	Andrich and Majd, 1992; Gillenwater, 1991; Roth and Gonzalez in Oski et al., 1994; Sherbotie and Cornfeld, 1991; Woodhead in Dershewitz, 1993	Prevent sepsis. Prevent renal scarring, renal hypertension, and chronic renal failure.	UTIs are rare in boys and are often associated with anatomic abnormalities.
20.	Any girl less than 3 years old with a first UTI or less than 10 years old with systemic symptoms** (and/or who has not had the following studies before) should have a VCUG or IC and one of the following within three months of diagnosis: – RUS, or – IVP, or – nuclear medicine renal scan.	III	Andrich and Majd, 1992; Gillenwater, 1991; Roth and Gonzalez in Oski et al., 1994; Sherbotie and Cornfeld, 1991; Woodhead in Dershewitz, 1993	Prevent sepsis. Prevent renal scarring, renal hypertension, and chronic renal failure.	Uncomplicated UTIs are not uncommon in older girls, so a radiologic work-up is not typically necessary.
21.	If a child with a diagnosis of UTI remains febrile for more than 48 hours on therapy, or if repeat urine culture is positive despite appropriate antibiotics, the child needs an immediate evaluation for urologic obstruction or abscess with renal ultrasound (RUS), intravenous pyelogram (IVP), or nuclear medicine renal scan.	III	Lebel in Oski et al., 1994	Prevent sepsis. Prevent renal scarring, renal hypertension, and chronic renal failure. Prevent damage to the urologic system.	Even with appropriate antibiotics, a UTI will often not resolve if there is an abscess or obstruction.
22.	Children who have a VCUG or IC following a UTI should be on prophylactic or therapeutic antibiotics continuously from the beginning of therapy for the UTI until the time of the study.	III	Woodhead in Dershewitz, 1993	Prevent sepsis. Prevent renal scarring, renal hypertension, and chronic renal failure.	Antibiotic treatment prevents reflux of *infected* urine. Reflux of infected urine is more likely to cause scarring than reflux of uninfected urine.
	Vesicoureteral Reflux (VUR)				
23.	Children diagnosed with Grade II or higher VUR should be on prophylactic antibiotics until the reflux has resolved.	III	Woodhead in Dershewitz, 1993; Lebel in Oski et al., 1994; Gillenwater, 1991; Andrich and Majd, 1992	Prevent sepsis. Prevent renal scarring, renal hypertension, and chronic renal failure.	Antibiotic treatment prevents reflux of *infected* urine. Reflux of infected urine is more likely to cause scarring than reflux of uninfected urine.

#	Indicator		Reference	Benefit	Comments
24.	Children with VUR should have annual monitoring with VCUG or nuclear cystogram.	III	Woodhead in Dershewitz, 1993	Prevent allergic reaction to antibiotics. Decrease antibiotic resistance.	The goal of annual monitoring is to detect early damage to kidneys as well as resolution of reflux. Determination of need for continued prophylaxis can be made based on monitoring test results.
25.	Children with high grade (Grade IV or higher) VUR or other anatomic abnormalities, such as posterior urethral valves, abnormal urethral implantation, or horse-shoe kidney, should be referred to a urologist.	III	Woodhead in Dershewitz, 1993; Gillenwater, 1991	Prevent allergic reaction to antibiotics. Decrease antibiotic resistance.	The references do not specify which grades count as "high grade," but common practice would count at least Grade III as high grade. Some clinicians would refer for Grade II. Clinicians who do not believe in surgical management of reflux may not consider it necessary to refer to a urologist. However, urologists have the best training and experience to determine whether surgical or medical treatment is most appropriate.
26.	Children with obstructive symptoms should be referred to a urologist.	III	Woodhead in Dershewitz, 1993	Prevent damage to the urologic system.	Specialist evaluation is important to ensure proper course of treatment.
27.	Children with VUR or other anatomic abnormalities who also have hypertension, decreased renal function, failure to thrive, or other related signs, should be referred to a pediatric nephrologist for treatment of renal insufficiency and hypertension.	III		Prevent renal failure.	Staff recommended this indicator.

*Indicators for laboratory tests in the presence of fever in children under 36 months of age can be found in Chapter 12.

Quality of Evidence Codes:

I:	RCT
II-1:	Nonrandomized controlled trials
II-2:	Cohort or case analysis
II-3:	Multiple time series
III:	Opinions or descriptive studies

REFERENCES - URINARY TRACT INFECTION

Andrich MP, and M Majd. September 1992. Diagnostic imaging in the evaluation of the first urinary tract infection in infants and young children. *Pediatrics* 90 (3): 436-41.

Gillenwater JY. March 1991. The role of the urologist in urinary tract infection. *Medical Clinics of North America* 75 (2): 471-9.

Kemper KJ, and ED Avner. March 1992. The case against screening urinalyses for asymptomatic bacteriuria in children. *American Journal of Diseases of Children* 146: 343-6.

Lebel MH. 1994. Urinary tract infections. In *Principles and Practice of Pediatrics*, Second ed. Editors Oski FA, CD DeAngelis, RD Feigin, et al., 532-3. Philadelphia, PA: J.B. Lippincott Company.

Marks MI, and AC Arrieta. 1 1992. Cystitis. In *Textbook of Pediatric Infectious Diseases*, Third ed. Editors Feigin RD, and JD Cherry, 480-7. Philadelphia, PA: W.B. Saunders Company.

Marks MI, and AC Arrieta. 2 1992. Pyelonephritis. In *Textbook of Pediatric Infectious Diseases*, Third ed. Editors Feigin RD, and JD Cherry, 487-94. Philadelphia, PA: W.B. Saunders Company.

O'Donnell B. 1990. The case for surgery. *British Medical Journal* 300: 1393-4.

Roth DR, and ET Gonzales. 1994. Urinary tract infection. In *Principles and Practice of Pediatrics*, Second ed. Editors Oski FA, CD DeAngelis, RD Feigin, et al., 1770-2. Philadelphia, PA: J.B. Lippincott Company.

Sherbotie JR, and D Cornfeld. March 1991. Management of urinary tract infections in children. *Medical Clinics of North America* 75 (2): 327-338.

Stull TL, and JJ LiPuma. March 1991. Epidemiology and natural history of urniary tract infections in children. *Medical Clinics of North America* 75 (2): 287-97.

Treves ST. October 1994. The ongoing challenge of diagnosis and treatment of urinary tract infection, vesicoureteral reflux and renal damage in children. *The Journal of Nuclear Medicine* 35 (10): 1608-11.

White RHR. 1990. Management of urinary tract infection and vesicoureteric reflux in children: Operative treatment has no advantage over medical management. *British Medical Journal* 300: 1391-2.

Woodhead JC. 1993. Genitourinary problems. In *Ambulatory Pediatric Care*, Second ed. Editor Dershewitz RA, 436-41. Philadelphia, PA: J.B. Lippincott Company.

Zelikovic I, RD Adelman, and PA Nancarrow. November 1992. Urinary tract infections in children: An update. *Western Journal of Medicine* 157 (5): 554-61.

21. VAGINITIS AND SEXUALLY TRANSMITTED DISEASES (DIAGNOSIS AND TREATMENT)[1]
Eve Kerr, M.D., M.P.H.

Approach

The general approach to reviewing vulvovaginitis and sexually transmitted diseases (STDs) was obtained from a general text on ambulatory medicine (Barker et al., 1991) and a text of diagnostic strategies for common medical problems (Panzer et al., 1991) and two textbooks on adolescent medicine (Friedman et al., 1992; McAnarney et al., 1992). Specific treatment recommendations were derived from the Centers for Disease Control 1993 Treatment Guidelines to Sexually Transmitted Diseases (CDC, 1993). The guidelines were based on systematic literature reviews by CDC staff and consensus opinions by experts. The literature reviews are summarized, in part, in the April 1995 Supplement to *Clinical Infectious Diseases*, which we reviewed to add greater detail to treatment controversies. Adolescents account for 3 to 6 million cases of sexually transmitted diseases annually.

VULVOVAGINITIS

IMPORTANCE

The most common causes of vulvovaginal infections are: *Gardnerella vaginalis, Candida albicans,* and *Trichomonas vaginalis.* An estimated 75 percent of women will experience at least one episode of vulvovaginal candidiasis in their lifetimes, and 40-45 percent will experience two or more episodes (CDC, 1993). There are an estimated 10 million visits to physicians' offices each year for vaginitis (Reef et al., 1995). *Vulvovaginal candidiasis* and bacterial vaginosis (*G. vaginalis*) are not considered sexually transmitted diseases, although women who are not

_____

[1]This chapter was originally written for the Women's Quality of Care Panel.

sexually active are rarely affected by bacterial vaginosis (CDC, 1993). *T. vaginalis* is transmitted through sexual activity and is a common cause of vaginitis among adolescents who are sexually active. Gonorrhea and chlamydial infections, although not causative of vulvovaginitis, sometimes present with an abnormal discharge. In fact, as many as 25 percent of women with a discharge have cervical infections (Panzer et al., 1991).

Candidal vaginitis does not have important medical sequlea but does cause discomfort that may impair the patient's quality of life. Bacterial vaginosis may be associated with pelvic inflammatory disease (PID) (Joesoef and Schmid, 1995). A recent randomized controlled trial (RCT) found a threefold decrease in the incidence of postabortion PID in women with bacterial vaginosis who had been treated with metronidazole (Joesoef and Schmid, 1995).

EFFICACY AND/OR EFFECTIVENESS OF INTERVENTIONS

Screening

There is no indication for general population screening for vaginitis.

Diagnosis

The approach to diagnosis is well summarized in Panzer et al. (1991). The history and physical examination have poor predictive value. For example, approximately 35 percent of symptomatic patients had no infection, 32 percent of asymptomatic patients had infection, and approximately 15 percent of infected patients had normal pelvic examinations. Risk factors for sexually transmitted diseases (STDs)-- such as the number of sexual partners in the past month, history of sexually transmitted disease, presence of genitourinary symptoms, and sexual contact with an infected partner--increase the prior probability of a sexually transmitted cause for vaginal discharge.

It is difficult to determine fully the operating characteristics of diagnostic tests for vaginitis. See Table 21.1 for details.

Table 21.1

**Operating Characteristics of Common Diagnostic Tests for
Vaginal and Cervical Infection**

Test	Sensitivity (Percent)	Specificity (Percent)
Vaginal infection		
Trichomonas vaginalis		
Saline wet mount	50-75	70-98
Direct fluorescent antibody	80-86	98
Vaginal candidiasis		
Potassium hydroxide preparation	30-84	90-99
Bacterial vaginosis		
Vaginal pH	81-97	...
Clue cells	85-90	80
"Whiff" test	38-84	...
Thin homogeneous discharge	80	...
Gram stain of vaginal wash	97	79
Abnormal amines by chromatography	98	...
Cervical infection		
Chlamydia trachomatis		
Direct fluorescent antibody	70-87	97-99
Enzyme immunoassay	80-85	98
Culture (single cervical swab)	70-80	98
Neisseria gonorrhoeae		
Cervix gram stain	50-79	98
Culture (single cervical swab)	85-90	98
Herpes simplex virus		
Tzanck smear: vesicular; pustular; crusted	67; 54; 17	85
Culture: vesicular; pustular; crusted	70; 67; 17	...

Source: Panzer et al., 1991.

Summary of diagnostic tests - Refer to Table 20.1

Trichomonas vaginalis

The wet mount is highly specific (70-98 percent) but not particularly sensitive (50-75 percent).

Candida albicans

The potassium hydroxide preparation has varied sensitivity (30-84 percent) compared with culture, but is highly specific (90-99 percent).

Bacterial vaginosis/Gardnerella vaginalis

Amsel et al. (1983) have developed criteria for diagnosis that are widely accepted (Panzer et al., 1991; Joesoef and Schmid, 1995). The diagnosis in a symptomatic patient is usually based on the presence of at least three of the four following criteria:

1) pH greater than 4.5;

2) positive whiff test;

3) clue cells on wet mount; and

4) thin homogeneous discharge.

See Table 20.1 for a summary of the sensitivity and specificity of these tests.

Diagnostic strategy in the evaluation of acute vulvovaginitis is often governed by the need to institute antimicrobial therapy. The first decision point lies in determining the source of infection (i.e., whether the infection is cervical or vaginal). An assessment of risk factors for sexually transmitted disease and a careful pelvic examination will help determine this. If the discharge is thought to be vaginal in origin, then a saline wet mount, potassium hydroxide wet mount, and the application of Amsel's criteria should be used to determine the cause of vaginitis.

A small proportion of women have recurrent vulvovaginal candidiasis (i.e., three or more episodes of symptomatic vulvovaginal candidiasis annually). These women should be evaluated for predisposing conditions, such as diabetes, immunosuppression, broad spectrum antibiotic use, corticosteroid use, and HIV infection. However, the majority of women with recurrent vulvovaginal candidiasis have no identifiable risk factors (Reef et al., 1995).

Treatment

Bacterial Vaginosis/Gardnerella vaginalis

These recommendations are based, in part, on randomized controlled studies and meta-analyses reviewed by the CDC (Joesoef and Schmid, 1995). Based on the CDC review, a 7-day treatment regimen is preferred over the single-dose regimen of metronidazole. The CDC notes that topical formulations require further study. However, all of the following have been rated as appropriate treatments for non-pregnant women (CDC, 1993):

- Metronidazole 500 mg orally 2 times per day for 7 days (95 percent overall cure rate); or
- Metronidazole 2 g orally in a single dose (84 percent overall cure rate); or
- Clindamycin cream at night for seven days; or
- Metronidazole cream twice a day for 5 days; or
- Clindamycin 300 mg orally twice a day for seven days.

These treatment recommendations are endorsed by the CDC (which provided the estimates of cure rates) and have been found effective in randomized controlled trials.[1]

T. Vaginalis

For *T. Vaginalis*, it is necessary to treat both the patient and sex partner(s) with:

- Metronidazole 2 g orally in a single dose; or
- Metronidazole 500 mg twice daily for 7 days;

Both regimens have been found to be equally effective in RCTs and result in a cure rate of approximately 95 percent (CDC, 1993; RCTs not reviewed).

---

[1]The individual randomized controlled trials were not reviewed.

Candida albicans

A number of topical formulations of the azole class (e.g., butoconazole, clotrimazole, miconazole, tioconazole, terconazole) provide effective treatment for vulvovaginal candidiasis with relief of symptoms and negative cultures among about 90 percent of patients after therapy is completed (CDC, 1993). These recommendations are based on clinical trials reviewed by the CDC (Reef et al., 1995).

In addition, several trials have demonstrated that oral azole drugs (e.g., fluconazole, ketoconazole, and itraconazole) may be as effective as topical agents. The FDA has approved single-dose fluconazole for the treatment of vulvovaginal candidiasis (*Wall Street Journal,* 1994). Practicing physicians report this therapy to be an effective treatment (Inman et al., 1994). Use of fluconazole is contraindicated for treatment of vaginal candidiasis in pregnancy. Optimal treatment for recurrent vulvovaginal candidiasis is not well established, but a role for oral agents is being investigated (Reef et al., 1995).

Follow-up Care

Follow-up is unnecessary for women whose symptoms resolve after treatment (CDC, 1993).

DISEASES CHARACTERIZED BY CERVICITIS

IMPORTANCE

Mucopurulent cervicitis is most often caused by *N. Gonorrhoea* and *C. trachomatis*--two sexually transmitted infections. *C. trachomatis* is the most common cause of cervical infection, with a prevalence ranging from about 9 to 35 percent in asymptomatic adolescents and 20 to 30 percent in women treated in sexually transmitted disease clinics. The incidence of chlamydia infection in 1988 was 215 per 100,000 (USDHHS, 1990). Approximately 13 percent of women with chlamydial infection have concurrent gonococcal infection and approximately 30 percent of women with gonococcal infection have chlamydial infection (Panzer et al., 1991). Transmission of gonorrhea from infected men to uninfected women occurs in 90 percent of exposures. The prevalence of gonorrhea infection among adolescents is 3 to 20 percent (Elster and Kuznets, 1994). Initially, both gonococcal and chlamydial infections may be asymptomatic, or present with vaginal symptoms (e.g., mucopurulent vaginal discharge, vaginal itching, dyspareunia, dysuria, vague lower abdominal pain), anorectal symptoms, and pharyngeal symptoms. However, both have the potential to cause pelvic inflammatory disease, the sequelae of which include ectopic pregnancy and infertility.

EFFICACY AND/OR EFFECTIVENESS OF INTERVENTIONS

Screening

Screening for both *N. gonorrhoea* and *C. trachomatis* should be performed with the yearly pelvic examination for all women with multiple sexual partners or with other sexually transmitted diseases (Barker, 1991), and perhaps for all sexually active women age 24 or younger (CDC, 1993).

Diagnosis

The presence of symptoms (i.e., mucopurulent vaginal discharge, vaginal itching, dyspareunia, dysuria, vague lower abdominal pain) in the right clinical context (i.e., a sexually active woman) would lead one to suspect cervicitis. Physical exam may reveal red, edematous and friable cervix with mucopurulent cervical discharge.

C. Trachomatis

Diagnosis in patients with symptoms of cervicitis is confirmed by direct fluorescent antibody testing (sensitivity 70-87 percent, specificity 97-99 percent; Panzer et al., 1991) or enzyme immunoassay (sensitivity 80-85 percent, specificity 98 percent; Panzer et al., 1991).

N. Gonorrhoea

Suspected gonococcal infection may be initially confirmed by gram stain (sensitivity 50-79 percent, specificity 98 percent; Panzer et al., 1991) and subsequently by culture (sensitivity 85-90 percent, specificity 98 percent; Panzer et al., 1991).

Treatment for Cervicitis

In patients with inconclusive symptoms and/or physical exam, one must take into account the pre-test probabilities of infection when determining the need for treatment. Therefore, in populations with a high prevalence of sexually transmitted diseases, and in women with known or suspected exposures, or if the patient is unlikely to return for treatment, one should treat without waiting for confirmatory cultures. Otherwise, results of tests should dictate the need for treatment (CDC, 1993).

According to the CDC, treatment for mucopurulent cervicitis should include the following:

- Treatment for gonorrhea and chlamydia in patient populations with high prevalence of both infections, such as patients seen at many STD clinics;
- Treatment for chlamydia only, if the prevalence of *N. gonorrhoea* is low but the likelihood of chlamydia is substantial;
- Await test results if the prevalence of both infections are low and if compliance with a recommendation for a return visit is likely.

Specific treatments

C. trachomatis

As recommended by the CDC based on RCTs (Weber and Johnson, 1995):

- Doxycylcine 100 mg orally twice a day for 7 days; or
- Azithromycin 1 g orally in a single dose.

Alternatives:

- Ofloxacin; Erythromycin; Sulfisoxazole

The partner(s) should be referred for therapy.

N. gonorrhoea

As recommended by the CDC based on RCTs (Moran and Levine, 1995). All women treated for gonorrhea should also be treated for chlamydia (see regimens for chlamydia).

Recommended regimens:

- Ceftriaxone 125 mg IM in single dose; or
- Cefixime 400 mg orally in a single dose; or
- Ciprofloxacin 500 mg orally in a single dose; or
- Ofloxacin 400 mg orally in a single dose.

Other effective antimicrobials may be used (e.g., spectinomycin, other cephalosporins, other quinolones).

Follow-up Care

For chlamydia, follow-up cultures are not necessary for women completing treatment with doxycycline or azithromycin unless symptoms persist or re-infection is suspected (CDC, 1993). For other antibiotic regimens, testing may be considered three weeks after completion of treatment. Similarly, women who are symptom free after treatment for gonorrhea with any recommended antibiotic do not need follow-up cultures (CDC, 1993).

PELVIC INFLAMMATORY DISEASE (PID)

IMPORTANCE

PID represents a spectrum of upper genital tract inflammatory disorder, including endometritis, salpingitis, tubo-ovarian abscess, and pelvic peritonitis. More than one million cases of PID are diagnosed and treated each year in the U.S. (US DHHS, 1990). Adolescents may be at greater risk than other groups for developing PID; estimates from one source suggest that a sexually active 15-year-old has a 1-in-8 chance of developing acute salpingitis as compared to 1-in-80 for a 24-year-old (Rosenfeld and Litman, in Friedman et al., 1992) The cost of PID and associated ectopic pregnancy and infertility exceed $2.7 billion (Walker et al., 1993). If one takes into account the medical consequences of PID, including infertility, ectopic pregnancy, and chronic pelvic pain, the direct and indirect costs of PID exceed $4.2 billion annually (Walker et al., 1993).

EFFICACY/EFFECTIVENESS OF INTERVENTIONS

Diagnosis

The diagnosis of PID is usually made on the basis of clinical findings. In some cases, women may have atypical PID, with abnormal bleeding, dyspareunia, or vaginal discharge. The CDC suggests that empiric treatment of PID should be instituted on the basis of the presence of all of the following clinical criteria for pelvic inflammation and in the absence of an established cause other than PID (e.g., ectopic pregnancy, acute appendicitis):

- Lower abdominal tenderness;
- Adnexal tenderness; and
- Cervical motion tenderness (CDC, 1993).

The specificity of the diagnosis can be increased if the following signs are also present:

- Oral temperature above 38.3° Centigrade;
- Abnormal cervical or vaginal discharge;
- Elevated erythrocyte sedimentation rate;
- Elevated C-reactive protein;
- Laboratory documentation of cervical infection with *N. gonorrhoea* or *C. Trachomatis* (CDC, 1993).

However, algorithms based only on clinical criteria fail to identify some women with PID and misclass by others (Walker et al., 1993). Assessment by endometrial biopsy, laparoscopy, or both is more specific but less sensitive (Walker et al., 1993).

Treatment

Hospitalization for antimicrobial treatment of PID is recommended by the CDC under the following circumstances:

- The diagnosis is uncertain and surgical emergencies such as appendicitis and ectopic pregnancy cannot be excluded;
- Pelvic abscess is suspected;
- The patient is pregnant;
- The patient is an adolescent;
- The patient has HIV infection;
- Severe illness or nausea and vomiting preclude outpatient management; or
- Clinical follow-up within 72 hours of starting antibiotic treatment cannot be arranged (CDC, 1993; MMWR, 1991).

These guidelines are based primarily on expert opinion.

Treatment with antibiotics has been well studied for inpatient regimens (Walker et al., 1993). Based on RCTs, the CDC supports the use of two antibiotic regimens for inpatient treatment of PID, both with cure rates above 90 percent (CDC, 1993; Walker et al., 1993).

Regimen 1

- Cefoxitin 2 g IV q 6 or cefotetan 2 g IV q 12 (for at least 48 hours) and
- Doxycycline 100 mg IV or orally every 12 hours (for 14 days).

or

Regimen 2

- Clindamycin 900 mg IV every 8 hours, and
- Gentamicin.

The above regimen should be continued for at least 48 hours, followed by oral doxycyline or clindamycin.

There is limited experience from clinical trials with outpatient regimens for PID (Walker et al., 1993). Further, no specific comparisons have been done on outpatient versus inpatient treatment.

The second regimen noted below provides broader coverage against anaerobic organisms (because of the addition of clindamycin or metronidazole) but is more expensive. Patients who do not respond to outpatient therapy within 72 hours should be hospitalized, since by 72 hours patients should have improvement of subjective complaints and be afebrile (Peterson et al., 1990).

Regimen 1

- Cefoxitin 2 g IM plus probenecid, 1 g orally in a single dose concurrently, or ceftriaxone 250 mg IM or other parenteral third-generation cephalosporin, and
- Doxycycline 100 mg orally 2 times a day for 14 days.

Regimen 2

- Ofloxacin 400 mg orally 2 times a day for 14 days, and
- Either clindamycin 450 mg orally 4 times a day, or metronidazole 500 mg orally 2 times a day for 14 days.

Further research must be done before the use of limited spectrum antibiotics (such as quinolone alone) can be recommended (Walker et al., 1993).

Follow-up Care

Patients receiving outpatient therapy should receive follow up within 72 hours to document clinical improvement and should have a microbiologic re-examination 7-10 days after completing therapy

Patients receiving inpatient therapy should have a microbiological re-examination 7-10 days after completing therapy to determine cure. Some experts advocate another microbiologic evaluation in 4-6 levels (USDHHS, 1991).

Sex partners should be empirically treated for *C. trachomatis* and *N. gonorrhoea*.

DISEASES CHARACTERIZED BY GENITAL ULCERS

IMPORTANCE

In the United States, most persons with genital ulcers have genital herpes, syphilis or chancroid, of which genital herpes is the most common. More than one of these disease may be present among at least 3-10 percent of patients with genital ulcers. Each of the conditions is associated with an increased risk for HIV infection (CDC, 1993).

GENITAL HERPES SIMPLEX INFECTION

On the basis of serologic studies, approximately 30 million persons in the United States may have genital herpes simplex virus (HSV) infection (CDC, 1993).

EFFICACY AND/OR EFFECTIVENESS OF INTERVENTIONS

Screening

There is no literature that suggests a useful role for screening.

Diagnosis

Diagnosis is most often made on the basis of history and physical exam and confirmed by HSV culture or antigen test. The sensitivity of the culture decreases with the age of the lesion (sensitivities for vesicular, pustular and crusted lesions are 70 percent, 67 percent, and 17 percent respectively) (Panzer et al., 1991). Further, specimens from primary lesions and cutaneous lesions are more likely to grow herpes simplex virus.

Treatment

As summarized by the CDC, RCTs demonstrate that acyclovir is effective in decreasing symptoms and signs of HSV in first clinical episodes and when used as a suppressive (daily) therapy (CDC, 1993; Stone and Whittington, 1990). The CDC does not generally recommend acyclovir treatment for recurrent episodes because early therapy can rarely be instituted. The CDC also recommends that after one year of continuous suppressive therapy, acyclovir should be discontinued to allow assessment of the patient's rate of recurrent episodes. If recurrence rate is low, suppressive treatment may be discontinued permanently or temporarily.

Other Management Issues

Patient education is important in preventing the transmission of HSV. Patients should abstain from sexual activity while lesions are present and use condoms during all sexual exposures.

All patients with genital ulcers should receive a serologic test for syphilis. HIV testing should be considered in the management of patients with known or suspected HSV.

CHANCROID

Chancroid is caused by the bacterium *Haemophilus ducreyi*. As many as 10 percent of patients with chancroid may be coinfected with *T. pallidum* or HSV (CDC, 1993).

EFFICACY AND/OR EFFECTIVENESS OF INTERVENTIONS

Screening

Screening is not indicated.

Diagnosis

With lack of readily available means to culture for *H. ducreyi*, the diagnosis rests on clinical grounds. The CDC states that a probable diagnosis can be made if the patient has one or more painful genital ulcers and:

1) no evidence of *T. Pallidum* infection by dark-field exam or by a serologic test for syphilis performed at least 7 days after onset of ulcers; and

2) the clinical presentation of the ulcer(s) is either not typical of HSV or the HSV test results are negative.

Treatment

The CDC recommends treatment with single-dose Azithromycin or IM Ceftriaxone or a 7-day course of Erythromycin.

Patients with Chancroid should be tested for HIV and syphilis, and retested three months later if initial results are negative (CDC, 1993).

Sexual partners (within 10 days before onset of the patient's symptoms) should be examined and treated.

Follow-up Care

Patients should be re-examined 3-7 days after initiation of treatment to assess clinical improvement.

PRIMARY AND SECONDARY SYPHILIS

IMPORTANCE

Syphilis is a systemic disease caused by *T. pallidum*. The incidence of primary and secondary syphilis in the United States has been steadily rising, with 118 cases per 100,000 reported in 1989 (USDHHS, 1990). In addition, there is an association between genital ulcer disease and the transmission of HIV through sexual contact.

EFFICACY AND/OR EFFECTIVENESS OF INTERVENTIONS

Screening

Screening of the general population is not indicated (except in pregnancy). At-risk populations (i.e., with other sexually transmitted diseases) should be screened using a non-treponemal test, as discussed below (CDC, 1993).

Diagnosis

Primary syphilis should be diagnosed on the basis of presence of (usually nonpainful) genital ulcer (or recent history of same), and laboratory testing for syphilis. Twenty percent of patients will have a negative non-treponemal test (VDRL or RPR) at the time of presentation, but direct examination of the chancer (dark-field microscopy or direct fluorescence antibody) will be positive (Panzer et al., 1991). Secondary syphilis is a systemic illness with a prominent rash, beginning six weeks to several months after exposure.

Treatment

Treatment for primary and secondary syphilis should be initiated with benzathine penicillin G (2.4 units IM in single dose) in the absence of allergy. One should not wait for test results to initiate treatment.

Follow-up Care

Treatment failures occur in approximately 5 percent of cases treated with penicillin regimens and more frequently with other regimens (Rofls, 1995). According to the CDC, patients should be re-examined clinically and serologically at three months and again at six months for evidence of successful treatment (CDC, 1993).

Management of sexual partners

Persons sexually exposed to a patient with syphilis in any stage should be evaluated clinically and serologically according the CDC recommendations.

RECOMMENDED QUALITY INDICATORS FOR VAGINITIS AND SEXUALLY TRANSMITTED DISEASES

The following criteria apply to nonpregnant, non-HIV-infected adolescents who are sexually active.

Diagnosis

	Indicator	Quality of evidence	Literature	Benefits	Comments
	Vaginitis				
1.	In adolescent girls presenting with complaint of vaginal discharge, the practitioner should perform a speculum exam to determine the source of discharge.	III	Panzer et al., 1991	Decrease discharge, itching and dysuria.	Since implications of and treatment for these two entities differ substantially, physical exam must be performed.
2.	At a minimum, the following tests should be performed on the vaginal discharge: normal saline wet mount for clue cells and trichomads; KOH wet mount for yeast hyphae.	III	Panzer et al., 1991	Decrease discharge, itching and dysuria.	pH determination is also sensitive, but its specificity is unknown. Therefore, at a minimum, the two wet mounts should be performed.
3.	A sexual history should be obtained from all women presenting with a vaginal discharge. The history should include: a. No. of sexual partners in previous 6 months; b. Absence or presence of symptoms in partners; c. Use of condoms; and d. Prior history of sexually transmitted diseases.	III	Panzer et al., 1991; CDC, 1993	Decrease discharge, itching and dysuria. Decrease PID and abdominal pain. Decrease infertility. Decrease mortality from ectopic pregnancy.	In patients with one or more risk factors, probability for a STD (i.e., chlamydia or gonorrhea) as a cause of discharge is increased and culture for the causative organisms may be appropriate. This is important because cervicitis has more significant long-term consequences than vaginitis, such as PID, infertility and ectopic pregnancy.
4.	If three of the following four criteria are met, a diagnosis of bacterial vaginosis or gardnerella vaginosis should be made: pH greater than 4.5; positive whiff test; clue cells on wet mount; thin homogenous discharge.	III	Panzer et al., 1991; Amsel et al., 1983	Decrease discharge, itching and dysuria.	Based on Amsel et al., the presence of three criteria is highly sensitive and specific for bacterial vaginosis.
	Cervicitis				
5.	Routine testing for gonorrhea and chlamydia trachomatis (culture and antigen detection, respectively) should be performed with the routine pelvic exam in all adolescent girls.	III	CDC, 1993; ACOG, 1993 (The Obstetrician Gynecologist Primary Preventive Healthcare)	Alleviate pain. Alleviate fever. Decrease infertility. Decrease mortality from ectopic pregnancy.	This recommendation is based upon epidemiologic studies of transmission and prevalence, as summarized by the CDC. Women with multiple sexual partners are at higher risk for STDs, and these may be asymptomatic. Because adolescent girls may not be honest about the number of sexual partners, and their partners are likely to have multiple partners, screening adolescents routinely is suggested.

PID					
6.	If a patient is given the diagnosis of PID, a speculum and bimanual pelvic exam should have been performed.	III	CDC, 1993	Alleviate pain. Alleviate fever. Decrease infertility. Decrease mortality from ectopic pregnancy.	The diagnosis of PID is based primarily on physical exam. In addition, one should obtain cervical specimens for culture. Therefore, a physical exam is mandatory before treatment can be initiated.
7.	If a patient is given the diagnosis of PID, at least 2 of the following signs should be present on physical exam: - lower abdominal tenderness - adnexal tenderness - cervical motion tenderness.	III	CDC, 1993	Alleviate pain. Alleviate fever. Decrease infertility. Decrease mortality from ectopic pregnancy.	It is important to correctly identify PID since symptoms may mimic appendicitis and ovarian torsion. The CDC states that all three signs should be present. We have stated that at least two must be present and documented.
Genital Ulcers					
8.	If a patient presents with genital ulcer(s) of any cause, HIV testing should be recommended.	III	CDC, 1993	Delay progression to AIDS. Prevention of HIV spread.*	Based on this observation, it is particularly important to recommend testing in patients with genital ulcers, although testing could be recommended in persons with any STD.
STDs—General					
9.	If a patient presents with any sexually transmitted disease (gonorrhea, chlamydia, trachomatis, herpes, chancroid, syphilis) a non-treponemal test (VDRL or RPR) for syphilis should be obtained.	III	CDC, 1993	Prevention of late complications of syphilis.**	Persons with one STD are at high risk for another. Since there is effective treatment to prevent late complications of syphilis, testing is recommended.

384

	Indicator	Quality of evidence	Literature	Benefits	Comments
	Vaginitis				
10.	Treatment for bacterial vaginosis should be with metronidazole (orally or vaginally) or clindamycin (orally or vaginally) per the CDC recommendations.	I	CDC, 1993	Decrease discharge, itching and dysuria.	These are the only proven effective regimens. RCTs reviewed by the CDC show that the evidence for efficacy of oral treatment is better than for topical treatment. CDC recommends the 7-day over the single-dose regimen.
11.	Treatment for *T. vaginalis* should be with oral metronidazole in the absence of allergy to metronidazole.	I	CDC, 1993	Decrease discharge, itching and dysuria.	Based on RCTs reviewed by the CDC, this is the only known effective treatment.
12.	Treatment for non-recurrent (three or fewer episodes in previous year) yeast vaginitis should be with topical "azole" preparations (e.g., clotrimazole, butoconazole, etc.) or fluconazole.	I	CDC, 1993; ADD REF.	Decrease discharge, itching and dysuria.	Based on RCTs reviewed by the CDC. These regimens are approved by the FDA.
	Cervicitis				
13.	All women treated for gonorrhea should also be treated for chlamydia per the CDC recommendations.	II-2; III	CDC, 1993	Prevent PID. Decrease infertility. Decrease mortality from ectopic pregnancy.	Women with gonorrhea are likely to be coinfected with chlamydia. Since the sensitivity of chlamydia assays is variable, concurrent treatment is recommended.
	PID				
14.	Patients with PID and any of the following conditions should be hospitalized: - appendicitis; - ectopic pregnancy; - pelvic abscess is present or suspected; - the patient is pregnant; - the patient is an adolescent (under age 18); - the patient has HIV infection; - uncontrolled nausea and vomiting; - clinical follow-up within 72 hours of starting antibiotic treatment cannot be arranged; or - the patient does not improve within 72 hours of starting therapy.	III	CDC, 1993	Alleviate pain. Alleviate fever. Prevent sepsis. Decrease infertility. Decrease mortality from ectopic pregnancy.	While other reasons for hospitalization may exist (i.e., cannot rule out appendicitis), these have been recommended by the CDC and should be discernable by chart review. The purpose of hospitalization is to ensure effective treatment in persons at risk of complications (e.g., HIV infection) or poor follow-up (e.g., adolescents).
15.	Total antibiotic therapy for PID should be for no less than 10 days (inpatient, if applicable, plus outpatient).	III	CDC, 1993; Peterson et al., 1991	Alleviate pain. Alleviate fever. Prevent sepsis. Decrease infertility. Decrease mortality from ectopic pregnancy.	The standard of care is 10-14 days, although RCTs have not specifically addressed duration of treatment. Shorter treatment periods may results in lower cure rates.
	Genital Ulcers				
16.	All patients with genital herpes should be counseled regarding reducing the risk of transmission to sexual partners.	III	CDC, 1993	Prevent spread of genital herpes.	Genital herpes is transmissible even in the absence of current outbreak. Unlike most other STDs, there is not effective cure for herpes. Therefore, prevention of transmission is of prime importance.

385

No.	Recommendation			Benefits	Comments
17.	In the absence of allergy, patients with chancroid should be treated with Azithromycin, Ceftriaxone, or Erythromycin.	CDC, 1993	I	Decrease pain. Heal ulcer. Limit transmission of chancroid.	These have been shown in RCTs reviewed by the CDC to be effective.
18.	In the absence of allergy, patients with primary and secondary syphilis should be treated with benzathine penicillin G (IM).	CDC, 1993	I	Prevention of late complications of syphilis.**	Penicillin is the best studied of all regimens and known to be effective through single IM administration. This recommendation is based on RCTs reviewed by the CDC.
19.	If a patient has a primary ulcer consistent with syphilis, treatment for syphilis should be initiated before laboratory test results are received.	CDC, 1993	III	Prevention of late complications of syphilis.**	Not all patients will return for follow-up. Because effective treatment exists and consequences of untreated syphilis are serious, treatment should be initiated at the time of first presentation. This is particularly important for adolescents.
	STDs—General				
20.	Sexual partners of patients with new diagnoses of gonorrhea, chlamydia, chancroid and primary or secondary syphilis should be referred for treatment.	CDC, 1993	III	Effective treatment and prevention of complications of STDs in partners. Prevention of STD spread.*	Patients with STDs have either contracted them from their current sexual partner or may have infected their current sexual partner. In either case, the most recent sexual partner should be referred for therapy. While there are specific guidelines for which partners should be referred, based on the time period from last sexual activity with the partner and infection, at least some indication that the patient was told to refer her sexual partner(s) for treatment should be in the chart.

386

Follow-up

Indicator	Quality of evidence	Literature	Benefits	Comments
PID				
21. Patients receiving outpatient therapy for PID should receive a follow-up visit within 72 hours of diagnosis.	III	CDC, 1993; Peterson et al., 1991	Alleviate pain. Alleviate fever. Prevent sepsis. Decrease infertility. Decrease mortality from ectopic pregnancy.	Early effective treatment is important in preventing complications.
22. All patients being treated for PID should have a microbiological re-examination (e.g., cultures) within 10 days of completing therapy.	III	CDC, 1993	Decrease infertility. Decrease mortality from ectopic pregnancy.	A small percentage of patients may not have complete resolution even after treatment (successes with various regimens vary, ranging from 80-99%).
Genital Ulcers				
23. Patients receiving treatment for chancroid should be re-examined within 7 days of treatment initiation to assess clinical improvement.	III	CDC, 1993	Prevention of complications of untreated syphilis.** Prevent transmission of chancroid, syphilis, and herpes.	Most patients will have improved by 7 days.
24. Patients with primary or secondary syphilis should be re-examined clinically and serologically within 6 months after treatment.	III	CDC, 1993	Prevention of complications of untreated syphilis.**	If a treatment failure has occurred, the patient requires re-treatment.

*HIV causes fatigue, diarrhea, neuropathic symptoms, fevers, and opportunistic infections (OIs). OIs cause a wide variety of symptoms, including cough, shortness of breath, and vomiting. Average life expectancy after HIV infection is less than 10 years. Other STDs include gonorrhea, syphilis, and chlamydia. They cause a wide variety of symptoms, including dysuria, genital ulcers, infertility, rashes, neurologic and cardiac problems and rarely contribute to mortality. Preventing HIV and STDs has the added benefit of interrupting the spread of disease and preventing morbidity and mortality in those who thus avoid infection.

**Untreated syphilis infection can lead to tertiary syphilis (neurosyphilis and cardiovascular syphilis) and congential syphilis among babies born to infected mothers.

Quality of Evidence Codes:

I: RCT
II-1:   Nonrandomized controlled trials
II-2:   Cohort or case analysis
II-3:   Multiple time series
III: Opinions or descriptive studies

REFERENCES - VAGINITIS AND SEXUALLY TRANSMITTED DISEASES

Amsel R, PA Totten, CA Spiegel, et al. January 1983. Nonspecific vaginitis: Diagnostic criteria and microbial and epidemiologic associations. *American Journal of Medicine* 74: 14-22.

Barker LR, JR Burton, and PD Zieve, Editors. 1991. *Principles of Ambulatory Medicine*, Third ed.Baltimore, MD: Williams and Wilkins.

Centers for Disease Control. 24 September 1993. 1993 sexually transmitted diseases treatment guidelines. *Morbidity and Mortality Weekly Report* 42 (RR-14): 1-102.

Centers for Disease Control. 26 April 1991. Pelvic inflammatory disease: Guidelines for prevention and management. *Morbidity and Mortality Weekly Report* 40 (RR-5): 1-25.

Centers for Disease Control. May 1991. *Sexually Transmitted Diseases: Clinical Practice Guidelines*. Atlanta, GA: U.S. Department of Health and Human Services.

Inman W, G Pearce, and L Wilton. 1994. Safety of fluconazole in the treatment of vaginal candidiasis: A prescription-event monitoring study, with special reference to the outcome of pregnancy. *European Journal of Clinical Pharmacology* 46: 115-8.

Joesoef MR, and GP Schmid. 1995. Bacterial vaginosis: Review of treatment options and potential clinical indications for therapy. *Clinical Infectious Diseases* 20 (Suppl. 1): S72-9.

Moran JS, and WC Levine. 1995. Drugs of choice for the treatment of uncomplicated gonococcal infections. *Clinical Infectious Diseases* 20 (Suppl. 1): S47-65.

Panzer RJ, ER Black, and PF Griner, Editors. 1991. *Diagnostic Strategies for Common Medical Problems*.Philadelphia, PA: American College of Physicians.

Peterson HB, EI Galaid, and JM Zenilman. July 1990. Pelvic inflammatory disease: Review of treatment options. *Reviews of Infectious Diseases* 12 (Suppl. 6): S656-64.

Peterson HB, CK Walker, JG Kahn, et al. 13 November 1991. Pelvic inflammatory disease: Key treatment issues and options. *Journal of the American Medical Association* 266 (18): 2605-2611.

Reef SE, WC Levine, MM McNeil, et al. 1995. Treatment options for vulvovaginal candidiasis, 1993. *Clinical Infectious Diseases* 20 (Suppl. 1): S80-90.

Rolfs RT. 1995. Treatment of syphilis, 1993. *Clinical Infectious Diseases* 20 (Suppl. 1): S23-38.

Stone KM, and WL Whittington. July 1990. Treatment of genital herpes. *Reviews of Infectious Diseases* 12 (Suppl. 6): S610-9.

U.S. Department of Health and Human Services. 1991. *Healthy People 2000: National Health Promotion and Disease Prevention Objectives*. U.S. Government Printing Office, Washington, DC.

Walker CK, JG Kahn, EA Washington, et al. October 1993. Pelvic inflammatory disease: Metaanalysis of antimicrobial regimen efficacy. *The Journal of Infectious Diseases* 168: 969-78.

Wall Street Journal. 1994. Pfizer one-dose drug for yeast infections gets FDA approval. (Food and Drug Administration approves Diflucan). *Wall Street Journal*, B, 4:6.

Weber JT, and RE Johnson. 1995. New treatments for chlamydia trachomatis genital infection. *Clinical Infectious Diseases* 20 (Suppl. 1): S66-71.

22. WELL CHILD CARE
Mark Schuster, M.D., Ph.D.

We reviewed: (1) textbooks on pediatrics (Cochran in Oski et al., 1994) and pediatric primary care (Grimm in Dershewitz, 1993; Dershewitz in Dershewitz, 1993; Keefer in Dershewitz, 1993; Cunningham in Hoekelman et al., 1992; Strahlman in Hoekelman et al., 1992; Hoekelman in Hoekelman et al., 1992); (2) the American Academy of Pediatrics (AAP) *Guidelines for Health Supervision II* (AAP, 1988); (3) *Bright Futures: Guidelines for Health Supervision of Infants, Children and Adolescents* (Green, 1994); and (4) the *Guide to Clinical Preventive Services* (United States Preventive Services Task Force [USPSTF], 1989). Several additional articles were identified from a MEDLINE search of English-language review articles on prevention and primary prevention published between January 1990 and March 1995. In addition, several AAP policy statements pertaining to well child care were identified through the AAP's Policy Reference Guide.

This review does not cover every aspect of well child care that is recommended by these sources. Rather, we have focused on topics that lend themselves to the development of quality indicators and that have broad support from clinicians. Many recommended components of well child care are the product of expert opinion and are not the result of findings from studies based on rigorous research designs. This is particularly true for the frequency and timing of certain aspects of the physical examination, topics for counseling, and tests. For example, there would probably be little disagreement that a child's weight should be measured periodically during the first year of life, but there would be much less agreement on the exact number of times it should be measured. Therefore, the indicators contain a fair amount of latitude on such issues.

Childhood immunizations (Chapter 14), tuberculosis screening (Chapter 18), sickle cell screening (Chapter 17), and developmental assessments (Chapter 8) are addressed in other reviews.

IMPORTANCE

Well child care is central to the practice of pediatrics. It accounts for 10.6 percent of visits for children under 15 years old (National Center for Health Statistics [NCHS], 1992). Well child care serves many purposes, including to: screen for disease, provide counseling about how to foster healthy development of the child and prevent disease and injury (anticipatory guidance), identify problems at a sufficiently early stage to intervene to prevent further problems, provide immunizations, answer questions, allow a physician to become familiar with a child and his/her family (Grimm in Dershewitz, 1993). While textbooks and guidelines universally recommend well child visits, they do not always specify the content of those visits. For example, they typically recommend that a complete physical examination should be conducted at each visit without detailing the specific components. Much is left to the discretion of the physician. Another characteristic of well child care that presents a challenge in the development of quality indicators is that much of the care that is provided is not routinely documented in the medical record. Clinicians who provide anticipatory guidance might not note it in the chart or might only make a general note that they provided anticipatory guidance without specifying what issues were covered. Therefore, in constructing quality indicators, we selected indicators for which there is general agreement that they should be both performed and documented.

INTERVENTIONS THAT CONSTITUTE WELL CHILD CARE

Recommended Components of a Newborn Examination

Cochran (in Oski et al., 1994) and the AAP (1988) recommend that newborns be examined within the first 24 hours of life. Several sources were used to determine important components of the newborn examination. The specific components mentioned in each source are listed in the table below. Failure by a source to mention a component does not necessarily mean that the component is considered unimportant or unnecessary. Likewise, some sources list components of the physical examination that are not important from a medical perspective (e.g., Mongolian spots) or that are unlikely to be documented if normal; thus, not all components mentioned in a source are included in the chart below.

Table 22.1

Comparison of Components of the Newborn Examination Recommended by Four Sources

Recommended Components	AAP	Cochran	Green	Unti
Weight	X	X	X	X
Length	X	X	X	X
Head circumference	X	X	X	X
Anterior fontanelle				X
Jaundice	X		X	
Red Reflex	X	X	X	
Palate		X	X	
Clavicles		X	X	X
Heart rate and exam (e.g., rhythm and murmurs)	X	X	X	X
Femoral pulses	X		X	X
Respiratory rate and lung exam		X		X
Abdominal exam (especially for masses)				X
Hip exam	X	X	X	X
Genital exam (including descended testes)	X	X	X	X
Anus		X		
Neural tube defects		X		
Pilonidal sinus tract		X		
Extremities and digits (including club feet, metatarsus adductus)	X	X	X	
Neurologic exam (including reflexes)	X	X	X	X
Muscle tone	X		X	

Screening for congenital hypothyroidism should be performed by the seventh day of life (AAP, 1993). Screening for phenylketonuria should be done as close to hospital discharge as possible. If performed prior to 24 hours, it should be repeated between the first and second weeks of life (AAP, 1992). Results for both should be recorded in the medical record (AAP, 1992).

Recommended Components of Well Child Care for Children Under 2 Years Old

The AAP (1988) recommends a well child visit at 2-4 weeks, and 2, 4, 6, 9, 12, 15, 18, and 24 months. It provides some recommendations for what should occur at each visit. This timetable has generally been accepted as the standard of care. Bright Futures (Green, 1994) recommends visits at 1 week and 1 month in place of the 2-4 week visit because children are frequently discharged from the hospital in less than 24 hours; however, the additional visit has not become the standard of care, so it will not be incorporated into an indicator at this time.

Birth and Pregnancy History

The first visit after birth should cover maternal illnesses during pregnancy, medications taken during pregnancy, labor process and associated complications (e.g., preterm labor, medications during labor, use of forceps) (Unti, 1994), history of tuberculosis or tuberculosis screening (See Chapter 18), and history of hepatitis or hepatitis screening (See Chapter 14). These should be noted in the child's medical record either at the time of the newborn visit or the first outpatient visit.

Physical Examination

The AAP (1988) recommends a complete physical examination at each well child visit, but it does not specify all components that should be included. Therefore, we have selected as indicators several components that are specifically mentioned.

The child's umbilicus should be examined at the 2-4 week exam (AAP, 1988) to make sure it is healing properly and is not infected. If the child has been circumcised at birth, his penis should be examined at 2-4 week visit (AAP, 1988). The heart (AAP, 1988) and femoral pulses need to be reexamined at the 2-4 week visit because the results of this exam can change after the first several days of life. Examination for hip dislocation should be noted throughout the first year (Unti, 1994). Hoekelman points out that, although screening for congenital dislocation of the hip is generally considered important, there is some evidence suggesting that clinicians may do more harm than good with the hip exam by causing dislocations that were not there already (Hoekelman in

Hoekelman et al., 1992). Strabismus should be checked throughout the first year of life (Green, 1994) to assure proper neurologic development. Reflexes should be examined throughout the first year of life.

Deviations in growth can reflect problems such as endocrinologic, metabolic, and gastrointestinal disease, family stress, and temperamental difficulties with the child (Keefer in Dershewitz, 1993). Weight, length, and head circumference should be measured at every well child visit during the first year of life (AAP, 1988; Unti, 1994). The AAP (1988) recommends measurement of weight and length at every well child visit during the second year, whereas Unti (1994) includes head circumference as well. Ideally, these measures should be plotted on growth curves (Keefer in Dershewitz, 1993; AAP, 1988) so that trends can be observed. However, recording the percentiles in the chart (without actually plotting measurements) may be acceptable since clinicians could compare percentiles from visit to visit.

Safety Issues

Accidents and injuries are a leading cause of morbidity and mortality in children (Dershewitz in Dershewitz, 1993). Half of all childhood and three-quarters of all adolescent deaths are attributable to injuries (Wilson in Oski, 1994). Because of the risk of mortality or serious morbidity, these topics should be documented to assure they are addressed.

a. **Child-Proofing:** Child-proofing involves making the home safe for the child, e.g., locking cabinets, gating stairs, protecting unused electrical outlets, removing from the child's reach small objects that can be aspirated, cleaning fluids and medications. Unti (1994) recommends addressing this topic at the six and nine month visits.

b. **Poison Control:** The phone number of a poison control center should be given by the 12-month visit (Grimm in Dershewitz, 1993), unless the city does not have a center. In that case, the caregiver should be given an alternative (e.g., emergency room) to use. The USPSTF (1989) includes the poison control number on its list of parent counseling topics for birth to 18 months. However, it would be more advisable to provide the number before the child can crawl (i.e., 6 months).

c. **Car Seat:** Car seats protect the child while in a car. In many states, car seats for children are required by law. It is customary to discuss the importance of a car seat at the initial visit and to confirm that one is being used. There should be documentation of whether or not a car seat is used by the time the child is one month old (AAP, 1990).

Screening for Anemia

Before their 18th birthday, about one-fifth of all children in the United States will be anemic. The AAP recommends a Hematocrit or Hemoglobin be obtained between the first outpatient visit and one year of age (AAP, 1988). The USPSTF (1989) recommends screening for anemia at least once between birth and 18 months. Because hematologic values vary with age, hemoglobin or hematocrit results must be compared to age-adjusted normal values (Martin and Pearson, in Oski, 1994). Cause of anemia also vary by age.

Hearing

Routine screening of hearing is recommended at three years old (Green, 1994; Grimm in Dershewitz, 1993). While Cunningham (in Hoekelman et al., 1992) recommends targeted screening in younger children, he recommends routine pure-tone audometric screening starting at four years old, with pure tones at frequencies of 1, 2, 4, and 6 KHz and intensity of 25 dB at each frequency. A 1993 National Institutes of Health (NIH) Consensus Statement recommended that a two-stage screening protocol be conducted during the first three months of life: initial screening with an evoked otoacoustic emissions (EOAC) test, with auditory brainstem response (ABR) screen for infants who failed the first test (NIH Consensus Statement, 1993). However, a commentary in *Pediatrics* (Bess and Paradise, 1994) criticized the statement and raised concerns that following its recommendations might produce more harm than good. Because these recommendations do not appear to have become the standard of care, no indicator was developed for routine screening for hearing impairment during the first three months.

Vision

Green (1994) recommends routine screening of vision starting at 3 years old. The Snellen Illiterate Eye Chart is appropriate for preschool children who are at least three years old (Strahlman in Hoekelman et al., 1992)

RECOMMENDED QUALITY INDICATORS FOR WELL CHILD CARE

The following criteria apply to well child care for newborns.

Indicator	Quality of evidence	Literature	Benefits	Comments
1. Within 24 hours of birth, every child not admitted to a neonatal intensive care unit should have a physical examination that determines and documents all of the following:	III	AAP, 1988; Unti, 1994; Green, 1994; Cochran, 1994		It might be preferable to provide a 36-48 hour grace period for the newborn exam. The newborn exam items may be difficult to implement for children in a NICU. These indicators generally measure whether the exam was done rather than proper response to abnormal findings.
a. whether the anterior fontanelle is normal;			Prevent neurologic deficits.	Detect increased or decreased intracranial pressure, either of which could be due to etiologies (e.g., hydrocephalus, cerebral edema, infection) that can lead to neurological and other damage if untreated.
b. whether jaundice is present;			Prevent neurologic deficits. Prevent severe anemia.	Detect hyperbilirubinemia due to hemolytic disease. High bilirubin can cause neurologic damage. Hemolytic disease can also cause severe anemia and circulatory collapse.
c. whether a red reflex is present;			Prevent visual deficits.	Detect cataracts, which should be treated so vision can develop normally. It might be adequate to wait until the 2 week visit.
d. whether the palate is intact;			Prevent dehydration. Prevent otitis media. Reduce speech problems.	Detect cleft palate, which can cause feeding problems, speech problems, and recurrent otitis media, and which can be treated surgically.
e. whether heart rate and rhythm are regular, whether a murmur is present;			Prevent heart failure.	Detect cardiac anomalies, which could lead to death if not treated.
f. whether femoral pulses are normal;			Prevent heart failure.	Detect cardiac anomalies, which could lead to death if not treated.
g. whether respiratory rate is normal;			Prevent anoxia, respiratory failure, and lung damage.	Detect such problems as pneumonia, pneumothorax, and tracheoesophageal fistula, which can cause severe morbidity or mortality and which can be treated.
h. whether lung sounds are normal;			Prevent anoxia, respiratory failure, and lung damage.	Detect such problems as pneumonia, pneumothorax, and tracheoesophageal fistula, which can cause severe morbidity or mortality and which can be treated.

					Detect diaphragmatic hernia, abnormally large abdominal organs, and altered bowel sounds, possibly suggestive of obstruction or ileus, all of which should be addressed quickly to prevent possible severe morbidity or death.
i.	whether abdominal exam is normal, including normal bowel sounds, absence of enlarged liver and spleen, and absence of abnormal masses;			Prevent gastrointestinal damage.	
j.	whether genitals are normal, whether testes are descended;			Prevent urologic damage. Prevent endocrinologic collapse. Prevent genital malfunction.	Detect abnormalities that may be surgically correctable, that may raise questions about the gender of the child, and that may indicate such problems as congenital adrenal hyperplasia, which can be fatal.
k.	whether the anus is patent;			Prevent gastrointestinal emergency.	Detect imperforate anus, which can lead to death without surgical correction. Passing stool may serve as sufficient evidence that the anus is patent.
l.	whether hips are dislocated;			Prevent hip disability.	Detect hip dysplasia, which can cause severe disability if not treated early.
m.	whether evidence of a possible a neural tube defect is present (e.g., sacral dimple, sacral mass, hair tuft, and pilonidal sinus tract);			Prevent bladder and lower extremity dysfunction. Prevent infection.	Detect problems (e.g., meningomyelocele) that can cause serious neurologic morbidity and may be associated with many other abnormalities (e.g., inability to move legs, lack of bladder control, infection), some of which can be corrected surgically.
n.	whether there are the proper number of fingers and toes and the extremities are formed normally;			Prevent permanent limb disabilities.	Detect abnormalities that could be associated with serious congenital syndrome.
o.	whether the child moves all four extremities;			Prevent permanent limb disability. Prevent neurologic problems.	Detect underlying neurologic problems. Detect meningomyelocele. Detect clavicle fracture.
p.	whether tone is normal;			Prevent neurologic deficits.	Abnormal tone can be due to congenital myasthenia, structural abnormalities of the brain, metabolic disease, etc. Detect neurologic problems such as hydrocephalus, brain malformation, and cerebral palsy.
q.	whether the Moro reflex is normal.			Prevent neurologic abnormalities.	Detect subtle weaknesses. Detect neurologic problems such as hydrocephalus, brain malformation, and cerebral palsy.
2.	Weight should be documented.	III	AAP, 1988; Cochran in Oski et al., 1994; Green, 1994; Unti, 1994	Prevent growth abnormalities.	Baseline weight helps to detect growth abnormalities, such as those due to potentially treatable conditions like chronic illness or malnutrition.

#	Indicator	Quality of evidence	Literature	Benefits	Comments
3.	Length should be documented.	III	AAP, 1988; Cochran in Oski et al., 1994; Green, 1994; Unti, 1994	Prevent growth abnormalities.	Baseline length helps to detect growth abnormalities, such as those due to potentially treatable conditions like chronic illness or malnutrition.
4.	Head circumference should be documented.	III	AAP, 1988; Cochran in Oski et al., 1994; Green, 1994; Unti, 1994	Prevent neurologic deficits. Prevent growth abnormalities.	Detect increased or decreased intracranial pressure so that treatment to limit neurologic damage can begin. Baseline head circumference helps to detect growth abnormalities, such as those due to potentially treatable conditions like chronic illness or malnutrition.
5.	Screening for congenital hypothyroidism should have been done by the seventh day of life.	III	AAP, 1993	Prevent neurologic deficits.	Allow for treatment of hypothyroidism before permanent neurologic damage occurs.
6.	Screening for phenylketonuria should have been done after 24 hours of age and before two weeks of age.	III	AAP, 1992	Prevent neurologic deficits.	Screening identifies phenylketonuria and allows treatment before permanent neurologic damage occurs. A test done before 24 hours of age must be repeated before two weeks of age.

The following criteria apply to well child care for infants and children.

#	Indicator	Quality of evidence	Literature	Benefits	Comments
7.	An inquiry should be made about the mother's pregnancy and delivery history (e.g., length of pregnancy; illnesses; use of medications; use of alcohol, drugs, or tobacco during pregnancy; complications) by the end of the first month of life.	III	Unti, 1994	Prevent multiple illnesses.	Pregnancy history could affect present or future illness, including neurologic problems. For example, knowing the child was premature will affect interpretation of growth parameters. These should be noted in the child's chart. Phrases like "full-term," "normal pregnancy," "normal delivery," and "no complications" are acceptable. Maternal medication use will guide the clinician in looking for their impact on the child, e.g., occult spina bifida due to maternal anticonvulsants.
8.	The child's weight should be measured at least four times during the first year of life. This information must either be plotted on a growth curve or be recorded with the age/gender percentile.	III	AAP, 1988; Keefer in Dershewitz, 1993; Green, 1994; Unti, 1994	Prevent growth abnormalities.	Detect growth abnormalities, such as those due to potentially treatable conditions like chronic illness or malnutrition. The standard AAP recommendation is for these to be done at the newborn visit, the 2 week visit, and the 2, 4, 6, 9, and 12 month visits.

#	Indicator	Quality of Evidence	Reference	Objective	Comments
9.	The child's length should be measured at least four times during the first year of life. This information must either be plotted on a growth curve or be recorded with the age/gender percentile.	III	AAP, 1988; Keefer in Dershewitz, 1993; Green, 1994; Unti, 1994	Prevent growth abnormalities.	Detect growth abnormalities, such as those due to potentially treatable conditions like chronic illness or malnutrition. The standard AAP recommendation is for these to be done at the newborn visit, the 2 week visit, and the 2, 4, 6, 9, and 12 month visits.
10.	The child's head circumference should be measured at least four times during the first year of life. This information must either be plotted on a growth curve or be recorded with the age/gender percentile.	III	AAP, 1988; Keefer in Dershewitz, 1993; Green, 1994; Unti, 1994	Prevent neurologic deficits. Prevent growth abnormalities.	Detect growth abnormalities, such as those due to potentially treatable conditions like chronic illness or malnutrition. Also, detect hydrocephalus and craniosynostosis, which can cause severe neurologic problems if not treated. The standard AAP recommendation is for these to be done at the newborn visit, the 2-week visit, and the 2-, 4-, 6-, 9-, and 12-month visits.
11.	If a boy has been circumcised, a follow-up examination of his penis should be conducted during the first month of life.	III	AAP, 1988	Prevent infection. Prevent cosmetic damage.	Detect infection or abnormal result requiring corrective surgery.
12.	The child's umbilicus should be examined after the newborn exam during the first month of life.	III	AAP, 1988	Prevent infection.	Detect and allow treatment of infection.
13.	The child's heart and femoral pulses should be examined at least once after the newborn exam during the first month of life.	III	AAP, 1988	Prevent heart failure.	Detects cardiac anomalies that can be fatal if not treated. The AAP (1988) does not specifically mention this exam when it mentions the heart exam, but femoral pulses are a standard part of the cardiovascular exam at this age.
14.	A child's hips should be examined at least four times during the first year of life.	III	Green, 1994; Unti, 1994	Prevent hip disability.	Detects hip dysplasia, which can cause severe disability if not treated early.
15.	A child should be checked for strabismus between the end of the second month of life and the end of the sixth month of life.	III	Green, 1994	Prevent visual deficits.	Green (1994) recommends multiple checks throughout the first year of life. The indicator gives a six month cut off to ensure that the child is examined for strabismus at least once during early infancy so that treatment can begin. The examination for strabismus is more reliable after the second month.
16.	A child's deep tendon reflexes should be examined at least once during the first year of life.	III	Green, 1994	Prevent neurologic deficits.	Detects neurologic abnormalities that may be treatable. For example, peripheral neuropathies can be caused by hypothyroidism, infections, renal failure, lead toxicity, malnutrition, etc.

#	Indicator		Citation		Comments
17.	An inquiry about use of a car seat should be made by the end of the first month.	III	Green, 1994	Prevent injury from motor vehicle accident.	Documentation of this information increases the chance that the issue will be addressed and that other providers who read the chart will know that it has been addressed. Proper use of a car seat can significantly increase the chance of survival in an auto accident. Car seat usage is required in all 50 states.
18.	An inquiry about use of a car seat should be made between the end of the sixth month and the end of the first year.	III	Green, 1994	Prevent injury from motor vehicle accident.	A second inquiry should be made as the child grows since some parents might not continue use of a car seat. Car seat usage is required in all 50 states.
19.	Child-proofing the home should be discussed by the end of the seventh month of life.	III	Unti, 1994	Prevent injury and death from accidents in the home.	This time period was selected to precede the age when the child is likely to be mobile and to give time for the sixth month visit to take place since this is a likely time at which to discuss child-proofing.
20.	The number for a poison center should have been given by the end of the seventh month of life.	III	Grimm in Dershewitz, 1993; USPSTF, 1989	Prevent morbidity and mortality from poisoning.	Once children become mobile, they are at greater risk of poisoning.
21.	A hemoglobin or hematocrit should be checked between the first outpatient visit and the end of the 18th month of life.	III	AAP, 1988; USPSTF, 1989	Prevent growth delay. Prevent neurologic deficits. Prevent severe anemia.	Severe anemia can cause growth problems. It can be evidence of lead toxicity, which can cause neurologic deficits.
22.	Hearing should be screened by an audiometer by the end of the fourth year of life.	III	Cunningham in Hoekelman et al., 1992; Green, 1994; Grimm in Dershewitz, 1993	Prevent permanent hearing loss.	There is variation in when routine screening is recommended. The latest that routine screening is usually recommended is during the fourth year.
23.	If the child fails to hear the stimulus at two frequencies in one ear, he/she should be referred to an audiologist within one month.	III	Cunnginham in Hoekelman et al., 1992	Prevent permanent hearing loss.	Standard office hearing tests serve as screening tools. If there is evidence of hearing loss, more sophisticated testing by an audiologist is warranted.
24.	Vision should be tested by the end of the fourth year of life.	III	Green, 1994	Prevent visual deficits.	This indicator provides a grace period beyond the recommendation in the source. Vision screening can detect refractive error or other visual problems.

Quality of Evidence Codes:

I: RCT
II-1:   Nonrandomized controlled trials
II-2:   Cohort or case analysis
II-3:   Multiple time series
III: Opinions or descriptive studies

REFERENCES - WELL CHILD CARE

American Academy of Pediatrics, and Committee on Psychosocial Aspects of Child and Family Health, 1985-1988. 1988. *Guidelines for Health Supervision II*, Second ed.Elk Grove Village, Illinois: American Academy of Pediatrics.

American Academy of Pediatrics, and Committee on Genetics. February 1992. Issues in newborn screening. *Pediatrics* 89 (2): 345-9.

American Academy of Pediatrics. 1993. Newborn screening for congenital hypothyroidism: Recommended guidelines. *Pediatrics* 91 (6): 1203-9.

American Academy of Pediatrics, and Committee on Accident and Poison Prevention. September 1990. Safe transportation of newborns discharged from the hospital. *Pediatrics* 86 (3): 486-7.

Bess FH, and JL Paradise. 1994. Universal screening for infant hearing impairment: Not simple, not risk-free, not necessarily beneficial, and not presently justified. *Pediatrics* 93 (2): 330-4.

Cochran WD. 1994. Management of the normal newborn. In *Principles and Practice of Pediatrics*, Second ed. Editors Oski FA, CD DeAngelis, RD Feigin, et al., 302-8. Philadelphia, PA: J.B. Lippincott Company.

Cunningham DR. 1992. Auditory screening. In *Primary Pediatric Care*, Second ed. Editor Hoekelman RA, 229-33. St. Louis, MO: Mosby-Year Book, Inc.

Dershewitz RA. 1993. Injury prevention. In *Ambulatory Pediatric Care*, Second ed. Editor Dershewitz RA, 85-9. Philadelphia, PA: J.B. Lippincott Company.

Green, M. 1994. *Bright Futures: Guidelines for Health Supervision of Infants, Children, and Adolescents*. Arlington, VA: National Center for Education in Maternal and Child Health.

Grimm KCT. 1993. The well-child visit. In *Ambulatory Pediatric Care*, Second ed. Editor Dershewitz RA, 44-55. Philadelphia, PA: J.B. Lippincott Company.

Hoekelman RA. 1992. The physical examination as a screening test. In *Primary Pediatric Care*, Second ed. Editor Hoekelman RA, 213-4. St. Louis, MO: Mosby-Year Book, Inc.

Keefer CH. 1993. Normal growth and development: An overview. In *Ambulatory Pediatric Care*, Second ed. Editor Dershewitz RA, 36-9. Philadelphia, PA: J.B. Lippincott Company.

Martin PL, and HA Pearson. 1994. The anemias. In *Principles and Practice of Pediatrics*, Second ed. Editors Oski FA, CD DeAngelis, RD Feigin, et al., 1657-1700. Philadelphia: J.B. Lippincott Company.

National Center for Health Statistics. April 1992. *National Ambulatory Medical Care Survey: 1989 summary*. U.S. Department of Health and Human Services, Hyattsville, MD.

National Institutes of Health Consensus Statement. 1993. *Early Identification of Hearing Impairment in Infants and Young Children. March 1-3, 1993*. U.S. Department of Health and Human Services. Volume 11, Number 1, Bethesda, MD.

Strahlman ER. 1992. Vision screening. In *Primary Pediatric Care*, Second ed. Editor Hoekelman RA, 233-4. St. Louis, MO: Mosby-Year Book, Inc.

U.S. Preventive Services Task Force. 1989. *Guide to Clinical Preventive Services: An Assessment of the Effectiveness of 169 Interventions*. Baltimore, MD: Williams and Wilkins.

Unti SM. October 1994. The critical first year of life: History, physical examination, and general developmental assessment. *Pediatric Clinics of North America* 41 (5): 859-73.

APPENDIX A: DEFINITIONS FOR INDICATOR TABLES

DEFINITIONS FOR ACNE
(CHAPTER 1)

There are no definitions for this chapter.

DEFINITIONS FOR ADOLESCENT PREVENTIVE SERVICES
(CHAPTER 2)

Blood pressure above the 95th percentile: We define both significant and severe hypertension for adolescents according to the following age-specific criteria:

Age	Significant Hypertension	Severe Hypertension
10-12	Systolic ≥ 126 mm Hg Diastolic ≥ 82 mm Hg	Systolic ≥ 134 mm Hg Diastolic ≥ 90 mm Hg
13-15	Systolic ≥ 136 mm Hg Diastolic ≥ 86 mm Hg	Systolic ≥ 144 mm Hg Diastolic ≥ 92 mm Hg
16-18	Systolic ≥ 142 mm Hg Diastolic ≥ 92 mm Hg	Systolic ≥ 150 mm Hg Diastolic ≥ 98 mm Hg

Normal Pap smear: one without atypia, dysplasia, CIS or invasive carcinoma.

Severely abnormal Pap smear: a note that indicates "moderate dysplasia" or "severe dysplasia" or "carcinoma in situ" or CIS or CIN II or CIN III, or "high grade SIL" or "squamous cell carcinoma" or "adenocarcinoma."

Counseling (for cigarette smoking): includes providing pamphlets, brief advice, specialized structured programs.

DEFINITIONS FOR ALLERGIC RHINITIS
(CHAPTER 3)

There are no definitions for this chapter.

DEFINITIONS FOR ASTHMA
(CHAPTER 4)

Chronic oral corticosteroids: Three or more (14-day or greater) corticosteroid tapers for exacerbations in the past year; or continuous treatment with any dose of prednisone; or three or more administrations of IM corticosteroids in the past year.

Frequent bursts of prednisone: Two to three (or more) 5 day courses, following an exacerbation, in a 6 month period.

Asthma exacerbation: characterized by acute obstruction to airflow; patients become acutely short of breath, tachycardic, and if severe, use accessory muscles of respiration.

Intensive care setting: A monitored setting with the capacity to monitor continuous O2 saturation at a minimum. For example, a step down unit would meet this definition.

DEFINITIONS FOR ATTENTION DEFICIT/HYPERACTIVITY
DISORDER (CHAPTER 5)

Comorbidities: Thyroid disease, sleep disorder, cognitive disorder, family dysfunction such as parent child conflict disorder, poor fit with the home or school environment, oppositional behavior disorder, conduct disorder, pervasive developmental disorder, any neurologic disorder, learning disorder, affective disorder such as depression, vision disorder, hearing disorder.

Risks (of pharmacotherapy): Effects on the cardiorespiratory system, on weight and height, as well as possibility of tics, decreased appetite, insomnia, headaches, stomach aches, irritability, anxiety, excessive sadness, social withdrawal, euphoria or dizziness.

Benefits (of pharmacotherapy): May lead to improved short-term abatement of the core symptom complex of inattention, impulsivity and overactivity compared to nonpharmacologic or no treatment. Also may improve child's performance on intelligence measures, achievement scores, and perceptual, motor and memory measures.

Development: Appropriateness of development should be based on standardized development tests such as the Denver II or development guidelines of the American Academy of Pediatrics (AAP, 1988).

Learning disorder (of family member): A physician notation in the chart that a family member had a learning disorder or an equivalent notation (e.g., "(family member) had problems in school" is sufficient). Physicians typically will not have adequate information to make a definitive diagnosis for a family member.

Behavior problem (of family member): A physician notation in the chart that a family member had a behavior problem or an equivalent notation is sufficient. Physicians typically will not have adequate information to make a definitive diagnosis for a family member.

Psychiatric disorder (of family member): A physician notation in the chart that a family member had a psychiatric disorder or an equivalent notation is sufficient. Physicians typically will not have adequate information to make a definitive diagnosis for a family member.

Isolated ADHD: ADHD with no comorbidities (see list under comorbidities).

Failure to respond (to a trialsof medication): lack of improvement in attention and impulsivity/hyperactivity, despite maximal therapeutic dosage of sufficient duration.

Parent rating scale: Examples include the ADHD Rating Scale; Swanson, Nolan, and Pelham Rating Scale; Child Behavior Check List; Conners Scales; Yale Children's Inventory; or Aggregate Neurobehavioral Student Health and Education Review.

Teacher rating scale: Examples include the ADHD Rating Scale; Swanson, Nolan, and Pelham Rating Scale; Child Behavior Check List; ADD-H Comprehensive Teacher Rating Scale; Conners Scales; Yale Children's Inventory; or Aggregate Neurobehavioral Student Health and Education Review.

Affective symptoms: include unexplained somatic complaints; drop in school performance; apathy and loss of interest; social withdrawal; increased irritability or tearfulness; sleep changes; appetite changes; suicidal ideation or behavior; substance use; promiscuous sexual behavior; or risk-taking behavior.

Oppositional Defiant Disorder: characterized by symptoms of negativistic, hostile, and defiant behavior.

Conduct Disorder: characterized by symptoms of aggression to people and animals, destruction of property, deceitfulness or theft, and serious violations of rules.

DEFINITIONS FOR CESAREAN DELIVERY (CHAPTER 6)

Antiobiotic Prophylaxis

There are no definitions for this portion of the chapter.

Failure to Progress in Labor

Failure to progress (FTP) in labor: Also known as "dystocia." Labor (as measured by cervical dilation and descent of the presenting part) has either stopped progressing or progresses at a rate below accepted norms. Accepted norms for cervical dilation range from 0.5 to 1.5 cm of cervical change per hour. *Also known as "cephalopelvic disproportion," "protracted or prolonged active phase," "protracted or prolonged first stage," "feto-pelvic disproportion," and "arrest of dilatation."*

Active phase of labor: a cervical dilatation of 3 cm for nulliparas and 4 cm for multiparas.

Fetal Distress

Electronic fetal monitoring (EFM): A method by which the fetal heart rate can be monitored continuously during labor. External EFM uses a doppler device strapped to the mother's abdomen. Internal EFM uses a clip attached to the fetal scalp to detect electrocardiographic impulses from the fetus. Certain patterns of EFM tracing may be indicative of fetal hypoxia.

Prior Cesarean

Trial of labor: This term implies that vaginal delivery is intended. Labor is allowed to procede until delivery, or until some indication for cesarean (such as fetal distress of failure to progress in labor) intervenes.

DEFINITIONS FOR DEPRESSION
(CHAPTER 7)

Risk factors for depression in adolescents include: parental divorce in past six months; death of family member or friend in past six months; school failure; history of depression; history of cigarette, alcohol, or other drug use; history of depression, substance abuse, or suicide attempts in family members; fired from job; parental marital discord, parental-patient discord; school suspension, expulsion, or dropping out.

Symptoms of depression: include depressed mood, diminished interest or pleasure in activities, weight loss/gain, impaired concentration, suicidality, fatigue, feelings of worthlessness and guilt, and psychomotor agitation/retardation.

Medical complications of substance abuse: include blackouts, seizures, delerium, liver failure (for alcohol); local infection, endocarditis, hepatitis and HIV, death from overdose (for IV drugs of any kind); seizures, myocardial infarction, and hypertensive crises (for cocaine and amphetamines).

DEFINITIONS FOR DEVELOPMENTAL SCREENING
(CHAPTER 8)

Social/personal development: An amalgamation of development in multiple streams, particularly cognition. Social dysfunction may be a symptom of neurodevelopmental abnormality assessed by looking at milestones such as play skills, domestic mimicry, and parallel play (up to 24 months) and associative play (up to 42 months). We will accept a note on social or personal development status (normal or delayed) as an indicator that this area was assessed.

Fine motor/visuomotor development: This is assessed to quantify the cognitive components of visual and fine motor manipulative tasks. May be abnormal secondary to visual impairment, gross or fine motor impairment, or outright refusal to perform task. Adequate cognitive abilities frequently overcome mild to moderate upper extremity limitations. We will accept a note on fine motor or visuomotor development status (normal or delayed) as an indicator that this area was assessed.

Language development: This is the best single measure of cognitive development both in infancy and childhood. Language can be used as an objective tool for early assessment via prelinguistic and linguistic milestones of later cognitive development. Recognition of language delay is probably the most sensitive indicator of subsequent mental retardation. We will accept a note on language development status (normal or delayed) as an indicator that this area was assessed.

Gross motor development: Gross motor development is the key to early detection of many disabilities. Significant early motor delay and abnormalities of the neuromotor examination are the hallmark of cerebral palsy. We will accept a note on gross motor development status (normal or delayed) as an indicator that this area was assessed.

Developmental delay: Refers to a performance signifiantly below average in a given area of skill. A developmental quotient below 70 constitutes delay;

$$\text{Developmental Quotient} = \text{DG} = \frac{\text{developmental age}}{\text{chonologic age}} \times 100$$

DEFINITIONS FOR DIABETES MELLITUS (CHAPTER 9)

Diabetic complications: Although the following list is not intended to be exhaustive, examples include visual loss, dysfunction of the heart, peripheral vasculature, peripheral nerves, and kidneys.

Failed dietary therapy: Adherence to ADA diet fails to improve glycemic control, as glycosylated hemoglobin measure remains above 6.05 mg/dl percent.

Failure of preferred agents: Failure to achieve glycemic control or reduce diabetic complications.

DEFINITIONS FOR ACUTE DIARRHEA (CHAPTER 10)

Note: These indicators are intended to apply to children up to age 3 years.

Acute diarrhea: Symptoms have lasted less than two weeks.

Frequency and volume (of fluid intake):   How much and how frequently child takes fluids.

Frequency and volume (of urinary output):   How much and how often urine is produced. (e.g. number of diapers with urine, notation of "less than normal", "having urine", etc.)

Recent weight obtained: A recent weight is age-specific and defined according to the National Center for Health Statistics Growth Curves as follows:

Age	Definition of Recency
<=3 months	Within 1 week of visit
3 months to <= 6 months	Within 2 weeks of visit
6 months to <= 9 months	Within 4 weeks of visit
9 months to <=15 months	Within 10 weeks of visit
15 months to <= 4 years	Within 4 months

Severity of dehydration is defined in terms of estimated fluid loss (percentages below multiplied by patient's recent weight) as shown below:

% Dehydration		Clinical Observation
5-6%	Mild Dehydration	HR (10-15% above baseline); slightly dry mucous membranes; concentration of urine; *poor tear production.
7-8%	Moderate Dehydration	Increase in severity of above signs; decreased skin turgor; oliguria; sunken eyeballs*; sunken anterior fonatanelle.
>9%	Severe Dehydration	Marked severity of above signs; decreased blood pressure for age; delayed capillary refill; acidosis (large base deficit).

Pulse rate was elevated: An elevated pulse rate at rest is age-specific and defined as greater than the upper limits of normal as follows:

Age	Elevated Pulse Rate
Newborn	>150/min
1-11 months	>160
1-2 years	>130
2-4 years	>120
4-6 years	>115
6-8 years	>110
8-12 years	>110 for girls, >105 for boys
12-14 years	>105 for girls, >100 for boys
14-16 years	>100 for girls, >95 for boys

Low blood pressure: A low blood pressure is age-specific and may be defined as follows:

Age	Low Blood Pressure (Systolic)
< 7 days to 30 days	< 65
30 days to 2 years	< 85
2-5 years	< 95 (diastolic < 60)

Immunocompromise: Person with immune disorders such as hematologic and solid tumors, congenital immunodeficiency, HIV and long-term immunosuppressive therapy.

Growth delay: Child younger than 2 years whose weight or height is below the fifth percentile for age on more than one occasion or who has dropped 2 major percentile lines (e.g., from the 90th percentile to below the 50th percentile), using the standard growth charts of the National Center for Health Statistics (NCHS):

Age	Length (in cm) Male	Female	Weight (in kg) Male	Female
Birth	46.4	45.4	2.54	2.36
1 month	50.4	49.2	3.16	2.97
3 months	56.7	55.4	4.43	4.18
6 months	63.4	61.8	6.20	5.79
9 months	68.0	66.1	7.52	7.00
12 months	71.7	69.8	8.43	7.84
18 months	77.5	76.0	9.59	8.92
24 months	82.3	81.3	10.54	9.87

For the purpose of the study, growth delay will be present if the health care provider documents in any problem list the general term growth delay or the specific term failure to thrive or short stature (not familial/genetic or constitutional).

Malnutrition: For the purpose of the study, malnutrition will be present if the health care provider documents in any problem list the general term malnutrition or a synonym, such as marasmus or protein malnutrition.

General condition: characterized by well, alert; restless, irritable; or lethargic or unconscious, floppy.

Appearance of eyes: characterized by normal; sunken; or very sunken and dry.

Degree of oral moisture: characterized by moist; dry; or very dry.

Degree of thirst: characterized by drinks normally, not thirsty; thirsty, drinks eagerly; or drinks poorly or not able to drink.

Degree of skin turgor: characterized by skin goes back quickly; skin goes back slowly; or skin goes back very slowly.

Condition of anterior fontanelle: characterized by normal/flat; slightly sunken; or severely sunken.

Young infant: an infant aged 3 months or less.

Morbidity (of untreated diarrhea): may include severe hydration, abdominal and rectal pain, weight loss, lost school days, and lost work days for the parent.

Complications of sepsis: include multi-organ failure and death.

DEFINITIONS FOR FAMILY PLANNING (CHAPTER 11)

Effective contraception: Any one of the following methods is considered an effective method of preventing contraception:

- Hormonal contraception (OC, injectable prostaglandins or implants)
- IUD
- Barrier + spermicide
- Sterilization
- Complete abstinence

At risk for unintended pregnancy: those who are sexually active without effective contraception and who do not desire pregnancy.

DEFINITIONS FOR FEVER IN CHILDREN UNDER 3 YEARS OF AGE (CHAPTER 12)

Cerebrospinal fluid studies are abnormal: Values for cerebrospinal fluid white blood count, protein, or glucose outside the normal range are age specific and will be defined as below:

Test	Abnormal
WBC	$\geq 22.4/\mu L$ (up to 1 month)
	$\geq 5/\mu L$ with 0% PMNs (over 1 month)
Serum glucose	≥ 119 mg/dL (term infant to 1 month)
	≥ 80 mg/dL (over 1 month)
Protein	≥ 90 mg/dL (term infant to 2 months)
	> 40 mg/dL (over 2 months)

Low risk *(infant 28 days to 3 months)*: All of the following criteria are true:

- appears generally well,

- previously healthy (see definition below)
- no evidence of skin, soft tissue, bone, joint, or ear infection found, and
- laboratory values negative
  - peripheral blood white blood count 5.0 to 15.0 x 10^3 cells/ml,
  - absolute band from count ≤ 1.5 x 10^3 cells/ml,
  - ≤ 10 WBC per high-power field (x 40) on microscopic examination of a spun urine sediment, and
  - < 5 WBC per high-power filed (x 40) on microscopic examination of a stool smear (only for infants with diarrhea).

High risk (infant 28 days to 3 months): Two or more of the following criteria are NOT true:

- appears generally well,
- previously healthy (see definition below)
- no evidence of skin, soft tissue, bone, joint, or ear infection found, and
- laboratory values negative
  - peripheral blood white blood count 5.0 to 15.0 x 10^3 cells/ml,
  - absolute band form count ≤ 1.5 x 10^3 cells/ml,
  - ≤ 10 WBC per high-power field (x 40) on microscopic examination of a spun urine sediment, and
  - < 5 WBC per high-power field (x 40) on microscopic examination of a stool smear (only for infants with diarrhea).

High risk in an infant/child 3 to 36 months of age would be indicated by: lethargy; poor perfusion; or marked hypoventilation, hyperventilation, hypotension/tachycardia, or cyanosis.

Low risk in an infant child 3 to 36 months of age is defined as a patient that meets none of the criteria for high risk.

Toxic appearing infant (28 to 90 days): signs of sepsis based on lethargy, poor perfusion, hypoventilation, hyperventilation, or cyanosis.

Previously healthy: An infant is considered to have been previously healthy if all the following apply:

- born at term (≥ 37 weeks' gestation)
- did not receive perinatal, antimicrobial therapy

- was not treated for unexplained hyperbilirubinemia,

- had not received and was not receiving antimicrobial agents,

- had not been previously hospitalized,

- had no chronic underlying illness, and

- was not hospitalized longer than the mother.

Afebrile: Without fever. For a child less than three months old, the diagnosis of fever should be based on a temperature measurement of 38 degrees centigrade or greater taken at home or in the medical setting. For children older than three months, the threshhold for defining fever is 39 degrees centigrade.

Positive urine culture: The following colony counts from a pure culture, by method of collection, are defined as a positive urine culture (Feld, et al. 1989):

- Suprapubic aspiration: gram-negative bacilli (any number), gram-positive cocci (> few thousand)

- Catheterization $>10^4$ (10^3-10^4 is suspicious, meriting a repeat test)

- Clean-voided $> 10^4$ (boy), $> 10^5$ (girl), (10^4-10^5 for girls is suspicious; repeat test)

Tachypnea: Respiratory rate above 60 for children less than 90 days; above 40 for children age 3 months to one year; and above 30 for children age 1 to 3 years.

Lower respiratory symptoms: *include tachypnea, grunting, flaring, retractions, decreased breath sounds, rales, or rhonchi.*

DEFINITIONS FOR HEADACHE (CHAPTER 13)

New patients: Patients who present for the first time to the physician, practice or health plan. In other words, patient for whom a history and physical has been performed and is available to the physician.

New onset headache: Patient has no prior history of presenting with headache complaint.

Abnormal neurological examination: any physician note that indicates the following are not normal: cranial nerves, including pupils and eye movements, examination of the deep tendon reflexes and of the fundi, focal neurologic signs, and cerebellar signs.

Constant headache: Unrelieved, persistent headache that may range from low-level to severe. Experts contend that such headaches are more indicative of intracanial neoplasm than intermittent headaches.

Moderate or Severe headache: Headache of a severity that prohibits daily activities.

Acute headache: Headache lasting less than one week.

Tension headaches: Tension headaches are likely to be described as dull, nagging and persistent, with tight and constricting pain, and are also referred to as contraction, stress or ordinary headaches. The pain of these headaches may be either unilateral or bilateral and may involve the frontal region. Pain is likely to be most severe in the neck, shoulders and occipital region.

Uncontrolled hypertension: Failure to control blood pressure to normal or stage 1 levels (sytolic less than 160, diastolic less than100).

Side effects of migraine therapeutic agents: Although not exhaustive, examples of side effects include the following:

- Ergotamines: vasoconstriction, nausea, abdominal pain, somnolence;
- Opiates: dependence, somnolence, withdrawal;
- Phenothiazines: distonic reactions, anticholinergic reactions, insomnia.

Migraine symptoms and headaches: Migraines typically last 4 to 72 hours, with the vast majority lasting less than 24 hours and involving headache-free periods between prostrating attacks. Migraine pain can occur anywhere in the head or face, but seems to occur most often in the temple. Common migraine symptoms include unilateral location, pulsating quality, moderate or severe intensity (inhibits or prohibits daily activities), aggravation by walking stairs or similar activity, nausea and/or vomiting, and/or photophobia and phonophobia. Classic migraine symptoms include homonymous visual disturbance, unilateral parasthesias, unilateral weakness and aphasia or unclassifiable speech difficulty.

Risk factors for depression in adolescents include: parental divorce in past six months; death of family member or friend in past six months; school failure; history of depression; history of cigarette, alcohol, or other drug use; history of depression, substance abuse, or suicide attempts in family members; fired from job; parental marital discord, parental-patient discord; school suspension, expulsion, or dropping out.

Symptoms of depression include : depressed mood, diminished interest or pleasure in activities, weight loss/gain, impaired concentration, suicidality, fatigue, feelings of worthlessness and guilt, and psychomotor agitation/retardation.

DEFINITIONS FOR IMMUNIZATIONS (CHAPTER 14)

IPV: Inactivated polio vaccine.

OPV: Oral polio vaccine.

Immunodeficiency: Immune disorders such as hematologic and solid tumors, congenital immunodeficiency, and long-term immunosuppressive therapy. For immunization recommendations, HIV infection generally is treated as distinct from other causes of immunodeficiency.

Immunocompromised contact: Immunocompromised person to whom the patient is frequently exposed.

Anaphylactic reaction: Allergic reaction to a vaccine or vaccine constituent involving angioedema of the airways and potential respiratory arrest.

DTP--Vaccine for Diphtheria-Tetanus-Pertussis.

DTaP: Diphtheria-Tetanus-Pertussis (DTP) vaccine formulation with acellular pertussis.

Td: Diphtheria-Tetanus-Pertussis (DTP) vaccine formulation with a smaller amount of diptheria toxoid.

Encephalopathy: Cerebropathy; diffuse disturbance of brain function resulting in behavioral changed, altered consciousness, and/or seizures.

PRP-OMP Hib: Formulation of the Haemophilus influenzae type b vaccine using PedvaxHIB[R].

Hib: Haemophilus influenza type b vaccine .

Adolescents: Age 13 through 17.

DEFINITIONS FOR OTITIS MEDIA
(CHAPTER 15)

Nonspecific behavioral changes and symtpoms: Includes irritability, lethargy, decreased appetite, vomiting, diarrhea.

DEFINITIONS FOR PRENATAL CARE
(CHAPTER 16)

Screened for anemia: A hemoglobin or hematocrit (blood test)

Smoking history: Interview asking the patient whether or not she smokes or has smoked during the pregnancy, and if so how much.

Drug history: Interview asking the patient whether or not she has used illicit drugs during the pregnancy or prior to pregnancy, and if so which drugs, how much and how often.

Alcohol history: Interview asking the patient whether she has used alcohol during the pregnancy, and if so how much and how often.

DEFINITIONS FOR SICKLE CELL SCREENING
(CHAPTER 17)

Sickle cell screening: Any of the following methods may be used; hemoglobin electrophoresis, isoelectric focusing, or high performance liquid chromatography.

Repeat sickle cell screen: Hemoglobin electrophoresis, immunologic testing, or DNA testing are acceptable. Involves reassessment of infant's hemoglobin phenotype, measurement of hemoglobin concentration and red cell indices, inspection of the red cell morphology, and correlation with clinical history. Globin DNA testing of infant may also be used. Parental assessment may also assist in making a definitive diagnosis.

DEFINITIONS FOR TUBERCULOSIS SCREENING
(CHAPTER 18)

Region of the world with high TB prevalence: Based on 1990 estimates of turberculosis incidence produced by the World Health Organization, high prevalence is defined to be greater than 100 infections per 100,000 population. High prevalence regions include

Mexico, Central America (excluding Panama), Ecuador, Peru, Bolivia, Paraguay, Africa (excluding Algeria, Libya and Egypt), Iraq, South Asia and East Asia (excluding Japan).

Frequently exposed: A notation or the equivalent is made of "frequent contact," when screening, diagnosis and/or treatment are merited.

Immunodeficiency: Immune disorders such as hematologic and solid tumors, congenital immunodeficiency, and long-term immunosuppressive therapy. For immunization recommendations, HIV infection generally is treated as distinct from other causes of immunodeficiency.

Risk factors: These include abnormalities on chest x-ray suggestive of TB; clinical evidence of TB; HIV-infection, Hodgkin's disease, lymphoma, diabetes mellitus, chronic renal failure, malnutrition, or another immunosuppressive condition; contact with an adult/adolescent with infectious TB; is from, or household contacts are from, a region of the world with high TB prevalence; or is frequently exposed to adults or adolescents who are HIV-infected, homeless, users of injection and other street drugs, poor and medically-indigent city dwellers, residents of nursing homes, or migrant farm workers.

DEFINITIONS FOR UPPER RESPIRATORY INFECTIONS (CHAPTER 19)

ARF: Acute rheumatic fever.

Nasal symptoms: Nasal congestion and/or discharge.

Preceding viral infection: Viral infection two weeks or less prior to onset. Viral infection examples include common cold and influenza.

Acute sinusitis: defined as lasting less than 3 weeks. If symptoms last longer, the patient may have chronic sinusitis, which is more difficult to treat and requires longer duration of antibiotic therapy.

Suppurative complications of strep throat: include otitis media, sinusitis, peritonsillar abscess, and suppurative cervical adentis.

Chronic sinusitis: symptoms include nasal congestions, fever, headache, facial pain, toothache, rhinorrhea, and purulent nasal discharge.

DEFINITIONS FOR URINARY TRACT INFECTION (CHAPTER 20)

Note: These indicators are intended to apply to children up to age 12 or puberty.

Failure to thrive (FTT): Child younger than 2 years whose weight or height is below the fifth percentile for age on more than one occasion or who has dropped 2 major percentile lines (e.g., from the 90th percentile to below the 50th percentile), using the standard growth charts of the National Center for Health Statistics (NCHS):

Age	Length (in cm) Male	Female	Weight (in kg) Male	Female
Birth	46.4	45.4	2.54	2.36
1 month	50.4	49.2	3.16	2.97
3 months	56.7	55.4	4.43	4.18
6 months	63.4	61.8	6.20	5.79
9 months	68.0	66.1	7.52	7.00
12 months	71.7	69.8	8.43	7.84
18 months	77.5	76.0	9.59	8.92
24 months	82.3	81.3	10.54	9.87

For the purpose of the study, FTT will be present if the health care provider documents in any problem list the general term growth delay or the specific term failure to thrive or short stature (not familial/genetic or constitutional).

Fever in an infant (or febrile): The diagnosis of fever should be based on a temperature measurement of 38 degrees centigrade or greater taken at home or in the medical setting if under 3 months old; if the infant is 3 months to one year, fever is defined as greater than or equal to 39 degrees centigrade. Afebrile or without fever is defined as temperatures under these threshholds.

Infant: Up to one year old.

Pyelonephritis: Nephropyelitis; inflammation of the renal parenchyma and pelvis due to local bacterial infection.

Systemic symptoms: Examples include fever, chills.

VCUG: Voiding cystourethrogram.

RUS: Renal ultrasound.

IVP: Intravenous pyelogram.

Obstructive symptoms: Examples include midline lower abdominal distention; flank mass; infrequent or prolonged voiding; weak, dribbling or threadline urinary stream; or ballooning of the penile urethra.

DEFINITIONS FOR VAGINITIS AND STDs (CHAPTER 21)

There are no definitions for this chapter.

DEFINITIONS FOR WELL CHILD CARE (CHAPTER 22)

There are no definitions for this chapter.

DEFINITION FOR THE USE OF MEDICATIONS (NO TEXT CHAPTER ACCOMPANYING INDICATIONS)

There are no definitions for these indicators.

APPENDIX B: PANEL RATING SHEETS

Chapter 1
QUALITY INDICATORS FOR ACNE

	Validity	Feasibility	

(DIAGNOSIS)

1. For all patients presenting with acne, the following history should be documented in their chart:

a. Location of lesions (back, face, neck, chest).
```
                    2        6                                    7 2
1 2 3 4 5 6 7 8 9      1 2 3 4 5 6 7 8 9
  (8.0, 0.8, A)          (8.0, 0.2, A)
        2 1 1 2 2              1 3 2 2
```
(1- 3)

b. Aggravating factors (stress, seasons, cosmetics, creams).
```
1 2 3 4 5 6 7 8 9      1 2 3 4 5 6 7 8 9
  (6.5, 1.9, I)          (6.0, 1.1, I)
        3 2 2                4 2 1 1
```
(4- 6)

c. Menstrual history and premenstrual worsening of acne for girls.
```
1 2 3 4 5 6 7 8 9      1 2 3 4 5 6 7 8 9
  (5.5, 1.1, I)          (5.0, 0.9, A)
            2 6              3 5 1
```
(7- 9)

d. Previous treatments.
```
1 2 3 4 5 6 7 8 9      1 2 3 4 5 6 7 8 9
  (8.0, 0.2, A)          (8.0, 0.4, A)
            2 6              7 1 1
```
(10- 12)

e. Medication use.
```
1 2 3 4 5 6 7 8 9      1 2 3 4 5 6 7 8 9
  (8.0, 0.2, A)          (7.0, 0.3, A)
```
(13- 15)

(TREATMENT)

2. If oral antibiotics are prescribed, papules and pustules must be present.
```
        2 1      1 5          2 2      2 3
1 2 3 4 5 6 7 8 9      1 2 3 4 5 6 7 8 9
  (9.0, 2.0, I)          (8.0, 1.4, I)
                2 7                  2 7
```
(16- 18)

3. Tetracycline should not be prescribed for adolescents less than 12 years of age.
```
1 2 3 4 5 6 7 8 9      1 2 3 4 5 6 7 8 9
  (9.0, 0.2, A)          (9.0, 0.2, A)
    2        2 4 1        1 1 1 4 2
```
(19- 21)

4. If tetracycline is prescribed, there must be documentation of the last menstrual period or a negative pregnancy test for all girls who have reached puberty.
```
1 2 3 4 5 6 7 8 9      1 2 3 4 5 6 7 8 9
  (8.0, 1.4, A)          (6.0, 1.2, I)
```
(22- 24)

5. If isotretinoin is prescribed, there must be documentation of severe acne (papules, pustules, cysts and nodules) and failure of previous therapy.
```
                2 6                  3 5
1 2 3 4 5 6 7 8 9      1 2 3 4 5 6 7 8 9
  (9.0, 0.2, A)          (9.0, 0.4, A)
```
(25- 27)

6. If isotretinoin is prescribed to post-pubescent girls, a negative pregnancy test should be obtained within two weeks of start of therapy.
```
        1        3 5          2 2      2 5
1 2 3 4 5 6 7 8 9      1 2 3 4 5 6 7 8 9
  (9.0, 0.8, A)          (9.0, 0.7, A)
```
(28- 30)

7. If isotretinoin is prescribed to post-pubescent girls, there should be documentation that counseling regarding use of an effective means of contraception (including abstinence) was provided.
```
    1 1 1 1 2 4          1        1 3 3 1
1 2 3 4 5 6 7 8 9      1 2 3 4 5 6 7 8 9
  (8.0, 1.1, A)          (7.0, 1.1, A)
```
(31- 33)

7. If tetracycline is prescribed to post-pubescent girls, there should be documentation that counseling regarding use of an effective means of contraception (including abstinence) was provided.
```
    1 2        3 1 2          2 2 2 2
1 2 3 4 5 6 7 8 9      1 2 3 4 5 6 7 8 9
  (7.0, 1.9, I)          (6.0, 1.3, I)
```
(34- 36)

(FOLLOW-UP)

8. If isotretinoin is prescribed, a pregnancy test should be performed at least every three months.
```
    2 1      1 4 1          1 3      2 1
1 2 3 4 5 6 7 8 9      1 2 3 4 5 6 7 8 9
  (8.0, 2.4, D)          (6.0, 1.8, I)
        2        2 3
```
(37- 39)

9. If isotretinoin is prescribed, liver function tests should be performed at least every three months.
```
1 2 3 4 5 6 7 8 9      1 2 3 4 5 6 7 8 9
  (7.0, 0.9, A)          (7.5, 1.0, A)
```
(40- 42)

Scales: 1 = low validity or feasibility; 9 = high validity or feasibility.

Chapter 1
QUALITY INDICATORS FOR ACNE

	Validity	Feasibility
10. If isotretinoin is prescribed, triglyceride levels should be performed at least every three months.	1 2 1 3 2 1 2 3 4 5 6 7 8 9 (7.0, 1.2, I)	1 1 4 1 2 1 2 3 4 5 6 7 8 9 (6.0, 1.1, I)	(43- 45)

Scales: 1 = low validity or feasibility;   9 = high validity or feasibility.

Chapter 2
QUALITY INDICATORS FOR ADOLESCENT PREVENTIVE SERVICES

                                                          Validity   Feasibility

(SCREENING)

General

1. Between the ages of 11 and 18 years, all adolescents should
have an annual visit at which risk assessment/preventive
services were discussed.

Validity: 1 1   1 2 1 3 ; 1 2 3 4 5 6 7 8 9   (7.0, 2.0, I)   (1- 3)
Feasibility: 1   1 3 4 ; 1 2 3 4 5 6 7 8 9   (8.0, 1.4, A)

2. Confidentiality should be discussed and documented by age 14
or at the first visit afterwards.

Validity: 1 1 1 5 ; 1 2 3 4 5 6 7 8 9   (8.0, 1.6, I)   (4- 6)
Feasibility: 1 1 1 3 1 1 ; 1 2 3 4 5 6 7 8 9   (5.0, 1.4, I)

2. Weight and height should be measured at least once a year and
plotted on a growth chart.

Validity: 1 1 1 6 ; 1 2 3 4 5 6 7 8 9   (9.0, 1.1, A)   (7- 9)
Feasibility: 1 1 5 3 ; 1 2 3 4 5 6 7 8 9   (8.0, 0.4, A)

Substance Abuse Screening

3. Documentation of discussion of substance use (tobacco,
alcohol, marijuana, other illicit drugs, anabolic steroids) or
of the adolescent's history should occur annually.

Validity: 1 1 1 5 ; 1 2 3 4 5 6 7 8 9   (9.0, 1.8, I)   (10- 12)
Feasibility: 2 2 2 ; 1 2 3 4 5 6 7 8 9   (7.0, 1.9, I)

3. There should be documentation that the risks of anabolic
steroid use were discussed or a history of anabolic steroid use
was taken for adolescent males participating in team sports or
weight-training at least once a year.

Validity: 1 2 3 4 5 6 7 8 9   (, ,)   (13- 15)
Feasibility: 1 2 3 4 5 6 7 8 9   (, ,)

Sexually Transmitted Diseases and HIV Prevention

4. Documentation of discussion of sexual activity and risk
reduction should occur annually.

Validity: 1   3 4 ; 1 2 3 4 5 6 7 8 9   (8.0, 1.6, A)   (16- 18)
Feasibility: 1 1   2 4 ; 1 2 3 4 5 6 7 8 9   (8.0, 2.1, I)

5. Patients for whom the medical records indicate that they have
ever been sexually active should be asked the following
questions: if they currently have a single sexual partner; if
they have had more than 2 sexual partners in the past 6 months;
and if they have had a history of any STDs.

Validity: 1   1 2 1 3 ; 1 2 3 4 5 6 7 8 9   (7.0, 1.8, I)   (19- 21)
Feasibility: 1 2 1 1 1 1 ; 1 2 3 4 5 6 7 8 9   (5.0, 2.1, D)

Injury Prevention

7. Documentation of discussion of injury prevention should occur
annually.

Validity: 1   3 4 ; 1 2 3 4 5 6 7 8 9   (8.0, 1.7, A)   (22- 24)
Feasibility: 1 1   2 3 1 ; 1 2 3 4 5 6 7 8 9   (7.0, 2.0, I)

8. Patients should receive counseling regarding the use of seat
belts annually.

Validity: 2   2 1 ; 1 2 3 4 5 6 7 8 9   (6.0, 2.2, I)   (25- 27)
Feasibility: 2 1 1   2 1 ; 1 2 3 4 5 6 7 8 9   (4.0, 1.7, I)

Hyperlipidemia Screening

9. Documentation of parental history of hypercholesterolemia
should be sought.

Validity: 2 3 2 1 1 ; 1 2 3 4 5 6 7 8 9   (3.0, 1.6, I)   (28- 30)
Feasibility: 2 3 2 1 ; 1 2 3 4 5 6 7 8 9   (2.0, 1.8, I)

10. Adolescents whose parents have a serum cholesterol level
greater than 240 mg/dl should receive a total blood cholesterol
screen.

Validity: 2 4   2 1 ; 1 2 3 4 5 6 7 8 9   (3.0, 2.2, D)   (31- 33)
Feasibility: 2 2 1 1 2 1 ; 1 2 3 4 5 6 7 8 9   (4.0, 2.4, D)

11. Documentation of parents', or grandparents' history of
coronary artery disease (CAD), peripheral vascular disease
(PVD), cerebrovascular disease, or sudden cardiac death at age
55 or younger should occur annually.

Validity: 1 3 1   2 1 ; 1 2 3 4 5 6 7 8 9   (4.0, 2.0, I)   (34- 36)
Feasibility: 1 1 1 2 1 1 1 ; 1 2 3 4 5 6 7 8 9   (4.0, 1.9, I)

Scales: 1 = low validity or feasibility;   9 = high validity or feasibility.

Chapter 2
QUALITY INDICATORS FOR ADOLESCENT PREVENTIVE SERVICES

12. Adolescents whose parents or grandparents have a positive history of CAD, PVD, cerebrovascular disease or sudden cardiac death at age 55 or younger should have a fasting lipoprotein analysis. (37- 39)

Validity:
```
  1 2 1 1     2 1
1 2 3 4 5 6 7 8 9
    (5.0, 2.2, D)
```
Feasibility:
```
  1 3 1 1     1 2
1 2 3 4 5 6 7 8 9
    (4.0, 2.0, D)
```

Hypertension Screening

13. Blood pressure should be measured at least once a year. (40- 42)

Validity:
```
1 1           2 5
1 2 3 4 5 6 7 8 9
    (9.0, 1.8, A)
```
Feasibility:
```
2             4 3
1 2 3 4 5 6 7 8 9
    (8.0, 1.7, A)
```

14. If a patient has an elevated blood pressure, at least 2 additional blood pressure readings on 2 separate occasions within 3 months are recorded in the chart. (43- 45)

Validity:
```
    1 1     4 3
1 2 3 4 5 6 7 8 9
    (8.0, 0.9, A)
```
Feasibility:
```
  1 1 1 4 2
1 2 3 4 5 6 7 8 9
    (8.0, 0.9, A)
```

Cervical Cancer Screening

15. All sexually active females, or those who present for contraception, should have an annual Pap smear within one year of becoming sexually active. (46- 48)

Validity:
```
          1 1 3 4
1 2 3 4 5 6 7 8 9
    (8.0, 0.8, A)
```
Feasibility:
```
            3 4 2
1 2 3 4 5 6 7 8 9
    (8.0, 0.9, I)
```

General

(TREATMENT)

Cigarette Use Counseling--Treatment

21. All current smokers should receive counseling to stop smoking. (49- 51)

Validity:
```
1         2 2 4
1 2 3 4 5 6 7 8 9
    (8.0, 1.0, A)
```
Feasibility:
```
1         1 2 1 4
1 2 3 4 5 6 7 8 9
    (8.0, 1.6, A)
```

Cervical Cancer Screening--Follow-up

25. All adolescents with a Pap smear consistent with HPV should have colposcopy performed. (52- 54)

Validity:
```
            2 1 4
1 2 3 4 5 6 7 8 9
    (9.0, 0.7, A)
```
Feasibility:
```
        1 3 2 1
1 2 3 4 5 6 7 8 9
    (7.0, 0.7, A)
```

Cigarette Use Counseling--Follow-up

28. Tobacco abuse should be added to the problem list of all current smokers or addressed during at least one subsequent visit. (55- 57)

Validity:
```
2 1 1 1   2 1 1
1 2 3 4 5 6 7 8 9
    (5.0, 2.2, D)
```
Feasibility:
```
2     2   2 1 2
1 2 3 4 5 6 7 8 9
    (6.0, 2.2, I)
```

Eating Disorders

29. Tanner staging recorded annually. (58- 60)

Validity:
```
1 3 1   1 2 1
1 2 3 4 5 6 7 8 9
    (4.0, 2.8, D)
```
Feasibility:
```
2 2 1 1   2 1
1 2 3 4 5 6 7 8 9
    (4.0, 2.4, D)
```

30. Abnormal height/weight velocity - additional visit. (61- 63)

Validity:
```
1       1 1 3 3
1 2 3 4 5 6 7 8 9
    (8.0, 1.4, A)
```
Feasibility:
```
1   1 2 1 1 4
1 2 3 4 5 6 7 8 9
    (8.0, 1.3, I)
```

31. Eating patterns (chronic dieting, binging, laxatives, purging, other drugs, #/type of meals). (64- 66)

Validity:
```
2 1   1 3 1 1 4 1 1
1 2 3 4 5 6 7 8 9
    (8.0, 2.2, I)
```
Feasibility:
```
2     1 1 4 1 1
1 2 3 4 5 6 7 8 9
    (7.0, 1.6, I)
```

Scales: 1 = low validity or feasibility; 9 = high validity or feasibility.

Chapter 3
QUALITY INDICATORS FOR ALLERGIC RHINITIS

	Validity	Feasibility
(DIAGNOSIS)		

1. If a diagnosis of allergic rhinitis is made, the search for a specific allergen by history should be documented in the chart (for initial history). (1- 3)	`        3 1 3 2`
	`1 2 3 4 5 6 7 8 9`
	(7.0, 1.0, I)
		`            1 2   2 4`
		`1 2 3 4 5 6 7 8 9`
		(6.0, 1.2, I)

2. If a diagnosis of allergic rhinitis is made, history should include whether the patient uses any topical nasal decongestants. (4- 6)	`    1 1 1 1 1 4`
	`1 2 3 4 5 6 7 8 9`
	(7.0, 1.6, I)
		`          1 2 3 1 2`
		`1 2 3 4 5 6 7 8 9`
		(6.0, 1.0, I)

(TREATMENT)		

3. Treatment for allergic rhinitis should include at least one of the following: recommendation for allergen avoidance, antihistamine, nasal steroids, nasal cromolyn. (7- 9)	`            3 5 1`
	`1 2 3 4 5 6 7 8 9`
	(8.0, 0.4, A)
		`            4 3 2`
		`1 2 3 4 5 6 7 8 9`
		(8.0, 0.7, A)

4. If topical nasal decongestants are prescribed, duration of treatment should be for no longer than 4 days. (10- 12)	`        1 5 1 2`
	`1 2 3 4 5 6 7 8 9`
	(7.0, 0.7, A)
		`        1 1   1 2 4`
		`1 2 3 4 5 6 7 8 9`
		(7.0, 1.6, I)

5. A specific discussion of environmental triggers and controls should be documented. (13- 15)	`1 1   1 2 1 1 3`
	`1 2 3 4 5 6 7 8 9`
	(7.0, 1.9, I)
		`1 1   1 3   2 2`
		`1 2 3 4 5 6 7 8 9`
		(5.0, 1.8, I)

Scales: 1 = low validity or feasibility;   9 = high validity or feasibility.

panelist 10; round 2;

Chapter 4
QUALITY INDICATORS FOR ASTHMA

	Validity	Feasibility	

1. All patients age 5 or older with the diagnosis of asthma should have baseline spirometry or PEFR performed (within six months of diagnosis).

Validity: 1 2 2 2 1 2 / 1 2 3 4 5 6 7 8 9 / (5.0, 1.6, I)
Feasibility: 3 4 1 / 1 2 3 4 5 6 7 8 9 / (7.0, 1.3, I)   (1- 3)

2. All patients with the diagnosis of asthma should have had a historical evaluation of asthma triggers (e.g., environmental exposures, exercise, allergens) within six months (before or after) of the initial diagnosis.

Validity: 1 1 2 2 3 / 1 2 3 4 5 6 7 8 9 / (8.0, 1.9, A)
Feasibility: 1 2 3 2 / 1 2 3 4 5 6 7 8 9 / (8.0, 1.4, A)   (4- 6)

3. PEFR should be measured in all patients > 5 years of age with chronic asthma (except for those with only exercise-induced asthma) at least annually in an office visit in which asthma is evaluated.

Validity: 1 1 1 2 3 1 / 1 2 3 4 5 6 7 8 9 / (7.0, 1.9, I)
Feasibility: 1 2 2 3 1 / 1 2 3 4 5 6 7 8 9 / (6.0, 1.1, I)   (7- 9)

(TREATMENT)

4. All patients > 5 years of age with the diagnosis of asthma should have been prescribed a beta2-agonist inhaler for symptomatic relief of exacerbations.

Validity: 1 1 3 1 3 / 1 2 3 4 5 6 7 8 9 / (7.0, 1.1, A)
Feasibility: 2 4 1 2 / 1 2 3 4 5 6 7 8 9 / (7.0, 0.8, A)   (10- 12)

5. Patients <= 5 years of age should be prescribed a nebulizer (for administering asthma medications).

Validity: 1 1 1 3 3 / 1 2 3 4 5 6 7 8 9 / (7.0, 1.8, I)
Feasibility: 1 1 1 1 1 3 / 1 2 3 4 5 6 7 8 9 / (6.0, 1.9, I)   (13- 15)

6. Patients who report using a beta2-agonist inhaler more than 3 times per day on a daily basis should be prescribed a longer acting bronchodilator (theophylline) and/or an anti-inflammatory agent (inhaled corticosteroids, cromolyn).

Validity: 1 1 3 2 2 / 1 2 3 4 5 6 7 8 9 / (7.0, 1.2, A)
Feasibility: 1 2 2 2 1 1 / 1 2 3 4 5 6 7 8 9 / (6.0, 1.6, I)   (16- 18)

7. Patients with asthma should not receive beta-blocker medications (e.g., atenolol, propanalol).

Validity: 1 5 3 / 1 2 3 4 5 6 7 8 9 / (8.0, 0.4, A)
Feasibility: 1 1 1 4 2 / 1 2 3 4 5 6 7 8 9 / (8.0, 1.1, A)   (19- 21)

8. In any patients requiring chronic treatment with oral corticosteroids a trial of inhaled corticosteroids should have been attempted.

Validity: 1 1 5 1 1 / 1 2 3 4 5 6 7 8 9 / (7.0, 0.7, A)
Feasibility: 1 2 3 2 1 / 1 2 3 4 5 6 7 8 9 / (7.0, 0.9, I)   (22- 24)

9. Any child with asthma who takes high doses of inhaled corticosteroids should have growth patterns monitored at least annually.

Validity: 1 5 3 / 1 2 3 4 5 6 7 8 9 / (7.0, 0.4, A)
Feasibility: 2 6 1 / 1 2 3 4 5 6 7 8 9 / (8.0, 0.3, A)   (25- 27)

10. Patients who require frequent bursts of prednisone (2-3 trials of 5-day therapy with oral corticosteroids after an exacerbation of asthma within the past 6 months) who are not already on inhaled corticosteroids or cromolyn sodium should be started on them.

Validity: 2 1 4 2 / 1 2 3 4 5 6 7 8 9 / (8.0, 0.8, A)
Feasibility: 1 1 2 3 2 / 1 2 3 4 5 6 7 8 9 / (8.0, 1.0, A)   (28- 30)

11. Patients on theophylline should have at least one theophylline level determination per year.

Validity: 1 3 1 2 1 1 / 1 2 3 4 5 6 7 8 9 / (5.0, 1.9, I)
Feasibility: 1 1 1 5 2 / 1 2 3 4 5 6 7 8 9 / (7.0, 1.2, A)   (31- 33)

13. Patients with the diagnosis of asthma that is moderate to severe should have a pneumococcal vaccination documented in the chart within one year of diagnosis.

Validity: 3 3 1 2 / 1 2 3 4 5 6 7 8 9 / (4.0, 0.9, I)
Feasibility: 1 1 1 2 1 3 / 1 2 3 4 5 6 7 8 9 / (7.0, 1.9, I)   (34- 36)

(TREATMENT OF EXACERBATIONS)

14. All patients > 5 years of age presenting to the physician's office with an asthma exacerbation or historical worsening of asthma symptoms should be evaluated with PEFR or FEV1.

Validity: 3 1 5 / 1 2 3 4 5 6 7 8 9 / (8.0, 0.8, I)
Feasibility: 5 1 3 / 1 2 3 4 5 6 7 8 9 / (6.0, 0.8, I)   (37- 39)

Scales: 1 = low validity or feasibility; 9 = high validity or feasibility.

Chapter 4
QUALITY INDICATORS FOR ASTHMA

	Validity	Feasibility	

15. At the time of exacerbation, symptomatic patients on theophylline should have a theophylline level measured.
Validity: 1 2 3 4 5 6 7 8 9   (7.0, 1.0, A)
Feasibility: 1 2 3 4 5 6 7 8 9   (7.0, 1.2, A)   (40– 42)

16. A physical exam of the chest should be performed in all patients presenting with an asthma exacerbation.
Validity: 1 2 3 4 5 6 7 8 9   (9.0, 0.8, A)
Feasibility: 1 2 3 4 5 6 7 8 9   (9.0, 0.4, A)   (43– 45)

17. All patients presenting to the physician's office or emergency department with an FEV1 or PEFR<=70 percent of baseline (or predicted) should be treated with beta2-agonists before discharge.
Validity: 1 2 3 4 5 6 7 8 9   (8.0, 0.6, A)
Feasibility: 1 2 3 4 5 6 7 8 9   (8.0, 0.3, A)   (46– 48)

18. Patients who receive treatment with beta2-agonists for FEV1 or PEFR <70 percent in the physician's office or emergency department (ED) should have an FEV1 or PEFR repeated prior to discharge.
Validity: 1 2 3 4 5 6 7 8 9   (8.0, 1.0, A)
Feasibility: 1 2 3 4 5 6 7 8 9   (7.0, 0.8, I)   (49– 51)

19. Patients with an FEV1 or PEFR <=70 percent of baseline (or predicted) after treatment for an asthma exacerbation in the physician's office should be placed on an oral corticosteroid taper.
Validity: 1 2 3 4 5 6 7 8 9   (7.0, 1.0, I)
Feasibility: 1 2 3 4 5 6 7 8 9   (8.0, 0.4, A)   (52– 54)

20. Patients who have persistent symptoms, diffuse wheezes on chest auscultation, and a PEFR or FEV1<=40 percent of baseline (or predicted) after treatment with beta2-agonists should be admitted to the hospital.
Validity: 1 2 3 4 5 6 7 8 9   (8.0, 1.3, I)
Feasibility: 1 2 3 4 5 6 7 8 9   (9.0, 1.0, A)   (55– 57)

(HOSPITAL TREATMENT)

21. All patients admitted to the hospital for asthma exacerbation should have oxygen saturation measured.
Validity: 1 2 3 4 5 6 7 8 9   (9.0, 1.1, A)
Feasibility: 1 2 3 4 5 6 7 8 9   (9.0, 0.4, A)   (58– 60)

22. All hospitalized patients with PEFR or FEV1 < 25 percent of predicted or personal best should receive arterial blood gas measurement.
Validity: 1 2 3 4 5 6 7 8 9   (8.0, 1.0, A)
Feasibility: 1 2 3 4 5 6 7 8 9   (9.0, 0.9, A)   (61– 63)

23. All hospitalized patients should receive systemic (IV) or oral steroids.
Validity: 1 2 3 4 5 6 7 8 9   (9.0, 1.0, A)
Feasibility: 1 2 3 4 5 6 7 8 9   (9.0, 0.6, A)   (64– 66)

24. All hospitalized patients should receive treatment with beta2-agonists.
Validity: 1 2 3 4 5 6 7 8 9   (9.0, 0.9, A)
Feasibility: 1 2 3 4 5 6 7 8 9   (9.0, 0.6, A)   (67– 69)

25. All hospitalized patients should receive treatment with methylxanthines.
Validity: 1 2 3 4 5 6 7 8 9   (3.0, 0.8, I)
Feasibility: 1 2 3 4 5 6 7 8 9   (7.0, 2.4, D)   (70– 72)

26. All hospitalized patients with oxygen saturation less than 92 percent should receive supplemental oxygen.
Validity: 1 2 3 4 5 6 7 8 9   (7.0, 1.6, I)
Feasibility: 1 2 3 4 5 6 7 8 9   (9.0, 1.0, A)   (73– 75)

27. All hospitalized patients with pCO2 of greater than 40 should receive at least one additional blood gas measurement to evaluate response to treatment.
Validity: 1 2 3 4 5 6 7 8 9   (8.0, 0.8, A)
Feasibility: 1 2 3 4 5 6 7 8 9   (9.0, 0.4, A)   (76– 78)

28. Hospitalized patients with pCO2 of greater than 40 should be monitored in an intensive care setting.
Validity: 1 2 3 4 5 6 7 8 9   (6.0, 1.4, I)
Feasibility: 1 2 3 4 5 6 7 8 9   (9.0, 1.2, A)   (79– 81)

29. Patients with 2 or more hospitalizations for asthma exacerbation in the previous year should receive (or should have received) consultation with an asthma specialist.
Validity: 1 2 3 4 5 6 7 8 9   (6.0, 2.6, D)
Feasibility: 1 2 3 4 5 6 7 8 9   (6.0, 1.6, I)   (82– 84)

Scales: 1 = low validity or feasibility; 9 = high validity or feasibility.

panelist 10; round 2;

Mon Mar 25 14:22:10 1996

Chapter 4
QUALITY INDICATORS FOR ASTHMA

	Validity	Feasibility	
30. Hospitalized patients not on a ventilator should not receive sedative drugs (e.g., benzodiazepines).	3 1 1 3 1 1 2 3 4 5 6 7 8 9 (7.0, 1.3, I)	4 2 3 1 2 3 4 5 6 7 8 9 (8.0, 0.8, A)	(85- 87)

(FOLLOW-UP)

	Validity	Feasibility	
31. Patients with the diagnosis of moderate to severe asthma should have at least 2 scheduled visits within a calendar year.	1 1 4 1 1 1 2 3 4 5 6 7 8 9 (7.0, 1.4, I)	1 2 3 2 1 1 2 3 4 5 6 7 8 9 (7.0, 1.0, I)	(88- 90)
32. Patients whose asthma medication is changed (new medication added, current dose decreased/increased) during one visit should have a follow-up within 3 weeks.	1 1 2 4 1 2 3 4 5 6 7 8 9 (7.0, 1.7, I)	1 6 1 1 2 3 4 5 6 7 8 9 (8.0, 0.9, A)	(91- 93)
33. Patients on chronic oral corticosteroids should have follow-up visits at least 4 times in a calendar year.	2 1 2 3 1 1 2 3 4 5 6 7 8 9 (7.0, 1.9, I)	1 2 2 3 1 1 2 3 4 5 6 7 8 9 (7.0, 1.4, I)	(94- 96)
34. Patients seen in the emergency department with an asthma exacerbation should have a follow-up reassessment within 72 hours.	1 1 6 1 1 2 3 4 5 6 7 8 9 (8.0, 1.1, A)	1 3 4 1 1 2 3 4 5 6 7 8 9 (8.0, 0.7, A)	(97- 99)
35. Patients with a hospitalization for an asthma exacerbation should receive follow-up assessment within 7 days.	1 1 5 2 1 2 3 4 5 6 7 8 9 (8.0, 1.1, A)	1 6 2 1 2 3 4 5 6 7 8 9 (8.0, 0.3, A)	(100-102)

Scales: 1 = low validity or feasibility; 9 = high validity or feasibility.

panelist 10; round 2;

Chapter 5
QUALITY INDICATORS FOR ATTENTION DEFICIT/HYPERACTIVITY
DISORDER

THESE INDICATORS COVER AGES 5-18 years old:

(DIAGNOSIS)

	Validity	Feasibility	

1. Before making the diagnosis of ADHD, the health care provider should document a history of inattention and impulsivity/hyperactivity, using input from a parent and from a teacher (if the child is in school). An effort to communicate with a teacher or have a teacher fill out a rating scale is acceptable.

Validity:
```
                    3   5
1 2 3 4 5 6 7 8 9
(9.0, 1.4, A)
```
Feasibility:
```
              2 1 2 3 1
1 2 3 4 5 6 7 8 9
(7.0, 1.1, I)
```
(1- 3)

2. Before making the diagnosis of ADHD, the health care provider should document:

a. That the core symptoms of inattention and impulsivity/hyperactivity happen in more than one setting.

Validity:
```
1 1           3 4
1 2 3 4 5 6 7 8 9
(7.0, 1.4, A)
```
Feasibility:
```
        1   1 2 5
1 2 3 4 5 6 7 8 9
(7.0, 0.9, I)
```
(4- 6)

b. That the core symptoms of inattention and impulsivity/hyperactivity have been of >= 6 months duration.

Validity:
```
1 1       1 5 1
1 2 3 4 5 6 7 8 9
(8.0, 1.6, I)
```
Feasibility:
```
        1   1 3 2 1
1 2 3 4 5 6 7 8 9
(6.0, 1.2, I)
```
(7- 9)

c. That the core symptoms of inattention and impulsivity/hyperactivity had been present prior to 7 years of age.

Validity:
```
1 1 1 1 1 1 3
1 2 3 4 5 6 7 8 9
(6.0, 2.1, I)
```
Feasibility:
```
          2 2 4
1 2 3 4 5 6 7 8 9
(6.0, 1.2, I)
```
(10- 12)

d. The child's social functioning, with regard to pervasive developmental disorder, by evaluating the following:
- impairment of social interaction,
- impairment in communication,
- restricted, repetitive and stereotyped patterns of behavior, interests, and activities.

Validity:
```
1 1         6 1
1 2 3 4 5 6 7 8 9
(7.0, 1.1, A)
```
Feasibility:
```
        1   3 4
1 2 3 4 5 6 7 8 9
(6.0, 1.2, I)
```
(13- 15)

e. The presence or absence of affective symptoms.***

Validity:
```
1 1 1 3 3
1 2 3 4 5 6 7 8 9
(7.0, 1.3, I)
```
Feasibility:
```
        1   2 2 4
1 2 3 4 5 6 7 8 9
(6.0, 1.0, I)
```
(16- 18)

f. The child's social functioning, with regard to:
- oppositional defiant disorder, and
- conduct disorder.

Validity:
```
1 1         3 4
1 2 3 4 5 6 7 8 9
(7.0, 1.4, A)
```
Feasibility:
```
        1   1 5 1 1
1 2 3 4 5 6 7 8 9
(6.0, 0.9, I)
```
(19- 21)

3. Through history, physical exam and lab, an effort was made to rule out organic and pharmacologic causes.

Validity:
```
1     2 3 3
1 2 3 4 5 6 7 8 9
(7.0, 1.2, I)
```
Feasibility:
```
        2   2 3 1 1
1 2 3 4 5 6 7 8 9
(7.0, 1.4, I)
```
(22- 24)

6. The health care provider should document the child's cognitive level and academic achievement levels, including:

a. Academic performance/achievement level (if in school).

Validity:
```
1 1   1 2 4
1 2 3 4 5 6 7 8 9
(8.0, 1.9, I)
```
Feasibility:
```
        1 1 2 1 4
1 2 3 4 5 6 7 8 9
(8.0, 1.2, A)
```
(25- 27)

b. Cognitive level ability/psychoeducational testing.

Validity:
```
1     1 1 1 4
1 2 3 4 5 6 7 8 9
(8.0, 2.0, I)
```
Feasibility:
```
          1 2 3
1 2 3 4 5 6 7 8 9
(7.0, 1.1, I)
```
(28- 30)

Scales: 1 = low validity or feasibility; 9 = high validity or feasibility.

panelist 10; round 2;   Mon Mar 25 14:22:10 1996

Chapter 5
QUALITY INDICATORS FOR ATTENTION DEFICIT/HYPERACTIVITY
DISORDER

	Validity	Feasibility	
7. The health care provider should document the structure of the family, home environment, and school environment. Such information should include:			
a. A list of parents or guardians and other household members.	1 1 2 3 1 1 2 3 4 5 6 7 8 9 (7.0, 1.6, I)	1 2 2 3 1 2 3 4 5 6 7 8 9 (7.0, 1.3, I)	(31- 33)
b. Environmental stressors.	1 2 2 2 1 1 2 3 4 5 6 7 8 9 (7.0, 1.7, I)	1 2 2 1 3 1 2 3 4 5 6 7 8 9 (6.0, 1.4, I)	(34- 36)
c. Family functioning.	1 1 2 2 1 2 1 2 3 4 5 6 7 8 9 (7.0, 1.7, I)	2 3 3 1 2 3 4 5 6 7 8 9 (7.0, 1.3, I)	(37- 39)
d. School features (if in school).	1 1 4 1 1 1 1 2 3 4 5 6 7 8 9 (7.0, 1.4, I)	1 2 1 1 1 3 1 2 3 4 5 6 7 8 9 (6.0, 2.1, I)	(40- 42)
8. The health care provider should document the presence or absence of any family history of:			
a. Psychiatric disorder.	1 1 4 2 1 2 3 4 5 6 7 8 9 (7.0, 1.6, I)	1 1 4 3 1 2 3 4 5 6 7 8 9 (6.0, 0.7, I)	(43- 45)
b. Attention deficit/hyperactivity disorder.	1 2 2 1 2 2 1 2 3 4 5 6 7 8 9 (7.0, 1.7, I)	2 1 4 2 1 2 3 4 5 6 7 8 9 (7.0, 0.8, I)	(46- 48)
c. Learning disorder.	1 1 2 3 1 1 2 3 4 5 6 7 8 9 (7.0, 1.4, I)	1 3 4 1 1 2 3 4 5 6 7 8 9 (7.0, 0.7, I)	(49- 51)
10. The physical examination should include a neurologic exam.	1 1 1 1 2 3 1 2 3 4 5 6 7 8 9 (7.0, 1.8, I)	4 1 4 1 2 3 4 5 6 7 8 9 (7.0, 0.9, I)	(52- 54)
10. The physical examination should include observation of mood and social interactions.	1 1 1 2 4 1 2 3 4 5 6 7 8 9 (7.0, 1.6, I)	1 2 2 1 2 1 1 2 3 4 5 6 7 8 9 (6.0, 1.7, I)	(55- 57)
11. The health care provider should document the child's current medications.	1 3 2 1 2 3 4 5 6 7 8 9 (8.0, 1.4, A)	1 1 1 2 1 2 3 4 5 6 7 8 9 (8.0, 1.1, A)	(58- 60)
15. The health care provider should document a vision screening test.	2 2 1 2 1 1 2 3 4 5 6 7 8 9 (5.0, 2.0, I)	1 2 3 2 1 1 2 3 4 5 6 7 8 9 (7.0, 1.2, I)	(61- 63)
17. The health care provider should document a hearing screening test.	1 1 2 2 1 1 2 3 4 5 6 7 8 9 (7.0, 1.8, I)	1 5 2 1 1 2 3 4 5 6 7 8 9 (7.0, 1.2, I)	(64- 66)
(TREATMENT)			
18. Medications specific to the treatment of ADHD should not be prescribed for children who do not meet criteria for ADHD.	2 1 2 4 1 2 3 4 5 6 7 8 9 (8.0, 1.0, A)	2 1 2 4 1 2 3 4 5 6 7 8 9 (8.0, 1.2, A)	(67- 69)

Scales: 1 = low validity or feasibility;   9 = high validity or feasibility.

Chapter 5
QUALITY INDICATORS FOR ATTENTION DEFICIT/HYPERACTIVITY
DISORDER

19. The health care provider should document counseling about
how to adjust the home and school environments. These
adjustments would include:

a. At home, work with parents to structure home environment:
- predictable schedule for bed time, meal times, play times,
and homework,
- breakdown of chores into smaller tasks,
- predictable, acceptable limits of behavior, or
- predictable and immediate consequences for inappropriate
behavior.   (70- 72)

Validity:
```
        1 1 5 1       1
1 2 3 4 5 6 7 8 9
(7.0, 1.2, I)
```
Feasibility:
```
3 1 1         3 1
1 2 3 4 5 6 7 8 9
(4.0, 2.2, D)
```

b. At school, communicate with school officials to structure
school environment:
- a seat with minimal distractions,
- allow child to get up periodically from seat,
- brief instructions,
- frequent reminders to stay on task with discrete cues or
signs,
- predictable and immediate consequences for inappropriate
behavior, or
- provide opportunities for success.   (73- 75)

Validity:
```
      1 2 1 2 2
1 2 3 4 5 6 7 8 9
(7.0, 1.8, I)
```
Feasibility:
```
4         1 1 1 1 1
1 2 3 4 5 6 7 8 9
(4.0, 2.0, I)
```

20. If the child has isolated ADHD, the health care provider
should initiate or refer for behavioral modification.   (76- 78)

Validity:
```
1       1 2 5
1 2 3 4 5 6 7 8 9
(7.0, 1.2, I)
```
Feasibility:
```
2 1     2 1 1 2
1 2 3 4 5 6 7 8 9
(5.0, 1.9, D)
```

21. If a child has another psychiatric disorder, the child
should be referred for psychiatric or psychologic evaluation
and/or therapy.   (79- 81)

Validity:
```
1       5 2
1 2 3 4 5 6 7 8 9
(8.0, 1.3, A)
```
Feasibility:
```
1     1 4 1 2
1 2 3 4 5 6 7 8 9
(7.0, 1.2, A)
```

23. If the child has a learning disorder, the child should be
referred to the school system or other setting for psychoeducational intervention.   (82- 84)

Validity:
```
      2 2 4
1 2 3 4 5 6 7 8 9
(8.0, 1.4, A)
```
Feasibility:
```
1     1 1 2 1 3
1 2 3 4 5 6 7 8 9
(7.0, 1.6, I)
```

25. If the child has ADHD without a comorbidity or with
oppositional defiant disorder, or conduct disorder or a
learning dosorder, and is started on pharmacotherapy, the
the initial medication choice should be methylphenidate,
dextroamphetamine, or pemoline.   (85- 87)

Validity:
```
1 1     1 5 1
1 2 3 4 5 6 7 8 9
(8.0, 1.2, A)
```
Feasibility:
```
1 3 3 2
1 2 3 4 5 6 7 8 9
(8.0, 0.8, A)
```

27. If the child has ADHD and Tourette Syndrome or a tic
disorder and is begun on pharmacotherapy, the initial medication
should be clonidine, methylphenidate, penoline, or
dextroamphetamine.   (88- 90)

Validity:
```
1     1 5 1 1 1
1 2 3 4 5 6 7 8 9
(7.0, 0.9, A)
```
Feasibility:
```
1 6 2
1 2 3 4 5 6 7 8 9
(8.0, 0.4, A)
```

28. If the child has ADHD and a mood disorder and is begun on
pharmacotherapy, the initial medication should be a tricyclic
antidepressant.   (91- 93)

Validity:
```
3 1 4 1
1 2 3 4 5 6 7 8 9
(7.0, 0.9, I)
```
Feasibility:
```
1 3 5
1 2 3 4 5 6 7 8 9
(8.0, 0.6, A)
```

31. Before a child is started on stimulant medication such as
methylphenidate, dextroamphetamine, or pemoline, the health care
provider should document the weight, height, heart rate, and
blood pressure of the child.   (94- 96)

Validity:
```
1   2 3 2
1 2 3 4 5 6 7 8 9
(8.0, 1.6, A)
```
Feasibility:
```
1   2 4 1
1 2 3 4 5 6 7 8 9
(8.0, 0.8, A)
```

Scales: 1 = low validity or feasibility; 9 = high validity or feasibility.

Chapter 5
QUALITY INDICATORS FOR ATTENTION DEFICIT/HYPERACTIVITY
DISORDER

	Validity	Feasibility	

32. If a child is started on pemoline, the health care provider should document the absence of hepatic disease prior to the start of therapy by history and baseline liver function tests. (97- 99)

```
                  1 1 1 4 2                        2 1 5 1
        1 2 3 4 5 6 7 8 9                1 2 3 4 5 6 7 8 9
          (8.0, 1.3, A)                    (8.0, 0.7, A)
```

33. If a child is started on a tricyclic antidepressant, the health care provider should take a cardiac history and obtain a baseline electrocardiogram. (100-102)

```
                      2   3 3                      1 1 5 1
        1 2 3 4 5 6 7 8 9                1 2 3 4 5 6 7 8 9
          (8.0, 1.6, I)                    (8.0, 1.0, A)
```

34. The primary health care provider who is not an ADHD specialist should not prescribe for treatment of ADHD:
- chlorpromazine,
- haloperidol,
- levodopa,
- lithium,
- monoamine oxidase inhibitors,
- thioridazine. (103-105)

```
                4 2   2                        4 1 1 3
        1 2 3 4 5 6 7 8 9                1 2 3 4 5 6 7 8 9
          (6.0, 1.4, I)                    (7.0, 1.2, I)
```

35. The primary health care provider should not simultaneously treat a child with ADHD with more than one medication for treatment of ADHD without the consultation of an ADHD specialist, e.g., a psychiatrist, neurologist, or behavioralist. (106-108)

```
            1 1 1 2 1 2                      3 2 1 3
        1 2 3 4 5 6 7 8 9                1 2 3 4 5 6 7 8 9
          (7.0, 1.9, I)                    (7.0, 1.1, I)
```

36. The primary health care provider should request consultation from an ADHD specialist (e.g., a multidisciplinary referral center or psychiatrist, neurologist, or behavioralist) if a child fails to respond to separate trials with methylphenidate, dextroamphetamine, pemoline, clonidine, and a single tricyclic antidepressant. (109-111)

```
            1   1 1 2 3                        1 2   3 3
        1 2 3 4 5 6 7 8 9                1 2 3 4 5 6 7 8 9
          (8.0, 1.9, I)                    (8.0, 1.2, I)
```

(FOLLOW-UP)

37. During the initial treatment period, the health care provider should maintain at least biweekly (every other week) contact with the family, either through office visits or by phone, for at least 4 contacts. (112-114)

```
            1 1 2 3 1                      3 3 1 2
        1 2 3 4 5 6 7 8 9                1 2 3 4 5 6 7 8 9
          (5.0, 1.9, I)                    (5.0, 0.9, A)
```

41. After the initial four visits for pharmacotherapeutic intervention, and once an improvement is seen in attention or impulsivity/hyperactivity, the provider of such therapy should see the child in the office at least every six months. (115-117)

```
            1   1 2 3 1                        4 4 1
        1 2 3 4 5 6 7 8 9                1 2 3 4 5 6 7 8 9
          (6.0, 1.6, I)                    (6.0, 0.7, A)
```

42. If a change in therapy has occurred, the health care provider initiating the change must:

a. Evaluate the effect of the change within two weeks, either by an office visit or by phone contact. (118-120)

```
                  1 4 3                        1 4 4
        1 2 3 4 5 6 7 8 9                1 2 3 4 5 6 7 8 9
          (7.0, 1.1, A)                    (7.0, 0.7, A)
```

43. At least every six months, the health care provider should document the child's behavior both at home and at school. (121-123)

```
                1 2 4 1                      1 2 4 2
        1 2 3 4 5 6 7 8 9                1 2 3 4 5 6 7 8 9
          (8.0, 1.3, A)                    (7.0, 0.8, I)
```

44. The health care provider should request and review the child's academic records, such as report cards or interviews with the child's teacher, at least once a year. (124-126)

```
              1 2 2   3                      1 1 2   3
        1 2 3 4 5 6 7 8 9                1 2 3 4 5 6 7 8 9
          (7.0, 1.8, I)                    (6.0, 2.7, D)
```

Scales: 1 = low validity or feasibility; 9 = high validity or feasibility.

Chapter 5
QUALITY INDICATORS FOR ATTENTION DEFICIT/HYPERACTIVITY
DISORDER

	Validity	Feasibility	

45. If stimulant medications have been prescribed, the following should be documented at least every six months:

a. Weight.
```
                1         6 1                        1         6 2
        1 2 3 4 5 6 7 8 9                    1 2 3 4 5 6 7 8 9
        (8.0, 1.1, A)                        (8.0, 0.4, A)
```
(127-129)

b. Height.
```
        1       15 1                          1         6 2
        1 2 3 4 5 6 7 8 9                    1 2 3 4 5 6 7 8 9
        (8.0, 1.7, A)                        (8.0, 0.4, A)
```
(130-132)

c. Heart rate.
```
          2   2 1 2 1                          1 1 2 4 1
        1 2 3 4 5 6 7 8 9                    1 2 3 4 5 6 7 8 9
        (6.0, 2.1, D)                        (8.0, 1.0, A)
```
(133-135)

d. Blood pressure.
```
        1   1 1 1 4 1                        1 1 1 1 5 1
        1 2 3 4 5 6 7 8 9                    1 2 3 4 5 6 7 8 9
        (8.0, 1.7, I)                        (8.0, 0.8, A)
```
(136-138)

46. If stimulant medications have been prescribed, the health care provider should document at least every six months the presence or absence of side effects.
```
        1     1 1 3 2                          1 3       3 2
        1 2 3 4 5 6 7 8 9                    1 2 3 4 5 6 7 8 9
        (8.0, 1.7, I)                        (8.0, 1.2, I)
```
(139-141)

47. If a tricyclic antidepressant has been prescribed, the health care provider should document at least every six months the presence or absence of side effects.
```
            1 1 4 2                              1 2     3 3
        1 2 3 4 5 6 7 8 9                    1 2 3 4 5 6 7 8 9
        (8.0, 1.3, A)                        (8.0, 1.1, I)
```
(142-144)

48. If clonidine has been prescribed, the health care provider should document at least every six months the presence or absence of side effects.
```
            1 1 3 3                              1 2     2 4
        1 2 3 4 5 6 7 8 9                    1 2 3 4 5 6 7 8 9
        (8.0, 1.4, A)                        (8.0, 1.2, I)
```
(145-147)

49. If the child is on pemoline, the health care provider should assess liver function every six months.
```
        2       1 4 2                          2       1 4 2
        1 2 3 4 5 6 7 8 9                    1 2 3 4 5 6 7 8 9
        (8.0, 1.9, A)                        (8.0, 0.8, A)
```
(148-150)

50. If the child is on a tricyclic antidepressant, the health care provider should order an electrocardiogram every six months.
```
        2 1   2 2 1   1                      1 2 1 2 1 1 1
        1 2 3 4 5 6 7 8 9                    1 2 3 4 5 6 7 8 9
        (5.0, 2.0, I)                        (6.0, 2.0, D)
```
(151-153)

Scales: 1 = low validity or feasibility;   9 = high validity or feasibility.

Chapter 7
QUALITY INDICATORS FOR DEPRESSION

	Validity	Feasibility

(DIAGNOSIS/DETECTION)

1. Clinicians should ask about the presence or absence of depression or depressive symptoms* in any person with any of the following risk factors for depression:
- parental divorce in past six months,
- school failure,
- history of depression,
- death of family member or friend in past six months,
- history of alcohol, cigarette or other drug use,
- history of depression, substance abuse or suicide attempts in family members,
- fired from job,
- parental marital discord,
- parental patient discord,
- school suspension, truancy, expulsion, or dropping out,
- encounters with criminal justice,
- breaking up with a girlfriend/boyfriend,
- homosexuality.

(1- 3)

```
              1   1 1 3 2              1 1 1 4 1 1
1 2 3 4 5 6 7 8 9          1 2 3 4 5 6 7 8 9
   (8.0, 2.0, I)              (7.0, 1.0, I)
```

2. If the diagnosis of depression is made, specific co-morbidities should be elicited and documented in the chart:
- presence or absence of substance abuse,
- medication use, and
- general medical disorder(s).

(4- 6)

```
            1     6 1                    1 1 2 5
1 2 3 4 5 6 7 8 9          1 2 3 4 5 6 7 8 9
   (8.0, 1.1, A)              (8.0, 0.8, A)
```

(TREATMENT)

3. If co-morbidity (substance abuse, contributing medication, general medical disorder) is present that contributes to depression, the initial treatment objective should be to remove the comorbidity or treat medical disorder.

(7- 9)

```
          1   3 1 2                      1 3 3 1
1 2 3 4 5 6 7 8 9          1 2 3 4 5 6 7 8 9
   (7.0, 1.2, A)              (7.5, 0.8, A)
```

4. Once diagnosis of major depression has been made, treatment with anti-depressant medication and/or psychotherapy should begin within 2 weeks.

(10- 12)

```
        1 1 1 5 1                          3 3 3
1 2 3 4 5 6 7 8 9          1 2 3 4 5 6 7 8 9
   (8.0, 0.8, A)              (8.0, 0.7, A)
```

5. Presence or absence of suicidal ideation should be documented during the first diagnostic visit.

(13- 15)

```
              1 3 5                        2 2 5
1 2 3 4 5 6 7 8 9          1 2 3 4 5 6 7 8 9
   (9.0, 0.6, A)              (9.0, 0.7, A)
```

6. Medication treatment visits or telephone contacts should occur weekly for a minimum of 4 weeks.

(16- 18)

```
      1 1 3 2 1                        1 1 3 4
1 2 3 4 5 6 7 8 9          1 2 3 4 5 6 7 8 9
   (7.0, 1.7, I)              (7.0, 1.1, A)
```

7. At least one of the following should occur if there is no or inadequate response to therapy for depression at 8 weeks:
- referral to psychotherapist if not already seeing one,
- change or increase in dose of medication if on medication,
- addition of medication if only using psychotherapy, or
- change in diagnosis documented in chart.

(19- 21)

```
          1 1 5 1                    2 1 2 3 1
1 2 3 4 5 6 7 8 9          1 2 3 4 5 6 7 8 9
   (8.0, 1.2, A)              (7.0, 1.1, I)
```

7. A follow-up family meeting should occur within 2 weeks of the initial evaluation.

(22- 24)

```
    1 2 2 1 1                            3 4
1 2 3 4 5 6 7 8 9          1 2 3 4 5 6 7 8 9
   (6.5, 1.6, I)              (6.5, 1.1, I)
```

8. Anti-depressants should be used at appropriate dosages.

(25- 27)

```
                1 8                        1 8
1 2 3 4 5 6 7 8 9          1 2 3 4 5 6 7 8 9
   (9.0, 0.2, A)              (9.0, 0.2, A)
```

Scales: 1 = low validity or feasibility; 9 = high validity or feasibility.

Chapter 7
QUALITY INDICATORS FOR DEPRESSION

	Validity	Feasibility	

9. Anti-anxiety agents should NOT be used (except alprazolam as the sole agent for treatment of depression), unless there is documentation of a comorbid anxiety disorder. (28- 30)

```
                1 2      6                    2 1      6
      1 2 3 4 5 6 7 8 9            1 2 3 4 5 6 7 8 9
        (9.0, 0.8, A)               (9.0, 0.9, A)
```

10. Persons who have suicidality should be asked if they have specific plans to carry out suicide, access to a gun, and access to prescription medicines. (31- 33)

```
            3      5                      1 2 1    5
      1 2 3 4 5 6 7 8 9            1 2 3 4 5 6 7 8 9
        (9.0, 1.4, A)               (9.0, 1.3, I)
```

11. Persons who have suicidality and have any of the following risk factors should be hospitalized:

a. Psychosis. (34- 36)

```
        1   1   3 4                        2 1      6
      1 2 3 4 5 6 7 8 9            1 2 3 4 5 6 7 8 9
        (8.0, 1.2, A)               (9.0, 0.9, A)
```

b. Current alcohol or drug abuse. (37- 39)

```
      1   3 2   3                      1   2 1 1 4
      1 2 3 4 5 6 7 8 9            1 2 3 4 5 6 7 8 9
        (7.0, 1.4, I)               (8.0, 1.6, I)
```

c. Specific plans to carry out suicide (e.g., obtaining a weapon, putting affairs in order, making a suicide note). (40- 42)

```
      1   2   1 5                        1   2      6
      1 2 3 4 5 6 7 8 9            1 2 3 4 5 6 7 8 9
        (9.0, 1.4, I)               (9.0, 1.1, A)
```

(FOLLOW-UP)

12. Once depression has resolved, visits should occur every 16 weeks at a minimum, while patient is still on medication, for the first year of treatment. (43- 45)

```
      1 1 1 1 3 1                      1 1 5 1
      1 2 3 4 5 6 7 8 9            1 2 3 4 5 6 7 8 9
        (7.5, 1.8, I)               (7.0, 0.5, A)
```

13. At each visit during which depression is discussed, degree of response/remission and side effects of medication should be assessed and documented during the first year of treatment. (46- 48)

```
            3 4                              7 1
      1 2 3 4 5 6 7 8 9            1 2 3 4 5 6 7 8 9
        (7.5, 1.2, A)               (7.0, 0.1, A)
```

14. Persons hospitalized for depression should have follow-up with a mental health specialist or their primary care doctor within one week of discharge. (49- 51)

```
          2 2 2 3                    1       3 4
      1 2 3 4 5 6 7 8 9            1 2 3 4 5 6 7 8 9
        (8.0, 1.5, A)               (8.5, 0.8, A)
```

Scales: 1 = low validity or feasibility; 9 = high validity or feasibility.

Chapter 8
QUALITY INDICATORS FOR DEVELOPMENTAL SCREENING

	Validity	Feasibility	

1. Social/personal development should be documented at least:

a. Three times during the first year of life.
```
                 1         2 2 3                          1         1 3 4
          1 2 3 4 5 6 7 8 9                        1 2 3 4 5 6 7 8 9
             (8.0, 1.8, A)                            (8.0, 0.9, A)          ( 1-  3)
```

b. Two times during the second year of life.
```
          1 1       1 2 1 3                        1         1 2 1 2
          1 2 3 4 5 6 7 8 9                        1 2 3 4 5 6 7 8 9
             (7.0, 1.9, I)                            (7.0, 1.0, A)          ( 4-  6)
```

c. One time during the third year of life.
```
          1 1       1 2 1 3                        1         1 3       4
          1 2 3 4 5 6 7 8 9                        1 2 3 4 5 6 7 8 9
             (7.0, 1.9, I)                            (7.0, 1.7, A)          ( 7-  9)
```

d. One time during the fourth year of life.
```
          1 1       1 2 1 3                        1 1       1 3 1 3
          1 2 3 4 5 6 7 8 9                        1 2 3 4 5 6 7 8 9
             (7.0, 1.9, I)                            (7.0, 1.6, A)          (10- 12)
```

e. One time during the fifth year of life.
```
          1 1       1 2 1 3                        2         3 1 3
          1 2 3 4 5 6 7 8 9                        1 2 3 4 5 6 7 8 9
             (7.0, 1.9, I)                            (7.0, 1.2, A)          (13- 15)
```

2. Fine motor/visuomotor/problem solving development should be documented at least:

a. Three times during the first year of life.
```
          1         2 3 2                          1         2 3 3
          1 2 3 4 5 6 7 8 9                        1 2 3 4 5 6 7 8 9
             (8.0, 1.7, A)                            (8.0, 0.9, A)          (16- 18)
```

b. Two times during the second year of life.
```
          1         1 3 1 3                        1         2 3 2
          1 2 3 4 5 6 7 8 9                        1 2 3 4 5 6 7 8 9
             (7.0, 1.8, A)                            (7.0, 1.1, A)          (19- 21)
```

c. One time during the third year of life.
```
          1 1       1 2 1 3                        1 1       1 3       4
          1 2 3 4 5 6 7 8 9                        1 2 3 4 5 6 7 8 9
             (7.0, 1.9, I)                            (7.0, 1.7, A)          (22- 24)
```

d. One time during the fourth year of life.
```
          1 1       1 2 1 3                        1 1       1 3 1 3
          1 2 3 4 5 6 7 8 9                        1 2 3 4 5 6 7 8 9
             (7.0, 1.9, I)                            (7.0, 1.6, A)          (25- 27)
```

e. One time during the fifth year of life.
```
          1         1 3 1 3                        2         3       4
          1 2 3 4 5 6 7 8 9                        1 2 3 4 5 6 7 8 9
             (7.0, 1.8, A)                            (7.0, 1.3, A)          (28- 30)
```

3. Language development should be documented at least:

a. Three times during the first year of life.
```
          1         4 2 1                          1 1       2 3 2
          1 2 3 4 5 6 7 8 9                        1 2 3 4 5 6 7 8 9
             (7.0, 1.3, A)                            (8.0, 1.0, A)          (31- 33)
```

b. Two times during the second year of life.
```
          1         1 1       3 4                  2         2 3 2
          1 2 3 4 5 6 7 8 9                        1 2 3 4 5 6 7 8 9
             (7.0, 1.8, A)                            (8.0, 1.1, A)          (34- 36)
```

c. One time during the third year of life.
```
          1         1 1       2       4            1         1 3       4
          1 2 3 4 5 6 7 8 9                        1 2 3 4 5 6 7 8 9
             (7.0, 1.1, A)                            (7.0, 1.3, A)          (37- 39)
```

d. One time during the fourth year of life.
```
          1 1       1 3 1 3                        1 1       2 2 3
          1 2 3 4 5 6 7 8 9                        1 2 3 4 5 6 7 8 9
             (7.0, 1.9, I)                            (7.0, 1.7, A)          (40- 42)
```

e. One time during the fifth year of life.
```
          1         2 3 1 3                        1 1       3 2 2
          1 2 3 4 5 6 7 8 9                        1 2 3 4 5 6 7 8 9
             (7.0, 1.7, A)                            (8.0, 1.8, A)          (43- 45)
```

Scales: 1 = low validity or feasibility; 9 = high validity or feasibility.

Chapter 8
QUALITY INDICATORS FOR DEVELOPMENTAL SCREENING

	Validity	Feasibility	
4. Gross motor development should be documented at least:			
a. Three times during the first year of life.	1 2 2 3 1 2 3 4 5 6 7 8 9 (8.0, 1.8, A)	1 1 4 3 1 2 3 4 5 6 7 8 9 (8.0, 0.8, A)	(46- 48)
b. Two times during the second year of life.	1 3 1 3 1 2 3 4 5 6 7 8 9 (7.0, 1.8, A)	2 2 1 4 1 2 3 4 5 6 7 8 9 (8.0, 1.3, A)	(49- 51)
c. One time during the third year of life.	1 3 1 3 1 2 3 4 5 6 7 8 9 (7.0, 1.8, A)	1 1 2 1 4 1 2 3 4 5 6 7 8 9 (8.0, 1.7, A)	(52- 54)
d. One time during the fourth year of life.	1 1 3 3 1 2 3 4 5 6 7 8 9 (7.0, 1.8, I)	1 1 2 1 4 1 2 3 4 5 6 7 8 9 (8.0, 1.8, A)	(55- 57)
e. One time during the fifth year of life.	1 1 5 1 1 2 3 4 5 6 7 8 9 (7.0, 1.3, I)	1 1 3 1 3 1 2 3 4 5 6 7 8 9 (8.0, 1.2, A)	(58- 60)
5. In children with suspected or known developmental delay, a follow-up plan should be documented.	1 1 2 2 1 2 3 4 5 6 7 8 9 (7.0, 1.3, I)	1 1 1 3 1 2 3 4 5 6 7 8 9 (7.0, 1.2, A)	(61- 63)
8. Age 6-12, school performance should be asked about during a health assessment visit.	1 1 1 4 2 1 2 3 4 5 6 7 8 9 (7.0, 1.9, I)	1 1 1 1 3 1 2 3 4 5 6 7 8 9 (8.0, 1.1, A)	(64- 66)

Scales: 1 = low validity or feasibility; 9 = high validity or feasibility.

Chapter 9
QUALITY INDICATORS FOR INSULIN DEPENDENT DIABETES MELLITUS IN
CHILDREN >= 7 YEARS OLD

	Validity	Feasibility	

(DIAGNOSIS)

1. Patients with the diagnosis of diabetes should have the following routine monitoring tests:

a. Glycosylated hemoglobin or fructosomine every 6 months.
   Validity: 1 2 3 4 5 6 7 8 9 (9.0, 0.4, A)
   Feasibility: 1 2 3 4 5 6 7 8 9 (9.0, 0.7, A)   (1- 3)

b. Eye and visual exam if more than 5 years since diagnosis at least once a year.
   Validity: 1 2 3 4 5 6 7 8 9 (8.0, 1.9, I)
   Feasibility: 1 2 3 4 5 6 7 8 9 (8.0, 0.9, A)   (4- 6)

d. Total cholesterol at least once a year.
   Validity: 1 2 3 4 5 6 7 8 9 (6.0, 1.8, I)
   Feasibility: 1 2 3 4 5 6 7 8 9 (8.0, 1.3, A)   (7- 9)

f. Urinalysis or protein in urine at least once a year.
   Validity: 1 2 3 4 5 6 7 8 9 (8.0, 1.3, I)
   Feasibility: 1 2 3 4 5 6 7 8 9 (8.0, 1.4, I)   (10- 12)

g. Examination of feet once a year.
   Validity: 1 2 3 4 5 6 7 8 9 (2.0, 1.1, A)
   Feasibility: 1 2 3 4 5 6 7 8 9 (5.0, 1.9, D)   (13- 15)

h. Measurement of blood pressure every six months.
   Validity: 1 2 3 4 5 6 7 8 9 (4.0, 2.0, D)
   Feasibility: 1 2 3 4 5 6 7 8 9 (8.0, 1.0, I)   (16- 18)

i. Height and weight on growth chart every six months.
   Validity: 1 2 3 4 5 6 7 8 9 (7.0, 1.7, I)
   Feasibility: 1 2 3 4 5 6 7 8 9 (8.0, 0.7, A)   (19- 21)

j. Tanner stage every six months after 10 years old until Tanner stage V.
   Validity: 1 2 3 4 5 6 7 8 9 (7.0, 2.3, I)
   Feasibility: 1 2 3 4 5 6 7 8 9 (5.0, 2.3, I)   (22- 24)

k. Psychosocial assessment at least annually.
   Validity: 1 2 3 4 5 6 7 8 9 (8.0, 1.9, A)
   Feasibility: 1 2 3 4 5 6 7 8 9 (8.0, 1.4, A)   (25- 27)

2. All patients taking insulin should monitor their glucose at home daily.
   Validity: 1 2 3 4 5 6 7 8 9 (8.0, 2.4, I)
   Feasibility: 1 2 3 4 5 6 7 8 9 (6.0, 1.2, I)   (28- 30)

(TREATMENT)

3. All diabetics should receive dietary counseling at least once a year.
   Validity: 1 2 3 4 5 6 7 8 9 (8.0, 0.9, A)
   Feasibility: 1 2 3 4 5 6 7 8 9 (6.0, 1.4, I)   (31- 33)

(FOLLOW-UP)

4. All patients with diabetes should have a follow-up visit at least every 6 months.
   Validity: 1 2 3 4 5 6 7 8 9 (8.0, 1.3, A)
   Feasibility: 1 2 3 4 5 6 7 8 9 (8.0, 0.4, A)   (34- 36)

5. If HgAlc or fructosomine indicates poor control, chart should indicate assessment of compliance and/or change in treatment regimen.
   Validity: 1 2 3 4 5 6 7 8 9 (8.0, 1.4, A)
   Feasibility: 1 2 3 4 5 6 7 8 9 (8.0, 0.7, A)   (37- 39)

Scales: 1 = low validity or feasibility; 9 = high validity or feasibility.

Chapter 10
QUALITY INDICATORS FOR ACUTE DIARRHEAL DISEASE

Indicator	Validity	Feasibility	
1. In all children up to age 3 presenting with acute diarrhea, history should be obtained regarding:			
a. The date of onset or duration of diarrheal stools.	1 2 3 4 5 6 7 8 9 (9.0, 1.7, A)	1 2 3 4 5 6 7 8 9 (8.0, 0.8, A)	(1- 3)
b. Stool consistency and frequency (e.g., number per day).	1 2 3 4 5 6 7 8 9 (8.0, 1.7, I)	1 2 3 4 5 6 7 8 9 (7.0, 1.1, I)	(4- 6)
c. Presence or absence of blood in the stool.	1 2 3 4 5 6 7 8 9 (8.0, 1.9, I)	1 2 3 4 5 6 7 8 9 (7.0, 1.2, I)	(7- 9)
d. Presence or absence of fever, as reported by the parent.	1 2 3 4 5 6 7 8 9 (7.0, 1.6, I)	1 2 3 4 5 6 7 8 9 (7.0, 1.0, A)	(10- 12)
e. Presence or absence of vomiting.	1 2 3 4 5 6 7 8 9 (9.0, 1.6, A)	1 2 3 4 5 6 7 8 9 (8.0, 0.9, A)	(13- 15)
f. Frequency or volume of fluid intake.	1 2 3 4 5 6 7 8 9 (8.0, 1.6, I)	1 2 3 4 5 6 7 8 9 (6.0, 1.6, I)	(16- 18)
g. Frequency of urinary output.	1 2 3 4 5 6 7 8 9 (8.0, 1.4, A)	1 2 3 4 5 6 7 8 9 (7.0, 1.0, I)	(19- 21)
3. The weight should be recorded and, if available, compared to a recent weight obtained prior to the onset of diarrhea.	1 2 3 4 5 6 7 8 9 (9.0, 1.1, A)	1 2 3 4 5 6 7 8 9 (9.0, 0.3, A)	(22- 24)
4. Documentation should also include:			
a. Heart rate.	1 2 3 4 5 6 7 8 9 (4.0, 1.7, I)	1 2 3 4 5 6 7 8 9 (5.0, 1.8, I)	(25- 27)
b. Respiratory rate.	1 2 3 4 5 6 7 8 9 (4.0, 1.2, I)	1 2 3 4 5 6 7 8 9 (5.0, 1.8, I)	(28- 30)
c. Blood pressure.	1 2 3 4 5 6 7 8 9 (6.0, 1.3, I)	1 2 3 4 5 6 7 8 9 (6.0, 1.6, I)	(31- 33)
d. Temperature.	1 2 3 4 5 6 7 8 9 (5.0, 1.8, I)	1 2 3 4 5 6 7 8 9 (8.0, 1.6, I)	(34- 36)
e. Capillary refill.	1 2 3 4 5 6 7 8 9 (4.0, 2.1, D)	1 2 3 4 5 6 7 8 9 (5.0, 2.3, D)	(37- 39)
5. At least two of the following findings regarding hydration status should be recorded:			
a. General condition, appearance of the eyes, presence or absence of tears, degree of oral moisture, degree of thirst, degree of skin turgor, or condition of anterior fontanelle.	1 2 3 4 5 6 7 8 9 (9.0, 1.7, I)	1 2 3 4 5 6 7 8 9 (8.0, 1.2, I)	(40- 42)
6. The exam should note the presence or absence of blood in the stools, either by visual inspection or by chemical means.	1 2 3 4 5 6 7 8 9 (7.0, 1.9, I)	1 2 3 4 5 6 7 8 9 (6.0, 1.2, I)	(43- 45)

Scales: 1 = low validity or feasibility; 9 = high validity or feasibility.

Chapter 10
QUALITY INDICATORS FOR ACUTE DIARRHEAL DISEASE

Validity

Feasibility

7. The assessment of hydration status should be recorded in
terms of percent dehydration or fluid deficit in milliliters per
kilogram or as:
- not dehydrated (less than 50 milliliters per kilogram fluid
  deficit),
- mild-moderate dehydration (50-100 milliliters per kilogram
  fluid deficit), or
- severe dehydration (greater than 100 milliliters per
  kilogram fluid deficit).

```
                1       3         5
          1 2 3 4 5 6 7 8 9
          (9.0, 1.8, I)
```
```
                        1       3           5
                  1 2 3 4 5 6 7 8 9
                  (9.0, 1.8, I)
```
(46- 48)

8. Serum electrolytes should have been obtained if the child's
dehydration was severe.
```
              2 1 5
          1 2 3 4 5 6 7 8 9
          (9.0, 1.3, A)
```
```
            1   2 2 4
          1 2 3 4 5 6 7 8 9
          (8.0, 0.9, A)
```
(49- 51)

9. Urinalysis should be ordered if the child's dehydration was
severe.
```
          2 2 1 1
          1 2 3 4 5 6 7 8 9
          (4.0, 1.8, D)
```
```
          2 2 2 1         1
          1 2 3 4 5 6 7 8 9
          (3.0, 1.7, I)
```
(52- 54)

10. Fecal leukocytes should have been obtained if the child with
diarrhea is less than 36 months of age and had fever or blood in
the stool.
```
                  6 3
          1 2 3 4 5 6 7 8 9
          (7.0, 0.3, A)
```
```
          1       2 5     1
          1 2 3 4 5 6 7 8 9
          (7.0, 0.9, I)
```
(55- 57)

11. Stool culture should be obtained if the child with diarrhea
is less than 36 months of age and had fever or blood in the
stool or > 5 fecal leukocytes per high power field.
```
                2 2 5
          1 2 3 4 5 6 7 8 9
          (9.0, 0.7, A)
```
```
          1           1 1 6
          1 2 3 4 5 6 7 8 9
          (9.0, 1.0, A)
```
(58- 60)

12. A stool examination for ova and parasites should be obtained
if the child had a history of recent travel to a developing
country, acquired or congenital immunocompromise, or exposure to
a potential carrier of parasitic diarrhea.
```
          1 1 3   1 2 1
          1 2 3 4 5 6 7 8 9
          (5.0, 1.7, I)
```
```
          1 1 1 3 2 1
          1 2 3 4 5 6 7 8 9
          (7.0, 1.1, I)
```
(61- 63)

13. If stool was obtained for ova and parasite examination,
three stool samples, obtained on three consecutive days, should
have been ordered.
```
          1 2 1 3 1           1
          1 2 3 4 5 6 7 8 9
          (5.0, 1.6, I)
```
```
          1 4 1 1           2
          1 2 3 4 5 6 7 8 9
          (2.0, 2.0, I)
```
(64- 66)

(TREATMENT)

14. If the child had diarrhea but was not dehydrated, the
practitioner should recommend additional fluid intake beyond
what is normal for the child.
```
              3       3 2
          1 2 3 4 5 6 7 8 9
          (7.0, 1.4, I)
```
```
          1 1       5 1
          1 2 3 4 5 6 7 8 9
          (7.0, 1.2, I)
```
(67- 69)

15. If the child had mild-moderate dehydration and is able to
take p/o fluids, oral rehydration therapy should be prescribed.
```
                  1   2 6
          1 2 3 4 5 6 7 8 9
          (9.0, 0.4, A)
```
```
          1       1 4 3
          1 2 3 4 5 6 7 8 9
          (8.0, 0.8, A)
```
(70- 72)

16. If the child had severe dehydration, intravenous rehydration
should be prescribed.
```
          1       2 5
          1 2 3 4 5 6 7 8 9
          (9.0, 1.1, A)
```
```
          1       1 7
          1 2 3 4 5 6 7 8 9
          (9.0, 0.3, A)
```
(73- 75)

17. If while healthy the child was being breast fed, the health
care provider should advise the parent to continue breast
feeding if the child is able to feed orally.
```
                2 2 5
          1 2 3 4 5 6 7 8 9
          (9.0, 0.7, A)
```
```
          1       2 5 1
          1 2 3 4 5 6 7 8 9
          (8.0, 1.0, I)
```
(76- 78)

18. If while healthy the child was formula fed or weaned, the
health care provider should have instituted refeeding within
twenty-four hours of the onset of hydration therapy if able to
take p/o.
```
          1 2 2 4
          1 2 3 4 5 6 7 8 9
          (8.0, 0.9, A)
```
```
          2 1 1 4 1
          1 2 3 4 5 6 7 8 9
          (8.0, 1.1, I)
```
(79- 81)

Scales: 1 = low validity or feasibility; 9 = high validity or feasibility.

Chapter 10
QUALITY INDICATORS FOR ACUTE DIARRHEAL DISEASE

| | Validity | Feasibility | |

19. Antimicrobial agents should be used in a child with:

a. Suspected or culture-proven shigella.

```
                    1 2 3 3                          3 2 4
1 2 3 4 5 6 7 8 9            1 2 3 4 5 6 7 8 9
    (8.0, 0.8, A)                (8.0, 0.8, A)
```
(82- 84)

b. Salmonella in patients with sickle cell anemia, lymphoma,
leukemia, other immune compromise (acquired or congenital),
positive stool culture for bacterial pathogen and less than 3
months of age, or bacteremia with salmonella and less than 6
months of age.

```
          1 2 2 2 2                      1   2 2 4
1 2 3 4 5 6 7 8 9            1 2 3 4 5 6 7 8 9
    (7.0, 1.1, I)                (8.0, 1.0, A)
```
(85- 87)

c. Giardia with symptoms of greater than 10-14 days duration
and with positive stool ova and parasite examination.

```
        2 1 3 1 2                        1   2 2 1 3
1 2 3 4 5 6 7 8 9            1 2 3 4 5 6 7 8 9
    (7.0, 1.1, I)                (7.0, 1.7, I)
```
(88- 90)

d. Amoeba with positive stool ova and parasite examination.

```
            1 2 2 4                        1 1 4 3
1 2 3 4 5 6 7 8 9            1 2 3 4 5 6 7 8 9
    (8.0, 0.9, A)                (8.0, 0.7, A)
```
(91- 93)

20. Antidiarrheal or antimotility medications are not used in
treatment of diarrhea in a child.

```
1 1       2 3 2                1 2       1 3 2
1 2 3 4 5 6 7 8 9            1 2 3 4 5 6 7 8 9
    (8.0, 1.9, A)                (8.0, 2.4, D)
```
(94- 96)

Scales: 1 = low validity or feasibility; 9 = high validity or feasibility.

Chapter 11
QUALITY INDICATORS FOR FAMILY PLANNING/CONTRACEPTION

	Validity	Feasibility

(SCREENING)

1. A history to determine risk for unintended pregnancy should be taken at a family planning visit on all women. In order to establish risk, the following elements of the history need to be documented:

a. Menstrual status, last menstrual period, or pregnancy test.   (1- 3)

```
            1 2 3 2                      2 4 1 2
1 2 3 4 5 6 7 8 9          1 2 3 4 5 6 7 8 9
   (8.0, 1.4, A)             (7.0, 0.8, A)
```

b. Sexual history (presence or absence of current sexual intercourse).   (4- 6)

```
            1 1 3 3                    1 1 1 2 3
1 2 3 4 5 6 7 8 9          1 2 3 4 5 6 7 8 9
   (8.0, 1.6, A)             (8.0, 1.8, I)
```

c. Current contraceptive practices.   (7- 9)

```
          1 1 2 4                      1   2 4 2
1 2 3 4 5 6 7 8 9          1 2 3 4 5 6 7 8 9
   (8.0, 1.7, A)             (8.0, 1.0, A)
```

d. Desire for pregnancy.   (10- 12)

```
  1 2       3 2            1 1 1   1 3 2
1 2 3 4 5 6 7 8 9          1 2 3 4 5 6 7 8 9
   (7.0, 2.1, I)             (7.0, 1.7, I)
```

e. Past pregnancies   (13- 15)

```
        1 1 3 3                    1 1 4 3
1 2 3 4 5 6 7 8 9          1 2 3 4 5 6 7 8 9
   (8.0, 1.4, A)             (8.0, 0.7, A)
```

(TREATMENT)

2. All adolescent girls at risk for unintended pregnancy (i.e., sexually active) should receive counseling about effective risk reduction for pregnancy.   (16- 18)

```
        1 2 1 4                1 1 1 1 2 3
1 2 3 4 5 6 7 8 9          1 2 3 4 5 6 7 8 9
   (8.0, 1.7, A)             (8.0, 1.6, I)
```

3. The smoking status of all women prescribed combination OCs should be documented in the medical record.   (19- 21)

```
1           4 3              1       2 4 2
1 2 3 4 5 6 7 8 9          1 2 3 4 5 6 7 8 9
   (8.0, 1.3, A)             (8.0, 1.2, I)
```

4. All women who smoke and are prescribed oral contraceptives should be counseled and encouraged to quit smoking.   (22- 24)

```
2 1   1 1 4              1 1       4 2 1
1 2 3 4 5 6 7 8 9          1 2 3 4 5 6 7 8 9
   (8.0, 2.2, I)             (7.0, 1.4, A)
```

5. Women prescribed contraceptives for the first time should have a follow-up visit within one month.   (25- 27)

```
    1 1 1 2 4                1       1 1 3
1 2 3 4 5 6 7 8 9          1 2 3 4 5 6 7 8 9
   (8.0, 1.7, A)             (8.0, 1.2, A)
```

6. Pelvic exam within 1 month of family planning visit.   (28- 30)

```
        3 2 3                    1 2 4 2
1 2 3 4 5 6 7 8 9          1 2 3 4 5 6 7 8 9
   (8.0, 1.4, A)             (8.0, 0.8, A)
```

7. Risks, benefits, alternatives to contraception have been discussed with patient and documented in chart.   (31- 33)

```
1 1 1       2 3            1 1 1 3 1
1 2 3 4 5 6 7 8 9          1 2 3 4 5 6 7 8 9
   (8.0, 2.1, I)             (6.0, 1.4, I)
```

8. Condoms should be made available to all women who are prescribed contraceptives.   (34- 36)

```
1 1 1 2 2 1              2 2 1 1 2 1
1 2 3 4 5 6 7 8 9          1 2 3 4 5 6 7 8 9
   (7.0, 2.0, I)             (6.0, 1.6, I)
```

9. Women who are prescribed contraceptives should have a follow-up every 6 months thereafter.   (37- 39)

```
1 1   3 1 3              1 1     2 3 2
1 2 3 4 5 6 7 8 9          1 2 3 4 5 6 7 8 9
   (7.0, 1.9, A)             (8.0, 1.6, A)
```

Scales: 1 = low validity or feasibility; 9 = high validity or feasibility.

Chapter 12
QUALITY INDICATORS FOR FEVER IN CHILDREN UNDER 3 YEARS OF AGE

	Validity	Feasibility	

(DIAGNOSIS)

1. The diagnosis of fever should be based on a temperature
measurement of 38 degrees centigrade or greater taken at home or
in the medical setting.

```
                    1 2   4 1 1              1     2 1 3 2
          1 2 3 4 5 6 7 8 9        1 2 3 4 5 6 7 8 9      ( 1-  3)
            (7.0, 1.1, I)            (8.0, 1.3, I)
```

2. The health care provider should document if the child had
received an antipyretic and, if so, the time and the dose.

```
              1   2 4 1              1 1 2 3 2
          1 2 3 4 5 6 7 8 9        1 2 3 4 5 6 7 8 9      ( 4-  6)
            (8.0, 1.3, A)            (7.0, 1.1, I)
```

3. The health care provider should document a temperature
measured by oral or rectal thermometry in the medical setting.

```
                    3 3 3              1   1 2 5
          1 2 3 4 5 6 7 8 9        1 2 3 4 5 6 7 8 9      ( 7-  9)
            (8.0, 0.7, A)            (9.0, 0.9, A)
```

(TREATMENT REGARDLESS OF AGE)

4. The child's age should be recorded in the chart.

```
            1     1 2 5              1 2   6
          1 2 3 4 5 6 7 8 9        1 2 3 4 5 6 7 8 9      (10- 12)
            (9.0, 1.2, A)            (9.0, 0.4, A)
```

5. In all children presenting with fever, the following should
be documented:

a. Heart rate.

```
          2 3 1 1   2              1   2 1 1   4
          1 2 3 4 5 6 7 8 9        1 2 3 4 5 6 7 8 9      (13- 15)
            (3.0, 1.4, I)            (7.0, 1.9, I)
```

b. Respiratory rate.

```
          1 1   3 1 2 1              1   2   3 3
          1 2 3 4 5 6 7 8 9        1 2 3 4 5 6 7 8 9      (16- 18)
            (5.0, 1.6, I)            (7.0, 1.6, I)
```

c. Blood pressure.

```
          1 3 1 2 1   1              4 1 1 2         1
          1 2 3 4 5 6 7 8 9        1 2 3 4 5 6 7 8 9      (19- 21)
            (3.0, 1.4, I)            (4.0, 1.6, I)
```

(TREATMENT FOR THE INFANT LESS THAN 28 DAYS OF AGE PRESENTING
WITH FEVER > 38.0)

6. If the infant has fever, a CBC & UA should be obtained.

```
                  2 2 4              2 2 5
          1 2 3 4 5 6 7 8 9        1 2 3 4 5 6 7 8 9      (22- 24)
            (8.0, 1.3, A)            (9.0, 0.7, A)
```

6. If the infant has fever and diarrhea, a fecal leucocyte
should be obtained.

```
          1   1 2 3 2              1 1 2 1 3 1
          1 2 3 4 5 6 7 8 9        1 2 3 4 5 6 7 8 9      (25- 27)
            (8.0, 1.3, A)            (7.0, 1.3, I)
```

6. If the infant has fever, and is not at low risk, the infant
should be hospitalized.

```
            1 1 2 2 3              1   1   3 5
          1 2 3 4 5 6 7 8 9        1 2 3 4 5 6 7 8 9      (28- 30)
            (8.0, 1.4, A)            (9.0, 0.7, A)
```

6. The assessment should document whether or not the infant
appears toxic, i.e., if the infant has signs of sepsis based on:
- lethargy,
- poor perfusion, or
- hypoventilation, hyperventilation, or cyanosis.

```
                  2 2 5              1 4 4
          1 2 3 4 5 6 7 8 9        1 2 3 4 5 6 7 8 9      (31- 33)
            (9.0, 0.7, A)            (8.0, 0.6, A)
```

6. The assessment should include whether or not the infant had
been healthy up to the point of this illness.

```
          1   1 2 1 4              1 1 4 3
          1 2 3 4 5 6 7 8 9        1 2 3 4 5 6 7 8 9      (34- 36)
            (8.0, 1.6, A)            (8.0, 0.7, A)
```

Scales: 1 = low validity or feasibility; 9 = high validity or feasibility.

Chapter 12
QUALITY INDICATORS FOR FEVER IN CHILDREN UNDER 3 YEARS OF AGE

	Validity	Feasibility	

7. If the infant is not at low risk, the assessment should include:

c. Cerebrospinal fluid, gram stain, cell count, cerebrospinal fluid culture studies.
Validity: 1 2 3 4 5 6 7 8 9 (9.0, 1.3, A)
Feasibility: 1 2 3 4 5 6 7 8 9 (9.0, 0.9, A)
(37- 39)

f. Blood culture.
Validity: 1 2 3 4 5 6 7 8 9 (8.0, 1.4, A)
Feasibility: 1 2 3 4 5 6 7 8 9 (9.0, 0.9, A)
(40- 42)

g. Urine culture.
Validity: 1 2 3 4 5 6 7 8 9 (8.0, 1.4, A)
Feasibility: 1 2 3 4 5 6 7 8 9 (9.0, 0.7, A)
(43- 45)

8. If the infant has lower respiratory signs or symptoms not explained by elevated fever, a chest radiograph should be obtained.
Validity: 1 2 3 4 5 6 7 8 9 (8.5, 1.0, A)
Feasibility: 1 2 3 4 5 6 7 8 9 (9.0, 0.6, A)
(46- 48)

9. If the infant has bloody diarrhea or a fecal leukocyte count >= 5 leukocytes per high power field, a stool culture should be obtained.
Validity: 1 2 3 4 5 6 7 8 9 (9.0, 0.7, A)
Feasibility: 1 2 3 4 5 6 7 8 9 (9.0, 1.0, A)
(49- 51)

10. If the infant is nontoxic and at low risk,** then the infant should be treated with empiric antibiotics.
Validity: 1 2 3 4 5 6 7 8 9 (3.0, 1.2, I)
Feasibility: 1 2 3 4 5 6 7 8 9 (8.0, 2.0, I)
(52- 54)

10. If the infant with fever is at low risk and is being managed as an outpatient, the infant's condition should be reassessed in 18-24 hours.
Validity: 1 2 3 4 5 6 7 8 9 (8.0, 1.9, A)
Feasibility: 1 2 3 4 5 6 7 8 9 (7.0, 1.2, I)
(55- 57)

10. The infant who was nontoxic and initially at low risk and was still nontoxic and at low risk on first follow-up should receive another follow-up within 24 hours.
Validity: 1 2 3 4 5 6 7 8 9 (6.0, 2.1, I)
Feasibility: 1 2 3 4 5 6 7 8 9 (6.0, 1.2, I)
(58- 60)

11. If the infant is toxic in appearance (e.g., lethargic; poor perfusion; or marked hypoventilation, hyperventilation, or cyanosis), or at high risk,** then the infant should be treated with empiric parenteral antibiotics pending the culture results.
Validity: 1 2 3 4 5 6 7 8 9 (9.0, 1.4, A)
Feasibility: 1 2 3 4 5 6 7 8 9 (9.0, 0.6, A)
(61- 63)

12. The infant should be treated with parenteral antimicrobials if:
- any culture is positive, the chest radiograph demonstrates effusion,
- the cerebrospinal fluid studies are abnormal,
- the chest radiograph demonstrates an infiltrate,
- cellulitis, soft tissue, bone, joint, or ear infection are present,
Validity: 1 2 3 4 5 6 7 8 9 (9.0, 0.6, A)
Feasibility: 1 2 3 4 5 6 7 8 9 (9.0, 0.3, A)
(64- 66)

- cellulitis, soft tissue, bone, joint, or ear infection are present.
Validity: 1 2 3 4 5 6 7 8 9 (7.0, 2.4, D)
Feasibility: 1 2 3 4 5 6 7 8 9 (7.0, 2.2, D)
(67- 69)

(TREATMENT FOR THE INFANT 28-TO-90 DAYS OF AGE WITH FEVER > 38.0)

13. The assessment should document whether or not the infant appears toxic, i.e., if the infant has signs of sepsis based on:
- lethargy,
- poor perfusion, or
- hypoventilation, hyperventilation, or cyanosis.
Validity: 1 2 3 4 5 6 7 8 9 (8.0, 0.9, A)
Feasibility: 1 2 3 4 5 6 7 8 9 (8.0, 0.8, A)
(70- 72)

Scales: 1 = low validity or feasibility; 9 = high validity or feasibility.

Chapter 12
QUALITY INDICATORS FOR FEVER IN CHILDREN UNDER 3 YEARS OF AGE

	Validity	Feasibility	
14. The assessment should include whether or not the infant had been healthy up to the point of this illness.	1 2 2 3 1 2 3 4 5 6 7 8 9 (8.0, 1.4, A)	1 1 5 2 1 2 3 4 5 6 7 8 9 (8.0, 0.6, A)	(73- 75)
15. All children who present with fever > 38C should receive:			
a. Complete blood count.	1 3 3 2 1 2 3 4 5 6 7 8 9 (7.0, 1.3, A)	2 2 5 1 2 3 4 5 6 7 8 9 (9.0, 0.7, A)	(76- 78)
b. Urinalysis.	3 3 2 1 1 3 3 1 1 2 3 4 5 6 7 8 9 (8.0, 1.2, A)	2 2 5 1 2 3 4 5 6 7 8 9 (9.0, 0.7, A)	(79- 81)
16. If the child has fever and diarrhea, a fecal leucocyte evaluation should be done.	1 3 2 3 1 1 3 3 1 1 2 3 4 5 6 7 8 9 (7.0, 1.2, A)	1 2 2 1 1 2 1 2 3 4 5 6 7 8 9 (6.0, 1.4, I)	(82- 84)
17. If the infant is toxic or at high risk, the infant should be hospitalized.	3 2 3 1 2 3 4 5 6 7 8 9 (8.0, 1.3, A)	2 2 5 1 2 3 4 5 6 7 8 9 (9.0, 0.7, A)	(85- 87)
18. If the infant is toxic or at high risk, the assessment should also include:			
a. Cerebrospinal fluid, gram stain, cell count, cerebrospinal fluid culture studies.	4 1 4 1 2 3 4 5 6 7 8 9 (8.0, 0.9, A)	2 2 5 1 2 3 4 5 6 7 8 9 (9.0, 1.1, A)	(88- 90)
d. Blood culture.	3 1 5 1 2 3 4 5 6 7 8 9 (9.0, 0.8, A)	1 1 7 1 2 3 4 5 6 7 8 9 (9.0, 0.8, A)	(91- 93)
e. Urine culture.	5 4 1 2 3 4 5 6 7 8 9 (7.0, 0.9, A)	1 3 5 1 2 3 4 5 6 7 8 9 (9.0, 1.2, A)	(94- 96)
19. If the infant is not toxic and is at low risk, the infant may be managed as an outpatient. One of the following courses should be followed:			
a. Obtain cerebrospinal fluid for glucose, protein, gram stain, and cell count determination; obtain blood, urine, and cerebrospinal fluid cultures; and, administer intramuscular ceftriaxone or equivalent.	1 2 1 1 1 2 1 1 2 3 4 5 6 7 8 9 (4.0, 1.9, I)	2 1 1 2 2 1 2 3 4 5 6 7 8 9 (7.0, 2.2, I)	(97- 99)
b. Obtain at least a urine culture and withhold antimicrobial treatment.	2 3 2 1 1 1 1 1 1 2 3 4 5 6 7 8 9 (6.0, 1.9, D)	1 1 1 3 2 1 2 3 4 5 6 7 8 9 (8.0, 2.0, I)	(100-102)
20. If the infant with fever is at low risk and is being managed as an outpatient, the infant's condition should be reassessed in 18-24 hours.	2 2 2 2 1 2 3 4 5 6 7 8 9 (7.0, 1.4, I)	1 3 3 2 1 2 3 4 5 6 7 8 9 (8.0, 0.9, A)	(103-105)
21. If the infant who was initially nontoxic and at low risk is still nontoxic at follow-up, then:			
a. Under the first course: - a second dose of ceftriaxone is administered, and - the culture results are reviewed.	2 1 1 2 2 1 1 2 3 4 5 6 7 8 9 (6.0, 2.0, I)	1 2 4 2 1 2 3 4 5 6 7 8 9 (8.0, 1.1, A)	(106-108)
b. Under the second course: - the culture result(s) are reviewed.	1 1 1 1 2 1 1 1 2 3 4 5 6 7 8 9 (6.0, 1.9, I)	1 1 2 3 2 1 2 3 4 5 6 7 8 9 (8.0, 1.3, A)	(109-111)
22. The infant who was nontoxic and initially at low risk and was still nontoxic and at low risk on first follow-up should receive another follow-up within 24 hours.	1 1 2 1 1 2 1 2 3 4 5 6 7 8 9 (5.0, 1.8, I)	1 2 3 1 1 1 2 3 4 5 6 7 8 9 (7.0, 1.2, I)	(112-114)

Scales: 1 = low validity or feasibility; 9 = high validity or feasibility.

Chapter 12
QUALITY INDICATORS FOR FEVER IN CHILDREN UNDER 3 YEARS OF AGE

	Validity	Feasibility

23. If the infant with fever has lower respiratory signs and symptoms not explained by elevated fever, a chest radiograph should be obtained. (115-117)

```
            1   1 4 3                          2 2 5
  1 2 3 4 5 6 7 8 9              1 2 3 4 5 6 7 8 9
     (8.0, 0.8, A)                  (9.0, 0.7, A)
```

24. If the infant with fever has bloody diarrhea or a fecal leukocyte count greater than 5 leukocytes per high power field, a stool culture should be obtained. (118-120)

```
              1 3 5                          1 2 6
  1 2 3 4 5 6 7 8 9              1 2 3 4 5 6 7 8 9
     (9.0, 0.6, A)                  (9.0, 0.4, A)
```

25. If at any point the blood culture is positive, and not felt to be a contaminant, the infant should be hospitalized for parenteral antibiotic treatment appropriate to the specific diagnosis except in the case of bacteremia due to Streptococcus pneumonia. (121-123)

```
    2 2       1 4                    2             7
  1 2 3 4 5 6 7 8 9              1 2 3 4 5 6 7 8 9
     (8.0, 2.4, I)                  (9.0, 1.3, A)
```

26. If at any point the urine culture is positive, and not felt to be a contaminant, the infant should be hospitalized for parenteral antibiotic treatment appropriate to the specific diagnosis except in the case of an afebrile and nontoxic infant. (124-126)

```
    2 1   2     4                      2     2   5
  1 2 3 4 5 6 7 8 9              1 2 3 4 5 6 7 8 9
     (6.0, 2.2, I)                  (9.0, 1.8, A)
```

27. If at any point the cerebrospinal fluid results are abnormal or the cerebrospinal fluid culture is positive, and not felt to be a contaminant, the infant should be hospitalized for parenteral antimicrobial treatment appropriate to the specific diagnosis. (127-129)

```
        1 1       6                        1 2 6
  1 2 3 4 5 6 7 8 9              1 2 3 4 5 6 7 8 9
     (9.0, 1.2, A)                  (9.0, 0.4, A)
```

28. If at any point pneumonia is diagnosed, the infant should be hospitalized for parenteral antimicrobial treatment appropriate to the specific diagnosis. (130-132)

```
    4   2       3                      2 1       5
  1 2 3 4 5 6 7 8 9              1 2 3 4 5 6 7 8 9
     (5.0, 2.2, D)                  (9.0, 2.1, I)
```

29. If at any point cellulitis or a soft tissue, bone, or joint infection is diagnosed, the infant should be hospitalized for parenteral antimicrobial treatment appropriate to the specific diagnosis. (133-135)

```
    1 2     1 1   4                    2     1 1 5
  1 2 3 4 5 6 7 8 9              1 2 3 4 5 6 7 8 9
     (7.0, 2.4, D)                  (9.0, 1.9, I)
```

(TREATMENT FOR THE CHILD 3 TO 36 MONTHS OF AGE)

30. The assessment should document:

a. Level of consciousness. (136-138)

```
        1   1 3   4                        1 2 1 4
  1 2 3 4 5 6 7 8 9              1 2 3 4 5 6 7 8 9
     (7.0, 1.4, A)                  (8.0, 1.3, I)
```

f. Perfusion. (139-141)

```
      1   1 1 3 2 1                      1 1 3 2 2
  1 2 3 4 5 6 7 8 9              1 2 3 4 5 6 7 8 9
     (7.0, 1.2, I)                  (6.0, 1.2, I)
```

g. Degree of cyanosis. (142-144)

```
      2 1   1 2 2 1                  1 2     2 1 1 1 1
  1 2 3 4 5 6 7 8 9              1 2 3 4 5 6 7 8 9
     (7.0, 1.8, I)                  (5.0, 1.9, D)
```

31. If the infant/child is at high risk for sepsis,** the infant should be hospitalized. (145-147)

```
    2     3 1 3                      2         1 1 5
  1 2 3 4 5 6 7 8 9              1 2 3 4 5 6 7 8 9
     (7.0, 1.4, A)                  (9.0, 1.2, A)
```

32. If the infant/child is at high risk for sepsis,** the assessment should include a complete blood count; urinalysis; cerebrospinal fluid analysis of glucose & protein; gram stain, and cell count; and, + blood, urine, and cerebrospinal fluid cultures. (148-150)

```
      1   1 2 5                          1 2 6
  1 2 3 4 5 6 7 8 9              1 2 3 4 5 6 7 8 9
     (9.0, 0.9, A)                  (9.0, 0.4, A)
```

Scales: 1 = low validity or feasibility; 9 = high validity or feasibility.

Chapter 12
QUALITY INDICATORS FOR FEVER IN CHILDREN UNDER 3 YEARS OF AGE

	Validity	Feasibility
33. If the infant/child is at low risk for sepsis** and the temperature is greater than or equal to 39C and there is no obvious source of infection, a urine culture should be obtained if the child is a female less than two years of age or a male less than six months of age, or uncircumcised male < 2 years. (151-153)	1 1 1 4 2 1 2 3 4 5 6 7 8 9 (8.0, 1.4, A)	1 2 2 4 1 2 3 4 5 6 7 8 9 (8.0, 1.2, A)
34. If the infant/child is at low risk for sepsis** and the temperature is greater than or equal to 39C and diarrhea is present, a stool culture should be obtained if there is blood and mucus in the stool or if there are 35 leukocytes per high power field in the stool. (154-156)	1 4 4 1 2 3 4 5 6 7 8 9 (8.0, 0.6, A)	1 3 5 1 2 3 4 5 6 7 8 9 (9.0, 0.6, A)
35. If the infant/child is at low risk for sepsis** and the temperature is greater than or equal to 39C, a chest radiograph should be obtained in a child with dyspnea, tachypnea, rales, or decreased breath sounds. (157-159)	2 1 2 2 2 1 2 3 4 5 6 7 8 9 (7.0, 2.0, I)	1 3 4 1 2 3 4 5 6 7 8 9 (8.0, 1.3, A)
36. If the infant/child is at low risk for sepsis** and the temperature is greater than or equal to 39C, then: b. The child should be treated empirically with parenteral antibiotics. (160-162)	2 1 2 2 1 2 3 4 5 6 7 8 9 (3.0, 1.2, I)	1 1 11 14 1 2 3 4 5 6 7 8 9 (7.0, 2.2, I)
37. If the infant/child is at low risk for sepsis** and the temperature is greater than or equal to 39C, then: - a blood culture should be obtained, if WBC is greater than or equal to 15,000, - a CBC should be obtained, and - (if the WBC is greater than or equal to 15,000) the child should be treated with antibiotics. (163-165)	2 2 2 2 1 1 2 3 4 5 6 7 8 9 (3.0, 2.2, D)	1 1 1 1 3 1 1 2 3 4 5 6 7 8 9 (7.0, 2.3, D)
38. If the infant/child is at low risk for sepsis** and the temperature is greater than or equal to 39C, then the infant/child should be reassessed in 24-48 hours. (166-168)	2 1 2 2 1 2 3 4 5 6 7 8 9 (6.0, 2.2, I)	5 2 1 1 2 3 4 5 6 7 8 9 (7.0, 1.1, A)
39. If the infant/child at low risk for sepsis** with an initial temperature greater than or equal to 39C, is well-appearing at follow-up, no further intervention is required; but, the parent should be advised to return if the fever persists greater than 48 hous. (169-171)	1 1 1 3 2 1 1 2 3 4 5 6 7 8 9 (7.0, 1.8, I)	2 1 1 2 3 1 2 3 4 5 6 7 8 9 (8.0, 1.3, I)
40. If at any point the blood culture is positive, and not felt to be a contaminant, the infant/child should be hospitalized for parenteral antibiotic treatment appropriate to the specific diagnosis except in the case of bacteremia due to Streptococcus pneumonia. (172-174)	2 1 2 1 3 1 2 3 4 5 6 7 8 9 (7.0, 2.2, I)	1 1 1 6 1 2 3 4 5 6 7 8 9 (9.0, 1.2, A)
41. If at any point the urine culture is positive, and not felt to be a contaminant, the infant/child should be hospitalized for parenteral antibiotic treatment appropriate to the specific diagnosis except in the case of an afebrile, nontoxic infant/child. (175-177)	2 1 2 1 1 2 1 2 3 4 5 6 7 8 9 (4.0, 2.4, D)	1 1 2 5 1 2 3 4 5 6 7 8 9 (9.0, 1.8, A)

Scales: 1 = low validity or feasibility;   9 = high validity or feasibility.

Chapter 12
QUALITY INDICATORS FOR FEVER IN CHILDREN UNDER 3 YEARS OF AGE

	Validity	Feasibility	

42. If at any point the cerebrospinal fluid results are abnormal
or the cerebrospinal fluid culture is positive, and not felt to
be a contaminant, the infant/child should be hospitalized for
parenteral antimicrobial treatment appropriate to the specific
diagnosis.   (178-180)

```
          1          1  7                    1          1  8
        1 2 3 4 5 6 7 8 9                  1 2 3 4 5 6 7 8 9
         (9.0, 0.9, A)                      (9.0, 0.2, A)
```

43. If at any point pneumonia is diagnosed, the infant/child
should be hospitalized for parenteral antimicrobial treatment
appropriate to the specific diagnosis.   (181-183)

```
        4 2 1   2                          2 1 1   1   1 2 1
        1 2 3 4 5 6 7 8 9                  1 2 3 4 5 6 7 8 9
         (2.0, 1.2, A)                      (5.0, 2.8, D)
```

44. If at any point cellulitis or a soft tissue, bone or joint
infection is diagnosed, the infant/child should be hospitalized
for parenteral antimicrobial treatment appropriate to the
specific diagnosis.   (184-186)

```
        2 1 2   2      1 1                 1 1 1 1        3 2
        1 2 3 4 5 6 7 8 9                  1 2 3 4 5 6 7 8 9
         (3.0, 2.2, I)                      (8.0, 2.7, D)
```

44. If at any point cellulitis or a soft tissue, bone or joint
infection is diagnosed, the infant/child should be hospitalized
for parenteral antimicrobial treatment appropriate to the
specific diagnosis.   (187-189)

```
        1 1   2   1 4                      1 1   1   3 4
        1 2 3 4 5 6 7 8 9                  1 2 3 4 5 6 7 8 9
         (8.0, 2.1, I)                      (8.0, 1.2, A)
```

Scales: 1 = low validity or feasibility; 9 = high validity or feasibility.

Chapter 13
QUALITY INDICATORS FOR HEADACHE

(DIAGNOSIS)

	Validity	Feasibility	

1. All patients with new onset headache should be asked about:

a. Location of the pain (e.g., frontal, bilateral).
```
          1 1           2 2 3                    1                 4 4
        1 2 3 4 5 6 7 8 9                      1 2 3 4 5 6 7 8 9
          (8.0, 1.7, A)                          (8.0, 0.9, A)
```
(1- 3)

b. Associated symptoms (e.g., aura).
```
            1   2 3 2                              1             4 4
        1 2 3 4 5 6 7 8 9                      1 2 3 4 5 6 7 8 9
          (8.0, 1.3, A)                          (8.0, 0.9, A)
```
(4- 6)

c. Temporal profile (e.g., new onset, constant).
```
            1   2 3 2                          1   1 1 3 4
        1 2 3 4 5 6 7 8 9                      1 2 3 4 5 6 7 8 9
          (8.0, 1.3, A)                          (8.0, 0.8, A)
```
(7- 9)

d. Severity.
```
          1     2 1 3 2                          1             5 3
        1 2 3 4 5 6 7 8 9                      1 2 3 4 5 6 7 8 9
          (8.0, 1.4, I)                          (8.0, 0.7, A)
```
(10- 12)

e. Family history.
```
          1 1 1 1 3 2                              2   5 2
        1 2 3 4 5 6 7 8 9                      1 2 3 4 5 6 7 8 9
          (8.0, 1.6, I)                          (8.0, 0.7, A)
```
(13- 15)

f. Risk factors or symptoms of depression.
```
        1 2 2 1 2 1                            2       3 3 1
        1 2 3 4 5 6 7 8 9                      1 2 3 4 5 6 7 8 9
          (5.0, 1.7, D)                          (6.0, 1.3, I)
```
(16- 18)

2. All patients with new onset headache should have an examination evaluating the:

a. Cranial nerves.
```
        2     1   2 2 2                        1       2   1 3 2
        1 2 3 4 5 6 7 8 9                      1 2 3 4 5 6 7 8 9
          (7.0, 2.2, I)                          (8.0, 1.8, I)
```
(19- 21)

b. Fundi.
```
          1     3 2 1                          1       1 2   3 2
        1 2 3 4 5 6 7 8 9                      1 2 3 4 5 6 7 8 9
          (7.0, 1.2, A)                          (8.0, 1.1, I)
```
(22- 24)

c. Deep tendon reflexes.
```
          1   3 2 1                            1     3 2 1 1
        1 2 3 4 5 6 7 8 9                      1 2 3 4 5 6 7 8 9
          (6.0, 1.4, I)                          (6.5, 1.2, I)
```
(25- 27)

d. Visual fields.
```
        1   1 1 1 4       1                    1 1   1 1 1 2 1 2
        1 2 3 4 5 6 7 8 9                      1 2 3 4 5 6 7 8 9
          (7.0, 1.4, I)                          (7.0, 1.9, I)
```
(28- 30)

e. Visual acuity.
```
        1     1 4 1 1 1                        1             5 1 2
        1 2 3 4 5 6 7 8 9                      1 2 3 4 5 6 7 8 9
          (7.0, 1.4, I)                          (7.0, 1.1, A)
```
(31- 33)

f. Extraocular movement.
```
        1   1 1 4 1 1 1                        1       2   2 2 2
        1 2 3 4 5 6 7 8 9                      1 2 3 4 5 6 7 8 9
          (7.0, 1.3, I)                          (7.0, 1.7, I)
```
(34- 36)

g. Blood pressure.
```
          1   3 2 2                              2       4 3
        1 2 3 4 5 6 7 8 9                      1 2 3 4 5 6 7 8 9
          (7.0, 1.3, A)                          (8.0, 0.6, A)
```
(37- 39)

Scales: 1 = low validity or feasibility; 9 = high validity or feasibility.

Chapter 13
QUALITY INDICATORS FOR HEADACHE

	Validity	Feasibility	

3. CT or MRI scanning is indicated in patients with new onset headache and any of the following circumstances:

a. Abnormal neurological examination.
Validity: 1 1 1 1 5 / 1 1 1 1 — 1 2 3 4 5 6 7 8 9 (9.0, 1.3, A)
Feasibility: 1 1 2 5 / 1 1 4 1 — 1 2 3 4 5 6 7 8 9 (9.0, 0.8, A)
(40- 42)

b. Constant headache.
Validity: 1 4 4 — 1 2 3 4 5 6 7 8 9 (6.0, 1.7, I)
Feasibility: 2 1 2 2 1 3 — 1 2 3 4 5 6 7 8 9 (7.0, 1.4, I)
(43- 45)

c. Severe headache.
Validity: 1 1 1 3 2 — 1 2 3 4 5 6 7 8 9 (4.0, 1.1, A)
Feasibility: 1 3 2 2 1 — 1 2 3 4 5 6 7 8 9 (6.0, 1.3, I)
(46- 48)

d. Migraine that is always on the same side.
Validity: 2 1 1 1 3 2 — 1 2 3 4 5 6 7 8 9 (6.0, 1.6, I)
Feasibility: 1 2 4 2 — 1 2 3 4 5 6 7 8 9 (6.0, 1.1, I)
(49- 51)

e. Morning headache with vomiting.
Validity: 1 3 5 — 1 2 3 4 5 6 7 8 9 (7.0, 1.9, I)
Feasibility: 1 2 6 — 1 2 3 4 5 6 7 8 9 (8.0, 1.4, I)
(52- 54)

4. Skull X-rays should not be part of an evaluation for headache.
Validity: 1 3 5 — 1 2 3 4 5 6 7 8 9 (9.0, 0.6, A)
Feasibility: 1 2 6 — 1 2 3 4 5 6 7 8 9 (9.0, 0.4, A)
(55- 57)

(TREATMENT)

5. If the patient has an acute mild migraine or tension headache, he or she should receive aspirin, tylenol, other non-steroidal anti-inflammatory agents, isometheptic compound (Midrin), or an ergot preparation.
Validity: 1 2 5 — 1 2 3 4 5 6 7 8 9 (9.0, 0.5, A)
Feasibility: 1 5 2 — 1 2 3 4 5 6 7 8 9 (8.0, 0.4, A)
(58- 60)

6. If the patient has an acute moderate or severe migraine headache, he or she should receive one of the following before being prescribed any other agent:

a. Parenteral ketorolac.
Validity: 1 1 2 2 1 — 1 2 3 4 5 6 7 8 9 (7.0, 1.9, I)
Feasibility: 1 2 4 1 — 1 2 3 4 5 6 7 8 9 (7.0, 0.8, I)
(61- 63)

b. Parenteral dihydroergotamine.
Validity: 3 3 1 — 1 2 3 4 5 6 7 8 9 (7.5, 1.4, A)
Feasibility: 1 2 4 1 — 1 2 3 4 5 6 7 8 9 (7.0, 0.8, I)
(64- 66)

c. Parenteral phenothiazines.
Validity: 1 4 2 1 — 1 2 3 4 5 6 7 8 9 (7.0, 1.2, A)
Feasibility: 1 2 4 1 — 1 2 3 4 5 6 7 8 9 (7.0, 0.8, I)
(67- 69)

d. Sumatriptan.
Validity: 4 2 2 — 1 2 3 4 5 6 7 8 9 (7.5, 0.8, A)
Feasibility: 1 6 1 — 1 2 3 4 5 6 7 8 9 (7.0, 0.4, A)
(70- 72)

e. Solumedrol.
Validity: 1 1 2 1 2 — 1 2 3 4 5 6 7 8 9 (3.0, 1.9, I)
Feasibility: 1 1 2 3 — 1 2 3 4 5 6 7 8 9 (6.0, 1.1, I)
(73- 75)

f. Butorphanol.
Validity: 1 2 1 1 1 1 — 1 2 3 4 5 6 7 8 9 (5.0, 2.1, I)
Feasibility: 3 3 1 — 1 2 3 4 5 6 7 8 9 (7.0, 1.0, I)
(76- 78)

Scales: 1 = low validity or feasibility;   9 = high validity or feasibility.

Chapter 13
QUALITY INDICATORS FOR HEADACHE

	Validity	Feasibility

8. If a patient has more than 2 moderate to severe migraine
headaches each month, then prophylactic treatment may be used
with one of the following agents:

```
                                          Validity                 Feasibility

a. Beta blockers.                       2 3 4                     4 1 4          ( 79- 81)
                              1 2 3 4 5 6 7 8 9         1 2 3 4 5 6 7 8 9
                                (8.0, 0.7, A)             (8.0, 0.9, A)
                                      4 2 2                     5 1 2

b. Calcium channel blockers.          4 2 2                     5 1 2          ( 82- 84)
                              1 2 3 4 5 6 7 8 9         1 2 3 4 5 6 7 8 9
                                (7.5, 0.8, A)             (7.0, 0.6, A)
                                  1 3 2 2                     5 1 2

c. Tricyclic antidepressants.       1 3 2 2                     5 1 2          ( 85- 87)
                              1 2 3 4 5 6 7 8 9         1 2 3 4 5 6 7 8 9
                                (7.5, 0.9, A)             (7.0, 0.6, A)
                                      5 1 2                     1 1 4

e. Fluoxitene.                        5 1 2                     1 1 4          ( 88- 90)
                              1 2 3 4 5 6 7 8 9         1 2 3 4 5 6 7 8 9
                                (7.0, 0.6, A)             (7.0, 0.9, A)
                                  1 4 2 1                       6 2

f. Valproate.                     1 4 2 1                       6 2            ( 91- 93)
                              1 2 3 4 5 6 7 8 9         1 2 3 4 5 6 7 8 9
                                (7.0, 0.6, A)             (7.0, 0.5, A)
                                      5 1 2                 1 4 1 2

g. Cyproheptadine.                    5 1 2                 1 4 1 2            ( 94- 96)
                              1 2 3 4 5 6 7 8 9         1 2 3 4 5 6 7 8 9
                                (7.0, 0.6, A)             (7.0, 0.8, A)
                                  1 1 3 2                   1 2 2 3

9. Opioid agonists and barbiturates should not be first-line
therapy for migraine or tension headaches.
                                  1 1 3 2                   1 2 2 3            ( 97- 99)
                              1 2 3 4 5 6 7 8 9         1 2 3 4 5 6 7 8 9
                                (8.0, 1.5, A)             (8.0, 1.0, A)
                                  1 4 1 2                 1 1 3 2 1

10. Sumatriptan and ergotamine should not be concurrently
administered.
                                  1 4 1 2                 1 1 3 2 1            (100-102)
                              1 2 3 4 5 6 7 8 9         1 2 3 4 5 6 7 8 9
                                (7.0, 0.9, A)             (7.0, 0.9, A)
                                  1 2 3 1                   1 2 2 1

11. Sumatriptan should not be used for hemiplegic migraines.
                                  1 2 3 1                   1 2 2 1            (103-105)
                              1 2 3 4 5 6 7 8 9         1 2 3 4 5 6 7 8 9
                                (8.0, 1.3, A)             (7.0, 1.6, A)
```

Scales: 1 = low validity or feasibility; 9 = high validity or feasibility.

Chapter 14
QUALITY INDICATORS FOR IMMUNIZATIONS

	Validity	Feasibility	

Polio

1. All children should have had two OPV/IPV between six weeks and the first birthday.*
Validity: 1 2 3 4 5 6 7 8 9 (9.0, 0.8, A) [1 1 6]
Feasibility: 1 2 3 4 5 6 7 8 9 (9.0, 0.3, A) [1 1 7]
(1- 3)

2. All children should have had three OPV/IPV between six weeks and the second birthday.*
Validity: 1 2 3 4 5 6 7 8 9 (9.0, 0.8, A) [1 1 6]
Feasibility: 1 2 3 4 5 6 7 8 9 (9.0, 0.4, A) [1 2 6]
(4- 6)

3. All children should have had four OPV/IPV between six weeks and the seventh birthday.*
Validity: 1 2 3 4 5 6 7 8 9 (9.0, 0.8, A) [1 1 6]
Feasibility: 1 2 3 4 5 6 7 8 9 (9.0, 0.4, A) [1 2 6]
(7- 9)

4. Children with immunocompromise (hematologic and solid tumors, congenital immunodeficiency, and long-term immunosuppressive therapy) or HIV infection should receive IPV rather than OPV (at the same ages as OPV).
Validity: 1 2 3 4 5 6 7 8 9 (9.0, 1.0, A) [1 1 2 5]
Feasibility: 1 2 3 4 5 6 7 8 9 (9.0, 1.6, A) [1 1 1 6]
(10- 12)

5. Before each OPV, guardians should be questioned about the presence of an immunocompromised contact in the household.
Validity: 1 2 3 4 5 6 7 8 9 (9.0, 1.6, A) [1 1 2 5]
Feasibility: 1 2 3 4 5 6 7 8 9 (5.0, 1.6, I) [2 1 4 1 1]
(13- 15)

6. If there is a household contact with immunocompromise, children should receive IPV instead of OPV.
Validity: 1 2 3 4 5 6 7 8 9 (9.0, 0.9, A) [1 1 6]
Feasibility: 1 2 3 4 5 6 7 8 9 (8.0, 2.4, D) [2 1 1 4]
(16- 18)

Diphtheria/Tetanus/Pertussis

7. All children should have had three DTP between six weeks and the first birthday.*
Validity: 1 2 3 4 5 6 7 8 9 (9.0, 0.7, A) [1 2 6]
Feasibility: 1 2 3 4 5 6 7 8 9 (9.0, 0.2, A) [2 7]
(19- 21)

8. All children should have had four DTP between six weeks and the second birthday, with at least six months between the third and fourth dose (the fourth may be DTaP if given after 15 months old).*
Validity: 1 2 3 4 5 6 7 8 9 (9.0, 0.8, A) [1 1 6]
Feasibility: 1 2 3 4 5 6 7 8 9 (9.0, 0.4, A) [1 2 6]
(22- 24)

9. All children should have had five DTP/DTaP between six weeks and the seventh birthday, with at least six weeks between the third and fourth doses (the fourth and fifth may be DTaP if given after 15 months).*
Validity: 1 2 3 4 5 6 7 8 9 (9.0, 0.8, A) [1 1 6]
Feasibility: 1 2 3 4 5 6 7 8 9 (9.0, 0.4, A) [1 2 6]
(25- 27)

10. By age 17, all children should have had one Td between age 7 and 17.
Validity: 1 2 3 4 5 6 7 8 9 (9.0, 0.7, A) [1 1 2 6]
Feasibility: 1 2 3 4 5 6 7 8 9 (9.0, 0.2, A) [2 7]
(28- 30)

11. Children who have had encephalopathy within 7 days of a prior dose of DTP should not receive any further vaccination with DTP.
Validity: 1 2 3 4 5 6 7 8 9 (9.0, 0.9, A) [1 1 2 5]
Feasibility: 1 2 3 4 5 6 7 8 9 (8.0, 1.4, A) [3 1 4]
(31- 33)

Haemophilus influenzae type B

12. All children should have had two PRP-OMP Hib or three Hib (any combination of formulations) between six weeks and the first birthday.*
Validity: 1 2 3 4 5 6 7 8 9 (9.0, 0.6, A) [1 1 7]
Feasibility: 1 2 3 4 5 6 7 8 9 (9.0, 0.3, A) [3 6]
(34- 36)

13. Between the ages of six weeks and 2 years, all children should have had either:
- four Hib vaccinations, or
- three Hib vaccinations if the first two were PRP-OMB Hib.*
Validity: 1 2 3 4 5 6 7 8 9 (9.0, 0.7, A) [1 1 7]
Feasibility: 1 2 3 4 5 6 7 8 9 (9.0, 0.4, A) [1 2 6]
(37- 39)

Scales: 1 = low validity or feasibility; 9 = high validity or feasibility.

Chapter 14
QUALITY INDICATORS FOR IMMUNIZATIONS

Measles/Mumps/Rubella

	Validity	Feasibility	
14. All children should have had one MMR between their first and second birthdays.*	1 1 7 1 2 3 4 5 6 7 8 9 (9.0, 0.8, A)	1 2 6 1 2 3 4 5 6 7 8 9 (9.0, 0.4, A)	(40- 42)
15. All children should have had a second MMR before their thirteenth birthday.*	1 1 6 1 2 3 4 5 6 7 8 9 (9.0, 1.1, A)	1 2 1 5 1 2 3 4 5 6 7 8 9 (9.0, 1.0, A)	(43- 45)
16. Children who are immunocompromised (with the exception of children with HIV infection) (hematologic and solid tumors, congenital immunodeficiency, and long-term immunosuppressive therapy) should not receive MMR.	1 1 7 1 2 3 4 5 6 7 8 9 (9.0, 0.7, A)	1 1 7 1 2 3 4 5 6 7 8 9 (9.0, 0.8, A)	(46- 48)

Hepatitis B

	Validity	Feasibility	
17. The mother's HBsAg status should be documented in the child's chart within one week of birth.	1 6 1 2 3 4 5 6 7 8 9 (9.0, 1.4, A)	1 1 3 2 2 1 2 3 4 5 6 7 8 9 (7.0, 1.2, A)	(49- 51)
18. All children whose mothers are known to be HBsAg-Negative should have had at least two HBV by the first birthday with at least one month between the first two doses.*	1 1 2 4 1 2 3 4 5 6 7 8 9 (8.0, 1.4, A)	1 2 2 4 1 2 3 4 5 6 7 8 9 (8.0, 1.2, I)	(52- 54)
19. All children whose mothers are known to be HBsAg-Negative should have had three HBV by the second birthday with at least one month between the first two doses.*	1 1 1 5 1 2 3 4 5 6 7 8 9 (9.0, 1.4, A)	1 2 2 4 1 2 3 4 5 6 7 8 9 (8.0, 1.2, I)	(55- 57)
20. All children whose mothers are known to be HBsAg-Positive at birth should receive HBIG and HBV by the beginning of the twelfth hour of life.	1 7 1 2 3 4 5 6 7 8 9 (9.0, 1.0, A)	1 1 2 5 1 2 3 4 5 6 7 8 9 (9.0, 0.8, A)	(58- 60)
21. All children whose mothers are known to be HBsAg-Positive should have had three HBV by the beginning of the ninth month of life.*	1 1 6 1 2 3 4 5 6 7 8 9 (9.0, 1.1, A)	1 3 5 1 2 3 4 5 6 7 8 9 (9.0, 0.6, A)	(61- 63)
22. All children whose mother's HBsAg status is not known should receive HBV by the beginning of the twelfth hour of life.	1 1 2 4 1 1 2 3 4 5 6 7 8 9 (8.0, 1.4, A)	1 3 3 2 1 2 3 4 5 6 7 8 9 (8.0, 0.9, A)	(64- 66)
23. All children whose mother's HBsAg status is not known by the end of the first week of life should receive HBIG.	1 1 1 2 2 1 1 2 3 4 5 6 7 8 9 (7.0, 1.7, I)	1 1 1 3 2 1 1 2 3 4 5 6 7 8 9 (7.0, 1.2, I)	(67- 69)
24. Adolescents with any of the following risk factors should recieve the full three-part HBV series within one year of the clinician becoming aware of the risk factor: - have a history of sexually transmitted infection, - have had more than one sexual partner in the previous six months, - use injection drugs, - are males who are sexually active with other males, - are sexual contacts of high-risk individuals, or - have tasks as employees, volunteers, or trainees that involve contact with blood or blood-contaminated body fluids.	1 2 5 1 2 3 4 5 6 7 8 9 (9.0, 1.3, A)	1 2 3 1 2 3 4 5 6 7 8 9 (7.0, 1.1, I)	(70- 72)

Scales: 1 = low validity or feasibility; 9 = high validity or feasibility.

Chapter 14
QUALITY INDICATORS FOR IMMUNIZATIONS

	Validity	Feasibility	

Influenza

25. Children with asthma and other chronic pulmonary diseases, hemodynamically significant cardiac disease, hemoglobinopathies (e.g., sickle cell disease) or undergoing immunosuppresssive therapy should receive a yearly influenza vaccine. Other children at high risk may also benefit from an annual influenza vaccine, including those with: HIV infection, diabetes mellitus, chronic renal disease, and chronic metabolic diseases.

```
            3 1 5                1 2 1 5
1 2 3 4 5 6 7 8 9      1 2 3 4 5 6 7 8 9
   (9.0, 0.8, A)          (9.0, 0.9, A)
```
(73- 75)

General Indicators

26. An inquiry should be made before each new set of immunizations (or after each prior set) about reactions to prior vaccines.

```
          1 2 5              1 1 2 1 2 2
1 2 3 4 5 6 7 8 9      1 2 3 4 5 6 7 8 9
   (9.0, 1.2, A)          (7.0, 1.6, I)
```
(76- 78)

27. Children who have had an anaphylactic reaction to a prior vaccine should not receive that vaccine again.

```
            1 8                      2 7
1 2 3 4 5 6 7 8 9      1 2 3 4 5 6 7 8 9
   (9.0, 0.1, A)          (9.0, 0.2, A)
```
(79- 81)

28. Each immunization given at that institution should be documented with the date of administration, manufacturer, lot number, and name of health care provider administering the vaccine.

```
        1 2   5            1   3 1 4
1 2 3 4 5 6 7 8 9      1 2 3 4 5 6 7 8 9
   (9.0, 1.6, A)          (8.0, 1.1, A)
```
(82- 84)

Catch-Up Immunizations

29. Children at least 8 months old but less than 5 years old who are behind on their immunizations should have received a total of three OPV/IPV, four DTP/DTaP/Td, three Hib, three HBV, and one MMR within one year of the first visit with the provider.

```
      2 1 1 4              1 2 2 3 1
1 2 3 4 5 6 7 8 9      1 2 3 4 5 6 7 8 9
   (8.0, 1.7, I)          (7.0, 1.0, I)
```
(85- 87)

30. Children at least 5 years old but less than 7 years old who are behind on their immunizations should have received a total of three OPV/IPV, four DTP/DTaP/Td, three HBV, and one MMR within one year of the first visit with the provider.

```
      3 1 1 3              1 1   3 3 1
1 2 3 4 5 6 7 8 9      1 2 3 4 5 6 7 8 9
   (7.0, 1.7, I)          (7.0, 1.1, A)
```
(88- 90)

31. Children who are at least 7 years old but less than 18 years old and who are behind on their immunizations should have received a total of three OPV/IPV, three Td, and two MMR within one year of the first visit with the provider.

```
    1 2 1 1 3              1 1   4 2 1
1 2 3 4 5 6 7 8 9      1 2 3 4 5 6 7 8 9
   (7.0, 1.8, I)          (7.0, 1.0, A)
```
(91- 93)

Prior Immunization Record

32. For children less than five years old who are new to the practice, there should be a notation of prior immunization history or a notation of an effort to obtain such information (e.g., parent will call in or bring it to next visit, letter will be sent to prior provider) at the first visit.

```
        1 2   5            2 1 1 5
1 2 3 4 5 6 7 8 9      1 2 3 4 5 6 7 8 9
   (9.0, 1.3, A)          (9.0, 1.4, I)
```
(94- 96)

33. If a prior immunization record for a child less than five years old has not been obtained within six months of the first visit, the child should be given catch-up immunizations.

```
      1 2 2 3              1 2 2 1 3
1 2 3 4 5 6 7 8 9      1 2 3 4 5 6 7 8 9
   (8.0, 1.6, A)          (7.0, 1.2, I)
```
(97- 99)

Scales: 1 = low validity or feasibility; 9 = high validity or feasibility.

Chapter 15
QUALITY INDICATORS FOR OTITIS MEDIA, AGES 1-3

A. OTITIS MEDIA WITH EFFUSION (SEROUS OTITIS MEDIA)

(DIAGNOSIS)

1. All patients with the diagnosis of suspected otitis media with effusion should be evaluated with pneumatic otoscopy. (1- 3)

	Validity	Feasibility
Distribution	1 1 1 1 3 2	1 1 3 1 2 1
Scale	1 2 3 4 5 6 7 8 9	1 2 3 4 5 6 7 8 9
Summary	(8.0, 2.1, I)	(3.0, 1.7, I)

2. Patients with persistent (>3 months duration) bilateral otitis media with effusion should have a hearing evaluation. (4- 6)

	Validity	Feasibility
Distribution	1 1 3 1 3	1 1 1 2 3 1
Scale	1 2 3 4 5 6 7 8 9	1 2 3 4 5 6 7 8 9
Summary	(7.0, 1.1, A)	(7.0, 1.6, I)

(TREATMENT)

3. All patients with the diagnosis of otitis media with effusion should receive either:
- antibiotics, or
- trial of observation. (7- 9)

	Validity	Feasibility
Distribution	6 1 2	5 1 3
Scale	1 2 3 4 5 6 7 8 9	1 2 3 4 5 6 7 8 9
Summary	(7.0, 0.6, A)	(7.0, 0.8, A)

4. For all patients with a diagnosis of otitis media with effusion, during the initial management period (up to 12 weeks), myringotomy with or without insertion of tympanostomy tubes should not be performed in an otherwise healthy child (no other complications). (10- 12)

	Validity	Feasibility
Distribution	1 3 5	2 2 5
Scale	1 2 3 4 5 6 7 8 9	1 2 3 4 5 6 7 8 9
Summary	(9.0, 0.6, A)	(9.0, 0.7, A)

5. All patients with the diagnosis of otitis media with effusion and a bilateral hearing loss (defined as 20 decibels hearing threshold level or worse in both ears) documented in the record, should have tymp tubes inserted. (13- 15)

	Validity	Feasibility
Distribution	1 1 3 2 1	1 2 1 2 2 1
Scale	1 2 3 4 5 6 7 8 9	1 2 3 4 5 6 7 8 9
Summary	(7.0, 1.6, I)	(6.0, 2.0, D)

6. Patients with persistent otitis media with effusion (at least 3 months duration) and hearing loss (bilateral hearing deficits of 20 decibels hearing threshold or worse) should receive:
a. One of the following:
- oral antibiotic therapy if child has not been on antibiotics,
- if on antibiotics, a change in antibiotics, or
- bilateral myringotomy with tube placement. (16- 18)

	Validity	Feasibility
Distribution	1 2 1 2 3	1 3 1 4
Scale	1 2 3 4 5 6 7 8 9	1 2 3 4 5 6 7 8 9
Summary	(8.0, 1.7, I)	(8.0, 1.0, A)

b. Environmental risk factor control counseling. (19- 21)

	Validity	Feasibility
Distribution	2 1 2 3	2 1 3 2 1
Scale	1 2 3 4 5 6 7 8 9	1 2 3 4 5 6 7 8 9
Summary	(7.0, 1.6, I)	(5.0, 1.3, I)

7. Management of patients with otitis media with effusion for 4-6 months and a history of significant bilateral hearing loss (at least 20 decibels) and a failure of adequate antibiotic therapy should include:

a. Bilateral myringotomy with tube placement. (22- 24)

	Validity	Feasibility
Distribution	1 3 1 2	1 1 5 2
Scale	1 2 3 4 5 6 7 8 9	1 2 3 4 5 6 7 8 9
Summary	(7.0, 1.6, I)	(7.0, 0.8, A)

b. Environmental risk factor counseling. (25- 27)

	Validity	Feasibility
Distribution	1 1 2 2 1	1 3 2 1 2
Scale	1 2 3 4 5 6 7 8 9	1 2 3 4 5 6 7 8 9
Summary	(7.0, 1.8, I)	(6.0, 1.2, I)

(FOLLOW-UP)

8. All patients identified as having otitis media with effusion must either have a recommendation for follow-up visit or have been seen for reevaluation within 12 weeks of diagnosis. (28- 30)

	Validity	Feasibility
Distribution	2 1 2 3 1	1 1 2 2 3
Scale	1 2 3 4 5 6 7 8 9	1 2 3 4 5 6 7 8 9
Summary	(7.0, 1.1, I)	(8.0, 1.1, A)

Scales: 1 = low validity or feasibility; 9 = high validity or feasibility.

Chapter 15
QUALITY INDICATORS FOR OTITIS MEDIA, AGES 1-3

	Validity	Feasibility

B. ACUTE OTITIS MEDIA

(DIAGNOSIS)

1. All children presenting to the clinician with fever,
nonspecific behavioral changes (e.g., irritability, lethargy,
decreased appetite, vomiting, diarrhea), or ear pain should
receive an ear examination using a pneumatic otoscope.   (31- 33)

Validity:
```
            1       4 1
1 2 3 4 5 6 7 8 9
(7.0, 2.1, D)
```

Feasibility:
```
1 2 1 1 1       1 1 1
1 2 3 4 5 6 7 8 9
(4.0, 2.3, D)
```

(TREATMENT)

2. For all patients with the diagnosis of acute otitis media, at
least 10 days of antibiotics should be prescribed.   (34- 36)

Validity:
```
1   1 5         1   1
1 2 3 4 5 6 7 8 9
(5.0, 1.3, I)
```

Feasibility:
```
                1 1 3 1 3
1 2 3 4 5 6 7 8 9
(7.0, 1.1, A)
```

(FOLLOW-UP)

3. Once a diagnosis of acute otitis media is made, follow-up
chart review should document a return visit after the course of
antibiotics within 8 weeks of diagnosis.   (37- 39)

Validity:
```
1 1 2 1 1 1 1 1 1
1 2 3 4 5 6 7 8 9
(4.0, 1.9, I)
```

Feasibility:
```
        2       4       2
1 2 3 4 5 6 7 8 9
(7.0, 1.4, I)
```

Scales: 1 = low validity or feasibility;   9 = high validity or feasibility.

Chapter 17
QUALITY INDICATORS FOR SICKLE CELL SCREENING AND SELECT
TOPICS IN PREVENTION OF COMPLICATIONS

(SCREENING)

	Validity	Feasibility	
1. All children in states with mandatory newborn sickle cell testing should be screened before hospital discharge or within 48 hours of birth, whichever comes first.	1 1 1 3 3 1 2 3 4 5 6 7 8 9 (8.0, 1.6, A)	1 2 2 4 1 2 3 4 5 6 7 8 9 (8.0, 1.0, A)	(1- 3)
2. In states without mandatory newborn sickle cell screening, African-American children should be tested for sickle cell disease by the end of the third month of life.	1 1 1 1 5 1 2 3 4 5 6 7 8 9 (9.0, 1.8, A)	2 2 5 1 2 3 4 5 6 7 8 9 (9.0, 1.3, A)	(4- 6)
3. Children with a positive sickle screen at less than or equal to one month of age should have a repeat screen after one month of age and prior to the end of six months of age.	1 1 6 1 2 3 4 5 6 7 8 9 (9.0, 1.7, A)	1 1 2 5 1 2 3 4 5 6 7 8 9 (9.0, 0.9, A)	(7- 9)
PREVENTION OF COMPLICATIONS			
4. Children with a positive sickle screen or children suspected of being positive for sickle cell disease should be placed on daily penicillin prophylaxis from at least six months of age until at least five years of age.	1 3 5 1 2 3 4 5 6 7 8 9 (9.0, 0.6, A)	1 2 2 2 1 2 3 4 5 6 7 8 9 (7.0, 1.1, I)	(10- 12)
5. Children with sickle cell disease should have a hematocrit or hemoglobin, and reticulocyte count performed at least every four months.	3 2 2 1 1 2 3 4 5 6 7 8 9 (6.0, 1.3, I)	1 1 4 2 1 1 2 3 4 5 6 7 8 9 (6.0, 1.0, I)	(13- 15)
6. Children with sickle cell disease should have received the pneumococcal vaccine between 2 years and 3 years of age.	1 1 1 2 4 1 2 3 4 5 6 7 8 9 (8.0, 1.6, A)	1 1 5 2 1 2 3 4 5 6 7 8 9 (8.0, 0.7, A)	(16- 18)
7. A new patient older than 3 years with sickle cell disease should have documention at the first visit of a prior pneumococcal vaccine or be vaccinated within one month of the first visit.	1 2 2 3 1 2 3 4 5 6 7 8 9 (8.0, 1.4, A)	1 2 1 2 3 1 2 3 4 5 6 7 8 9 (8.0, 1.2, I)	(19- 21)

Scales: 1 = low validity or feasibility;   9 = high validity or feasibility.

Chapter 18
QUALITY INDICATORS FOR TUBERCULOSIS SCREENING

1. By the time a child is four months old, there should be documentation of whether or not the child has tuberculosis risk factors* or documentation that the child has had a Mantoux test. (1- 3)

Validity:
```
        1 1 1 4       1
1 2 3 4 5 6 7 8 9, I
(6.0, 1.7, I)
```
Feasibility:
```
            2 3 2 2
1 2 3 4 5 6 7 8 9, A
(5.0, 0.9, A)
```

3. If a child has any of the TB risk factors listed below, he/she should receive an annual Mantoux skin test within one week of documenting the risk factor:

a. has abnormalities on chest X-ray suggestive of TB. (4- 6)

Validity:
```
        1 1 1     5
1 2 3 4 5 6 7 8 9, A
(9.0, 1.7, A)
```
Feasibility:
```
        1     3 1 4
1 2 3 4 5 6 7 8 9, A
(8.0, 1.1, A)
```

b. has clinical evidence of TB. (7- 9)

Validity:
```
        1 1       2     5
1 2 3 4 5 6 7 8 9, A
(9.0, 2.1, A)
```
Feasibility:
```
          4 1 4
1 2 3 4 5 6 7 8 9, A
(8.0, 0.9, A)
```

c. has HIV-infection, Hodgkin's disease, lymphoma, diabetes mellitus, chronic renal failure, malnutrition, or another immunosuppressive condition. (10- 12)

Validity:
```
        1 1 2 1 3
1 2 3 4 5 6 7 8 9, I
(7.0, 1.8, I)
```
Feasibility:
```
        1 1 1   3
1 2 3 4 5 6 7 8 9, A
(8.0, 1.0, A)
```

d. has had contact with an adult/adolescent with confirmed or suspected infectious TB. (13- 15)

Validity:
```
          1 4 3
1 2 3 4 5 6 7 8 9, A
(7.0, 1.4, A)
```
Feasibility:
```
          1 5 1 2
1 2 3 4 5 6 7 8 9, A
(7.0, 0.7, A)
```

e. has emigrated from, has traveled to, or has significant contact with indigenous persons from a region of the world with high TB prevalance. (16- 18)

Validity:
```
          1 3 2 1
1 2 3 4 5 6 7 8 9, A
(7.0, 1.4, A)
```
Feasibility:
```
          1 3   3 1
1 2 3 4 5 6 7 8 9, A
(7.5, 0.9, A)
```

3. Children who have been frequently exposed to adults or adolescents who are HIV-infected, homeless, users of injection and other street drugs, poor and medically-indigent city dwellers, incarcerated, institutionalized, residents of nursing homes, or migrant farm workers, should be Mantoux tested at least every 3 years. (19- 21)

Validity:
```
        1 1 3 1 2
1 2 3 4 5 6 7 8 9, I
(7.0, 1.6, I)
```
Feasibility:
```
        1 1 2 2 1
1 2 3 4 5 6 7 8 9, I
(7.0, 1.2, I)
```

4. Children with immunodeficiency or HIV-infection should have anergy testing (e.g., Candida or Mumps antigen) at the same time as TB testing. (22- 24)

Validity:
```
          2 3 3
1 2 3 4 5 6 7 8 9, A
(8.0, 1.3, A)
```
Feasibility:
```
          5 2 2
1 2 3 4 5 6 7 8 9, A
(7.0, 0.7, A)
```

5. Mantoux skin tests in children with risk factors should be read by a health professional or other trained personnel within 48-72 hours. (25- 27)

Validity:
```
        2     3 3
1 2 3 4 5 6 7 8 9, I
(8.0, 1.6, I)
```
Feasibility:
```
        1     3 2 3
1 2 3 4 5 6 7 8 9, A
(8.0, 1.2, A)
```

6. Results of tuberculin skin tests in children with risk factors should be documented within 96 hours of placing the test. (28- 30)

Validity:
```
        1 1 1 1 4
1 2 3 4 5 6 7 8 9, I
(8.0, 1.9, I)
```
Feasibility:
```
        1 3 1 2 2
1 2 3 4 5 6 7 8 9, I
(7.0, 1.2, I)
```

7. All Mantoux skin tests read as positive should document that there was induration and should document the diameter of the induration in milimeters. (31- 33)

Validity:
```
        1     2 5
1 2 3 4 5 6 7 8 9, A
(9.0, 1.3, A)
```
Feasibility:
```
        1     3 5
1 2 3 4 5 6 7 8 9, A
(9.0, 0.8, A)
```

8. A Mantoux skin test with greater than or equal to 15 mm should be read as positive. (34- 36)

Validity:
```
      1     1 6
1 2 3 4 5 6 7 8 9, A
(9.0, 1.0, A)
```
Feasibility:
```
      2     1 6
1 2 3 4 5 6 7 8 9, A
(9.0, 0.6, A)
```

8. A child with HIV infection should be Mantoux tested annually for TB. (37- 39)

Validity:
```
        1 1 1 2 4
1 2 3 4 5 6 7 8 9, A
(8.0, 1.6, A)
```
Feasibility:
```
        3 1   5
1 2 3 4 5 6 7 8 9, A
(9.0, 0.8, A)
```

8. An initial Mantoux test should be performed prior to initiation of immunosuppressive therapy. (40- 42)

Validity:
```
        1 2 2 3
1 2 3 4 5 6 7 8 9, A
(8.0, 1.7, A)
```
Feasibility:
```
        1 3 1 4
1 2 3 4 5 6 7 8 9, A
(8.0, 1.0, A)
```

Scales: 1 = low validity or feasibility; 9 = high validity or feasibility.

panelist 10; round 2;

Chapter 18
QUALITY INDICATORS FOR TUBERCULOSIS SCREENING

	Validity	Feasibility

9. A Mantoux skin test should be read as positive if there is
induration that is at least 10 mm in a child who:
- is less than 4 years old,
- has other medical risk factors for developing TB disease
  (Hodgkin's disease, lymphoma, diabetes mellitus, chronic
  renal failure, malnutrition),
- who was born, or whose parents were born, in regions of the
  world where TB is highly prevalent, or who have traveled to
  such regions, or
- who is frequently exposed to adults who are HIV-infected,
  homeless, users of intravenous and other street drugs, poor
  and medically indigent city dwellers, residents of nursing
  homes, incarcerated or institutionalized persons, and migrant
  farm workers.

```
                    1 1   2 4            1   1 2 3 2
          1 2 3 4 5 6 7 8 9      1 2 3 4 5 6 7 8 9     ( 43- 45)
            (8.0, 1.9, I)         (8.0, 1.2, A)
```

10. A Mantoux skin test should be read as positive if there is
induration that is at least 5 mm in a child who:
- is in close contact with someone with a known or suspected
  infectious case of TB (households with active or previously
  active cases), if treatment cannot be verified as adequate
  before exposure, treatment was initiated after the period of
  the child's contact began, or reactivation is suspected,
- is suspected of having TB disease clinically or by chest
  X-ray, or
- has an immunosuppressive condition (including HIV infection)
  or is receiving immunosuppressive treatment.

```
                1       3 4                1 2 3 3
          1 2 3 4 5 6 7 8 9      1 2 3 4 5 6 7 8 9     ( 46- 48)
            (8.0, 1.4, A)         (8.0, 0.8, A)
            1 4 1 2                1 1 2 3 2
          1 2 3 4 5 6 7 8 9      1 2 3 4 5 6 7 8 9     ( 49- 51)
            (7.0, 1.2, A)         (8.0, 1.0, A)
```

11. All children with positive Mantoux skin tests should have a
chest x-ray within two weeks.

```
            1     1 4 3                1 1 3 4
          1 2 3 4 5 6 7 8 9      1 2 3 4 5 6 7 8 9     ( 52- 54)
            (8.0, 1.1, A)         (8.0, 0.8, A)
```

12. Children with a positive Mantoux test and negative chest
x-ray and no other symptoms of TB should receive prophylaxis
with INH and/or Rifampin.

```
            1   2 3   2                2 5   2
          1 2 3 4 5 6 7 8 9      1 2 3 4 5 6 7 8 9     ( 55- 57)
            (7.0, 1.8, I)         (7.0, 0.9, A)
```

13. Children with a positive Mantoux test and negative chest
x-ray and no other symptoms of TB, whose presumed index case
(source of infection) has TB resistant to INH and Rifampin,
should have a referral made to an infectious disease specialist.

```
            1 1 1 1 4 1                2 3 3 1
          1 2 3 4 5 6 7 8 9      1 2 3 4 5 6 7 8 9     ( 58- 60)
            (8.0, 1.4, I)         (7.0, 0.8, A)
```

14. Prophylaxis with INH should be given for 9 months to
asymptomatic children without HIV and 12 months to asymptomatic
children with HIV.

```
            1 1 3 2   1                1   3 4   1
          1 2 3 4 5 6 7 8 9      1 2 3 4 5 6 7 8 9     ( 61- 63)
            (5.0, 1.4, I)         (6.0, 1.0, A)
```

15. Children receiving TB chemoprophylaxis should see a
clinician at least once every 5 weeks during therapy.

Scales: 1 = low validity or feasibility; 9 = high validity or feasibility.

Chapter 19
QUALITY INDICATORS FOR UPPER RESPIRATORY INFECTIONS

Validity   Feasibility

(DIAGNOSIS)

Pharyngitis

1. All patients with sore throat should be asked about presence or absence of fever.   (1- 3)
Validity: 1 4 1 1 2 / 1 2 3 4 5 6 7 8 9 (5.0, 1.6, I)
Feasibility: 1 3 2 3 / 1 2 3 4 5 6 7 8 9 (7.0, 1.2, I)

2. All patients with sore throat should be asked about nasal symptoms.   (4- 6)
Validity: 1 1 3 1 / 1 2 3 4 5 6 7 8 9 (5.0, 1.7, I)
Feasibility: 1 1 4 1 1 / 1 2 3 4 5 6 7 8 9 (7.0, 1.4, I)

3. Children with sore throat should have their temperature measured.   (7- 9)
Validity: 1 2 2 1 2 / 1 2 3 4 5 6 7 8 9 (6.0, 2.0, I)
Feasibility: 1 1 1 3 2 / 1 2 3 4 5 6 7 8 9 (8.0, 1.7, I)

4. If a rapid streptococcal test is negative, a culture should be sent within 24 hours.   (10- 12)
Validity: 1 1 2 2 2 / 1 2 3 4 5 6 7 8 9 (7.0, 2.3, D)
Feasibility: 1 1 4 2 / 1 2 3 4 5 6 7 8 9 (7.0, 1.7, I)

5. Diagnosis of GABHS, N. gonorrhoeae, or C. haemolyticum by gram stain in the absence of culture or rapid test is not appropriate.   (13- 15)
Validity: 1 3 1 2 1 / 1 2 3 4 5 6 7 8 9 (5.0, 4.0, I)
Feasibility: 1 / 1 2 3 4 5 6 7 8 9 (5.0, 4.0, I)

Bronchitis/Cough

5. The history of patients presenting with cough of less than 3 weeks duration should document presence or absence of preceding viral infection (e.g., common cold, influenza).   (16- 18)
Validity: 1 3 1 2 1 / 1 2 3 4 5 6 7 8 9 (4.0, 1.4, I)
Feasibility: 1 2 2 3 1 / 1 2 3 4 5 6 7 8 9 (5.0, 1.9, D)

6. The history of patients presenting with cough of less than 3 weeks duration should document presence or absence of fever and shortness of breath (dyspnea), chest pain.   (19- 21)
Validity: 2 3 1 2 / 1 2 3 4 5 6 7 8 9 (7.0, 1.9, I)
Feasibility: 1 1 3 1 3 / 1 2 3 4 5 6 7 8 9 (7.0, 1.4, A)

7. Patients presenting with acute cough should receive a physical examination of the chest for evidence of pneumonia.   (22- 24)
Validity: 1 1 2 5 / 1 2 3 4 5 6 7 8 9 (9.0, 1.8, I)
Feasibility: 2 1 1 5 / 1 2 3 4 5 6 7 8 9 (9.0, 1.0, A)

8. Patients presenting with acute cough and with evidence of consolidation on physical exam of the chest (dullness to percussion, egophony, etc.) should receive a chest x-ray.   (25- 27)
Validity: 1 1 3 3 / 1 2 3 4 5 6 7 8 9 (8.0, 1.4, A)
Feasibility: 1 2 1 5 / 1 2 3 4 5 6 7 8 9 (9.0, 1.0, A)

Nasal Congestion

9. If a patient presents with the complaint of nasal congestion and/or rhinorrhea not attributed to the common cold, the history should include: seasonality of symptoms, presence or absence of sneezing, facial pain, fever, specific irritants, use of topical nasal decongestants.   (28- 30)
Validity: 1 2 1 2 1 / 1 2 3 4 5 6 7 8 9 (6.0, 2.2, D)
Feasibility: 1 2 3 2 1 / 1 2 3 4 5 6 7 8 9 (4.0, 1.6, I)

Acute Sinusitis

10. If the diagnosis of acute sinusitis is made, symptoms should be present for a duration of less than 3 weeks (e.g., fever, malaise, cough, nasal congestion, purulent nasal discharge, ear pain or blockage, post-nasal drip, dental pain, headache, or facial pain).   (31- 33)
Validity: 1 1 1 1 2 / 1 2 3 4 5 6 7 8 9 (6.0, 2.1, I)
Feasibility: 2 1 2 2 1 1 / 1 2 3 4 5 6 7 8 9 (6.0, 1.7, I)

Scales: 1 = low validity or feasibility; 9 = high validity or feasibility.

Chapter 19
QUALITY INDICATORS FOR UPPER RESPIRATORY INFECTIONS

(TREATMENT)

Pharyngitis

	Validity	Feasibility	

11. Antibiotics should only be prescribed in a patient with nasal congestion and pharyngitis if a rapid strep test or throat culture is obtained, or if there is documentation of other bacterial infections.	`        1 1 3 2 2`
	`1 2 3 4 5 6 7 8 9`
	`(7.0, 1.0, A)`
		`            1 1 2 3`
		`1 2 3 4 5 6 7 8 9`
		`(8.0, 2.1, I)`
			(34- 36)

12. Tetracyclines and sulfonamides should not be used for treating GABHS pharyngitis.	`          1 1 1 6`
	`1 2 3 4 5 6 7 8 9`
	`(9.0, 0.8, A)`
		`              1 2 6`
		`1 2 3 4 5 6 7 8 9`
		`(9.0, 0.4, A)`
			(37- 39)

13. No antibiotics should be used for a patient with a diagnosis of viral pharyngitis (unless antibiotics were prescribed before culture results were obtained).	`1 1 1   1 4`
	`1 2 3 4 5 6 7 8 9`
	`(8.0, 2.7, D)`
		`1 2   1 1 1 2 1`
		`1 2 3 4 5 6 7 8 9`
		`(6.0, 2.1, D)`
			(40- 42)

14. Antibiotics should only be prescribed in a patient with conjunctivitis and pharyngitis if a rapid streptococcal test or throat culture is obtained.	`1 2   2 1   3`
	`1 2 3 4 5 6 7 8 9`
	`(5.0, 2.4, D)`
		`1 1   1   2 1 3`
		`1 2 3 4 5 6 7 8 9`
		`(7.0, 2.0, I)`
			(43- 45)

15. Patients who have had four episodes of documented or presumed and treated strep throat in a one-year period should not have penicillin prescribed for the next episode.	`  2 4 2`
	`1 2 3 4 5 6 7 8 9`
	`(6.0, 1.0, I)`
		`  2   1 4 2`
		`1 2 3 4 5 6 7 8 9`
		`(6.0, 1.0, I)`
			(46- 48)

16. Aspirin should not be used in children and teenagers with pharyngitis.	`1 1   3 2 2`
	`1 2 3 4 5 6 7 8 9`
	`(7.0, 1.6, A)`
		`1 1 1   1 4 1`
		`1 2 3 4 5 6 7 8 9`
		`(7.0, 2.0, D)`
			(49- 51)

17. If a diagnosis of infectious mononucleosis is made, it should be on the basis of a positive heterophil antibody test or other EBV antibody tests.	`    2 3 3`
	`1 2 3 4 5 6 7 8 9`
	`(8.0, 1.2, A)`
		`    1 1 1 6`
		`1 2 3 4 5 6 7 8 9`
		`(9.0, 0.7, A)`
			(52- 54)

Nasal Congestion

	Validity	Feasibility	

20. If topical nasal decongestants are prescribed, duration of treatment should be for no longer than 4 days.	`      3 4 2`
	`1 2 3 4 5 6 7 8 9`
	`(7.0, 1.7, I)`
		`        3 2 2 1`
		`1 2 3 4 5 6 7 8 9`
		`(7.0, 1.2, I)`
			(55- 57)

Acute Sinusitis

	Validity	Feasibility	

21. Treatment for acute sinusitis should be with antibiotics for at least 10 days.	`  2 1 3   2`
	`1 2 3 4 5 6 7 8 9`
	`(7.0, 1.7, I)`
		`          1 4 1 3`
		`1 2 3 4 5 6 7 8 9`
		`(7.0, 0.9, A)`
			(58- 60)

23. In the absence of symptoms of allergic rhinitis (thin, watery rhinorrhea, and sneezing), antihistamines should not be prescribed for acute sinusitis.	`1 1   6   1`
	`1 2 3 4 5 6 7 8 9`
	`(7.0, 1.2, A)`
		`1   1 1 3 1 2`
		`1 2 3 4 5 6 7 8 9`
		`(7.0, 1.3, I)`
			(61- 63)

24. If symptoms fail to improve after 48 hours of antibiotic treatment, clinical re-evaluation and therapy with another antibiotic should be instituted.	`1 3   2 1 1 1`
	`1 2 3 4 5 6 7 8 9`
	`(5.0, 1.7, I)`
		`  2   2 3   1 1`
		`1 2 3 4 5 6 7 8 9`
		`(6.0, 1.4, I)`
			(64- 66)

25. If the patient does not improve after two courses of antibiotics, referal to an otolaryngologist or for a diagnostic test (CT, x-ray, ultrasound of the sinuses) is indicated.	`1 2   1 2 1   1 1`
	`1 2 3 4 5 6 7 8 9`
	`(5.0, 2.1, I)`
		`1   1 1 5   1`
		`1 2 3 4 5 6 7 8 9`
		`(7.0, 1.4, I)`
			(67- 69)

Chronic Sinusitis

	Validity	Feasibility	

26. If a diagnosis of chronic sinusitis is made, the patient should be treated with at least 3 weeks of antibiotics.	`    3 4 1`
	`1 2 3 4 5 6 7 8 9`
	`(6.0, 1.0, A)`
		`1   1 1 5   1`
		`1 2 3 4 5 6 7 8 9`
		`(7.0, 1.0, I)`
			(70- 72)

Scales: 1 = low validity or feasibility; 9 = high validity or feasibility.

panelist 10; round 2:

Chapter 19
QUALITY INDICATORS FOR UPPER RESPIRATORY INFECTIONS

	Validity	Feasibility
27. If patient has repeated symptoms after 2 separate 3 week trials of antibiotics, a referral to an otolaryngologist should be ordered.	1 2 2 3 1 1 2 3 4 5 6 7 8 9 (4.0, 1.8, I)	1 2 1 3 2 1 2 3 4 5 6 7 8 9 (7.0, 1.8, D)	(73- 75)
28. If topical decongestants are prescribed, duration of treatment should be for no longer than 4 days.	1 1 3 4 1 2 3 4 5 6 7 8 9 (7.0, 1.4, A)	1 3 3 2 1 2 3 4 5 6 7 8 9 (7.0, 1.2, I)	(76- 78)
29. In the absence of symptoms of allergic rhinitis (thin, watery rhinorrhea, and sneezing), antihistamines should not be prescribed.	1 1 4 1 1 1 1 2 3 4 5 6 7 8 9 (7.0, 1.6, I)	1 2 2 1 1 2 1 2 3 4 5 6 7 8 9 (6.0, 1.7, I)	(79- 81)

Scales: 1 = low validity or feasibility; 9 = high validity or feasibility.

Chapter 20
QUALITY INDICATORS FOR URINARY TRACT INFECTIONS

(DIAGNOSIS)

	Validity	Feasibility	

1. If an infant or child presents with any of the following symptoms/signs,* either a urine culture should be performed or a urinalysis should be performed; if urinalysis is positive, a urine culture should be performed:

a. Malodorous urine, abnormal urinary stream, or change in urinary stream in an infant or child.

```
Validity                     Feasibility
1 2 3 4 5 6 7 8 9             1 2 3 4 5 6 7 8 9
(7.0, 2.3, I)                 (8.0, 1.3, I)            ( 1- 3)
```

b. Failure to thrive in an infant or child.

```
1 2 3 4 5 6 7 8 9             1 2 3 4 5 6 7 8 9
(8.0, 2.0, I)                 (9.0, 1.2, A)            ( 4- 6)
```

c. Vomiting associated with fever in an infant.

```
1 2 3 4 5 6 7 8 9             1 2 3 4 5 6 7 8 9
(3.0, 1.6, I)                 (6.0, 2.2, I)            ( 7- 9)
```

d. Jaundice associated with fever in a neonate.

```
1 2 3 4 5 6 7 8 9             1 2 3 4 5 6 7 8 9
(8.0, 1.6, A)                 (9.0, 0.9, A)            (10-12)
```

e. Pain/discomfort with urination (dysuria), frequency, urgency, flank pain (unrelated to trauma) in a child.

```
1 2 3 4 5 6 7 8 9             1 2 3 4 5 6 7 8 9
(9.0, 0.8, A)                 (9.0, 0.7, A)            (13-15)
```

f. Hematuria unrelated to trauma in infant or child.

```
1 2 3 4 5 6 7 8 9             1 2 3 4 5 6 7 8 9
(8.0, 1.1, A)                 (9.0, 1.0, A)            (16-18)
```

g. Secondary enuresis in a child.

```
1 2 3 4 5 6 7 8 9             1 2 3 4 5 6 7 8 9
(7.0, 1.1, A)                 (7.0, 1.0, A)            (19-21)
```

2. In order to diagnose UTI, a positive culture from one of the following methods of urine collection is necessary:
- bladder tap,
- catheterization, or
- clean catch.

3. In order to rule out UTI, a negative UA or culture from one of the following methods of urine collection is necessary:
- bladder tap,
- catheterization,
- clean catch, or
- urine bag.

```
1 2 3 4 5 6 7 8 9             1 2 3 4 5 6 7 8 9
(9.0, 1.6, A)                 (9.0, 1.1, A)            (22-24)
```

4. If the culture shows greater than 100,000 colonies/ml urine of a single organism, then the patient should be diagnosed and treated for UTI.

```
1 2 3 4 5 6 7 8 9             1 2 3 4 5 6 7 8 9
(9.0, 1.6, I)                 (9.0, 0.8, A)            (25-27)
```

5. If there is bacterial growth of a single organism with at least 10,000 colonies/ml urine from a catherized specimen, then UTI should be diagnosed and treated.

```
1 2 3 4 5 6 7 8 9             1 2 3 4 5 6 7 8 9
(9.0, 0.6, A)                 (9.0, 0.6, A)            (28-30)
```

6. Growth of 10,000 to 100,000 colonies/ml urine from clean catch should be followed up with a repeat urine culture if the patient has not already been treated.

```
1 2 3 4 5 6 7 8 9             1 2 3 4 5 6 7 8 9
(7.0, 1.7, I)                 (9.0, 1.1, A)            (31-33)
```

7. If there is any bacterial growth from a specimen obtained from a bladder tap then a UTI should be diagnosed and treated.

```
1 2 3 4 5 6 7 8 9             1 2 3 4 5 6 7 8 9
(7.0, 2.0, D)                 (7.0, 2.1, D)            (34-36)
1 2 3 4 5 6 7 8 9             1 2 3 4 5 6 7 8 9
(9.0, 1.0, A)                 (9.0, 0.7, A)            (37-39)
```

Scales: 1 = low validity or feasibility; 9 = high validity or feasibility.

Chapter 20
QUALITY INDICATORS FOR URINARY TRACT INFECTIONS

Scale positions are `1 2 3 4 5 6 7 8 9`. Summary given as (median, mad, agreement).

8. Urine culture must be obtained by clean catch, catheterization, or bladder tap before antibiotics are given. (40- 42)
- Validity: `2 1          1 1 4` → (8.0, 2.4, D)
- Feasibility: `1 1 1        1 1 4` → (8.0, 2.2, I)

(TREATMENT)

9. All infants under 3 months of age with a diagnosis of UTI must initially receive parenteral antibiotics. (43- 45)
- Validity: `1           2   3 3` → (8.0, 1.3, I)
- Feasibility: `1         1 3 4` → (8.0, 0.9, A)

10. Parenteral antibiotics may be switched to oral antibiotics if the infant has had at least 3 days without fever, a negative repeat urine culture, and negative blood and CSF culture. (46- 48)
- Validity: `5 1 1       1       4 3` → (1.0, 1.7, A)
- Feasibility: `1 1     1 1` → (3.0, 2.7, I)

11. Infants with UTI should receive a total of at least 10 days of antibiotics (parenteral and oral). (49- 51)
- Validity: `1 1              4 3` → (8.0, 1.4, A)
- Feasibility: `1 2     4 2` → (8.0, 0.7, A)

11. Children with a diagnosed UTI should be reassessed at 48 hours to determine if there is clinical improvement. (52- 54)
- Validity: `1 1 1 2 1 2` → (7.0, 1.8, I)
- Feasibility: `1 1 1 2 1 3` → (7.5, 1.2, A)

12. Infants with UTI who are not clinically improved should have a repeat urine culture between 48 hours and 72 hours of antibiotic therapy. (55- 57)
- Validity: `1         3 2 2` → (7.0, 1.6, A)
- Feasibility: `3         2 3 1` → (7.0, 1.2, I)

13. Children with UTI and systemic symptoms such as hypotension, poor perfusion, anorexia, or emesis, should be treated initially with IV antibiotics. (58- 60)
- Validity: `1 1     2 5` → (9.0, 1.0, A)
- Feasibility: `1 1     4 3` → (8.0, 0.9, A)

14. If the child is being treated with oral antibiotics and is not clinically improved by 48 hours, either (1) antibiotic sensitivities must be determined, or (2) a repeat culture must be sent. (61- 63)
- Validity: `1 2     2 3` → (8.0, 1.9, I)
- Feasibility: `1     4 1 3` → (6.0, 1.4, I)

15. When antibiotic sensitivities are checked, if the organism is not sensitive to the antibiotic, the antibiotic should be switched to one to which the organism is sensitive within 1 day. (64- 66)
- Validity: `3 2 3` → (6.0, 1.2, I)
- Feasibility: `1 1 3 2 2` → (6.0, 1.0, I)

16. All children with the diagnosis of UTI should receive at least 7 days of antibiotics. (67- 69)
- Validity: `1 1 2 1 3` → (6.0, 2.1, I)
- Feasibility: `1     2 2 4` → (7.0, 1.6, I)

17. All children with the diagnosis of pyelonephritis should be treated initially with parenteral antibiotics. (70- 72)
- Validity: `2 1 1   3   2` → (7.0, 2.7, D)
- Feasibility: `1 4 2 2` → (7.0, 1.3, A)

18. A child with four UTIs in a single year should receive prophylactic antibiotics for at least six months. (73- 75)
- Validity: `1 1 1 3 1 2` → (7.0, 1.8, I)
- Feasibility: `2 1 1 1 2 2` → (7.0, 1.7, I)

Radiologic Work-up

19. Any boy less than 10 years old with a first UTI or with systemic symptoms** (and/or who has not had the following study before) should have a VCUG and one of the following within three months of diagnosis: (76- 78)
- RUS,
- IVP, or
- nuclear medicine renal scan.
- Validity: `3 5` → (9.0, 1.6, A)
- Feasibility: `1   3 1 4` → (8.0, 1.1, A)

Scales: 1 = low validity or feasibility; 9 = high validity or feasibility.

Chapter 20
QUALITY INDICATORS FOR URINARY TRACT INFECTIONS

	Validity	Feasibility	

20. Any girl less than 3 years old with a first UTI or less than
10 years old with systemic symptoms** (and/or who has not had
the following studies before) should have a VCUG or IC and one
of the following within three months of diagnosis:
- RUS,
- IVP, or
- nuclear medicine renal scan.

Validity:
```
        1 1   1 2 2 2
1 2 3 4 5 6 7 8 9
(7.0, 2.0, I)
```
Feasibility:
```
        1   1 1 3 1 2
1 2 3 4 5 6 7 8 9
(7.0, 1.3, I)
```
(79- 81)

21. If a child with a diagnosis of UTI is not improving in 48
hours on therapy, and repeat urine culture is positive despite
appropriate antibiotics, the child should have an evaluation for
urologic obstruction or abscess with renal ultrasound (RUS),
intravenous pyelogram (IVP), or nuclear medicine renal scan
within 24 hours.

Validity:
```
            1 1 5 2
1 2 3 4 5 6 7 8 9
(8.0, 0.6, A)
```
Feasibility:
```
                5 2 2
1 2 3 4 5 6 7 8 9
(7.0, 0.7, A)
```
(82- 84)

22. Children who have a VCUG or IC following a UTI should be on
continuous antibiotics (prophylactic should follow therapeutic
antibiotics) from the beginning of therapy for the UTI until
the time of the study.

Validity:
```
1   2 4 1         2 2 1
1 2 3 4 5 6 7 8 9
(6.0, 1.2, I)
```
Feasibility:
```
1 1           2 2 1   2
1 2 3 4 5 6 7 8 9
(6.0, 1.8, I)
```
(85- 87)

Vesicoureteral Reflux (VUR)

23. Children diagnosed with Grade II or higher VUR should be on
prophylactic antibiotics until the reflux has resolved.

Validity:
```
1 1   2 1 2 1 1
1 2 3 4 5 6 7 8 9
(6.0, 1.9, I)
```
Feasibility:
```
            1   3   1 4
1 2 3 4 5 6 7 8 9
(8.0, 2.0, I)
```
(88- 90)

24. Children with VUR should have annual monitoring with VCUG or
nuclear cystogram.

Validity:
```
1     1 1 2 1 2
1 2 3 4 5 6 7 8 9
(7.0, 2.0, I)
```
Feasibility:
```
            3 1 3 2
1 2 3 4 5 6 7 8 9
(8.0, 1.3, I)
```
(91- 93)

25. Children with high grade (Grade IV or higher) VUR or other
anatomic abnormalities, such as posterior urethral valves,
abnormal urethral implantation, or horse-shoe kidney, should be
referred to a urologist.

Validity:
```
        1 1 1   5
1 2 3 4 5 6 7 8 9
(9.0, 1.6, A)
```
Feasibility:
```
        1   2 1 5
1 2 3 4 5 6 7 8 9
(9.0, 0.9, A)
```
(94- 96)

27. Children with VUR or other anatomic abnormalities who also
have hypertension, decreased renal function, failure to thrive,
or other related signs, should be referred to a pediatric
nephrologist for treatment of renal insufficiency and
hypertension.

Validity:
```
1 1         3 4
1 2 3 4 5 6 7 8 9
(8.0, 1.7, A)
```
Feasibility:
```
1           2 2 4
1 2 3 4 5 6 7 8 9
(8.0, 1.2, A)
```
(97- 99)

Scales: 1 = low validity or feasibility; 9 = high validity or feasibility.

Chapter 21
QUALITY INDICATORS FOR VAGINITIS AND SEXUALLY TRANSMITTED
DISEASES

	Validity	Feasibility	

(DIAGNOSIS)

Vaginitis

1. In sexually active adolescent girls presenting with complaint
of vaginal discharge, the practitioner should perform a speculum
exam to determine the source of discharge. (1- 3)

```
              1 4 3                    3 2 4
1 2 3 4 5 6 7 8 9, A      1 2 3 4 5 6 7 8 9, A
(8.0, 1.1, A)            (8.0, 0.8, A)
```

2. At a minimum, the following tests should be performed on the
vaginal discharge: normal saline wet mount for clue cells and
trichomonds; KOH wet mount for yeast hyphae. (4- 6)

```
            1 4 3                    1 4 3
1 2 3 4 5 6 7 8 9, A      1 2 3 4 5 6 7 8 9, A
(8.0, 0.8, A)            (8.0, 0.8, A)
```

3. A sexual history should be obtained from all women presenting
with a vaginal discharge. The history should include:

a. Number of sexual partners in previous 6 months. (7- 9)

```
          1 1 2 4                  1 2 1 1 2 2
1 2 3 4 5 6 7 8 9, A      1 2 3 4 5 6 7 8 9, I
(8.0, 1.4, A)            (7.0, 1.6, I)
```

b. Absence or presence of symptoms in partners. (10- 12)

```
        1 1 1 3                  1 1 3 1 1 2
1 2 3 4 5 6 7 8 9, A      1 2 3 4 5 6 7 8 9, I
(8.0, 1.2, A)            (5.0, 1.8, I)
```

c. Use of condoms. (13- 15)

```
          1 3 4                  2 1 2 1 3
1 2 3 4 5 6 7 8 9, A      1 2 3 4 5 6 7 8 9, I
(8.0, 1.2, A)            (7.0, 1.3, I)
```

d. Prior history of sexually transmitted diseases. (16- 18)

```
        3 1 2 4                  5 1 1 2
1 2 3 4 5 6 7 8 9, A      1 2 3 4 5 6 7 8 9, I
(8.0, 1.0, A)            (6.0, 1.0, I)
```

4. If three of the following four criteria are met, a diagnosis
of bacterial vaginosis or gardnerella vaginosis should be made:
pH greater than 4.5; positive whiff test; clue cells on wet
mount; thin homogenous discharge. (19- 21)

```
        1 1 3 1 3                2 1 1   2 1 2
1 2 3 4 5 6 7 8 9, A      1 2 3 4 5 6 7 8 9, D
(7.0, 1.4, A)            (6.0, 2.0, D)
```

Cervicitis

5. Routine testing for gonorrhea and chlamydia trachomatis
(culture and antigen detection, respectively) should be
performed with the routine pelvic exam in all adolescent girls. (22- 24)

```
      1 2   2 3                  1 2 1 2 3
1 2 3 4 5 6 7 8 9, I      1 2 3 4 5 6 7 8 9, I
(8.0, 1.9, I)            (8.0, 1.2, I)
```

PID

6. If a patient is given the diagnosis of PID, a speculum and
bimanual pelvic exam should have been performed. (25- 27)

```
        1 3 4                    3 2 4
1 2 3 4 5 6 7 8 9, A      1 2 3 4 5 6 7 8 9, A
(8.0, 1.2, A)            (8.0, 0.8, A)
```

7. If a patient is given the diagnosis of PID, at least 2 of the
following signs should be present on physical exam:
- lower abdominal tenderness,
- adnexal tenderness, or
- cervical motion tenderness. (28- 30)

```
        3 1 4                  1 3   5
1 2 3 4 5 6 7 8 9, A      1 2 3 4 5 6 7 8 9, A
(8.0, 1.4, A)            (9.0, 1.0, A)
```

STDs--General

7. If a patient has symptoms of urethritis, he should at least
be tested for both chlamydia and gonorrhea or receive treatment
for both (per CDC recommendations). (31- 33)

```
                                      9
1 2 3 4 5 6 7 8 9,  )     1 2 3 4 5 6 7 8 9
( , , )                  ( , , )
```

Scales: 1 = low validity or feasibility; 9 = high validity or feasibility.

panelist 10; round 2;   Mon Mar 25 14:22:10 1996

Chapter 21
QUALITY INDICATORS FOR VAGINITIS AND SEXUALLY TRANSMITTED
DISEASES

	Validity	Feasibility	
7. If a patient has evidence of asymptomatic urethritis, he should at least be tested for both chlamydia and gonorrhea or receive treatment for both (per CDC recommendations).	1 2 3 4 5 6 7 8 9	1 2 3 4 5 6 7 8 9	(34- 36)
8. If a patient presents with any STD, HIV testing should be offered.	2 2 4 (,) (,) 1 2 3 4 5 6 7 8 9	3 5 1 (,) (,) 1 2 3 4 5 6 7 8 9 (8.0, 0.4, A)	(37- 39)
9. If a patient presents with any sexually transmitted disease (gonorrhea, chlamydia, trachomatis, herpes, chancroid, syphilis) a non-treponemal test (VDRL or RPR) for syphilis should be obtained.	2 3 3 1 2 3 4 5 6 7 8 9 (8.0, 1.4, I)	4 1 4 1 2 3 4 5 6 7 8 9 (8.0, 0.9, A)	(40- 42)

(TREATMENT)

Vaginitis

	Validity	Feasibility	
10. Treatment for bacterial vaginosis should be with metronidazole (orally or vaginally) or clindamycin (orally or vaginally) per the CDC recommendations.	1 8 1 2 3 4 5 6 7 8 9 (9.0, 0.1, A)	3 6 1 2 3 4 5 6 7 8 9 (9.0, 0.3, A)	(43- 45)
11. Treatment for T. vaginalis should be with oral metronidazole in the absence of allergy to metronidazole.	1 8 1 2 3 4 5 6 7 8 9 (9.0, 0.1, A)	2 7 1 2 3 4 5 6 7 8 9 (9.0, 0.2, A)	(46- 48)
12. Treatment for non-recurrent (three or fewer episodes in previous year) yeast vaginitis should be with topical "azole" preparations (e.g., clotrimazole, butoconazole, etc.) or fluconazole.	1 8 1 2 3 4 5 6 7 8 9 (9.0, 0.1, A)	3 6 1 2 3 4 5 6 7 8 9 (9.0, 0.3, A)	(49- 51)

Cervicitis/Urethritis

	Validity	Feasibility	
13. All patients treated for gonorrhea should also be treated for chlamydia per the CDC recommendations.	1 3 5 1 2 3 4 5 6 7 8 9 (9.0, 0.7, A)	1 2 6 1 2 3 4 5 6 7 8 9 (9.0, 0.4, A)	(52- 54)

PID

	Validity	Feasibility	
14. Patients with PID and any of the following conditions should be hospitalized: - appendicitis, - ectopic pregnancy, - pelvic abscess is present or suspected, - the patient is pregnant, - the patient has HIV infection, - uncontrolled nausea and vomiting, - clinical follow-up within 72 hours of starting antibiotic treatment cannot be arranged, or - the patient does not improve within 72 hours of starting therapy.	1 1 3 3 1 1 2 3 4 5 6 7 8 9 (7.0, 1.4, A)	1 1 2 2 1 2 1 2 3 4 5 6 7 8 9 (7.0, 1.8, I)	(55- 57)
15. Total antibiotic therapy for PID should be for no less than 10 days (inpatient, if applicable, plus outpatient).	1 1 1 2 1 3 1 2 3 4 5 6 7 8 9 (7.0, 1.4, I)	1 2 2 4 1 2 3 4 5 6 7 8 9 (8.0, 0.9, A)	(58- 60)

Genital Ulcers

	Validity	Feasibility	
16. All patients with genital herpes should be counseled regarding reducing the risk of transmission to sexual partners.	1 1 1 3 3 1 2 3 4 5 6 7 8 9 (8.0, 1.1, A)	1 1 1 3 3 1 2 3 4 5 6 7 8 9 (8.0, 1.3, I)	(61- 63)

Scales: 1 = low validity or feasibility; 9 = high validity or feasibility.

Chapter 21
QUALITY INDICATORS FOR VAGINITIS AND SEXUALLY TRANSMITTED
DISEASES

	Validity	Feasibility	

17. In the absence of allergy, patients with chancroid should be treated with azithromycin, ceftriaxone, or erythromycin.   (64- 66)

```
            3 5                      1 3 4
1 2 3 4 5 6 7 8 9        1 2 3 4 5 6 7 8 9
  (9.0, 1.2, A)            (8.0, 1.3, A)
```

18. In the absence of allergy, patients with primary and secondary syphilis should be treated with benzathine penicillin G (IM).   (67- 69)

```
            2 7                        2 7
1 2 3 4 5 6 7 8 9        1 2 3 4 5 6 7 8 9
  (9.0, 0.2, A)            (9.0, 0.2, A)
```

19. If a patient has a primary ulcer consistent with syphilis, treatment for syphilis should be initiated before laboratory test results are received.   (70- 72)

```
          2 2 3                      1 2 6
1 2 3 4 5 6 7 8 9        1 2 3 4 5 6 7 8 9
  (8.0, 1.2, A)            (9.0, 0.4, A)
```

STDs--General

20. Sexual partners of patients with new diagnoses of T. vaginalis, gonorrhea, chlamydia, chancroid, and primary or secondary syphilis should be referred for treatment.   (73- 75)

```
          1 2 5                  2 1 2      3
1 2 3 4 5 6 7 8 9        1 2 3 4 5 6 7 8 9
  (9.0, 0.9, A)            (7.0, 1.7, I)
```

(FOLLOW-UP)

PID

21. Patients receiving outpatient therapy for PID should receive a follow-up visit within 72 hours of diagnosis.   (76- 78)

```
1    1    1 4 2          1    1 2 4    1
1 2 3 4 5 6 7 8 9        1 2 3 4 5 6 7 8 9
  (8.0, 1.4, A)            (7.0, 1.3, I)
```

22. All patients being treated for PID should have a microbiological re-examination (e.g., cultures) within 10 days of completing therapy.   (79- 81)

```
1 1    3 1 2    1        1 1    2 3    1
1 2 3 4 5 6 7 8 9        1 2 3 4 5 6 7 8 9
  (7.0, 2.0, I)            (6.0, 1.8, I)
```

Genital Ulcers

23. Patients receiving treatment for chancroid should be re-examined within 7 days of treatment initiation to assess clinical improvement.   (82- 84)

```
2 1 1    1    2 2        2 1 1 1 1 1    1 1
1 2 3 4 5 6 7 8 9        1 2 3 4 5 6 7 8 9
  (6.0, 2.9, D)            (4.0, 2.3, I)
```

24. Patients with primary or secondary syphilis should be re-examined clinically and serologically within 6 months after treatment.   (85- 87)

```
1 1         3 4              1 1 2 3 2
1 2 3 4 5 6 7 8 9        1 2 3 4 5 6 7 8 9
  (8.0, 1.6, A)            (8.0, 1.2, A)
```

25. Patients with a sexually transmitted disease should have a follow-up within 4 weeks of the diagnosis.   (88- 90)

```
1    1 1 2 1 2              4 1 1 2 1
1 2 3 4 5 6 7 8 9        1 2 3 4 5 6 7 8 9
  (7.0, 2.0, I)            (6.0, 1.3, I)
```

Scales: 1 = low validity or feasibility; 9 = high validity or feasibility.

Chapter 22
QUALITY INDICATORS FOR WELL CHILD CARE

HISTORY AND ANTICIPATORY GUIDANCE

1. The mother's pregnancy and delivery history (e.g., length of pregnancy; illnesses; use of medications; use of alcohol, drugs, or tobacco during pregnancy; complications) should be documented by the end of the first month of life.
Validity: 2 3 3 / 1 2 3 4 5 6 7 8 9 (8.0, 1.3, A)
Feasibility: 1 1 3 4 / 1 2 3 4 5 6 7 8 9 (8.0, 0.9, A)
(1- 3)

3. Discussion of feeding and nutritional issues should be documented at least once during the first two months of life.
Validity: 2 3 3 / 1 2 3 4 5 6 7 8 9 (8.0, 0.9, A)
Feasibility: 1 3 2 1 / 1 2 3 4 5 6 7 8 9 (7.0, 1.0, I)
(4- 6)

4. Discussion of transition to foods other than breast milk or formula should be documented at least once during the first six months of life.
Validity: 1 2 3 3 / 1 2 3 4 5 6 7 8 9 (8.0, 0.9, A)
Feasibility: 1 3 2 1 / 1 2 3 4 5 6 7 8 9 (7.0, 1.0, I)
(7- 9)

7. Discussion of age-appropriate injury prevention (per TIPP) should be documented at least twice during the first year of life.
Validity: 1 3 4 / 1 2 3 4 5 6 7 8 9 (8.0, 0.9, A)
Feasibility: 1 1 2 2 1 2 / 1 2 3 4 5 6 7 8 9 (7.0, 1.0, I)
(10- 12)

8. Discussion of age-appropriate injury prevention (per TIPP) should be documented at least once a year during the second-sixth year of life.
Validity: 1 3 4 / 1 2 3 4 5 6 7 8 9 (8.0, 1.3, A)
Feasibility: 1 1 2 2 1 2 / 1 2 3 4 5 6 7 8 9 (7.0, 1.7, I)
(13- 15)

9. Discussion of age-appropriate injury prevention (per TIPP) should be documented at least once every other year during the seventh-twelfth year of life.
Validity: 1 3 4 / 1 2 3 4 5 6 7 8 9 (8.0, 1.3, A)
Feasibility: 1 1 2 2 1 2 / 1 2 3 4 5 6 7 8 9 (7.0, 1.7, I)
(16- 18)

PHYSICAL EXAMINATION

10. Before discharge from the hospital, the newborn's weight should be documented.
Validity: 2 6 / 1 2 3 4 5 6 7 8 9 (9.0, 0.9, A)
Feasibility: 2 7 / 1 2 3 4 5 6 7 8 9 (9.0, 0.2, A)
(19- 21)

11. The child's weight should be documented at least four times between the end of the first week and the end of the first year of life. This information must either be plotted on a growth curve or be recorded with the age/gender percentile.
Validity: 2 6 / 1 2 3 4 5 6 7 8 9 (9.0, 0.9, A)
Feasibility: 2 7 / 1 2 3 4 5 6 7 8 9 (9.0, 0.2, A)
(22- 24)

12. The child's weight should be documented at least twice during the second year of life. This information must either be plotted on a growth curve or be recorded with the age/gender percentile.
Validity: 2 6 / 1 2 3 4 5 6 7 8 9 (9.0, 0.9, A)
Feasibility: 2 7 / 1 2 3 4 5 6 7 8 9 (9.0, 0.2, A)
(25- 27)

13. The child's weight should be documented at least once a year during the third-sixth year of life. This information must either be plotted on a growth curve or be recorded with the age/gender percentile.
Validity: 2 6 / 1 2 3 4 5 6 7 8 9 (9.0, 0.9, A)
Feasibility: 2 7 / 1 2 3 4 5 6 7 8 9 (9.0, 0.2, A)
(28- 30)

14. The child's weight should be documented at least once every other year during the seventh-twelfth year of life. This information must either be plotted on a growth curve or be recorded with the age/gender percentile.
Validity: 2 6 / 1 2 3 4 5 6 7 8 9 (9.0, 0.9, A)
Feasibility: 2 7 / 1 2 3 4 5 6 7 8 9 (9.0, 0.2, A)
(31- 33)

15. Before discharge from the hospital, the newborn's height should be documented.
Validity: 2 6 / 1 2 3 4 5 6 7 8 9 (9.0, 0.9, A)
Feasibility: 2 7 / 1 2 3 4 5 6 7 8 9 (9.0, 0.2, A)
(34- 36)

Scales: 1 = low validity or feasibility; 9 = high validity or feasibility.

Chapter 22
QUALITY INDICATORS FOR WELL CHILD CARE

	Validity	Feasibility	
16. The child's height should be documented at least four times between the end of the first week and the end of the first year of life. This information must either be plotted on a growth curve or be recorded with the age/gender percentile.	1 2 6 1 2 3 4 5 6 7 8 9 (9.0, 0.9, A)	2 7 1 2 3 4 5 6 7 8 9 (9.0, 0.2, A)	(37- 39)
17. The child's height should be documented at least twice during the second year of life. This information must either be plotted on a growth curve or be recorded with the age/gender percentile.	2 6 1 2 3 4 5 6 7 8 9 (9.0, 0.9, A)	2 7 1 2 3 4 5 6 7 8 9 (9.0, 0.2, A)	(40- 42)
18. The child's height should be documented at least once a year during the third-sixth year of life. This information must either be plotted on a growth curve or be recorded with the age/gender percentile.	2 6 1 2 3 4 5 6 7 8 9 (9.0, 0.9, A)	2 7 1 2 3 4 5 6 7 8 9 (9.0, 0.2, A)	(43- 45)
19. The child's height should be documented at least once every other year during the seventh-twelfth year of life. This information must either be plotted on a growth curve or be recorded with the age/gender percentile.	2 6 1 2 3 4 5 6 7 8 9 (9.0, 0.9, A)	2 7 1 2 3 4 5 6 7 8 9 (9.0, 0.2, A)	(46- 48)
20. Before discharge from the hospital, the newborn's head circumference should be documented.	2 6 1 2 3 4 5 6 7 8 9 (9.0, 0.9, A)	2 7 1 2 3 4 5 6 7 8 9 (9.0, 0.2, A)	(49- 51)
21. The child's head circumference should be documented at least four times between the end of the first week and the end of the first year of life. This information must either be plotted on a growth curve or be recorded with the age/gender percentile.	2 6 1 2 3 4 5 6 7 8 9 (9.0, 0.9, A)	2 7 1 2 3 4 5 6 7 8 9 (9.0, 0.2, A)	(52- 54)
22. The child's head circumference should be documented at least twice during the second year of life. This information must either be plotted on a growth curve or be recorded with the age/gender percentile.	2 6 1 2 3 4 5 6 7 8 9 (9.0, 0.9, A)	2 7 1 2 3 4 5 6 7 8 9 (9.0, 0.2, A)	(55- 57)
23. A heart examination should be documented during the first 24 hours of life.	1 1 5 1 2 3 4 5 6 7 8 9 (9.0, 1.8, I)	1 1 6 1 2 3 4 5 6 7 8 9 (9.0, 0.9, A)	(58- 60)
24. Examination of the femoral pulses should be documented during the first 24 hours of life.	1 1 2 2 1 1 2 3 4 5 6 7 8 9 (7.0, 2.0, I)	1 1 3 1 2 1 2 3 4 5 6 7 8 9 (7.0, 1.7, I)	(61- 63)
25. An abdominal examination should be documented during the first 24 hours of life.	1 2 3 1 2 3 4 5 6 7 8 9 (8.0, 1.6, I)	2 1 1 5 1 2 3 4 5 6 7 8 9 (9.0, 1.0, A)	(64- 66)
28. The newborn's feeding pattern should be documented before discharge.	1 2 3 1 2 3 4 5 6 7 8 9 (8.0, 0.9, A)	1 3 2 2 1 1 2 3 4 5 6 7 8 9 (7.0, 1.0, I)	(67- 69)
29. Heart rate should be documented during the first 24 hours of life.	1 1 5 1 2 3 4 5 6 7 8 9 (9.0, 1.8, I)	1 1 1 6 1 2 3 4 5 6 7 8 9 (9.0, 0.9, A)	(70- 72)
30. Respiratory rate should be documented during the first 24 hours of life.	1 2 1 1 3 1 2 3 4 5 6 7 8 9 (7.0, 1.9, I)	2 1 1 5 1 2 3 4 5 6 7 8 9 (9.0, 1.3, I)	(73- 75)
32. An eye examination (e.g., red reflex) should be documented at least once during the first two months of life.	2 1 1 1 4 1 1 2 3 4 5 6 7 8 9 (8.0, 2.4, D)	1 4 2 1 1 2 3 4 5 6 7 8 9 (7.0, 1.2, A)	(76- 78)
33. A hip examination should be documented at least once during the first two months of life.	1 1 1 2 4 1 2 3 4 5 6 7 8 9 (8.0, 1.6, A)	1 1 1 1 5 1 2 3 4 5 6 7 8 9 (9.0, 1.1, A)	(79- 81)

Scales: 1 = low validity or feasibility; 9 = high validity or feasibility.

Chapter 22
QUALITY INDICATORS FOR WELL CHILD CARE

	Validity	Feasibility	

34. A heart examination should be documented at least once between 72 hours and two months of life.

Validity: 1 2 3 4 5 6 7 8 9 (9.0, 1.8, I)
Feasibility: 1 2 3 4 5 6 7 8 9 (9.0, 0.9, A)
(82- 84)

35. A lung examination should be documented at least once during the first two months of life.

Validity: 1 2 3 4 5 6 7 8 9 (8.0, 2.0, I)
Feasibility: 1 2 3 4 5 6 7 8 9 (9.0, 0.9, A)
(85- 87)

36. An abdominal examination should be documented at least once between the end of the first week and two months of life.

Validity: 1 2 3 4 5 6 7 8 9 (8.0, 1.6, I)
Feasibility: 1 2 3 4 5 6 7 8 9 (9.0, 1.0, A)
(88- 90)

37. Examination of the femoral pulses should be documented between the end of the first week and two months of life.

Validity: 1 2 3 4 5 6 7 8 9 (9.0, 1.8, I)
Feasibility: 1 2 3 4 5 6 7 8 9 (9.0, 0.9, A)
(91- 93)

38. A neurologic examination (e.g., tone, reflexes) should be documented at least once during the first two months of life.

Validity: 1 2 3 4 5 6 7 8 9 (8.0, 1.7, I)
Feasibility: 1 2 3 4 5 6 7 8 9 (7.0, 1.3, I)
(94- 96)

39. A genital examination (e.g., descended testes) should be documented at least once during the first 2 months of life.

Validity: 1 2 3 4 5 6 7 8 9 (8.0, 1.6, A)
Feasibility: 1 2 3 4 5 6 7 8 9 (9.0, 0.8, A)
(97- 99)

40. A physical examination should be documented at least twice during the second six months of life.

Validity: 1 2 3 4 5 6 7 8 9 (8.0, 1.4, A)
Feasibility: 1 2 3 4 5 6 7 8 9 (8.0, 1.1, I)
(100-102)

41. A physical examination should be documented at least twice during the second year of life.

Validity: 1 2 3 4 5 6 7 8 9 (8.0, 1.4, A)
Feasibility: 1 2 3 4 5 6 7 8 9 (8.0, 1.1, I)
(103-105)

42. A physical examination should be documented at least once a year during the third-sixth year of life.

Validity: 1 2 3 4 5 6 7 8 9 (8.0, 1.4, A)
Feasibility: 1 2 3 4 5 6 7 8 9 (8.0, 1.1, I)
(106-108)

43. A physical examination should be documented at least once every other year during the sixth-twelfth year of life.

Validity: 1 2 3 4 5 6 7 8 9 (8.0, 1.4, A)
Feasibility: 1 2 3 4 5 6 7 8 9 (8.0, 1.1, I)
(109-111)

44. Hearing should be screened by an audiometer by the end of the fourth year of life.

Validity: 1 2 3 4 5 6 7 8 9 (8.0, 1.3, A)
Feasibility: 1 2 3 4 5 6 7 8 9 (7.0, 1.8, I)
(112-114)

45. If the child fails to hear the stimulus at two frequencies in one ear further evaluation/work-up should be ordered within one month.

Validity: 1 2 3 4 5 6 7 8 9 (7.0, 1.6, I)
Feasibility: 1 2 3 4 5 6 7 8 9 (7.0, 1.3, I)
(115-117)

46. Vision screening should be performed by the end of the fourth year of life.

Validity: 1 2 3 4 5 6 7 8 9 (8.0, 1.7, A)
Feasibility: 1 2 3 4 5 6 7 8 9 (8.0, 1.2, A)
(118-120)

LABORATORY SCREENING

47. Screening for congenital hypothyroidism should have been done by the seventh day of life.

Validity: 1 2 3 4 5 6 7 8 9 (8.0, 1.6, A)
Feasibility: 1 2 3 4 5 6 7 8 9 (8.0, 1.0, A)
(121-123)

48. Screening for phenylketonuria should have been done after 24 hours of age and before two weeks of age.

Validity: 1 2 3 4 5 6 7 8 9 (8.0, 1.6, A)
Feasibility: 1 2 3 4 5 6 7 8 9 (8.0, 1.0, A)
(124-126)

49. A hemoglobin or hematocrit should be checked by the end of the 18th month of life.

Validity: 1 2 3 4 5 6 7 8 9 (8.0, 1.6, A)
Feasibility: 1 2 3 4 5 6 7 8 9 (8.0, 1.0, A)
(127-129)

Scales: 1 = low validity or feasibility; 9 = high validity or feasibility.

Chapter 23
QUALITY INDICATORS FOR PRESCRIPTION OF MEDICATIONS

Note: There is no text chapter corresponding to the indicators
in this section.

	Validity	Feasibility	
1. The chart should have a clearly specified place to mark all medication allergies.	1 1 1 5 1 2 3 4 5 6 7 8 9 (9.0, 1.6, A)	3 5 1 2 3 4 5 6 7 8 9 (9.0, 0.8, A)	(1- 3)
2. All allergies found in the chart must be listed in the allergy list discussed in the preceding indicator.	1 1 4 3 1 2 3 4 5 6 7 8 9 (8.0, 1.4, A)	1 2 1 5 1 2 3 4 5 6 7 8 9 (9.0, 1.0, A)	(4- 6)
3. When prescribed a medication, the patient's allergy status should be notated in the progress notes and/or on the designated allergy list.	3 3 2 1 2 3 4 5 6 7 8 9 (8.0, 1.3, A)	2 3 3 1 2 3 4 5 6 7 8 9 (8.0, 1.8, I)	(7- 9)
4. People with an allergy to a medication should only receive it if they have a notation in their chart stating why.	2 1 5 1 2 3 4 5 6 7 8 9 (9.0, 1.4, A)	3 2 4 1 2 3 4 5 6 7 8 9 (8.0, 0.8, A)	(10- 12)

Scales: 1 = low validity or feasibility; 9 = high validity or feasibility.

APPENDIX C: INDICATOR CROSSWALK TABLE

Chapter 1 — Acne

Original Indicator	Modified Indicator	Comments
(DIAGNOSIS)	**(DIAGNOSIS)**	
1. For patients presenting with acne, the following history should be documented in their chart: a. location of lesions (back, face, neck, chest); b. aggravating factors (stress, seasons, cosmetics, creams); c. menstrual history and premenstrual worsening of acne; d. previous treatments; and e. medications and drug use	1. For **all** patients presenting with acne, the following history should be documented in their chart: **a.** location of lesions (back, face, neck, chest); **b.** aggravating factors (stress, seasons, cosmetics, creams); ~~c. menstrual history and premenstrual worsening of acne;~~ **c.** previous treatments; and **d.** medications and drug use	Menstrual history only applies to females. 1(e) wording changed to clarify original indicator. **•MODIFIED•** **dropped (c)** [menstrual history and premenstrual worsening of acne **for girls] due to low validity score from panelists.**
(TREATMENT)	**(TREATMENT)**	
2. If oral antibiotics are prescribed, there must be documentation of moderate to severe acne (papules and pustules).	2. If oral antibiotics are prescribed, there must be documentation of moderate to severe acne (papules **and/or pustules must be present.**	Panelists wanted to be specific about which symptoms need oral antibiotics.
3. Tetracycline should not be prescribed for adolescents less than 12 years of age.	3. Tetracycline should not be prescribed for adolescents less than 12 years of age.	**•UNCHANGED•**
4. If tetracycline is prescribed, there must be documentation of the last menstrual period or a negative pregnancy test for all girls who have reached puberty.	4. If tetracycline is prescribed, there must be documentation of the last menstrual period or a negative pregnancy test for all girls who have reached puberty.	**•UNCHANGED•**
5. If isotretinoin is prescribed, there must be documentation of severe acne (papules, pustules, cysts and nodules) and failure of previous therapy.	5. If isotretinoin is prescribed, there must be documentation of severe acne (papules, pustules, cysts and nodules) and failure of previous therapy.	**•UNCHANGED•**
6. If isotretinoin is prescribed, a negative serum pregnancy test should be obtained within two weeks of start of therapy.	6. If isotretinoin is prescribed **to post-pubescent girls,** a negative **serum** pregnancy test should be obtained within two weeks of start of therapy.	Wording changed to clarify that a pregnancy test is only necessary after menarche. Wording changed to clarify that serum or urine pregnancy test is adequate.
7. If isotretinoin is prescribed, there should be documentation that counseling regarding use of an effective means of contraception (including abstinence) was provided.	7. If isotretinoin is prescribed **to post-pubescent girls,** there should be documentation that counseling regarding use of an effective means of contraception (including abstinence) was provided.	Wording changed to clarify that a pregnancy test is only necessary after menarche.
7.5 **•NEW•**	8. **If tetracycline is prescribed to post-pubescent girls, there should be documentation that counseling regarding use of an effective means of contraception (including abstinence) was provided.**	**•NEW•** Panelists felt that use of tetracycline warranted counseling because of its potential to harm the fetus.

cont'd

	Original Indicator		Modified Indicator	Comments
	(FOLLOW-UP)		(FOLLOW-UP)	
8.	If isotretinoin is prescribed, monthly serum pregnancy tests should be performed.	--	If isotretinoin is prescribed, monthly serum a pregnancy test should be performed **at least every three months.**	Panelists indicated that a three month time interval was sufficient. Wording changed to clarify that serum or urine pregnancy test is adequate. •**DROPPED• due to disagreement among panelists.**
9.	If isotretinoin is prescribed, monthly liver function tests should be performed.	9.	If isotretinoin is prescribed, monthly liver function tests should be performed **at least every three months.**	Panelists indicated that a three-month time interval was sufficient.
10.	•NEW•	10.	**If isotretinoin is prescribed, triglyceride levels should be performed at least every three months.**	•**NEW•** PDR recommends monitoring until response to isotretinoin is established, and panelists felt this was important.

Pediatric Quality Indicators

Chapter 2 — Adolescent Preventive Services

Original Indicator	Modified Indicator	Comments
(SCREENING)	**(SCREENING)**	
General	*General*	
1. Between the ages of 13 and 18 years, all adolescents should have at least one clinician visit.	1. Between the ages of 11 and 18 years, all adolescents should have **an annual visit at which risk assessment/preventive services were provided.**	Panelists felt that more frequent visits were necessary, and revised indicator to be consistent with AMA GAPS, AAP and Bright Futures recommendations.
2. Confidentiality should be discussed and documented by age 14 or at the first visit afterwards.	2. Confidentiality should be discussed and documented by age 14 or at the first visit afterwards.	•UNCHANGED• •DROPPED• due to operationalization difficulties.
2.5 Weight and height should be measured at least once a year or at every visit, if visits occur less frequently.	3. Weight and height should be measured at least once a year **and plotted on a growth chart or be recorded with the age/gender percentile.**	[moved from #20 up to here as 2.5, since now included under "General" section] Panelists felt that plotting on a growth chart is necessary for tracking changes in growth velocity. Visit frequency modified to reflect indicator #1's requirement of an annual visit.
Substance Use	*Substance Use*	
3. Documentation of discussion of substance use (tobacco, alcohol, marijuana, other illicit drugs, anabolic steroids) or of the adolescent's history should occur by age 14 or the first well visit afterwards.	4. Documentation of discussion of substance use (tobacco, alcohol, marijuana, other illicit drugs, anabolic-steroids) or of the adolescent's history should occur **annually.**	Periodicity revised to be consistent with annual visit requirement; and panelists felt substance use needs to be discussed repeatedly throughout adolescence. Anabolic steroids were removed from the list of substances as a result of the creation of indicator #5.
3a. •NEW•	5. **There should be documentation that the risks of anabolic steroid use were discussed or a history of anabolic steroid use was taken for adolescent males participating in team sports or weight-training at least once a year.**	•NEW• Panelists requested the addition of an indicator on anabolic steroid use and resubmission to them for final review.
Sexually Transmitted Diseases and HIV Prevention	*Sexually Transmitted Diseases and HIV Prevention*	
4. Documentation of discussion of sexual activity and risk reduction or the adolescent's sexual history should occur by age 14 or the first well visit afterwards.	6. Documentation of discussion of sexual activity and risk reduction or the adolescent's sexual history should occur **annually.**	Panelists felt sexual activity needs to be discussed repeatedly throughout adolescence. Wording changed to clarify original indicator.
5. Patients for whom the medical records indicate that they have ever been sexually active should be asked the following questions: if they currently have a single sexual partner; if they have had more than 2 sexual partners in the past 6 months; and if they have had a history of any STDs.	7. Patients for whom the medical records indicate that they have ever been sexually active should be asked the following questions: if they currently have a single sexual partner; **about the number of partners in the past;** and if they have had a history of any STDs.	•UNCHANGED• Wording changed to improve operationalization.

Original Indicator	Modified Indicator	Comments
6. Patients for whom the medical records indicate that they are sexually active and not in a monogamous relationship, have had more than 2 sexual partners in the past six months, have a history of STDs, or have used intravenous drugs, should be counseled regarding the prevention and transmission of HIV and other STDs.	--	•DELETED•
Injury Prevention	*Injury Prevention*	
7. Documentation of discussion of injury prevention should occur by age 14 or the first well child visit afterwards.	8. Documentation of discussion of injury prevention should occur **annually**.	Panelists felt injury prevention needs to be discussed repeatedly throughout adolescence.
8. Patients should receive counseling regarding the use of seat belts on at least one occasion.	-- Patients should receive counseling regarding the use of seat belts **annually**.	Panelists felt seat belt use needs to be discussed repeatedly throughout adolescence. •DROPPED• **due to low validity score from panelists.**
Hyperlipidemia Screening	*Hyperlipidemia Screening*	
9. Documentation of parental history of hypercholesteremia should occur by 14 years of age or the first well visit afterwards.	-- Documentation of parental history of hypercholesteremia should **be sought.**	Parents may not be available and adolescents may not be able to provide this information. •DROPPED• **due to low validity score from panelists.**
10. Adolescents whose parents have a serum cholesterol level greater than 240 mg/dl should receive a total blood cholesterol screen.	-- Adolescents whose parents have a serum cholesterol level greater than 240 mg/dl should receive a total blood cholesterol screen.	•UNCHANGED•
11. Documentation of parents' or grandparents' history of coronary artery disease (CAD), peripheral vascular disease (PVD), cerebrovascular disease, or sudden cardiac death occur by 14 years of age or the first well visit afterwards.	-- Documentation of parents' or grandparents' history of coronary artery disease (CAD), peripheral vascular disease (PVD), cerebrovascular disease, or sudden cardiac death at age 55 or younger should occur **annually.**	Panelists felt history needs to be discussed repeatedly throughout adolescence. •DROPPED• **due to low validity score from panelists.**
12. Adolescents whose parents or grandparents have a positive history of CAD, PVD, cerebrovascular disease or sudden cardiac death at age 55 or younger should have a fasting lipoprotein analysis.	-- Adolescents whose parents or grandparents have a positive history of CAD, PVD, cerebrovascular disease or sudden cardiac death at age 55 or younger should have a fasting lipoprotein analysis.	•UNCHANGED• •DROPPED• **due to low validity score from panelists.**
Hypertension	*Hypertension*	
13. Blood pressure should be measured at least once a year or at every visit, if visits occur less frequently than once a year.	9. Blood pressure should be measured at least once a year or at every visit, if visits occur less frequently than once a year.	Panelists felt blood pressure needs to be measured repeatedly throughout adolescence.
14. If a patient has 3 or more blood pressure readings above the 95th percentile for age, a full work-up for hypertension should be conducted.	10. If a patient has **an elevated blood pressure, at least 2 additional blood pressure readings on 2 separate occasions within 3 months should be recorded in the chart.**	Panelists felt "full work-up" was too comprehensive for a single indicator. They preferred a revised indicator focusing on confirmation of elevated blood pressure.
Cervical Cancer	*Cervical Cancer*	

Pediatric Quality Indicators

Original Indicator	Modified Indicator	Comments
15. The medical record should contain the date and result of the last Pap smear for all females under 18 years of age, for whom there is documentation of a history of vaginal intercourse, if it has been at least one year since they first had vaginal intercourse.	11. **All sexually active females or those who present for contraception should have an annual Pap smear within one year of becoming sexually active.**	Wording changed to clarify original indicator.
16. All females under 18 years of age, for whom there is documentation of a history of vaginal intercourse, who have not had 3 consecutive normal smears and who have not had a Pap smear within the last year should have one performed.	--	•DELETED• Merged with original indicator #15.
17. All females under 18 years of age, for whom there is documentation of a history of vaginal intercourse, who have had three consecutive normal smears and subsequently have not had a Pap smear within the last 3 years should have one performed.	--	•DELETED• Merged with original indicator #15.
18. All females under 18 with a history of cervical dysplasia or carcinoma-in-situ who have not had a Pap smear within the last year should have one performed.	--	•DELETED• Merged with original indicator #15.
19. Adolescent girls presenting for contraception who have not previously had a Pap test should have one.	--	•DELETED• Merged with original indicator #15.
Eating Disorders– General	*General*	
20. Weight and height should be measured at least once a year or at every visit, if visits occur less frequently.	Weight and height should be measured at least once a year and plotted on a growth chart.	[moved up to #2.5, under the "General" section]
(TREATMENT) *Cigarette Use Counseling*	(TREATMENT) *Cigarette Use Counseling*	
21. All current smokers should receive counseling to stop smoking.	12. All current smokers should receive counseling to stop smoking.	•UNCHANGED•
22. If counseling alone fails to help the patient quit smoking, the patient should be offered nicotine replacement therapy (gum or patch).	--	•DELETED•
23. Nicotine replacement should only be prescribed in conjunction with counseling.	--	•DELETED•
24. Nicotine replacement should not be prescribed if the patient: 1) is pregnant or nursing 2) has temporomandibular joint disease 3) continues to smoke	--	•DELETED•
(FOLLOW-UP) *Cervical Cancer Screening*	(FOLLOW-UP) *Cervical Cancer Screening*	
25. All adolescents with severely abnormal Pap smear should have colposcopy performed.	13. All adolescents with a Pap smear **consistent with HPV** should have colposcopy performed.	Panelists felt colposcopy requirement was only necessary for adolescents with suspected HPV.
26. If an adolescent has a Pap smear that is not normal but is not severely abnormal, then one of the following should occur within 1 year of the initial Pap: 1) repeat Pap smear; or 2) colposcopy.	--	•DELETED• Merged into modified indicator #13.

	Original Indicator	Modified Indicator	Comments
27.	All adolescents with a Pap smear that is not "normal" but is not severely abnormal and who have had the abnormality documented on at least 2 Pap smears in a 2-year period should have colposcopy performed.	--	•DELETED• Merged into modified indicator #13.
	Cigarette Use Counseling	*Cigarette Use Counseling*	
28.	Tobacco abuse should be added to the problem list of all current smokers or addressed during at least one subsequent visit.	--	•UNCHANGED•
		Tobacco abuse should be added to the problem list of all current smokers or addressed during at least one subsequent visit.	•DROPPED• due to low validity score from panelists.
	Growth	*Growth*	
29.	•NEW•	--	•NEW• Panelists wanted this topic added to track the adolescent's development.
		Tanner staging should be recorded annually.	•DROPPED• due to low validity score from panelists.
30.	•NEW•	14. If abnormal height/weight velocity is found, a follow-up visit should occur.	•NEW• Panelists felt that adolescents with growth abnormalities should be followed more closely.
	Eating Disorders	*Eating Disorders*	
31.	•NEW•	15. Eating patterns (e.g., chronic dieting, binging, laxatives, purging, other drugs, number and type of meals) should be discussed annually.	•NEW• Panelists felt eating disorders are an important problem that providers should address regularly.

Chapter 3 — Allergic Rhinitis

	Original Indicator		Modified Indicator	Comments
	(DIAGNOSIS)		**(DIAGNOSIS)**	
1.	If a diagnosis of allergic rhinitis is made, the search for a specific allergen by history should be documented in the chart (for initial history).	1.	If a diagnosis of allergic rhinitis is made, the search for a specific allergen by history should be documented in the chart (for initial history).	**•UNCHANGED•**
2.	If a diagnosis of allergic rhinitis is made, history should include whether the patient uses any topical or systemic nasal decongestants.	2.	If a diagnosis of allergic rhinitis is made, history should include whether the patient uses any topical or systemic nasal decongestants.	**•UNCHANGED•**
	(TREATMENT)		**(TREATMENT)**	
3.	Treatment for allergic rhinitis should include at least one of the following: antihistamine, nasal steroids, nasal cromolyn.	3.	Treatment for allergic rhinitis should include at least one of the following: **recommendation for allergen avoidance,** antihistamine, nasal steroids, nasal cromolyn.	Panelists felt that allergen avoidance can be an appropriate treatment.
4.	If nasal decongestants are prescribed, duration of treatment should be for no longer than 4 days.	4.	If **topical** nasal decongestants are prescribed, duration of treatment should be for no longer than 4 days.	Topical added because it was a typographical error in original indicator.
5.	**•NEW•**	5.	**A specific discussion of environmental triggers and controls should be documented.**	**•NEW•** Panelists felt this topic should be discussed with all patients.

Chapter 4 — Asthma

	Original Indicator		Modified Indicator	Comments
	(DIAGNOSIS)		**(DIAGNOSIS)**	
1.	All patients age 5 or older with the diagnosis of asthma should have baseline spirometry performed (within six months of diagnosis).	--	All patients age 5 or older with the diagnosis of asthma should have baseline spirometry **or PEFR** performed (within six months of diagnosis).	Panelists felt PEFR is also an adequate measure of control in known asthmatics. •**DROPPED• due to low validity score from panelists.**
2.	All patients with the diagnosis of asthma should have had a historical evaluation of asthma triggers (e.g., environmental exposures, exercise, allergens) within six months (before or after) of the initial diagnosis.	1.	All patients with the diagnosis of asthma should have had a historical evaluation of asthma triggers (e.g., environmental exposures, exercise, allergens) within six months (before or after) of the initial diagnosis.	•**UNCHANGED•**
3.	PEFR should be measured in all patients > 5 years of age with chronic asthma (except for those with only exercise-induced asthma) at least annually in an office visit in which asthma is evaluated.	2.	PEFR should be measured in all patients > 5 years of age with chronic asthma (except for those with only exercise-induced asthma) at least annually in an office visit in which asthma is evaluated.	•**UNCHANGED•**
	(CHRONIC — TREATMENT)		**(CHRONIC — TREATMENT)**	
4.	All patients > 5 years of age with the diagnosis of asthma should have been prescribed a beta₂-agonist inhaler for symptomatic relief of exacerbations.	3.	All patients > 5 years of age with the diagnosis of asthma should have been prescribed a beta₂-agonist inhaler for symptomatic relief of exacerbations.	•**UNCHANGED•**
5.	Patients ≤ 5 years of age should be prescribed a nebulizer (for administering asthma medications).	4.	Patients ≤ 5 years of age should be prescribed a nebulizer (for administering asthma medications).	•**UNCHANGED•**
6.	Patients who report using a beta₂-agonist inhaler more than 3 times per day on a daily basis should be prescribed a longer acting bronchodilator (theophylline) and/or an anti-inflammatory agent (inhaled corticosteroids, cromolyn).	5.	Patients who report using a beta₂-agonist inhaler more than 3 times per day on a daily basis should be prescribed a longer acting bronchodilator (theophylline) and/or an anti-inflammatory agent (inhaled corticosteroids, cromolyn).	•**UNCHANGED•**
7.	Patients with asthma should not receive beta-blocker medications (e.g., atenolol, propanalol).	6.	Patients with asthma should not receive beta-blocker medications (e.g., atenolol, propanalol).	•**UNCHANGED•**
8.	In any patients requiring chronic treatment with oral corticosteroids a trial of inhaled corticosteroids should have been attempted.	7.	In any patients requiring chronic treatment with oral corticosteroids a trial of inhaled corticosteroids should have been attempted.	•**UNCHANGED•**
9.	Any child with asthma who takes high doses of inhaled corticosteroids should have growth patterns monitored annually.	8.	Any child with asthma who takes high doses of inhaled corticosteroids should have growth patterns monitored **at least** annually.	Wording changed to clarify original indicator.
10.	Patients who require frequent bursts of prednisone (2-3 trials of 5-day therapy with oral corticosteroids after an exacerbation of asthma within the past 6 months) who are not already on inhaled corticosteroids or chromolyn sodium should be started on them.	9.	Patients who require frequent bursts of prednisone (2-3 trials of 5-day therapy with oral corticosteroids after an exacerbation of asthma within the past 6 months) who are not already on inhaled corticosteroids or chromolyn sodium should be started on them.	•**UNCHANGED•**
11.	Patients on theophylline should have at least one theophylline level determination per year.	--	Patients on theophylline should have at least one theophylline level determination per year.	•**UNCHANGED•** •**DROPPED• due to low validity score from panelists.**

cont'd

#	Original Indicator	#	Modified Indicator	Comments
12.	Patients with the diagnosis of asthma that is moderate to severe who are at least six months of age should have a documented flu vaccination in the fall/winter of the previous year (September–January).	--		•DELETED• Duplicates immunization chapter #25.
13.	Patients with the diagnosis of asthma that is moderate to severe should have a pneumoccal vaccination documented in the chart.	--	Patients with the diagnosis of asthma that is moderate to severe should have a pneumoccal vaccination documented in the chart **within one year of diagnosis.**	Panelists felt that the vaccine should be given within a reasonable period of time after diagnosis. •DROPPED• due to low validity score from panelists.
	(FLARE-UP — DIAGNOSIS AND TREATMENT)		*(FLARE-UP — DIAGNOSIS AND TREATMENT)*	
14.	All patients > 5 years of age presenting to the physician's office with an asthma exacerbation or historical worsening of asthma symptoms should be evaluated with PEFR or FEV1.	10.	All patients > 5 years of age presenting to the physician's office with an asthma exacerbation or historical worsening of asthma symptoms should be evaluated with PEFR or FEV1.	•UNCHANGED•
15.	At the time of exacerbation, symptomatic patients on theophylline should have a theophylline level measured.	11.	At the time of exacerbation, symptomatic patients on theophylline should have a theophylline level measured.	•UNCHANGED•
16.	A physical exam of the chest should be performed in all patients presenting with an asthma exacerbation.	12.	A physical exam of the chest should be performed in all patients presenting with an asthma exacerbation **in the physician's office or emergency room.**	Wording changed to improve operationalization on indicator.
17.	All patients presenting to the physician's office or emergency department with an FEV1 or PEFR<=70 percent of baseline (or predicted) should be treated with beta₂-agonists before discharge.	13.	All patients presenting to the physician's office or emergency department with an FEV1 or PEFR<=70 percent of baseline (or predicted) should be treated with beta₂-agonists before discharge.	•UNCHANGED•
18.	Patients who receive treatment with beta₂-agonists for FEV1<70 percent in the physician's office or emergency department (ED) should have an FEV1 or PEFR repeated prior to discharge.	14.	Patients who receive treatment with beta₂-agonists for FEV1 **or PEFR** <70 percent in the physician's office or emergency department (ED) should have an FEV1 or PEFR repeated prior to discharge.	Omission in original indicator was an editing error.
19.	Patients with an FEV1 or PEFR <=70 percent of baseline (or predicted) after treatment for an asthma exacerbation in the physician's office should be placed on an oral corticosteroid taper.	15.	Patients with an FEV1 or PEFR <=70 percent of baseline (or predicted) after treatment for an asthma exacerbation in the physician's office should be placed on an oral corticosteroid taper.	•UNCHANGED•
20.	Patients who have persistent symptoms, diffuse wheezes on chest auscultation, or a PEFR or FEV1<=40 percent of baseline (or predicted) after treatment with beta₂-agonist should be admitted to the hospital.	16.	Patients who have persistent symptoms, diffuse wheezes on chest auscultation, **and** a PEFR or FEV1<=40 percent of baseline (or predicted) after treatment with beta₂-agonist should be admitted to the hospital.	Panelists felt that admission is not always necessary if only some of these signs and symptoms are present.
	(HOSPITAL — DIAGNOSIS AND TREATMENT)		*(HOSPITAL — DIAGNOSIS AND TREATMENT)*	
21.	All patients admitted to the hospital for asthma exacerbation should have oxygen saturation measured.	17.	All patients admitted to the hospital for asthma exacerbation should have oxygen saturation measured.	•UNCHANGED•
22.	All hospitalized patients with PEFR or FEV1 < 25 percent of predicted or personal best should receive arterial blood gas measurement.	18.	All hospitalized patients with PEFR or FEV1 < 25 percent of predicted or personal best should receive arterial blood gas measurement.	•UNCHANGED•
23.	All hospitalized patients should receive systemic (IV) or oral steroids.	19.	All hospitalized patients should receive systemic (IV) or oral steroids.	•UNCHANGED•
24.	All hospitalized patients should receive treatment with beta₂-agonists.	20.	All hospitalized patients should receive treatment with beta₂-agonists.	•UNCHANGED•

cont'd

	Original Indicator		Modified Indicator	Comments
25.	All hospitalized patients should receive treatment with methylxanthines.	--	All hospitalized patients should receive treatment with methylxanthines.	•UNCHANGED• •DROPPED• due to low validity score from panelists.
26.	All hospitalized patients with oxygen saturation less than 92 percent should receive supplemental oxygen.	21.	All hospitalized patients with oxygen saturation less than 92 percent should receive supplemental oxygen.	•UNCHANGED•
27.	All hospitalized patients with pCO2 of greater than 40 should receive at least one additional blood gas measurement to evaluate response to treatment.	22.	All hospitalized patients with pCO2 of greater than 40 should receive at least one additional blood gas measurement to evaluate response to treatment, UNLESS PC02 > 40 PREVIOUSLY DOCUMENTED??? [ASK MARK].	WORDING ADDED TO IMPROVE OPERATIONALIZATION OF INDICATOR.
28.	Hospitalized patients with pCO2 of greater than 40 should be monitored in an intensive care setting.	--	Hospitalized patients with pCO2 of greater than 40 should be monitored in an intensive care setting.	•UNCHANGED• •DROPPED• due to low validity score from panelists.
29.	Patients with 2 or more hospitalizations for asthma exacerbation in the previous year should receive (or should have received) consultation with an asthma specialist.	--	Patients with 2 or more hospitalizations for asthma exacerbation in the previous year should receive (or should have received) consultation with an asthma specialist.	•UNCHANGED• •DROPPED• due to low validity score from panelists.
30.	Hospitalized patients should not receive sedative drugs (e.g., benzodiazapines). (FOLLOW-UP)	23.	Hospitalized patients not on a ventilator should not receive sedative drugs (e.g., benzodiazapines). (FOLLOW-UP)	Sedative drugs are appropriate for patients on a ventilator.
31.	Patients with the diagnosis of asthma should have at least 2 visits within a calendar year.	24.	Patients with the diagnosis of moderate to severe asthma should have at least 2 scheduled visits within a calendar year.	Panelists felt indicator should be tied to severity and that there should be planned visits in addition to acute visits.
32.	Patients whose asthma medication is changed (new medication added, current dose decreased/increased) during one visit should have a follow-up visit within 3 weeks.	25.	Patients whose asthma medication is changed (new medication added, current dose decreased/increased) during one visit should have a follow-up visit within 3 weeks.	Panelists felt that telephone contact is an acceptable form of follow-up.
33.	Patients on chronic oral corticosteroids should have follow-up visits at least 4 times in a calendar year.	26.	Patients on chronic oral corticosteroids should have follow-up visits at least 4 times in a calendar year.	•UNCHANGED•
34.	Patients seen in the emergency department with an asthma exacerbation should have a follow-up reassessment within 72 hours.	27.	Patients seen in the emergency department with an asthma exacerbation should have a follow-up reassessment within 72 hours.	•UNCHANGED•
35.	Patients with a hospitalization for an asthma exacerbation should receive outpatient follow-up within 14 days.	28.	Patients with a hospitalization for an asthma exacerbation should receive follow-up assessment within 7 days.	Panelists felt that telephone contact is an acceptable form of follow-up, and that follow-up assessment is needed sooner.

Pediatric Quality Indicators

Chapter 5 — ADHD (Attention Deficit/Hyperactivity Disorder)

[Note: These indicators only apply to children/adolescents 5-18 years old.]

Original Indicator	Modified Indicator	Comments
(DIAGNOSIS)	(DIAGNOSIS)	
1. Before making the diagnosis of ADHD, the health care provider should document a history of inattention or impulsivity/hyperactivity, using input from all of the following: • a rating scale by the parent; • an interview with the parent; • a rating scale by the teacher; • communication with the teacher (phone or in person); and • physician observation.	1. Before making the diagnosis of ADHD, the health care provider should document a history of inattention **and** impulsivity/hyperactivity, using input from **a parent and from a teacher (if the child is in school). An effort to communicate with a teacher or have a teacher fill out a rating scale is acceptable.**	Panelists agreed that soliciting input from the specified sources was necessary in making the diagnosis, but wanted to allow more leeway with respect to the specific method employed.

2. Before making the diagnosis of ADHD, the health care provider should document:
a. that the core symptoms of inattention and impulsivity/hyperactivity happen in more than one setting;
b. that the core symptoms of inattention and impulsivity/hyperactivity have been of >= 6 months duration;
c. that the core symptoms of inattention and impulsivity/hyperactivity had been present prior to 7 years of age;
d. the child's social functioning, especially with regard to Pervasive Developmental Disorder, by evaluating at least one of the following:
  – impairment of social interaction,
  – impairment in communication, or
  – restricted repetitive and stereotyped patterns of behavior, interests, and activities;
e. the presence or absence of affective symptoms;
f. the child's social functioning, especially with regard to:
  – Oppositional Defiant Disorder
  – Conduct Disorder.
	2. Before making the diagnosis of ADHD, the health care provider should document:
	a. that the core symptoms of inattention and impulsivity/hyperactivity happen in more than one setting;
	b. that the core symptoms of inattention and impulsivity/hyperactivity have been of >= 6 months duration;
	-- that the core symptoms of inattention and impulsivity/hyperactivity had been present prior to 7 years of age;
	c. the child's social functioning, ~~especially~~ with regard to Pervasive Developmental Disorder, by evaluating ~~at least one~~ of the following:
	  – impairment of social interaction,
	  – impairment in communication, ~~or~~
	  – restricted repetitive and stereotyped patterns of behavior, interests, and activities;
	d. the presence or absence of affective symptoms;
	e. the child's social functioning, ~~especially~~ with regard to:
	  – Oppositional Defiant Disorder
	  – Conduct Disorder.
		•MODIFIED•
		
		Dropped (c) due to low validity score from panelists.
		
		2(d) wording changed because it was felt that all three topics were important in assessing Pervasive Development Disorder.
		
		2(f) wording changed to clarify original indicator.

3. The health care provider should document that past medical history was reviewed, including birth history, and history of accidents.	3. The health care provider should document that past medical history was reviewed, including birth history, and history of accidents.	**•UNCHANGED•**
3.5 **•NEW•**	4. **Through history, physical examination, and/or laboratory testing, an effort was made to rule out organic and pharmacologic causes.**	Panelists felt other causes should be explored. Created from panel indicators 4, 5, 9.
4. The health care provider should document that a review of systems was done.	--	**•DELETED•** Merged into new indicator #4.

Original Indicator	Modified Indicator	Comments
5. The health care provider should document the child's overall development. This may be based on parental-reported developmental milestones, such as social, fine motor/adaptive, language, and gross motor.	--	•DELETED• Merged into new indicator #4.
6. The health care provider should document the child's cognitive level and academic achievement levels, including: a. academic performance, b. cognitive level, c. achievement level (only for school-age children).	5. The health care provider should document the child's cognitive level and academic achievement levels, including: a. academic performance/**achievement level (if in school)**; b. cognitive level **ability, psychoeducational testing** c. ~~achievement level (only for school-age children)~~.	6(a) and 6(c) combined to clarify indicator. Psychoeducational testing added to clarify how cognitive ability might be measured.
7. The health care provider should document the structure of the family, home environment, and school environment. Such information should include: a. Parents or guardians and other household members, b. environmental stressors, c. family functioning, and d. school features.	6. The health care provider should document the structure of the family, home environment, and school environment. Such information should include: a. **A list of** parents or guardians and other household members, b. environmental stressors, c. family functioning, and d. school features **(if in school)**.	7(a) wording changed to clarify original indicator. 7(d) wording changed to clarify that it is not applicable if patient not in school.
8. The health care provider should document the presence or absence of any family history of: • psychiatric disorder, specifically – depression, – anxiety, – psychosis, – substance abuse, or – antisocial behavior; • attention deficit hyperactivity disorder; or • learning disorder	7. The health care provider should document the presence or absence of any family history of: **a.** psychiatric disorder, specifically ~~depression, anxiety, psychosis, substance abuse, or antisocial behavior~~; attention deficit hyperactivity disorder;~~or~~ , **c.** learning disorder.	Panelists felt that types of psychiatric disorders were too detailed for the indicators and were best addressed when operationalizing the indicator. Panelists wanted to rate each history item separately.
9. The health care provider should document a family history of medical conditions.	--	•DELETED• Merged into new indicator #4.
10a. The physical examination should include a neurologic exam and observation of mood and social interactions.	8. The physical examination should include a neurologic exam ~~and observation of mood and social interactions~~.	Original indicator split into two because panelists felt these components were distinct enough to rate separately.
10b. •NEW•	9. **The physical examination should include observation of mood and social interactions.**	Original indicator split into two because panelists felt these components were distinct enough to rate separately.
11. The health care provider should document the child's current medications.	10. The health care provider should document the child's current medications.	•UNCHANGED•
12. The health care provider should document the presence or absence of alcohol and illicit drug use by the child.	--	•DELETED•
13. If the child is on theophylline, the health care provider should check a theophylline level.	--	•DELETED•
14. If the theophylline level is high (>15 mg/ml), the dose should be reduced.	--	•DELETED•

Pediatric Quality Indicators

cont'd

	Original Indicator		Modified Indicator	Comments
15.	The health care provider should document a vision screening test.	--	The health care provider should document a vision screening test.	•UNCHANGED•
16.	If a vision problem exists, the health care provider should refer for evaluation and treatment, e.g., ophthalmologic or optometric care.	--		•DROPPED• due to low validity score from panelists. •DELETED•
17.	The health care provider should document a hearing screening test.	11.	The health care provider should document a hearing screening test.	•UNCHANGED•
18.	If a hearing problem exists, the health care provider should refer for evaluation and treatment, e.g., audiologic and/or otolaryngologic care.	--		•DELETED•
	(TREATMENT)		(TREATMENT)	
18.5	•NEW•	12.	Medications specific to the treatment of ADHD should not be prescribed for children who do not meet criteria for ADHD.	Panelists requested additional indicator to address overutilization of ADHD medications.
19.	The health care provider should document efforts to adjust the home and school environments. These adjustments would include: a. at home - predictable schedule for bed time, meal times, play times, and homework, - breakdown of chores into smaller tasks, - predictable acceptable limits of behavior, and - predictable and immediate consequences for inappropriate behavior; and b. at school (any 1) - a seat with minimal distractions, - allow child to get up periodically from seat, - brief instructions, - frequent reminders to stay on task with discrete cues or signs, - predictable and immediate consequences for inappropriate behavior, and - provide opportunities for success.	13.	The health care provider should document counseling about how to adjust the home and school environments. These adjustments would include: a. at home, work with parents to structure home environment: - predictable schedule for bed time, meal times, play times, and homework, - breakdown of chores into smaller tasks, - predictable acceptable limits of behavior, or - predictable and immediate consequences for inappropriate behavior; and b. at school (any 1), communicate with school officials to structure school environment: - a seat with minimal distractions, - allow child to get up periodically from seat, - brief instructions, - frequent reminders to stay on task with discrete cues or signs, - predictable and immediate consequences for inappropriate behavior, and or - provide opportunities for success.	Panelists felt it was most important for providers to teach how to make adjustments. 19(a) and 19(b) wording changed to clarify original indicator.
20.	If the child has isolated ADHD, the health care provider should initiate or refer for behavioral modification including any of the following techniques: • positive reinforcement, • negative consequences, or • response cost.	14.	If the child has isolated ADHD, the health care provider should initiate or refer for behavioral modification including any of the following techniques: • positive reinforcement, • negative consequences, or • response cost.	It was felt that there was no need to specify particular types of behavioral modifications in the indicator.
21.	If a child has oppositional-defiant disorder or conduct disorder, the child should be referred for psychiatric or psychologic therapy.	15.	If a child has another psychiatric disorder, the child should be referred for psychiatric or psychologic evaluation and/or therapy.	Panelists felt that any psychiatric disorder warranted a referral for evaluation as well as therapy.
22.	If the child has a mood disorder, the child should be referred for psychiatric or psychologic therapy.	--		•DELETED• Merged with original indicator #21.

Pediatric Quality Indicators

Original Indicator		Modified Indicator		Comments
23.	If the child has a learning disorder, the child should receive psychoeducational intervention.	16.	If the child has a learning disorder, the child should receive or be referred to the school system or other setting for psychoeducational intervention.	Panelists indicated that referral for treatment is appropriate and reflects actual practice.
24.	The health care provider should never prescribe stimulant pharmacotherapy for a child less than three years of age.	--		•DELETED•
25.	If the child has ADHD without a comorbidity and is started on pharmacotherapy, the initial medication choice should be a stimulant such as methylphenidate, dextroamphetamine, or pemoline.	17.	If the child has ADHD without a comorbidity, or with oppositional defiant disorder or conduct disorder, or with a learning disorder, and is started on pharmacotherapy, the initial medication choice should be a stimulant such as methylphenidate, dextroamphetamine, or pemoline.	Merged indicators 25, 26 and 29. Wording felt to be clearer because the listed medications represented all current first-order treatments for these disorders.
26.	If a child has ADHD and oppositional-defiant disorder or conduct disorder and is begun on pharmacotherapy, the child should be started on a stimulant medication, such as methylphenidate, pemoline, or dextroamphetamine.	--		•DELETED•

Merged with indicator 25. |
| 27. | If the child has ADHD and Tourette Syndrome or a tic disorder and is begun on pharmacotherapy, the child should be started on clonidine or stimulant medication (methylphenidate, pemoline, or dextroamphetamine). | 18. | If the child has ADHD and Tourette Syndrome or a tic disorder and is begun on pharmacotherapy, the initial medication should be started on clonidine, or stimulant medication (methylphenidate, pemoline, or dextroamphetamine). | Wording felt to be clearer because the listed medications represented all current first-order treatments for these disorders. |
| 28. | If the child has ADHD and a mood disorder and is begun on pharmacotherapy, the child should be started on a tricyclic antidepressant. | 19. | If the child has ADHD and a mood disorder and is begun on pharmacotherapy, the initial medication should be started on a tricyclic antidepressant. | Wording changed to clarify original indicator. |
| 29. | If the child has ADHD and a learning disorder and is begun on pharmacotherapy, the child should be started on a stimulant medication, such as methylphenidate, pemoline, or dextroamphetamine. | -- | | •DELETED•

Merged with indicator 25. |
30.	If the child is started on pharmacotherapy, the health care provider should document that the risks and benefits have been explained to the child, guardian, and teacher.	--		•DELETED•
31.	Before a child is started on stimulant medication such as methylphenidate, dextroamphetamine, or pemoline, the health care provider should document the weight, height, pulse, and blood pressure of the child.	20.	Before a child is started on stimulant medication such as methylphenidate, dextroamphetamine, or pemoline, the health care provider should document the weight, height, heart rate, and blood pressure of the child.	Baseline heart rate is also important.
32.	If a child is started on pemoline, the health care provider should document the absence of hepatic disease prior to the start of therapy by history and baseline liver function tests.	21.	If a child is started on pemoline, the health care provider should document the absence of hepatic disease prior to the start of therapy by history and baseline liver function tests.	•UNCHANGED•
33.	If a child is started on a tricyclic antidepressant, the health care provider should document the absence of cardiac disease by history and by a baseline electrocardiogram.	22.	If a child is started on a tricyclic antidepressant, the health care provider should take a cardiac disease by history and obtain a baseline electrocardiogram.	Wording changed to clarify original indicator.

cont'd

	Original Indicator	Modified Indicator	Comments
34.	The primary health care provider who is not an ADHD specialist should not prescribe for treatment of ADHD medications other than: • methylphenidate, • pemoline, • dextroamphetamine, • clonidine, or • tricyclic antidepressant.	--	The primary health care provider who is not an ADHD specialist should not prescribe as medications other than: • chlorpromazine, • haloperidol, • levodopa, • lithium • monoamine oxidase inhibitors • thioridazine.	It was preferable to list medications the provider should not prescribe as opposed to acceptable medications. •DROPPED• due to low validity score from panelists.
35.	The primary health care provider should not simultaneously treat a child with ADHD with more than one medication for treatment of ADHD without the consultation of an ADHD specialist, e.g., a psychiatrist, neurologist, or behavioralist.	23.	The primary health care provider should not simultaneously treat a child with ADHD with more than one medication for treatment of ADHD without the consultation of an ADHD specialist, e.g., a psychiatrist, neurologist, or behavioralist.	•UNCHANGED•
36.	The primary health care provider should request consultation from an ADHD specialist (e.g., a multidisciplinary referral center or psychiatrist, neurologist, or behavioralist) if a child fails to respond to separate trials with methylphenidate, dextroamphetamine, pemoline, clonidine, and a single tricyclic antidepressant.	24.	The primary health care provider should request consultation from an ADHD specialist (e.g., a multidisciplinary referral center or psychiatrist, neurologist, or behavioralist) if a child fails to respond to separate trials with methylphenidate, dextroamphetamine, pemoline, clonidine, and a single tricyclic antidepressant.	•UNCHANGED•
	(FOLLOW-UP)	(FOLLOW-UP)		
37.	During the initial evaluation and treatment, the health care provider coordinating care should maintain at least biweekly contact with the family, either through office visits or by phone, for at least 4 contacts.	--	During the initial evaluation ~~and treatment~~ **period**, the health care provider ~~coordinating care~~ should maintain at least biweekly **(every other week)** contact with the family, either through office visits or by phone, for at least 4 contacts.	Wording changed to clarify original indicator. •DROPPED• due to low validity score from panelists.
38.	During the initial implementation of behavioral or psychologic treatment, the provider of such services should see the child for office visits on a weekly basis for at least 4 visits.	--		•DELETED•
39.	For children receiving behavior or psychologic treatment, after the initial four visits, the health care provider coordinating care should see the child in the office every four months.	--		•DELETED•
40.	During the initial implementation of pharmacotherapy, the provider of such services should maintain biweekly contact with the family, either through office visits or by phone, for at least 4 contacts. Office visits should be at least at monthly intervals until improvement is seen in attention or impulsivity/hyperactivity by parent report or rating scale and, if in school, teacher report or rating scale.	--		•DELETED•
41.	After the initial four visits for pharmacotherapeutic intervention, the provider of such therapy should see the child in the office at least every four months once an improvement is seen in attention or impulsivity/hyperactivity by parent report or rating scale and, if in school, teacher report or rating scale.	--	After the initial four visits for pharmacotherapeutic intervention ~~and once an **improvement is seen in attention or impulsivity/hyperactivity**~~, the provider of such therapy should see the child in the office at least every **six** months ~~by parent report or rating scale and, if in-school, teacher report or rating scale~~.	It was felt that semi-annual follow-up is adequate and numerous methods are appropriate. Wording changed to clarify original indicator. •DROPPED• due to low validity score from panelists.

Pediatric Quality Indicators

cont'd

	Original Indicator		Modified Indicator	Comments
42.	If a change in therapy has occurred, the health care provider initiating the change must document at each follow-up visit the presence or absence of side effects. a. Evaluate the effect of the change within two weeks, either by an office visit or by phone contact, b. Inform the provider coordinating care about the change.	25.	If a change in therapy has occurred, the health care provider initiating the change must: a. ~~E~~ evaluate the effect of the change within two weeks, either by an office visit or by phone contact, b. ~~Inform the provider coordinating care about the change.~~	It was felt that this is not always necessary if a specialist is responsible for ADHD care.
43.	At each follow-up visit, the health care provider should document the child's behavior both at home and at school by parent report or rating scale and, if in school, teacher report or rating scale.	26.	At **least every six months**, the health care provider should document the child's behavior both at home and at school by parent report or rating scale and, ~~if in school, teacher report or rating scale.~~	It was felt that semi-annual follow-up is adequate and numerous methods are appropriate.
44.	The health care provider should request and review the child's academic records, such as report cards or interviews with the child's teacher, at least once a year.	27.	The health care provider should request and review the child's academic records, such as report cards or interviews with the child's teacher, at least once a year.	•UNCHANGED•
45.	If medications have been prescribed, at each follow-up visit the health care provider should document: a. weight b. height c. pulse d. blood pressure.	28.	If **stimulant** medications have been prescribed, **the following should be documented at least every six months:** **a.** a. weight **b.** b. height -- c. **heart rate** **c.** d. blood pressure.	It was felt that semi-annual follow-up is needed and type of medication should be clarified. Wording of (c) changed to clarify original indicator. •MODIFIED• **(c) Dropped due to low validity score from panelists.**
46.	If stimulant medications have been prescribed, the health care provider should document at each follow-up visit the presence or absence of side effects.	29.	If stimulant medications have been prescribed, the health care provider should document **at least every six months** the presence or absence of side effects.	It was felt that semi-annual follow-up is needed.
47.	If a tricyclic antidepressant has been prescribed, the health care provider should document at each follow-up visit the presence or absence of side effects.	30.	If a tricyclic antidepressant has been prescribed, the health care provider should document **at least every six months** the presence or absence of side effects.	It was felt that semi-annual follow-up is needed.
48.	If clonidine has been prescribed, the health care provider should document at each follow-up visit the presence or absence of side effects.	31.	If clonidine has been prescribed, the health care provider should document **at least every six months** the presence or absence of side effects.	It was felt that semi-annual follow-up is needed.
49.	If the child is on pemoline, the health care provider should assess liver function every six months.	32.	If the child is on pemoline, the health care provider should assess liver function every six months.	•UNCHANGED•
50.	If the child is on a tricyclic antidepressant, the health care provider should order an electrocardiogram every six months.	--	If the child is on a tricyclic antidepressant, the health care provider should order an electrocardiogram every six months.	•UNCHANGED• •DROPPED• **due to low validity score from panelists.**

Chapter 6 — Cesarean Delivery

[note: Scoring and modification of this chapter was deferred to the Women's Quality of Care Panel. See Chapter 6 of Women's Quality Indicators crosswalk table.]

Original Indicator		Modified Indicator		Comments
A. Prior Cesarean Delivery		**A. Prior Cesarean Delivery**		
(TREATMENT)		(TREATMENT)		
	1.	For women who have delivered by cesarean, the type of uterine incision used (transverse lower segment or vertical) should be noted in the medical record.	1.	For women who have delivered by cesarean, the type of uterine incision used (transverse lower segment or vertical) should be noted in the medical record.	•**UNCHANGED•** Note: This indicator applies to a cesarean section delivery that occurred during the study period, not to a prior cesarean section as the section heading implies.
	2.	For women with a cesarean delivery in a prior pregnancy, the number and type of previous uterine scar(s) should be noted in the current delivery medical record. (If this information is not available, an attempt to locate it should be documented in the chart.)	2.	For women with a cesarean delivery in a prior pregnancy, the number and type of previous uterine scar(s) should be noted in the current delivery medical record. (If this information is not available, an attempt to locate it should be documented in the chart.)	•**UNCHANGED•**
	3.	Women with one prior transverse lower segment cesarean should undergo a trial of labor unless another indication for cesarean delivery is present.	3.	Women with one prior transverse lower segment cesarean should undergo a trial of labor unless another indication for cesarean delivery is present **(including refusal of a trial of labor)**.	Women can not be forced to undergo a trial of labor if they do not desire it.
	4.	Women with a prior vertical cesarean should have a scheduled repeat cesarean delivery.	4.	Women with a prior **classical** vertical cesarean should have a scheduled repeat cesarean delivery.	Classical added because incidence of uterine rupture is highest with this type of vertical incision.
(DIAGNOSIS)		(DIAGNOSIS)		
B. Failure To Progress In Labor		**B. Failure To Progress In Labor**		
	1.	When the diagnosis of failure to progress in labor is made, a woman should be in the active phase of labor.	5.	When the diagnosis of failure to progress in labor is made, a woman should be in the active phase of labor.	•**UNCHANGED•**
	2.	When the diagnosis of failure to progress in labor is made, at least two exams of cervical dilatation separated in time by at least 2 hours should have been done and recorded in the medical record.	6.	When the diagnosis of failure to progress in labor is made, at least two exams of cervical dilatation separated in time by at least 2 hours should have been done and recorded in the medical record.	•**UNCHANGED•**
(TREATMENT)		(TREATMENT)		
	3.	Before a cesarean delivery is used to treat failure to progress in labor, at least one of the following therapeutic interventions should have been tried after the time of the diagnosis of FTP: • Amniotomy • Oxytocin • Ambulation	7.	Before a cesarean delivery is used to treat failure to progress in labor, at least **two** of the following therapeutic interventions should have been tried after the time of the diagnosis of FTP: • Amniotomy, • Oxytocin, or • Ambulation.	Changed to two of the following because more should be done before going to a C-section.
C. Fetal Distress		**C. Fetal Distress**		
(DIAGNOSIS)		(DIAGNOSIS)		

cont'd

	Original Indicator		Modified Indicator	Comments
1.	Fetuses should be monitored during active labor. The forms of monitoring are: • intermittent auscultation with a stethoscope or doppler device, or • continuous electronic fetal monitoring (EFM).	--	Fetuses should be monitored during active labor. The forms of monitoring are: • intermittent auscultation with a stethoscope or doppler device **as recommended by ACOG for low risk**, or • continuous electronic fetal monitoring (EFM).	ACOG minimum standard is every 30 minutes during first stage of labor for low risk. Added to define intermittent. **DROPPED due to operationalization difficulties.**
D. Antibiotic Prophylaxis			**D. Antibiotic Prophylaxis**	
(TREATMENT)			(TREATMENT)	
1.	Women who give birth by cesarean should receive at least one dose of antibiotic prophylaxis.	8.	Women who give birth by cesarean should receive at least one dose of antibiotic prophylaxis.	•**UNCHANGED•**
2.	Prophylactic antibiotic regimens should include one of the following: • broad spectrum penicillins, • broad spectrum cephalosporins, or • metronidazole.	9.	Prophylactic antibiotic regimens should include one of the following: • broad spectrum penicillins, • broad spectrum cephalosporins, or • metronidazole.	•**UNCHANGED•**
3.	Aminoglycosides should not be used, alone or in combination, for antibiotic prophylaxis.	10.	Aminoglycosides should not be used, alone or in combination, for antibiotic prophylaxis.	•**UNCHANGED•**
4.	Prophylactic antibiotics should be administered after the umbilical cord is clamped.	--	Prophylactic antibiotics should be administered after the umbilical cord is clamped.	**DROPPED due to operationalization difficulties**

Chapter 7 — Depression

	Original Indicator		Modified Indicator	Comments
	(SCREENING)		**(SCREENING)**	
1.	Clinicians should ask about the presence or absence of depression or depressive symptoms in any person with any of the following risk factors for depression: • divorce in past six months, • unemployment, • history of depression, • death in family in past six months, and • alcohol or other drug abuse.	1.	Clinicians should ask about the presence or absence of depression or depressive symptoms in any person with any of the following risk factors for depression: • **parental divorce in past six months,** • **school failure,** • history of depression, • death **of family member or friend** in past six months, **and** • **history of** alcohol, **cigarette,** or other drug abuse • **history of depression, substance abuse, or suicide attempts in family members** • **fired from job** • **parental marital discord** • **parental patient discord** • **school suspension, truancy, expulsion, or dropping out** • **Encounters with criminal justice** • **Breaking up with girlfriend/boyfriend** • **Homosexuality**	Panelists felt that additional risk factors should be assessed. Also, wording changed to clarify original indicator.
	(DIAGNOSIS)		**(DIAGNOSIS)**	
2.	If the diagnosis of depression is made, specific co-morbidities should be elicited and documented in the chart: - presence or absence of substance abuse - medication use - general medical disorder(s)	2.	If the diagnosis of depression is made, specific co-morbidities should be elicited and documented in the chart: - presence or absence of substance abuse - medication use - general medical disorder(s)	•UNCHANGED•
	(TREATMENT)		**(TREATMENT)**	
3.	If co-morbidity (substance abuse, contributing medication, general medical disorder) is present that contributes to depression, the initial treatment objective should be to remove the comorbidity or treat medical disorder.	--	If co-morbidity (substance abuse, contributing medication, general medical disorder) is present that contributes to depression, the initial treatment objective should be to remove the comorbidity or treat medical disorder.	•UNCHANGED• •DROPPED• due to operationalization difficulties.
4.	Once diagnosis of major depression has been made, treatment with anti-depressant medication and/or psychotherapy should begin within 2 weeks.	3.	Once diagnosis of major depression has been made, treatment with anti-depressant medication and/or psychotherapy should begin within 2 weeks.	•UNCHANGED•
5.	Presence or absence of suicidal ideation should be documented during the first or second diagnostic visit.	4.	Presence or absence of suicidal ideation should be documented during the first ~~or second~~ diagnostic visit.	It was felt that this could not wait until the second diagnostic visit.
6.	Medication treatment visits or telephone contacts should occur weekly for a minimum of 4 weeks.	5.	Medication treatment visits or telephone contacts should occur weekly for a minimum of 4 weeks.	•UNCHANGED•
7.	At least one of the following should occur if there is no or incomplete response to therapy for depression at 6 weeks: • Referral to psychotherapist if not already seeing one; or • Change or increase in dose of medication if on medication; or • Addition of medication if only using psychotherapy; or • Change in diagnosis documented in chart.	6.	At least one of the following should occur if there is no or **inadequate** response to therapy for depression at **8** weeks: • Referral to psychotherapist if not already seeing one; or • Change or increase in dose of medication if on medication; or • Addition of medication if only using psychotherapy; or • Change in diagnosis documented in chart.	It was felt that a time period of six weeks was too short. Also, wording changed to clarify original indicator.

Original Indicator	Modified Indicator	Comments
7.5 •NEW•	**7.** A follow-up family meeting should occur within 2 weeks of the initial evaluation.	•NEW• Panelists requested an additional indicator for follow-up to ensure patient is stable and to assess other health needs.
8. Anti-depressants should be used at appropriate dosages.	**8.** Anti-depressants should be used at appropriate dosages.	•UNCHANGED•
9. Anti-anxiety agents should generally NOT be used (except alprazolam).	**9.** Anti-anxiety agents should generally NOT be used (except alprazolam) **as the sole agent for treatment of depression, unless there is documentation of a comorbid anxiety disorder.**	Wording changed to clarify that anti-anxiety agents may be appropriate to treat comorbid anxiety.
10. Persons who have suicidality should be asked if they have specific plans to carry out suicide.	**10.** Persons who have suicidality should be asked if they have specific plans to carry out suicide, **access to a gun, and access to prescription medications.**	It was felt that physicians should assess enabling conditions as well as intent.
11. Persons who have suicidality and have any of the following risk factors should be hospitalized: a. psychosis, b. current alcohol or drug abuse, or c. specific plans to carry out suicide (e.g., obtaining a weapon, putting affairs in order, making a suicide note).	**11.** Persons who have suicidality and have any of the following risk factors should be hospitalized: a. psychosis, b. current alcohol or drug abuse, or c. specific plans to carry out suicide (e.g., obtaining a weapon, putting affairs in order, making a suicide note).	•UNCHANGED•
(FOLLOW-UP)	(FOLLOW-UP)	
12. Once depression has resolved, visits should occur every 16 weeks at a minimum, while patient is still on medication, for the first year of treatment.	-- Once depression has resolved, visits should occur every 16 weeks at a minimum, while patient is still on medication, for the first year of treatment.	•UNCHANGED• •DROPPED• due to operationalization difficulties.
13. At each visit during which depression is discussed, degree of response/remission and side effects of medication should be assessed and documented during the first year of treatment.	**12.** At each visit during which depression is discussed, degree of response/remission and side effects of medication should be assessed and documented during the first year of treatment.	•UNCHANGED•
14. Persons hospitalized for depression should have follow-up with a mental health specialist or their primary care doctor within two weeks of discharge.	**13.** Persons hospitalized for depression should have follow-up with a mental health specialist or their primary care doctor within **one week** of discharge.	Panelists felt that two weeks was too long to wait for follow-up.

Chapter 8 — Developmental Screening

	Original Indicator		Modified Indicator	Comments
1.	Social/personal development should be documented: a. Three times during the first year of life. b. Two times during the second year of life. c. One time during the third year of life. d. One time during the fourth year of life. e. One time during the fifth year of life.	1.	Social/personal development should be documented **at least:** a. **three** times during the first year of life. b. **two** times during the second year of life. c. one time during the third year of life. d. one time during the fourth year of life. e. one time during the fifth year of life.	Wording changed to clarify original indicator.
2.	Fine motor/visuomotor/problem solving development should be documented at least: a. Three times during the first year of life. b. Two times during the second year of life. c. One time during the third year of life. d. One time during the fourth year of life. e. One time during the fifth year of life.	2.	Fine motor/visuomotor/problem solving development should be documented at least: a. Three times during the first year of life. b. Two times during the second year of life. c. One time during the third year of life. d. One time during the fourth year of life. e. One time during the fifth year of life.	•UNCHANGED•
3.	Language development should be documented at least: a. Three times during the first year of life. b. Two times during the second year of life. c. One time during the third year of life. d. One time during the fourth year of life. e. One time during the fifth year of life.	3.	Language development should be documented at least: a. Three times during the first year of life. b. Two times during the second year of life. c. One time during the third year of life. d. One time during the fourth year of life. e. One time during the fifth year of life.	•UNCHANGED•
4.	Gross motor development should be documented at least: a. Three times during the first year of life. b. Two times during the second year of life. c. One time during the third year of life. d. One time during the fourth year of life. e. One time during the fifth year of life.	4.	Gross motor development should be documented at least: a. Three times during the first year of life. b. Two times during the second year of life. c. One time during the third year of life. d. One time during the fourth year of life. e. One time during the fifth year of life.	•UNCHANGED•
5.	In children with known developmental delay, referral to a specialist for early intervention should be documented.	5.	In children with **suspected or** known developmental delay, **a follow-up plan** should be documented.	Panelists felt that suspected developmental delay should be monitored, and that referral is not always necessary, depending on the type of delay and the context.
6.	In children with diagnosed language delay, referral to a specialist for speech therapy should be documented.	--		•DELETED• Merged into modified indicator #5.
7.	In children with gross or fine motor development delay, referral to a specialist for physical therapy should be documented.	--		•DELETED• Merged into modified indicator #5.
8.	•NEW•	6.	**For children ages 6-12, school performance should be asked about during a health assessment visit.**	•NEW• Panelists felt that school performance is a good measure of some components of development in this age group.

Chapter 9 — Diabetes Mellitus

[note: These indicators only apply to insulin-dependent diabetic children ≥ 7 years old.]

Original Indicator	Modified Indicator	Comments
(DIAGNOSIS)	(DIAGNOSIS)	
1. Patients with the diagnosis of diabetes should have the following routine monitoring tests:	1. Patients with the diagnosis of diabetes should have the following routine monitoring tests:	Fructosamine is an adequate substitute in (a).
a. Glycosylated hemoglobin every 6 months.	a. Glycosylated hemoglobin every 6 months.	Triglycerides (c) and HDL cholesterol (e) deleted pre-panel.
b. Eye and visual exam if more than 5 years since diagnosis at least once a year.	b. Eye and visual exam if more than 5 years since diagnosis at least once a year.	Urine protein is adequate in (f).
c. Triglycerides at least once a year.	c. ~~Triglycerides at least once a year.~~	Revision in (g) corrected a typographical error in original indicator.
d. Total cholesterol at least once a year.	d. Total cholesterol at least once a year.	Panelists felt six months was an appropriate interval for blood pressure in (h).
e. HDL cholesterol at least once a year.	-- ~~HDL cholesterol at least once a year.~~	(i) added because panelists wanted to ensure monitoring took place for normal growth.
f. Urinalysis at least once a year.	-- ~~Urinalysis at least once a year.~~	(j) added because Tanner stage can affect insulin dosing.
g. Examination of feet at every visit.	f. Urinalysis **or protein in urine** at least once a year.	(k) added because diabetes can be associated with psychosocial morbidity.
h. Measurement of blood pressure at every visit.	c. Examination of feet **once a year.**	•MODIFIED•
	-- ~~Measurement of blood pressure at every visit.~~	Dropped (d) (g) and (h) due to low validity score from panelists.
	h. Measurement of blood pressure every 6 months.	•UNCHANGED•
	i. Height and weight on growth chart every six months.	
	d. j. Tanner stage every six months after 10 years old until	
	e. Tanner stage V.	
	k. Psychosocial assessment at least annually	
	f.	
(TREATMENT)	(TREATMENT)	
2. All patients taking insulin should monitor their glucose at home daily.	2. All patients taking insulin should monitor their glucose at home daily.	
3. All diabetics should receive dietary and exercise counseling.	3. All diabetics should receive dietary and ~~exercise~~ counseling **at least once a year.**	Panelists felt annual requirement of exercise counseling for all diabetics does not reflect standard practice, and panelists felt that dietary counseling should occur repeatedly for reinforcement and to address changes in the patient's needs.

cont'd

Original Indicator	Modified Indicator	Comments
(FOLLOW-UP)	**(FOLLOW-UP)**	
4. All patients with diabetes should have a follow-up visit at least every 6 months.	4. All patients with diabetes should have a follow-up visit at least every 6 months.	•**UNCHANGED•**
5. •**NEW•**	5. **If HgA$_{1c}$ or ~~fructosamine~~ indicates poor control, the chart should indicate assessment of compliance and/or a change in treatment regimen.**	•**NEW•** Panelists request the addition of an indicator to address poor control of blood sugar. "fructosamine" dropped as the test was added to the peds indicator in error. The test is not performed in children.

Pediatric Quality Indicators

Chapter 10 — Diarrheal Disease, Acute

[note: **These indicators only apply to children up to 3 years old.**]

	Original Indicator		Modified Indicator	Comments
	(DIAGNOSIS)		(DIAGNOSIS)	
1.	In all children presenting with acute diarrhea, history should be obtained regarding:	1.	In all children presenting with acute diarrhea, history should be obtained regarding:	Volume deleted from 1(b) because it is difficult to assess accurately.
	a. The date of onset or duration of diarrheal stools.		a. The date of onset or duration of diarrheal stools.	
	b. Stool consistency, frequency (e.g., number per day), and volume.		b. Stool consistency **and** frequency (e.g., number per day), and volume.	1(f) changed from "and" to "or" because volume difficult to assess accurately.
	c. Presence or absence of blood in the stool.		c. Presence or absence of blood in the stool.	1(g) was moved up from #2.
	d. Presence or absence of fever, as reported by the parent.		d. Presence or absence of fever, as reported by the parent.	
	e. Presence or absence of vomiting.		e. Presence or absence of vomiting.	
	f. Frequency and volume of fluid intake.		f. Frequency **or** volume of fluid intake.	
			g. **Frequency of urinary output.**	
2.	History should be obtained regarding the frequency and volume of urinary output.		--	•DELETED• [moved up to #1g.]
3.	The weight should be recorded and, if available, compared to a recent weight obtained prior to the onset of diarrhea.	2.	The weight should be recorded and, if available, compared to a recent weight obtained prior to the onset of diarrhea.	•UNCHANGED•
4.	Documentation should also include:	---	Documentation should also include:	Capillary refill added as a measure of hydration status.
	a. Heart rate.		a. Heart rate.	
	b. Respiratory rate.		b. Respiratory rate.	•DROPPED• **(a), (b), (c), (d), and (e) due to low validity score from panelists.**
	c. Blood pressure.		c. Blood pressure.	
	d. Temperature.		d. Temperature.	
			e. **Capillary refill.**	
5.	All of the following findings regarding hydration status should be recorded:	3.	**At least two** of the following findings regarding hydration status should be recorded:	Panelists did not feel that is was necessary to document the full list, and they wanted to rate all of the hydration status findings together.
	a. General condition.		- general condition,	
	b. Appearance of eyes.		- appearance of eyes,	
	c. Presence or absence of tears.		- presence or absence of tears,	
	d. Degree of oral moisture.		- degree of oral moisture,	
	e. Degree of thirst.		- degree of thirst,	
	f. Degree of skin turgor.		- degree of skin turgor, or	
	g. Condition of anterior fontanelle.		- condition of anterior fontanelle.	
6.	The exam should note the presence or absence of blood in the stools, either by visual inspection or by chemical means.	4.	The exam should note the presence or absence of blood in the stools, either by visual inspection or by chemical means.	•UNCHANGED•
7.	The assessment of hydration status should be recorded in terms of percent dehydration or fluid deficit in milliliters per kilogram or as:	5.	The assessment of hydration status should be recorded in terms of percent dehydration or fluid deficit in milliliters per kilogram or as:	•UNCHANGED•
	• not dehydrated (less than 50 milliliters per kilogram fluid deficit)		• not dehydrated (less than 50 milliliters per kilogram fluid deficit),	
	• mild-moderate dehydration (50-100 milliliters per kilogram fluid deficit), or		• mild-moderate dehydration (50-100 milliliters per kilogram fluid deficit), or	
	• severe dehydration (greater than 100 milliliters per kilogram fluid deficit).		• severe dehydration (greater than 100 milliliters per kilogram fluid deficit).	

	Original Indicator		Modified Indicator	Comments
8.	Serum electrolytes should have been obtained if the child's dehydration was severe or if the pulse rate was elevated and the blood pressure was low.	6.	Serum electrolytes should have been obtained if the child's dehydration was severe or if the pulse rate was elevated and the blood pressure was low.	It was felt that severe dehydration was the salient issue and that the other signs did not necessitate this work-up in its absence.
9.	Urinalysis should have been obtained if the child's dehydration was severe or if the pulse rate was elevated and the blood pressure was low.	--	Urinalysis should be ordered if the child's dehydration was severe or if the pulse rate was elevated and the blood pressure was low.	It was felt that severe dehydration was the salient issue and that the other signs did not necessitate this work-up in its absence. •DROPPED• due to low validity score from panelists.
10.	Fecal leukocytes should have been obtained if the child with diarrhea is less than 36 months of age and had fever or blood in the stool.	7.	Fecal leukocytes should have been obtained if the child with diarrhea is less than 36 months of age and had fever or blood in the stool.	•UNCHANGED•
11.	Stool culture should be obtained if the child with diarrhea is less than 36 months of age and had fever or blood in the stool or > 5 fecal leukocytes per high power field.	8.	Stool culture should be obtained if the child with diarrhea is less than 36 months of age and had fever or blood in the stool or > 5 fecal leukocytes per high power field.	•UNCHANGED•
12.	A stool examination for ova and parasites should be obtained if the child had a history of recent travel to a developing country, acquired or congenital immunocompromise, or exposure to a potential carrier of parasitic diarrhea.	--	A stool examination for ova and parasites should be obtained if the child had a history of recent travel to a developing country, acquired or congenital immunocompromise, or exposure to a potential carrier of parasitic diarrhea.	•UNCHANGED• •DROPPED• due to low validity score from panelists.
13.	If stool was obtained for ova and parasite examination, three stool samples, obtained on three consecutive days, should have been ordered.	--	If stool was obtained for ova and parasite examination, three stool samples, obtained on three consecutive days, should have been ordered.	•UNCHANGED• •DROPPED• due to low validity score from panelists.
14.	(TREATMENT) If the child had diarrhea but was not dehydrated, the practitioner should recommend additional fluid intake beyond what is normal for the child.	9.	(TREATMENT) If the child had diarrhea but was not dehydrated, the practitioner should recommend additional fluid intake beyond what is normal for the child.	•UNCHANGED•
15.	If the child had mild-moderate dehydration, is not comatose, and is without intractable vomiting, has evidence of ileus, and moderate or severe purging upon administration of oral electrolyte-sugar solution, oral rehydration therapy should be prescribed and consist of: a. Electrolyte, sugar solution as specified by the American Academy of Pediatrics (1993) or the World Health Organization (Richards et al., 1993). b. Correction of the initial fluid deficit in the first 6 hours of treatment. c. Be monitored in the office or emergency room setting during entire period of rehydration.	10.	If the child had mild-moderate dehydration **and is able to take oral fluids**, oral rehydration therapy should be prescribed. and consist of: a. Electrolyte, sugar solution as specified by the American Academy of Pediatrics (1993) or the World Health Organization (Richards et al., 1993). b. Correction of the initial fluid deficit in the first 6 hours of treatment. c. Be monitored in the office or emergency room setting during entire period of rehydration.	Wording changed to clarify that oral rehydration is not feasible if a child cannot take oral fluids. Panelists felt that the original indicator was too detailed and specific.

Original Indicator	Modified Indicator	Comments
16. If the child had severe dehydration, intravenous rehydration should be prescribed and consist of: a. Replacement of the fluid deficit with either isotonic fluid, such as normal-saline or Ringer's Lactate solution as specified by the World Health Organization, or electrolyte solution based on serum electrolyte deficits. b. The pulse and blood pressure should be stabilized within normal limits for age within 6 hours of initiation of treatment. c. Replacement of the fluid deficit within 48 hours of initiation of treatment. d. Monitoring of input and output. e. Completion of all rehydration in the inpatient setting or observation unit.	11. If the child had severe dehydration, intravenous rehydration should be prescribed. ~~and consist of:~~ ~~a. Replacement of the fluid deficit with either isotonic fluid, such as normal-saline or Ringer's Lactate solution as specified by the World Health Organization, or electrolyte solution based on serum electrolyte deficits.~~ ~~b. The pulse and blood pressure should be stabilized within normal limits for age within 6 hours of initiation of treatment.~~ ~~c. Replacement of the fluid deficit within 48 hours of initiation of treatment.~~ ~~d. Monitoring of input and output.~~ ~~e. Completion of all rehydration in the inpatient setting or observation unit.~~	Panelists felt that the original indicator was too detailed and specific.
17. If while healthy the child was being breast fed, the health care provider should advise the parent to continue breast feeding if the child is able to feed orally.	12. If while healthy the child was being breast fed, the health care provider should advise the parent to continue breast feeding if the child is able to feed orally.	•UNCHANGED•
18. If while healthy the child was formula fed or weaned, the health care provider should have instituted refeeding within twenty-four hours of the onset of hydration therapy.	13. If while healthy the child was formula fed or weaned, the health care provider should have instituted refeeding within twenty-four hours of the onset of hydration therapy **if able to take oral fluids.**	Wording changed to clarify that this indicator is only appropriate if patient is able to take oral fluids.
19. Antimicrobial agents should be used in a child with: a. Suspected or culture-proven cholera with severe dehydration. b. Salmonella in patients with sickle cell anemia, lymphoma, leukemia, other immune compromise (acquired or congenital), positive stool culture for bacterial pathogen and less than 3 months of age, or bacteremia with salmonella and less than 6 months of age. c. Giardia with symptoms of greater than 10-14 days duration and with positive stool ova and parasite examination. d. Amoeba with positive stool ova and parasite examination.	14. Antimicrobial agents should be used in a child with: a. Suspected or culture-proven **shigella.** b. Salmonella in patients with sickle cell anemia, lymphoma, leukemia, other immune compromise (acquired or congenital), positive stool culture for bacterial pathogen and less than 3 months of age, or bacteremia with salmonella and less than 6 months of age. c. Giardia with symptoms of greater than 10-14 days duration and with positive stool ova and parasite examination. d. Amoeba with positive stool ova and parasite examination.	Cholera changed to shigella because panelists felt that cholera was too rare in the U.S. to warrant an indicator, but that shigella was prevalent enough to warrant an indicator.
20. Antidiarrheal or antimotility medications should never be used in treatment of diarrhea in a child.	15. Antidiarrheal or antimotility medications **are not** used in treatment of diarrhea in a child.	Wording changed to clarify original indicator.
(FOLLOW-UP)	(FOLLOW-UP)	
21. The young infant less than three months of age with acute diarrhea should have follow-up by the health care provider within: a. Three days of intervention for diarrhea without dehydration. b. One week after rehydration (either inpatient or outpatient) of mild-moderate or severe diarrhea.	--	•DELETED•

Original Indicator	Modified Indicator	Comments
22. The child with growth delay or malnutrition should have follow-up by the health care provider within: a. Three days of intervention for diarrhea without dehydration. b. One week after rehydration (either inpatient or outpatient) of mild-moderate or severe diarrhea.	--	•DELETED•
23. The child with immunocompromise should have follow-up by the health care provider within: a. Three days of intervention for diarrhea without dehydration. b. One week after rehydration (either inpatient or outpatient) of mild-moderate or severe diarrhea.	--	•DELETED•
24. Any child with severe dehydration should have follow-up by the health care provider within one week after discharge for intervention.	--	•DELETED•
25. Any child with inflammatory or invasive diarrhea should have follow-up by the health care provider within: a. Three days of intervention for diarrhea without dehydration. b. One week after discharge for intervention of mild-moderate or severe diarrhea.	--	•DELETED•
26. Any child with diarrhea and culture positive for parasites should have follow-up by the health care provider within: a. Three days of intervention for diarrhea without dehydration. b. One week after discharge for intervention of mild-moderate or severe diarrhea.	--	•DELETED•
27. If there is no improvement in diarrhea after 3 days of hydration therapy, the following work-up should be performed: a. Serum electrolytes. b. Urinalysis. c. Fecal leukocyte examination. d. Stool culture.	--	•DELETED•

Chapter 11 — Family Planning/Contraception

Original Indicator	Modified Indicator	Comments
(SCREENING)	**(SCREENING)**	
1. A history to determine risk for unintended pregnancy should be taken yearly on all women. In order to establish risk, the following elements of the history need to be documented:	1. A history to determine risk for unintended pregnancy should be taken at a **family planning visit** on all women. In order to establish risk, the following elements of the history need to be documented:	Panelists felt indicator should be limited to females interested in family planning and/or contraception.
a. Menstrual status (e.g., pre- or post-menopausal, history of hysterectomy, etc.), last menstrual period, or pregnancy test.	a. Menstrual status (e.g., pre- or post-menopausal, history of hysterectomy, etc.), last menstrual period, or pregnancy test.	Wording changed to be applicable to adolescent female population.
b. Sexual history (presence or absence of current sexual intercourse).	b. Sexual history (presence or absence of current sexual intercourse).	Past pregnancies were added because they are related to current risk of unintended pregnancy.
c. Current contraceptive practices.	c. Current contraceptive practices.	
d. Desire for pregnancy.	d. Desire for pregnancy.	
	e. **Past pregnancies**	
(TREATMENT)	**(TREATMENT)**	
2. All adolescent girls and boys at risk for unintended pregnancy (i.e., sexually active) should receive counseling about effective contraceptive methods.	2. All adolescent girls ~~and boys~~ at risk for unintended pregnancy (i.e., sexually active) should receive counseling about effective **risk reduction for pregnancy.**	Boys was deleted because it was a typographical error in the original indicator. Indicator broadened to cover counseling on all types of risk reduction methods.
3. The smoking status of all women prescribed combination OCs should be documented in the medical record.	3. The smoking status of all women prescribed combination OCs should be documented in the medical record.	•UNCHANGED•
4. All women who smoke and are prescribed oral contraceptives should be counseled and encouraged to quit smoking.	4. All women who smoke and are prescribed oral contraceptives should be counseled and encouraged to quit smoking.	•UNCHANGED•
5. •NEW•	5. Women prescribed contraceptives for the first time should have a follow-up visit within one month.	•NEW• Panelists felt follow-up is needed to monitor use and effectiveness.
6. •NEW•	6. Women prescribed contraceptives for the first time should have a pelvic exam within 1 month.	•NEW• Panelists wanted an indicator for pelvic exam.
7. •NEW•	7. Women prescribed contraceptives for the first time should have risks, benefits, and alternatives to contraception discussed with them and documented in chart.	•NEW• Patients should be fully informed.
8. •NEW•	8. Condoms should be made available to all women who are prescribed contraceptives.	•NEW• Indicator added because panelists felt that condoms are an important supplement to other contraceptives because they add protection against sexually transmitted diseases.

cont'd

Original Indicator	Modified Indicator	Comments
9. •NEW•	9. Women who are prescribed contraceptives should have a follow-up visit every 6 months thereafter.	•NEW• Panelists felt six month follow-up is needed to monitor contraceptive use.

Chapter 12 — Fever

[Note: These indicators only apply to children under 3 years old]

Original Indicator		Modified Indicator		Comments
(DIAGNOSIS)		(DIAGNOSIS)		
1.	The diagnosis of fever should be based on a temperature measurement of 38 degrees centigrade or greater taken at home or in the medical setting.	1.	The diagnosis of fever should be based on a temperature measurement of 38 degrees centigrade or greater taken at home or in the medical setting.	•UNCHANGED•
2.	The health care provider should document if the child had received an antipyretic and, if so, the time and the dose.	2.	The health care provider should document if the child had received an antipyretic and, if so, the time and the dose.	•UNCHANGED•
3.	The health care provider should document a temperature measured by oral or rectal thermometry in the medical setting.	3.	The health care provider should document a temperature measured by oral or rectal thermometry in the medical setting.	•UNCHANGED•
(TREATMENT)		(TREATMENT)		
Treatment regardless of age		*Treatment regardless of age*		
4.	In all children presenting with fever, the child's age should be recorded.	4.	In all children presenting with fever, The child's age should be recorded in the chart.	Child's age should be documented regardless of reason for visit.
5.	In all children presenting with fever, the following should be documented: a. Heart rate. b. Respiratory rate. c. Blood pressure.	--	In all children presenting with fever, the following should be documented: a. Heart rate. b. Respiratory rate. c. Blood pressure.	•UNCHANGED•
				•DROPPED• due to low validity score from panelists.
Treatment for the newborn infant less than 28 days of age presenting with fever (T>38.0)		*Treatment for the newborn infant less than 28 days of age presenting with fever (T>38.0)*		
6.	If the infant has fever, the infant should be hospitalized.	5.a.	If the infant has fever, a CBC and UA should be obtained.	Panelists wanted more detailed indicators for infants with fever.
		b.	If the infant has fever and diarrhea, a fecal leukocyte smear should be obtained.	CBC and UA are necessary to detect whether patient is at low risk (5a).
		c.	If the infant has fever and is not at low risk, the infant should be hospitalized.	Added fecal leukocyte from Rochester criteria to determine presence of a serious bacterial infection (5b).
		d.	The assessment should document whether or not the infant appears toxic, i.e., if the infant has signs of sepsis based on: • lethargy, • poor perfusion, or • hypoventilation, hyperventilation, or cyanosis.	Panelists felt only high-risk patients should be hospitalized (5c). Original indicator #6 became modified indicator #5c.
		e.	The assessment should include whether or not the infant had been healthy up to the point of this illness.	Based on Rochester criteria and need to determine risk level (5d). Based on Rochester criteria (5e).

	Original Indicator		Modified Indicator	Comments
7.	The assessment should include: a. A complete blood count. b. Urinalysis. c. Cerebrospinal fluid analysis of glucose and protein. d. Gram stain. e. Cell count. f. Blood culture. g. Urine culture. h. Cerebrospinal fluid culture.	6.	If the infant is not at low risk, the assessment should include: — a. A complete blood count. — b. Urinalysis. a. c. Cerebrospinal fluid studies — d. Gram stain. — e. Cell count. b. f. Blood culture. c. g. Urine culture. — h. Cerebrospinal fluid culture.	Panelists felt this indicator should be limited to high risk patients. CBC and UA moved to 5a above. Others combined into cerebrospinal fluid studies.
8.	If the infant has lower respiratory symptoms, a chest radiograph should be obtained.	7.	If the infant has lower respiratory **signs or** symptoms **not explained by elevated fever**, a chest radiograph should be obtained.	Panelists indicated that signs not explained by elevated fever are sufficient to necessitate a chest radiograph.
9.	If the infant has bloody diarrhea or a fecal leukocyte count >= 5 leukocytes per high power field, a stool culture should be obtained.	8.	If the infant has bloody diarrhea or a fecal leukocyte count >= 5 leukocytes per high power field, a stool culture should be obtained.	•UNCHANGED•
10.	If the infant is nontoxic and at low risk, then the infant should be treated with empiric antibiotics.	--	If the infant is nontoxic and at low risk, then the infant should be treated with empiric antibiotics.	•UNCHANGED• •DROPPED• **due to low validity score from panelists.**
10a.	•NEW•	9.	**If the infant with fever is at low risk and is being managed as an outpatient, the infant's condition should be reassessed in 18-24 hours.**	•NEW• It was felt that follow-up is important to prevent morbidity due to untreated serious bacterial infection.
10b.	•NEW•	--	**The infant who was nontoxic and initially at low risk and was still nontoxic and at low risk on first follow-up should receive another follow-up within 24 hours.**	•NEW• In many labs, final readings of tests do not occur until two days after collection of specimen. Intended to prevent morbidity due to untreated serious bacterial infection. •DROPPED• **due to low validity score from panelists.**
11.	If the infant is toxic in appearance (e.g., lethargic; poor perfusion; or marked hypoventilation, hyperventilation, or cyanosis), or at high risk, then the infant should be treated with empiric parenteral antibiotics pending the culture results.	10.	If the infant is toxic in appearance (e.g., lethargic; poor perfusion; or marked hypoventilation, hyperventilation, or cyanosis), or at high risk, then the infant should be treated with empiric parenteral antibiotics pending the culture results.	•UNCHANGED•

cont'd

	Original Indicator		Modified Indicator	Comments
12.	The infant should be treated with parenteral antimicrobials if: • any culture is positive, • the cerebrospinal fluid studies are abnormal, • the chest radiograph demonstrates an infiltrate or effusion, or • skin, soft tissue, bone, joint, or ear infection are present.	11.	The infant should be treated with parenteral antimicrobials if: • any culture is positive, • the cerebrospinal fluid studies are abnormal, • the chest radiograph demonstrates an infiltrate ~~or effusion~~, or • **the chest radiograph demonstrates an effusion,** • **cellulitis**, soft tissue, bone~~,~~ **or** joint~~, or ear~~ infection are present.	Panelists indicated that infiltrate and effusion should be separated. Skin changed to cellulitis to clarify original indicator. Panelists indicated that ear infections should be considered separately. Panelists rated cellulitis, soft tissue, bone, joint infection as one in indicator #11; ear infection rated separately in indicator 12a.
12a.	**•NEW•**	--	**The infant should be treated with parenteral antimicrobials if:** • **ear infection is present.**	•NEW• Panelists indicated that ear infections should be considered separately. Panelists rated cellulitis, soft tissue, bone, joint infection as one in indicator #11; ear infection rated separately in indicator 12a. **•DROPPED• due to low validity score from panelists.**
	Diagnosis and treatment for the infant 28 to 90 days of age with fever (>38°C)		***Diagnosis and treatment for the infant 28 to 90 days of age with fever (>38°C)***	
13.	The assessment should document whether or not the infant appears toxic, i.e., if the infant has signs of sepsis based on: • lethargy, • poor perfusion, or • hypoventilation, hyperventilation, or cyanosis.	12.	The assessment should document whether or not the infant appears toxic, i.e., if the infant has signs of sepsis based on: • lethargy, • poor perfusion, or • hypoventilation, hyperventilation, or cyanosis.	•UNCHANGED•
14.	The assessment should include whether or not the infant had been healthy up to the point of this illness.†	13.	The assessment should include whether or not the infant had been healthy up to the point of this illness.†	•UNCHANGED•
15.	All children who present with fever > 39°C should receive: a) Complete blood count. b) Urinalysis.	14.	All children who present with fever > **38**°C should receive: a) Complete blood count. b) Urinalysis.	Temperature changed because it was a typographical error in original indicator.
16.	If the child has fever and diarrhea, a fecal leukocyte evaluation should be done.	15.	If the child has fever and diarrhea, a fecal leukocyte evaluation should be done.	•UNCHANGED•
17.	If the infant is at high risk, the infant should be hospitalized.	16.	If the infant is **toxic or** at high risk, the infant should be hospitalized.	Panelists felt that toxic patients should be admitted for sepsis evaluation and parenteral antibiotics.

Original Indicator	Modified Indicator	Comments
18. If the infant is toxic or at high risk, the assessment should also include: a. Cerebrospinal fluid analysis of glucose and protein. b. Gram stain. c. Cell count. d. Blood culture. e. Urine culture. f. Cerebrospinal fluid culture.	17. If the infant is toxic or at high risk, the assessment should also include: a. Cerebrospinal fluid **studies.** -- ~~b. Gram stain.~~ -- ~~c. Cell count.~~ b. ~~d.~~ Blood culture. c. ~~e.~~ Urine culture. -- ~~f. Cerebrospinal fluid culture.~~	Wording of (a) changed to incorporate (b), (c), and (f).
19. If the infant is not toxic and is at low risk, the infant may be managed as an outpatient. One of the following courses should be followed: a. Obtain cerebrospinal fluid for glucose, protein, gram stain, and cell count determination; obtain blood, urine, and cerebrospinal fluid cultures; and, administer intramuscular ceftriaxone. b. Obtain at least a urine culture and withhold antimicrobial treatment.	-- If the infant is not toxic and is at low risk, the infant may be managed as an outpatient. One of the following courses should be followed: a. Obtain cerebrospinal fluid for glucose, protein, gram stain, and cell count determination; obtain blood, urine, and cerebrospinal fluid cultures; and, administer intramuscular ceftriaxone **or equivalent.** b. Obtain at least a urine culture and withhold antimicrobial treatment.	Clarified that treatment comparable to intramuscular ceftriaxone would be acceptable as an alternative. •DROPPED• (a) and (b) [all] due to low validity score from panelists.
20. If the infant with fever is at low risk and is being managed as an outpatient, the infant's condition should be reassessed in 18-24 hours in the medical care setting.	18. If the infant with fever is at low risk and is being managed as an outpatient, the infant's condition should be reassessed in ~~18-24 hours in the medical care setting.~~	Panelists felt that telephone assessment or other setting should count as appropriate.
21. If the infant who was initially nontoxic and at low risk is still nontoxic at follow-up in the outpatient setting, then: a. Under the first course: - a second dose of ceftriaxone is administered, and - the culture results are reviewed. b. Under the second course - the culture result(s) are reviewed.	-- If the infant who was initially nontoxic and at low risk is still nontoxic at follow-up ~~in the outpatient setting,~~ then: a. Under the first course: - a second dose of ceftriaxone is administered, and - the culture results are reviewed. b. Under the second course - the culture result(s) are reviewed.	Panelists felt that telephone assessment or other setting should count as appropriate. •DROPPED• due to low validity score from panelists.
22. The infant who was nontoxic and initially at low risk and was still nontoxic and at low risk on first follow-up in the outpatient setting should receive another follow-up in the medical care setting within 24 hours.	-- The infant who was nontoxic and initially at low risk and was still nontoxic and at low risk on first follow-up ~~in the outpatient setting~~ should receive another follow-up ~~in the medical care setting~~ within 24 hours.	Panelists felt that telephone assessment or other setting should count as appropriate. •DROPPED• due to low validity score from panelists.
23. If the infant with fever has lower respiratory symptoms, a chest radiograph should be obtained.	19. If the infant with fever has lower respiratory **signs and symptoms not explained by elevated fever,** a chest radiograph should be obtained.	Panelists indicated that a chest radiograph is only necessary if the patient has lower respiratory signs and symptoms not explained by fever.
24. If the infant with fever has bloody diarrhea or a fecal leukocyte count greater than 5 leukocytes per high power field, a stool culture should be obtained.	20. If the infant with fever has bloody diarrhea or a fecal leukocyte count greater than 5 leukocytes per high power field, a stool culture should be obtained.	•UNCHANGED•
25. If at any point the blood culture is positive, the infant should be hospitalized for parenteral antibiotic treatment appropriate to the specific diagnosis except in the case of bacteremia due to *Streptococcus pneumonia.*	21. If at any point the blood culture is positive, **and not felt to be a contaminant,** the infant should be hospitalized for parenteral antibiotic treatment appropriate to the specific diagnosis except in the case of bacteremia due to *Streptococcus pneumonia.*	Panelists wanted to rule out specimen contamination.

	Original Indicator		Modified Indicator	Comments
26.	If at any point the urine culture is positive, the infant should be hospitalized for parenteral antibiotic treatment appropriate to the specific diagnosis except in the case of an afebrile and nontoxic infant.	--	If at any point the urine culture is positive, **and not felt to be a contaminant**, the infant should be hospitalized for parenteral antibiotic treatment appropriate to the specific diagnosis except in the case of an afebrile and nontoxic infant.	Panelists wanted to rule out specimen contamination. •DROPPED• **due to low validity score from panelists.**
27.	If at any point the cerebrospinal fluid results are abnormal or the cerebrospinal fluid culture is positive, the infant should be hospitalized for parenteral antimicrobial treatment appropriate to the specific diagnosis.	22.	If at any point the cerebrospinal fluid results are abnormal or the cerebrospinal fluid culture is positive, **and not felt to be a contaminant**, the infant should be hospitalized for parenteral antimicrobial treatment appropriate to the specific diagnosis.	Panelists wanted to rule out specimen contamination. •UNCHANGED•
28.	If at any point pneumonia is diagnosed, the infant should be hospitalized for parenteral antimicrobial treatment appropriate to the specific diagnosis.	--	If at any point pneumonia is diagnosed, the infant should be hospitalized for parenteral antimicrobial treatment appropriate to the specific diagnosis.	•DROPPED• **due to low validity score from panelists.**
29.	If at any point a skin, soft tissue, bone, or joint infection is diagnosed, the infant should be hospitalized for parenteral antimicrobial treatment appropriate to the specific diagnosis.	--	If at any point **cellulitis or a** soft tissue, bone, or joint infection is diagnosed, the infant should be hospitalized for parenteral antimicrobial treatment appropriate to the specific diagnosis.	Skin changed to cellulitis to clarify original indicator. •DROPPED• **due to low validity score from panelists.**
	Treatment for the child 3 to 36 months of age		*Treatment for the child 3 to 36 months of age*	
30.	The assessment should document: a. Level of consciousness. b. Temperature. c. Heart rate. d. Respiratory rate. e. Blood pressure. f. Perfusion. g. Degree of cyanosis.	23. a. -- -- -- -- b. c.	The assessment should document: a. Level of consciousness. ~~b. Temperature.~~ ~~c. Heart rate.~~ ~~d. Respiratory rate.~~ ~~e. Blood pressure.~~ f. Perfusion. g. Degree of cyanosis.	30(b) deleted because it is a repeat of indicator #3. 30(c), (d), and (e) were deleted because they are repeats of indicator 5 (which was dropped due to low validity score from panelists).
31.	If the infant/child is at high risk for sepsis, the infant should be hospitalized.	24.	If the infant/child is at high risk for sepsis, the infant should be hospitalized.	•UNCHANGED•
32.	If the infant/child is at high risk for sepsis, the assessment should include a complete blood count; urinalysis; cerebrospinal fluid analysis of glucose, protein, gram stain, and cell count; and, blood, urine, and cerebrospinal fluid cultures.	25.	If the infant/child is at high risk for sepsis, the assessment should include a complete blood count; urinalysis; cerebrospinal fluid analysis of glucose **and** protein, gram stain, and cell count; and blood, urine, and cerebrospinal fluid cultures.	Wording changed to clarify original indicator.
33.	If the infant/child is at low risk for sepsis and the temperature is greater than or equal to 39°C and there is no obvious source of infection, a urine culture should be obtained if the child is a female less than two years of age or a male less than six months of age.	26.	If the infant/child is at low risk for sepsis and the temperature is greater than or equal to 39°C and there is no obvious source of infection, a urine culture should be obtained if the child is a female less than two years of age or a male less than six months of age **or an uncircumcised male less than 2 years of age.**	Panelists felt that uncircumcised males up to two years of age are at greater risk for infection.
34.	If the infant/child is at low risk for sepsis and the temperature is greater than or equal to 39°C and diarrhea is present, a stool culture should be obtained if there is blood and mucus in the stool or if there are ≥5 leukocytes per high power field in the stool.	27.	If the infant/child is at low risk for sepsis and the temperature is greater than or equal to 39°C and diarrhea is present, a stool culture should be obtained if there is blood and mucus in the stool or if there are ≥5 leukocytes per high power field in the stool.	•UNCHANGED•

	Original Indicator		Modified Indicator	Comments
35.	If the infant/child is at low risk for sepsis and the temperature is greater than or equal to 39°C, a chest radiograph should be obtained in a child with dyspnea, rales, or decreased breath sounds.	28.	If the infant/child is at low risk for sepsis and the temperature is greater than or equal to 39°C, a chest radiograph should be obtained in a child with dyspnea, **tachypnea**, rales, or decreased breath sounds.	Tachypnea added because it was a typographical error in original indicator.
36.	If the infant/child is at low risk for sepsis and the temperature is greater than or equal to 39°C, then: a. A blood culture should be obtained. b. The child should be treated empirically with parenteral antibiotics.	--	If the infant/child is at low risk for sepsis and the temperature is greater than or equal to 39°C, then: a. A blood culture should be obtained. b. The child should be treated empirically with parenteral antibiotics.	Panelists indicated that obtaining a blood culture is not standard practice. •DROPPED• (b) due to low validity score from panelists.
37.	If the infant/child is at low risk for sepsis and the temperature is greater than or equal to 39°C, then: a. A blood culture should be obtained. b. A CBC should be obtained. c. The child should be treated with antibiotics only if the WBC is ≥15,000.	--	If the infant/child is at low risk for sepsis and the temperature is greater than or equal to 39°C, then: • a blood culture should be obtained **if WBC ≥15,000,** • a CBC should be obtained, **and** • **if the WBC is ≥15,000, the child should be treated with antibiotics.**	WBC is needed to determine whether child is high risk (37a). Wording of 37(c) changed to clarify original indicator. •DROPPED• due to low validity score from panelists.
38.	If the infant/child is at low risk for sepsis and the temperature is greater than or equal to 39°C, then the infant/child should be reassessed in 24-48 hours in the medical setting.	--	If the infant/child is at low risk for sepsis and the temperature is greater than or equal to 39°C, then the infant/child should be reassessed in 24-48 hours in the medical setting.	Panelists felt that telephone assessment should count as appropriate. •DROPPED• due to low validity score from panelists.
39.	If the infant/child at low risk for sepsis with an initial temperature greater than or equal to 39°C is well-appearing at outpatient follow-up, no further intervention is required; but, the parent should be advised to return if the fever persists greater than 48 hours.	29.	If the infant/child at low risk for sepsis with an initial temperature greater than or equal to 39°C is well-appearing at outpatient follow-up, no further intervention is required; but, the parent should be advised to return if the fever persists greater than 48 hours.	Panelists felt that telephone assessment should count as appropriate.
40.	If at any point the blood culture is positive, the infant/child should be hospitalized for parenteral antibiotic treatment appropriate to the specific diagnosis except in the case of bacteremia due to Streptococcus pneumonia.	30.	If at any point the blood culture is positive, **and not felt to be a contaminant,** the infant/child should be hospitalized for parenteral antibiotic treatment appropriate to the specific diagnosis except in the case of bacteremia due to Streptococcus pneumonia.	Panelists wanted to rule out specimen contamination.
41.	If at any point the urine culture is positive, the infant/child should be hospitalized for parenteral antibiotic treatment appropriate to the specific diagnosis except in the case of an afebrile, nontoxic infant/child.	--	If at any point the urine culture is positive, **and not felt to be a contaminant,** the infant/child should be hospitalized for parenteral antibiotic treatment appropriate to the specific diagnosis except in the case of an afebrile, nontoxic infant/child.	Panelists wanted to rule out specimen contamination. •DROPPED• due to low validity score from panelists.
42.	If at any point the cerebrospinal fluid results are abnormal or the cerebrospinal fluid culture is positive, the infant/child should be hospitalized for parenteral antimicrobial treatment appropriate to the specific diagnosis.	31.	If at any point the cerebrospinal fluid results are abnormal or the cerebrospinal fluid culture is positive **and not felt to be a contaminant,** the infant/child should be hospitalized for parenteral antimicrobial treatment appropriate to the specific diagnosis.	Panelists wanted to rule out specimen contamination.
43.	If at any point pneumonia is diagnosed, the infant/child should be hospitalized for parenteral antimicrobial treatment appropriate to the specific diagnosis.	--	If at any point pneumonia is diagnosed, the infant/child should be hospitalized for parenteral antimicrobial treatment appropriate to the specific diagnosis.	•UNCHANGED• •DROPPED• due to low validity score from panelists.

cont'd

	Original Indicator	Modified Indicator	Comments
44.	If at any point a skin, soft tissue, bone, or joint infection is diagnosed, the infant/child should be hospitalized for parenteral antimicrobial treatment appropriate to the specific diagnosis.	--	If at any point **cellulitis or a** soft tissue, bone, or joint infection is diagnosed, the infant/child should be hospitalized for parenteral antimicrobial treatment appropriate to the specific diagnosis.	Panelists wanted to rate cellulitis/soft tissue and bone/joint infection separately. •**DROPPED• due to low validity score from panelists.**
44a.	•NEW•	33.	If at any point cellulitis or a soft tissue, a bone or joint infection is diagnosed, the infant/child should be hospitalized for parenteral antimicrobial treatment appropriate to the specific diagnosis.	Panelists wanted to rate cellulitis/soft tissue and bone/joint infection separately.

Pediatric Quality Indicators

Chapter 13 — Headache

Original Indicator	Modified Indicator	Comments
(DIAGNOSIS)	(DIAGNOSIS)	
1. All patients with new onset headache should be asked about: a. Location of the pain (e.g., frontal, bilateral). b. Associated symptoms (e.g., aura). c. Temporal profile (e.g., new onset, constant). d. Severity. e. Family history.	1. All patients with new onset headache should be asked about: a. Location of the pain (e.g., frontal, bilateral). **b. Associated symptoms (e.g., aura).** c. Temporal profile (e.g., new onset, constant). d. Severity. e. Family history. **-- f. Risk factors or symptoms of depression.**	Panelists felt that depression can cause headaches. •MODIFIED• **Dropped (f) due to low validity score from panelists.**
2. All patients with new onset headache should have a neurological examination evaluating the: a. Cranial nerves. b. Fundi. c. Deep tendon reflexes.	2. All patients with new onset headache should have a neurological an examination evaluating the: a. Cranial nerves. b. Fundi. -- c. Deep tendon reflexes. **d. Visual fields.** **e. Visual acuity.** **f. Extraocular movement.** **g. Blood pressure.**	Wording changed to eliminate redundancy. Additional components of a neurologic examination important for the headache work-up were added. •MODIFIED• **Dropped (c) due to low validity score from panelists.**
3. CT or MRI scanning is indicated in patients with new onset headache and any of the following circumstances: a. Abnormal neurological examination b. Constant headache c. Severe headache	3. CT or MRI scanning is indicated in patients with new onset headache and any of the following circumstances: a. Abnormal neurological examination -- b. Constant headache -- c. Severe headache **d. Migraine that is always on the same side.** **e. Morning headache with vomiting.**	Symptoms that could indicate intracranial tumors or other mass lesions were added. •MODIFIED• **Dropped (b), (c), and (d) due to low validity score from panelists.**
4. Skull X-rays should not be part of an evaluation for headache.	4. Skull X-rays should not be part of an evaluation for headache.	•UNCHANGED•
(TREATMENT)	(TREATMENT)	
5. If the patient has an acute mild migraine or tension headache, he or she should receive aspirin, tylenol, or other nonsteroidal anti-inflammatory agents before being prescribed any other medication.	5. If the patient has an acute mild migraine or tension headache, he or she should receive aspirin, tylenol, or other nonsteroidal anti-inflammatory agents, **isometheptic compound (Midrin), or an ergot preparation** before being prescribed any other medication.	Additional treatments considered appropriate were added.
6. If the patient has an acute moderate or severe migraine headache, he or she should receive one of the following before being prescribed any other agent: a. Intramuscular ketorolac. b. Intravenous dihydroergotamine. c. Intravenous chlorpromazine. d. Intravenous metaclopramide.	6. If the patient has an acute moderate or severe migraine headache, he or she should receive one of the following before being prescribed any other agent: a. **Parenteral** ketorolac. b. **Parenteral** dihydroergotamine. c. **Parenteral phenothiazines.** d. **Sumatriptan.** -- e. Solumedrol -- f. Butorphanol	Parenteral added to clarify original indicator. Changes in medication list were made to be consistent with standard practice. •MODIFIED• **Dropped (e) and (f) due to low validity score from panelists.**
7. Recurrent moderate or severe tension headaches should be treated with a trial of tricyclic antidepressant agents.	--	•DELETED•

cont'd

	Original Indicator	Modified Indicator	Comments
8.	If a patient has more than 2 migraine headaches each month, then prophylactic treatment is indicated with one of the following agents: a. Beta blockers. b. Calcium channel blockers. c. Tricyclic antidepressants. d. Naproxen. e. Fluoxetine. f. Valproate. g. Cyproheptadine.	7. If a patient has more than 2 **moderate to severe** migraine headaches each month, then prophylactic treatment **may be used** with one of the following agents: **a.** Beta blockers. **b.** Calcium channel blockers. **c.** Tricyclic antidepressants. ~~d. Naproxen.~~ **d.** Fluoxetine. **e.** Valproate. **f.** Cyproheptadine.	It was felt that this indicator should be limited to moderate to severe headaches. It was felt that prophylactic treatment is not always required but that this list of medications is appropriate for prophylaxis. Naproxen was not considered standard treatment for this indication.
9.	Opioid agonists and barbiturates should not be first-line therapy for migraine or tension headaches.	8. Opioid agonists and barbiturates should not be first-line therapy for migraine or tension headaches.	•UNCHANGED•
10.	•NEW•	9. **Sumatriptan and ergotamine should not be concurrently administered.**	•NEW• Omission of this indicator was a typographical error. This indicator was included in the literature review.
11.	•NEW•	10. **Sumatriptan should not be used for hemiplegic migraines.**	•NEW• This indicator was added because it was identified as an important contraindication.

-517-

Pediatric Quality Indicators

Chapter 14 — Immunizations

Original Indicator	Modified Indicator	Comments
Polio	**Polio**	
1. All children should have had two OPV/IPV between six weeks and the first birthday.	1. All children should have had two OPV/IPV between six weeks and the first birthday.	•UNCHANGED•
2. All children should have had three OPV/IPV between six weeks and the second birthday.	2. All children should have had three OPV/IPV between six weeks and the second birthday.	•UNCHANGED•
3. All children should have had four OPV/IPV between six weeks and the seventh birthday.	3. All children should have had four OPV/IPV between six weeks and the seventh birthday.	•UNCHANGED•
4. Children with immunocompromise (hematologic and solid tumors, congenital immunodeficiency, and long-term immunosuppressive therapy) or HIV infection should receive IPV rather than OPV (at the same ages as OPV).	4. Children with immunocompromise (hematologic and solid tumors, congenital immunodeficiency, and long-term immunosuppressive therapy) or HIV infection should receive IPV rather than OPV (at the same ages as OPV).	•UNCHANGED•
5. Before each OPV, guardians should be questioned about the presence of an immunocompromised contact in the household.	5. Before each OPV, guardians should be questioned about the presence of an immunocompromised contact in the household.	
6. If there is a household contact with immunocompromise, children should receive IPV instead of OPV.	6. If there is a household contact with immunocompromise, children should receive IPV instead of OPV.	•UNCHANGED•
Diphtheria/Tetanus/Pertussis	**Diphtheria/Tetanus/Pertussis**	
7. All children should have had three DTP between six weeks and the first birthday.	7. All children should have had three DTP/**DTaP/DT** between six weeks and the first birthday.	•UNCHANGED• **Added DTaP to reflect current recommendations.** **Added DT for clarification purposes.**
8. All children should have had four DTP between six weeks and the second birthday, with at least six months between the third and fourth dose (the fourth may be DTaP if given after 15 months old).	8. All children should have had four DTP/**DTaP/DT** between six weeks and the second birthday, with at least six months between the third and fourth dose (the fourth may be DTaP if given after 15 months old).	•UNCHANGED• **Added DTaP to reflect current recommendations.** **Added DT for clarification purposes.**
9. All children should have had five DTP/DTaP between six weeks and the seventh birthday, with at least six weeks between the third and fourth doses (the fourth and fifth may be DTaP if given after 15 months).	9. All children should have had five DTP/DTaP/**DT** between six weeks and the seventh birthday, with at least six weeks between the third and fourth doses (the fourth and fifth may be DTaP if given after 15 months).	•UNCHANGED• **Added DT for clarification purposes.**
10. By age 17, all children should have had one Td between age 7 and 17. A formulation that includes pertussis is acceptable.	10. By age 17, all children should have had one Td between age 7 and 17. A formulation that ~~includes pertussis is acceptable~~.	Panelists felt that pertussis is generally not given in this age group and did not need to be included in the indicator.
11. Children who have had encephalopathy within 7 days of a prior dose of DTP should not receive any further vaccination with DTP.	11. Children who have had encephalopathy within 7 days of a prior dose of DTP should not receive any further vaccination with DTP.	•UNCHANGED•
Haemophilus influenzae type B	**Haemophilus influenzae type B**	
12. All children should have had two PRP-OMP Hib or three Hib (any combination of formulations) between six weeks and the first birthday.	12. All children should have had two PRP-OMP Hib or three Hib (any combination of formulations) between six weeks and the first birthday.	•UNCHANGED•

cont'd

	Original Indicator	Modified Indicator	Comments
13.	Between the ages of six weeks and 2 years, all children should have had either: – four Hib vaccinations, or – three Hib vaccinations if the first two were PRP-OMB Hib.	Between the ages of six weeks and 2 years, all children should have had either: – four Hib vaccinations, or – three Hib vaccinations if the first two were PRP-OMB Hib.	•UNCHANGED•
Measles/Mumps/Rubella			
14.	All children should have had one MMR between their first and second birthdays.	All children should have had one MMR between their first and second birthdays.	•UNCHANGED•
15.	All children should have had an MMR between their fourth and thirteenth birthdays.	All children should have had **a second** MMR **before their** thirteenth birthday.	Panelists felt second MMR is acceptable if given before fourth birthday.
16.	Children who are immunocompromised (with the exception of children with HIV infection) (hematologic and solid tumors, congenital immunodeficiency, and long-term immunosuppressive therapy) should not receive MMR.	Children who are immunocompromised (with the exception of children with HIV infection) (hematologic and solid tumors, congenital immunodeficiency, and long-term immunosuppressive therapy) should not receive MMR.	•UNCHANGED•
Hepatitis B			
17.	The mother's HBsAg status should be documented in the child's chart within one week of birth.	The mother's HBsAg status should be documented in the child's chart within one week of birth.	•UNCHANGED•
18.	All children whose mothers are known to be HBsAg-Negative should have had at least two HBV by the first birthday with at least one month between the first two doses.	All children whose mothers are known to be HBsAg-Negative should have had at least two HBV by the first birthday with at least one month between the first two doses.	•UNCHANGED•
19.	All children whose mothers are known to be HBsAg-Negative should have had three HBV by the second birthday with at least one month between the first two doses.	All children whose mothers are known to be HBsAg-Negative should have had three HBV by the second birthday with at least one month between the first two doses.	•UNCHANGED•
20.	All children whose mothers are known to be HBsAg-Positive at birth should receive HBIG and HBV by the beginning of the twelfth hour of life.	All children whose mothers are known to be HBsAg-Positive at birth should receive HBIG and HBV by the beginning of the twelfth hour of life.	•UNCHANGED•
21.	All children whose mothers are known to be HBsAg-Positive should have had three HBV by the beginning of the ninth month of life.	All children whose mothers are known to be HBsAg-Positive should have had three HBV by the beginning of the ninth month of life.	•UNCHANGED•
22.	All children whose mother's HBsAg status is not known should receive HBV by the beginning of the twelfth hour of life.	All children whose mother's HBsAg status is not known should receive HBV by the beginning of the twelfth hour of life.	•UNCHANGED•
23.	All children whose mother's HBsAg status is not known by the end of the first week of life should receive HBIG.	All children whose mother's HBsAg status is not known by the end of the first week of life should receive HBIG.	•UNCHANGED•
24.	Adolescents with any of the following risk factors should receive the full three-part HBV series within one year of the clinician becoming aware of the risk factor: – have a history of sexually transmitted infection; – have had more than one sexual partner in the previous six months; – use injection drugs; – are males who are sexually active with other males; – are sexual contacts of high-risk individuals; or – have tasks as employees, volunteers, or trainees that involve contact with blood or blood-contaminated body fluids.	Adolescents with any of the following risk factors should receive the full three-part HBV series within one year of the clinician becoming aware of the risk factor: – have a history of sexually transmitted infection; – have had more than one sexual partner in the previous six months; – use injection drugs; – are males who are sexually active with other males; – are sexual contacts of high-risk individuals; or – have tasks as employees, volunteers, or trainees that involve contact with blood or blood-contaminated body fluids.	•UNCHANGED•
Influenza			

Pediatric Quality Indicators

Original Indicator	Modified Indicator	Comments
25. Children with asthma and other chronic pulmonary diseases, hemodynamically significant cardiac disease, hemoglobinopathies (e.g., sickle cell disease) or undergoing immunosuppressive therapy should receive a yearly influenza vaccine. Other children at high risk may also benefit from an annual influenza vaccine, including those with: HIV infection, diabetes mellitus, chronic renal disease, and chronic metabolic diseases.	25. Children with asthma and other chronic pulmonary diseases, hemodynamically significant cardiac disease, hemoglobinopathies (e.g., sickle cell disease) or undergoing immunosuppressive therapy should receive a yearly influenza vaccine. ~~Other children at high risk may also benefit from an annual influenza vaccine, including those with: HIV infection, diabetes mellitus, chronic renal disease, and chronic metabolic diseases.~~	•UNCHANGED• "other children..." deleted to clarify intent of indicator.
General Indicators	**General Indicators**	
26. An inquiry should be made before each new set of immunizations (or after each prior set) about reactions to prior vaccines.	26. An inquiry should be made before each new set of immunizations (or after each prior set) about reactions to prior vaccines.	•UNCHANGED•
27. Children who have had an anaphylactic reaction to a prior vaccine should not receive that vaccine again.	27. Children who have had an anaphylactic reaction to a prior vaccine should not receive that vaccine again.	•UNCHANGED•
28. Each immunization given at that institution should be documented with the date of administration, manufacturer, lot number, and name of health care provider administering the vaccine.	28. Each immunization given at that institution should be documented with the date of administration, manufacturer, lot number, and name of health care provider administering the vaccine.	•UNCHANGED•
Catch-Up Immunizations	**Catch-Up Immunizations**	
29. Children at least 8 months old but less than 5 years old who are behind on their immunizations should receive three OPV/IPV, four DTP/DTaP/Td, three Hib, three HBV, and one MMR within one year of the first visit with the managed care provider.	29. Children at least 8 months old but less than 5 years old who are behind on their immunizations should **have received a total of** three OPV/IPV, four DTP/DTaP/**DT**, three Hib, three HBV, and one MMR within one year of the first visit with the managed care provider.	Wording changed to clarify original indicator.
30. Children at least 5 years old but less than 7 years old who are behind on their immunizations should receive three OPV/IPV, four DTP/DTaP/Td, three HBV, and one MMR within one year of the first visit with the managed care provider.	30. Children at least 5 years old but less than 7 years old who are behind on their immunizations should **have received a total of** three OPV/IPV, four DTP/DTaP/**DT**/Td, three HBV, and one MMR within one year of the first visit with the managed care provider.	Wording changed to clarify original indicator. Added "DT" for clarification purposes.
31. Children who are at least 7 years old but less than 18 years old and who are behind on their immunizations should have had three OPV/IPV, three Td, and two MMR within one year of the first visit with the managed care provider.	31. Children who are at least 7 years old but less than 18 years old and who are behind on their immunizations should **have received a total of** three OPV/IPV, three **DTP/DTaP/DT/**Td, and two MMR within one year of the first visit with the managed care provider.	Wording changed to clarify original indicator. Added "DTaP" to reflect current recommendations. Added "DTP/DT" for clarification purposes.
Prior Immunization Record	**Prior Immunization Record**	
32. For children less than five years old who are new to the practice, there should be a notation of prior immunization history or a notation of an effort to obtain such information (e.g., parent will call in or bring it to next visit, letter will be sent to prior provider) at the first visit.	32. For children less than five years old who are new to the practice, there should be a notation of prior immunization history or a notation of an effort to obtain such information (e.g., parent will call in or bring it to next visit, letter will be sent to prior provider) at the first visit.	•UNCHANGED•
33. If a prior immunization record for a child less than five years old has not been obtained within six months of the first visit, the child should be given catch-up immunizations.	33. If a prior immunization record for a child less than five years old has not been obtained within six months of the first visit, the child should be given catch-up immunizations.	•UNCHANGED• •DROPPED• due to operationalization difficulties.

Chapter 15 — Otitis Media

[Note: These indicators only apply to children 1-3 years old.]

Original Indicator	Modified Indicator	Comments
A. OTITIS MEDIA WITH EFFUSION (SEROUS OTITIS MEDIA)	**A. OTITIS MEDIA WITH EFFUSION (SEROUS OTITIS MEDIA)**	•UNCHANGED•
(DIAGNOSIS)	(DIAGNOSIS)	
1. All patients with the diagnosis of suspected otitis media with effusion should be evaluated with pneumatic otoscopy.	--	•DROPPED• due to low feasibility score from panelists.
2. Patients with persistent (≥3 months duration) bilateral otitis media with effusion should have a hearing evaluation.	1. Patients with persistent (≥3 months duration) bilateral otitis media with effusion should have a hearing evaluation.	Correction of typographical error in original indicator.
(TREATMENT)	(TREATMENT)	
3. All patients with the diagnosis of otitis media with effusion should receive either: – antibiotics, or – trial of observation.	2. All patients with the diagnosis of otitis media with effusion should receive either: – antibiotics, or – trial of observation.	•UNCHANGED•
4. For all patients with a diagnosis of otitis media with effusion, during the initial management period (up to 12 weeks), myringotomy with or without insertion of tympanostomy tubes should not be performed in an otherwise healthy child (no other complications).	3. For all patients with a diagnosis of otitis media with effusion, during the initial management period (up to 12 weeks), myringotomy with or without insertion of tympanostomy tubes should not be performed in an otherwise healthy child (no other complications).	•UNCHANGED•
5. All patients with the diagnosis of otitis media with effusion who have tympanostomy tubes should have a bilateral hearing loss (defined as 20 decibels hearing threshold level or worse in both ears) documented in the record.	4. All patients with the diagnosis of otitis media with effusion **and a bilateral hearing loss (defined as 20 decibels hearing threshold level or worse in both ears) documented in the record should have tympanostomy tubes inserted.**	Wording changed to clarify original indicator. •DELETED• because covered in indicators #5 and 6.
6. Patients with persistent otitis media with effusion (≥3 months duration) and hearing loss (bilateral hearing deficits of 20 decibels hearing threshold or worse) should receive: a. One of the following: - oral antibiotic therapy if child has not been on antibiotics, - if on antibiotics, a change in antibiotics, or - bilateral myringotomy with tube placement. b. Environmental risk factor control counseling.	5. Patients with persistent otitis media with effusion (≥3 months duration) and hearing loss (bilateral hearing deficits of 20 decibels hearing threshold or worse) should receive: a. One of the following: - oral antibiotic therapy if child has not been on antibiotics, - if on antibiotics, a change in antibiotics, or - bilateral myringotomy with tube placement. b. Environmental risk factor control counseling.	•UNCHANGED•
7. Management of patients with otitis media with effusion for 4-6 months and a history of significant bilateral hearing loss (at least 20 decibels) and a failure of adequate antibiotic therapy should include: a. Bilateral myringotomy with tube placement. b. Environmental risk factor counseling.	6. Management of patients with otitis media with effusion for 4-6 months and a history of significant bilateral hearing loss (at least 20 decibels) and a failure of adequate antibiotic therapy should include: a. Bilateral myringotomy with tube placement. b. Environmental risk factor counseling.	•UNCHANGED•
(FOLLOW-UP)	(FOLLOW-UP)	

cont'd

	Original Indicator	Modified Indicator	Comments
8.	All patients identified as having otitis media with effusion must either have a recommendation for follow-up visit or have been seen for reevaluation within 8 weeks of diagnosis.	9. All patients identified as having otitis media with effusion must either have a recommendation for a follow-up visit or have been seen for reevaluation within **12** weeks of diagnosis.	Panelists felt that a 12 week follow-up was sufficient.
	B. ACUTE OTITIS MEDIA	***B. ACUTE OTITIS MEDIA***	
	(DIAGNOSIS)	(DIAGNOSIS)	
1.	All children presenting to the clinician with fever, nonspecific behavioral changes (e.g., irritability, lethargy, decreased appetite, vomiting, diarrhea), or ear pain should receive an ear examination using a pneumatic otoscope.	--	•UNCHANGED• •DROPPED• due to validity and feasibility disagreement among panelists.
	(TREATMENT)	(TREATMENT)	
2.	For all patients with the diagnosis of acute otitis media, at least 10 days of antibiotics should be prescribed.	--	•UNCHANGED• •DROPPED• due to low validity score from panelists.
	(FOLLOW-UP)	(FOLLOW-UP)	
3.	Once a diagnosis of acute otitis media is made, follow-up chart review should document a return visit after the course of antibiotics within 8 weeks of diagnosis.	--	•UNCHANGED• •DROPPED• due to low validity score from panelists.

Chapter 16 — Prenatal Care

[Note: Scoring and modification of this chapter was deferred to the Women's Quality of Care Panel. See Chapter 16 of Women's Quality Indicators crosswalk table.]

Original Indicator	Modified Indicator	Comments
(SCREENING)		
Routine Prenatal Care		
1. The first prenatal visit should occur in the first trimester.	1. The first prenatal visit should occur in the first trimester.	•UNCHANGED•
2. The physician should make an accurate determination of gestational age using: • An ultrasound in the 1st or 2nd trimester, or • Reliable LMP and size within 2 wks indicated by dates in the 1st trimester, or • No 1st trimester exam, but reliable LMP & 2 of the following: 1) size w/in 2 wks. of dates in 2d trimester; 2) quickening by 20 wks.; 3) fetal heart tones by fetoscope before 20 weeks, or • If unreliable LMP, then an ultrasound is required.	2. The physician should make an accurate determination of gestational age using **any one of the following:** a. • An ultrasound in the 1st or 2nd trimester; or • Reliable LMP and size within 2 wks indicated by dates in the 1st trimester; or • No 1st trimester exam, but reliable LMP & 2 of the following: 1) size w/in 2 wks. of dates in 2d trimester, 2) quickening by 20 wks., 3) fetal heart tones by fetoscope before 20 weeks; or b. • If **unknown** LMP, then an ultrasound is required.	Panelists wanted to rate (a) and (b) separately. Wording changed to clarify the original indicator.
3. Pregnant women should be screened for anemia at the first prenatal visit.	3. Pregnant women should be screened for anemia at the first prenatal visit.	•UNCHANGED•
4. Pregnant women should be rescreened for anemia after 24 weeks.	4. Pregnant women should be rescreened for anemia after 24 weeks.	•UNCHANGED•
Substance Abuse	**Substance Abuse**	
5. A smoking history should be obtained at the first prenatal visit.	5. A smoking history should be obtained at the first prenatal visit.	•UNCHANGED•
6. An alcohol history should be obtained at the first prenatal visit.	6. An alcohol history should be obtained at the first prenatal visit.	•UNCHANGED•
7. A drug history should be obtained during the first prenatal visit.	7. A drug history should be obtained during the first prenatal visit.	•UNCHANGED•
Infections and Sexually Transmitted Diseases (STDs)	*Infections and Sexually Transmitted Diseases (STDs)*	
7.5 •NEW•	8. A history should be taken at the first prenatal visit to elicit risk factors for STDs and Hepatitis B.	•NEW• Added because panelists felt this indicator was important for assessment of quality of prenatal care.
Asymptomatic Bacteriuria	*Asymptomatic Bacteriuria*	
8. Women should receive a urine culture at the first prenatal visit.	9. Women should receive a urine **screen** at the first prenatal visit.	A full culture is not necessary according to the literature. A urine screen is sufficient.
Rubella	*Rubella*	
9. Women should receive a serologic test for rubella immunity before delivery.	10. Women should receive a serologic test for rubella immunity before delivery.	•UNCHANGED•
Hepatitis B Carriers	*Hepatitis B Carriers*	

cont'd

Original Indicator	Modified Indicator	Comments
10. Women should be screened for HBsAg before delivery.	11. Women should be screened for HBsAg before delivery.	•UNCHANGED• Panelists preferred to only screen women at risk, but this change was impossible to operationalize.
Syphilis	*Syphilis*	
11. A non-treponemal screening test (e.g., VDRC) should be performed on women at the first prenatal visit.	12. A non-treponemal screening test (e.g., VDRL) should be performed on women at the first prenatal visit.	VDRC changed to VDRL to correct a typographical error in the original indicator. Panelists preferred to only screen women at risk, but this change was impossible to operationalize.
Gonorrhea	*Gonorrhea*	
12. A cervical gonorrhea culture should be performed on women at the first prenatal visit.	13. A cervical gonorrhea culture should be performed on women at the first prenatal visit.	•UNCHANGED• Panelists preferred to only screen women at risk, but this change was impossible to operationalize.
Chlamydia	*Chlamydia*	
13. Women at high risk (adolescents, unmarried, those with multiple sex partners, low SES, other STD diagnosed) should receive a cervical chlamydia culture or antigen detection at the first prenatal visit.	14. Women at high risk (adolescents, unmarried, those with multiple sex partners, low SES, other STD diagnosed) should receive a cervical chlamydia culture or antigen detection at the first prenatal visit.	•UNCHANGED•
Human Immunodeficiency Virus	*Human Immunodeficiency Virus*	
14. Pregnant women should be counseled about their individual risk for HIV infection at the first prenatal visit.	15. Pregnant women should be counseled about their individual risk for HIV infection at the first prenatal visit.	•UNCHANGED•
15. Pregnant women should be offered HIV testing at the first prenatal visit.	16. Pregnant women should be offered HIV testing at the first prenatal visit.	•UNCHANGED•
Inherited Disorders		
Neural Tube Defects (NTDs)		
16. Women under age 35 should be offered serum AFP; this should be performed between 15 and 20 weeks.	17. Women under age 35 should be offered serum AFP testing; this should be performed between 15 and 20 weeks.	All women, regardless of age, should be offered an AFP test.
17. Women who have had a previous NTD infant should receive amniocentesis or should explicitly decline such a test after genetic counseling.	18. Women who have had a previous NTD infant should receive amniocentesis or should explicitly decline such a test after genetic counseling.	Panelists felt that genetic counseling was not necessary.
17.5 •NEW•	19. **Women with a prior NTD infant should have folic acid supplementation recommended in the preconceptual period.**	•NEW• Panelists felt this indicator should be added because of recent studies showing benefit of folic acid.
Sickle Cell Disease		
18. Women who are African American or have a family history of sickle cell disease should be screened at the first prenatal visit.	20. Women who are African American or have a family history of sickle cell disease should be **offered screening** at the first prenatal visit, **if status unknown.**	Medical record should indicate that screening was offered. Women cannot be forced to undergo the test.
19. For women with the sickle cell trait, the baby's father should be screened.	21. For women with the sickle cell trait, the baby's father should be **offered screening.**	Medical record should indicate that screening was offered. Women cannot be forced to undergo the test.
Rh Isoimmunization		

Original Indicator	Modified Indicator	Comments
20. Women should receive an Rh factor and antibody screen at the first prenatal visit.	22. Women should receive an Rh factor and antibody screen at the first prenatal visit.	•UNCHANGED•
Common Pregnancy Complications	*Common Pregnancy Complications*	
Intrauterine Growth Retardation	*Intrauterine Growth Retardation*	
21. Measurements of the symphysis-fundal height should be made at each visit from 20-32 weeks.	23. Measurements of the symphysis-fundal height should be made at each visit from 20-32 weeks.	•UNCHANGED•
Post-term Pregnancy	*Post-term Pregnancy*	
22. Weekly fetal monitoring should begin at 41.5 weeks and continue until labor (spontaneous or induced) begins.	24. Weekly Fetal **assessment** should begin at 41.5 weeks and continue until labor (spontaneous or induced) begins.	Weekly deleted because many practitioners will not allow a women to go beyond 42 weeks. Assessment need not include continuous or intermittent monitoring of heart rate.
Pregnancy-Induced Hypertension (PIH)	*Pregnancy-Induced Hypertension (PIH)*	
23. Blood pressure measurements should be taken at each visit.	25. Blood pressure measurements should be taken at each visit.	•UNCHANGED•
Gestational Diabetes Mellitus	*Gestational Diabetes Mellitus*	
24. A one-hour, 50g glucose challenge test should be performed on women with risk factors at 24-28 weeks.	26. A one-hour, 50g glucose challenge test should be performed on women with risk factors at 24-28 weeks.	•UNCHANGED•
(DIAGNOSIS)	(DIAGNOSIS)	
Infections and STDs	*Infections and STDs*	
Hepatitis B Carriers	*Hepatitis B Carriers*	
25. For women carrying HBsAg, carrier status should be documented in delivery record.	27. For women carrying HBsAg, carrier status should be documented in delivery record.	•UNCHANGED•
Syphilis	*Syphilis*	
26. Women whose non-treponemal tests are weakly reactive or reactive should receive a treponemal test to confirm presence of syphilis.	28. Women whose non-treponemal tests are weakly reactive or reactive should receive a treponemal test to confirm presence of syphilis.	•UNCHANGED•

Original Indicator	Modified Indicator	Comments
Inherited Disorders		
Neural Tube Defects		
27. Women with an abnormal serum AFP should receive an ultrasound to evaluate gestational age and possible multiple gestation.	29. Women with an abnormal serum AFP should receive an ultrasound to evaluate gestational age and possible multiple gestation.	•UNCHANGED•
Sickle Cell Disease	*Sickle Cell Disease*	
28. Women with the sickle cell trait should receive either amniocentesis or chorionic villus sampling, unless the baby's father is known to be negative for the sickle trait.	30. Women with the sickle cell trait should **be offered** either amniocentesis or chorionic villus sampling, unless the baby's father is known to be negative for the sickle trait.	Medical record should indicate that screening was offered. Women cannot be forced to undergo the test.
Common Pregnancy Complications	***Common Pregnancy Complications***	
Intrauterine Growth Retardation	*Intrauterine Growth Retardation*	
29. Women whose symphysis-fundal height is 4 cm less than indicated by their gestational age between 20-32 weeks should have an ultrasound.	31. Women whose symphysis-fundal height is 4 cm less than indicated by their gestational age between 20-32 weeks should have an ultrasound.	•UNCHANGED•
Pregnancy-induced Hypertension (PIH)		
30. For elevated BPs (systolic > 140mm Hg, or diastolic > 90mm Hg, OR systolic rise >30mm Hg or diastolic rise > 15mm Hg), proteinuria and peripheral edema should be assessed.	32. **In women without a prior diagnosis of chronic hypertension, who have** elevated BPs (systolic > 140mm Hg **at 20 weeks or later,** or diastolic > 90mm Hg **at 20 weeks or later,** OR systolic rise >30mm Hg or diastolic rise > 15mm Hg), proteinuria and peripheral edema should be assessed.	Women with chronic hypertension were excluded to be comparable with the prior RAND study of prenatal care. "At 20 weeks or later" was added because PIH is not very common prior to 20 weeks.
31. For patients with elevated BP and either proteinuria (1+ or more) or edema (> trace), PIH diagnosis should be made.	33. **In women without a prior diagnosis of chronic hypertension, who have** elevated BP and either proteinuria (1+ or more) or edema (> trace), PIH diagnosis should be made.	Women with chronic hypertension were excluded to be comparable with the prior RAND study of prenatal care.
Gestational Diabetes Mellitus		
32. Pregnant women with abnormal glucose challenge tests (≥140 mg/dL or 7.8 mmol/L) should have a 3-hour plasma glucose tolerance test performed.	34. Pregnant women with abnormal glucose challenge tests (≥140 mg/dL or 7.8 mmol/L) should have a 3-hour plasma glucose tolerance test performed.	•UNCHANGED•
(TREATMENT)		
Substance Use		
33. Pregnant women identified as smokers should receive counseling to stop smoking from their physician.	35. Pregnant women identified as smokers should receive counseling to stop smoking from their physician.	•UNCHANGED•
34. Pregnant women identified as smokers should be referred to a smoking cessation clinic, group, or counselor.	--. Pregnant women identified as smokers should be referred to a smoking cessation clinic, group, or counselor.	•UNCHANGED• •DROPPED• due to low validity score from panelists.
35. Pregnant women who indicate they use any amount of alcohol should be counseled to eliminate alcohol consumption during pregnancy.	36. Pregnant women who indicate they use any amount of alcohol should be counseled to eliminate alcohol consumption during pregnancy **and should be referred for treatment if appropriate.**	Referral necessary if practitioner feels abuse is excessive.
36. Pregnant women who indicate they use cocaine or heroin should be counseled by their physician to cease use during pregnancy.	37. Pregnant women who indicate they use **drugs** should be counseled by their physician to cease use during pregnancy **and should be referred for treatment if appropriate.**	Changed to include drug use of any kind. Merged with original indicator #38.

Original Indicator	Modified Indicator	Comments
37. Pregnant women who indicate they use drugs should be referred to a drug treatment clinic, group, or counselor.	--	•DELETED• Merged with original indicator #37.
Infections and Sexually Transmitted Diseases		
Asymptomatic Bacteriuria		
38. Pregnant women with positive cultures (>100,000 bacteria/cc) should receive an appropriate antibiotic.	38. Pregnant women with positive cultures (>100,000 bacteria/cc) should receive an appropriate antibiotic.	•UNCHANGED•
Rubella		
39. Pregnant women not immune to rubella should receive postpartum immunization.	39. Pregnant women not immune to rubella should receive postpartum immunization **within 6 weeks.**	Timeframe added for operationalization.
Syphilis		
40. Pregnant women with confirmed positive serology should be treated with penicillin appropriate for the stage of disease; tetracycline and doxycycline are contraindicated.	40. Pregnant women with confirmed positive serology should be treated with penicillin, **if not allergic,** appropriate for the stage of disease; tetracycline and doxycycline are contraindicated.	Penicillin is contraindicated in some patients.
Gonorrhea		
41. Pregnant women with positive cultures should be treated as recommended by the PHS Guidelines on STD (250 mg IM once of ceftriaxone and erythromycin base 500 mg orally 4x/day for 7 days).	41. Pregnant women with positive cultures should **receive appropriate treatment.**	Panelists did not want to stipulate the exact treatment, so the indicator was changed to allow more general operationalization.
Human Immunodeficiency Virus		
42. Pregnant women known to be HIV positive with CD4+ counts of 200 or greater should be treated with zidovudine during pregnancy and intrapartum.	42. Pregnant women known to be HIV positive with CD4+ counts of 200 or greater should be **offered treatment** with zidovudine during pregnancy and intrapartum	Medical record should indicate that screening was offered. Women cannot be forced to undergo the treatment.
Inherited Disorders		
Down Syndrome		
43. Pregnant women whose amniocentesis shows infant with abnormal karyotype should receive additional genetic counseling.	43. Pregnant women whose amniocentesis shows infant with abnormal karyotype should receive additional genetic counseling.	Genetic counseling not necessary. Any appropriate counseling is sufficient.
Neural Tube Defects (NTDs)		
44. Pregnant women with abnormal serum AFP and normal ultrasound should be offered an amniocentesis and genetic counseling.	44. Pregnant women with abnormal serum AFP **for gestational age** and normal ultrasound should be offered an amniocentesis and genetic counseling.	Added gestational age for clarification. "Genetic counseling not necessary. Any appropriate counseling is sufficient.
45. Pregnant women whose amniotic fluid AFP shows infant with probable NTD should be offered additional genetic counseling.	45. Pregnant women whose amniotic fluid AFP shows infant with probable NTD should be offered additional genetic counseling.	Genetic counseling not necessary. Any appropriate counseling is sufficient.
Sickle Cell Disease		
46. Pregnant women whose amniocentesis shows an infant with sickle cell disease should be offered genetic counseling.	46. Pregnant women whose amniocentesis shows an infant with sickle cell disease should be offered genetic counseling.	Genetic counseling not necessary. Any appropriate counseling is sufficient.
Rh Isoimmunization		
47. Pregnant women who are Rh negative should receive Rhogam between 26 and 30 weeks antenatally and postpartum.	47. Pregnant women who are Rh negative should receive Rhogam between 26 and 30 weeks antenatally and postpartum.	•UNCHANGED•
Common Pregnancy Complications		

Pediatric Quality Indicators

	Original Indicator		Modified Indicator	Comments
	Post-Term Pregnancy		*Post-Term Pregnancy*	
48.	Labor should be induced when fetus shows signs of distress or oligohydramnios.	48.	Labor should be induced when **monitoring** shows **non-reassuring fetal status** or oligohydramnios.	Wording changed to clarify original indicator.
49.	Pregnancies with reliable dates should not extend beyond 44 weeks.	49.	Pregnancies with reliable dates should not extend beyond 44 weeks.	•UNCHANGED•
	Pregnancy-Induced Hypertension (PIH)		*Pregnancy-Induced Hypertension (PIH)*	
50.	If PIH diagnosed and patient is not admitted, bedrest should be recommended & a return visit should occur w/in 1 week.	50.	If PIH diagnosed and patient is not admitted, bedrest should be recommended & a return visit should occur w/in 1 week.	•UNCHANGED•
51.	If PIH diagnosed and pregnancy is at term (≥ 37 weeks), either labor should be induced or delivery by cesarean section should take place.	51.	If PIH diagnosed and pregnancy is at term (≥ 37 weeks), either labor should be induced or delivery by cesarean section should take place.	•UNCHANGED•
52.	If severe PIH is diagnosed by any of the following: systolic >160 mm Hg, diastolic >110 mm Hg, 3-4+ proteinuria, pulmonary edema, oliguria, RUQ pain or seizures, then patient should be admitted to induce labor or deliver by cesarean section.	52.	If severe PIH is diagnosed by any of the following: systolic >160 mm Hg, diastolic >110 mm Hg, 3-4+ proteinuria, pulmonary edema, oliguria, RUQ pain or seizures, then patient should be admitted to induce labor or deliver by cesarean section.	•UNCHANGED•
	Gestational Diabetes Mellitus		*Gestational Diabetes Mellitus*	
53.	Pregnant women with abnormal 3-hour glucose tolerance tests should receive dietary counseling from a dietician.	53.	Pregnant women with abnormal 3-hour glucose tolerance tests should receive dietary counseling **and have glucose monitoring.**	Panelists felt glucose monitoring was necessary in addition to dietary counseling.
54.	Pregnant women on dietary therapy with 2 or more consecutive abnormal fasting (>105 mg/dL) or postprandial (>120 mg/dL one-hour post) plasma glucose tests should be placed on insulin therapy.	54.	Pregnant women on dietary therapy with 2 or more consecutive abnormal fasting (>105 mg/dL) or postprandial (>120 mg/dL one-hour post) plasma glucose tests should be placed on insulin therapy.	•UNCHANGED•
55.	An oral agent should not be used in diabetic pregnant women.	55.	An oral agent should not be used in diabetic pregnant women.	•UNCHANGED•
	(FOLLOW-UP)			
	Infections and Sexually Transmitted Diseases			
	Asymptomatic Bacteriuria			
56.	Women treated for positive cultures should receive a post-treatment follow-up culture within one month of completing treatment.	56.	Women treated for positive cultures should receive a post-treatment follow-up culture within one month of completing treatment.	•UNCHANGED•
	Syphilis		*Syphilis*	
57.	Women diagnosed with syphilis in pregnancy should be followed up with monthly serology and retreated if necessary.	57.	Women diagnosed with syphilis in pregnancy should be followed up with monthly serology and retreated if necessary.	•UNCHANGED•
	Gonorrhea		*Gonorrhea*	
58.	Women with positive cultures should receive a post-treatment follow-up culture 4-7 days after treatment is completed.	58.	Women with positive cultures should receive a post-treatment follow-up culture **2 weeks** after treatment is completed.	Changed to 2 weeks because studies show that some cultures still show up positive 7-10 days after treatment.
	Chlamydia		*Chlamydia*	
59.	Women with positive cultures should receive a post-treatment follow-up culture 4-7 days after treatment is completed.	59.	Women with positive cultures should receive a post-treatment follow-up culture 4-7 days after treatment is completed.	•UNCHANGED•
	Common Pregnancy Complications			
	Gestational Diabetes Mellitus			

cont'd

	Original Indicator		Modified Indicator	Comments
60.	Women with abnormal 3-hour plasma glucose tolerance tests who are on dietary therapy should have biweekly fasting or postprandial glucose tests.	60.	Women with abnormal 3-hour plasma glucose tolerance tests who are on dietary therapy should have biweekly fasting or postprandial glucose tests.	•UNCHANGED•

Chapter 17 — Sickle Cell Screening for Newborns And Prevention of Complications

	Original Indicator		Modified Indicator	Comments
	(SCREENING)		(SCREENING)	
1.	All children in states with mandatory newborn sickle cell testing should be screened before hospital discharge or within 48 hours of birth, whichever comes later.	1.	All children in states with mandatory newborn sickle cell testing should be screened before hospital discharge or within 48 hours of birth, whichever comes later.	•UNCHANGED•
2.	African-American children should be tested for sickle cell disease by the end of the third month of life.	2.	In states without mandatory newborn sickle cell screening, African-American children should be tested for sickle cell disease by the end of the third month of life.	Wording changed to clarify original indicator.
3.	Children with a positive sickle screen at less than or equal to one month of age should have a repeat screen after one month of age and prior to the end of six months of age.	3.	Children with a positive sickle screen at less than or equal to one month of age should have a repeat screen after one month of age and prior to the end of six months of age.	•UNCHANGED•
	(PREVENTION OF COMPLICATIONS) (TREATMENT)		(TREATMENT)	
4.	Children with a positive sickle screen or children suspected of being positive for sickle cell disease should be placed on daily penicillin prophylaxis from at least six months of age until at least five years of age.	4.	Children with a positive sickle screen or children suspected of being positive for sickle cell disease should be placed on daily penicillin prophylaxis from at least six months of age until at least five years of age.	•UNCHANGED•
5.	Children with sickle cell disease should have a hematocrit or hemoglobin, and reticulocyte count performed at least every four months.	--	Children with sickle cell disease should have a hematocrit or hemoglobin, and reticulocyte count performed at least every four months.	•UNCHANGED• •DROPPED• due to low validity score from panelists.
6.	Children with sickle cell disease should have received the pneumococcal vaccine between 2 years and 3 years of age.	5.	Children with sickle cell disease should have received the pneumococcal vaccine between 2 years and 3 years of age.	•UNCHANGED•
7.	A child older than 2 years with sickle cell disease should have documented at the first visit whether or not he/she has ever had a pneumococcal vaccine or that efforts are being made to determine the vaccine history.	6.	A child older than 3 years with sickle cell disease should have documented at the first visit of a prior pneumococcal vaccine or be vaccinated within one month of the first visit.	Panelists felt that the prior indicator adequately applied to children up to age three years. They felt that if a new patient's prior vaccine history could not be determined quickly, it was better to revaccinate than to risk leaving a child unvaccinated for an extended period.
8.	The patient should receive the vaccination within one month of this visit if the patient or the patient's caregiver does not know if the vaccine has been given and it has not been confirmed by other means. If the patient or patient's caregiver does not believe the vaccine had been given before, the vaccine should be given at that visit.	--		•DELETED•

Chapter 18 — Tuberculosis Screening

Original Indicator		Modified Indicator		Comments
1.	By the time a child is four months old, there should be documentation of whether or not the child has tuberculosis risk factors or documentation that the child has had a Mantoux test.	--	By the time a child is four months old, there should be documentation of whether or not the child has tuberculosis risk factors or documentation that the child has had a Mantoux test.	•UNCHANGED•
2.	If no contacts have evidence of current TB disease but at least one has a positive tuberculin skin test, newborns should be Mantoux tested by the end of the fourth month of life.	--		•DROPPED• due to low validity score from panelists. •DELETED•
3.	If a child has any of the TB risk factors listed below, he/she should receive an annual Mantoux skin test during the duration of the risk factor:	1.	If a child has any of the TB risk factors listed below, he/she should receive an ~~annual~~ a Mantoux skin test **within one week of documenting the risk factor:**	Panelists wanted to revise the TB screening indicator to be consistent with current recommendations.
a.	has abnormalities on chest X-ray suggestive of TB.	a.	has abnormalities on chest X-ray suggestive of TB.	
b.	has clinical evidence of TB.	b.	has clinical evidence of TB.	
c.	has HIV-infection, Hodgkin's disease, lymphoma, diabetes mellitus, chronic renal failure, malnutrition, or another immunosuppressive condition.	c.	has HIV-infection, Hodgkin's disease, lymphoma, diabetes mellitus, chronic renal failure, malnutrition, or another immunosuppressive condition.	
d.	has had contact with an adult/adolescent with infectious TB.	d.	has had contact with an adult/adolescent with **confirmed or suspected** infectious TB.	
e.	is from, or household contacts are from, a region of the world with high TB prevalence.	e.	**has emigrated from, has traveled to, or has significant contact with indigenous persons from** a region of the world with high TB prevalence.	
f.	is frequently exposed to adults or adolescents who are HIV-infected, homeless, users of injection and other street drugs, poor and medically-indigent city dwellers, residents of nursing homes, or migrant farm workers.	--	~~is frequently exposed to adults or adolescents who are HIV-infected, homeless, users of injection and other street drugs, poor and medically-indigent city dwellers, residents of nursing homes, or migrant farm workers.~~	
3.5a	•NEW•	2.	**Children who have been frequently exposed to adults or adolescents who are HIV-infected, homeless, users of injection and other street drugs, poor and medically-indigent city dwellers, incarcerated, institutionalized, residents of nursing homes, or migrant farm workers should be Mantoux tested when the risk factor initially is identified ~~and at least every 3-years.~~**	•NEW• Modification of original indicator #3. Panelists wanted to revise the TB screening indicators to be consistent with current recommendations. "and at least every 3 years" dropped because it spans a 3-year time period beyond initial diagnosis within the study period.
3.5b	•NEW•	3.	**A child with HIV infection should be Mantoux tested annually for tuberculosis.**	•NEW• Panelists wanted to revise the TB screening indicators to be consistent with current recommendations.

cont'd

	Original Indicator		Modified Indicator	Comments
3.5c	•NEW•	4.	An initial Mantoux test should be performed prior to initiation of immunosuppressive therapy.	•NEW• Panelists wanted to revise the TB screening indicators to be consistent with current recommendations.
4.	Children with immunodeficiency or HIV-infection should have anergy testing (e.g., Candida or Mumps antigen) at the same time as TB testing.	5.	Children with immunodeficiency or HIV-infection should have anergy testing (e.g., Candida or Mumps antigen) at the same time as TB testing.	•UNCHANGED•
5.	Mantoux skin tests in children with risk factors should be read by a health professional or other trained personnel within 48-72 hours.	6.	Mantoux skin tests in children with risk factors should be read by a health professional or other trained personnel within 48-72 hours.	•UNCHANGED•
6.	Results of tuberculin skin tests in children with risk factors should be documented within 96 hours of placing the test.	7.	Results of tuberculin skin tests in children with risk factors should be documented within 96 hours of placing the test.	•UNCHANGED•
7.	All Mantoux skin tests read as positive should document that there was induration and should document the diameter of the induration in millimeters.	8.	All Mantoux skin tests read as positive should document that there was induration and should document the diameter of the induration in millimeters.	•UNCHANGED•
8.	A Mantoux skin test with ≥15 mm should be read as positive.	9.	A Mantoux skin test with ≥15 mm should be read as positive.	•UNCHANGED•
9.	A Mantoux skin test should be read as positive if there is induration that is at least 10 mm in a child who: - is less than 4 years old; - has other medical risk factors for developing TB disease (Hodgkin's disease, lymphoma, diabetes mellitus, chronic renal failure, malnutrition); - who was born, or whose parents were born, in regions of the world where TB is highly prevalent; or - who is frequently exposed to adults who are HIV-infected, homeless, users of intravenous and other street drugs, poor and medically indigent city dwellers, residents of nursing homes, incarcerated or institutionalized persons, and migrant farm workers.	10.	A Mantoux skin test should be read as positive if there is induration that is at least 10 mm in a child who: - is less than 4 years old; - has other medical risk factors for developing TB disease (Hodgkin's disease, lymphoma, diabetes mellitus, chronic renal failure, malnutrition); - who was born, or whose parents were born, in regions of the world where TB is highly prevalent; - **who has traveled to regions of the world where TB is highly prevalent;** - who is frequently exposed to adults who are HIV-infected, homeless, users of intravenous and other street drugs, poor and medically indigent city dwellers, residents of nursing homes, incarcerated or institutionalized persons, and migrant farm workers.	Expanded indicator because patients travelling to TB-prevalent regions also are at higher risk.
10.	A Mantoux skin test should be read as positive if there is induration that is at least 5 mm in a child who: - is in close contact with someone with a known or suspected infectious case of TB (households with active or previously active cases) if (a) treatment cannot be verified as adequate before exposure, (b) treatment was initiated after the period of the child's contact began, or (c) reactivation is suspected; - is suspected of having TB disease clinically or by chest X-ray; or - has an immunosuppressive condition or HIV infection or is receiving immunosuppressive treatment	11.	A Mantoux skin test should be read as positive if there is induration that is at least 5 mm in a child who: - is in close contact with someone with a known or suspected infectious case of TB (households with active or previously active cases) if (a) treatment cannot be verified as adequate before exposure, (b) treatment was initiated after the period of the child's contact began, or (c) reactivation is suspected; - is suspected of having TB disease clinically or by chest X-ray; or - has an immunosuppressive condition (**including HIV infection**) or is receiving immunosuppressive treatment	Wording changed to clarify original indicator.
11.	All children with positive Mantoux skin tests should have a chest x-ray within two weeks.	12.	All children with positive Mantoux skin tests should have a chest x-ray within two weeks.	•UNCHANGED•

Pediatric Quality Indicators

cont'd

	Original Indicator		Modified Indicator	Comments
12.	Children with a positive Mantoux test and negative chest x-ray and no other symptoms of TB should receive prophylaxis with INH and/or Rifampin.	13.	Children with a positive Mantoux test and negative chest x-ray and no other symptoms of TB should receive prophylaxis with INH and/or Rifampin.	•UNCHANGED•
13.	Children with a positive Mantoux test and negative chest x-ray and no other symptoms of TB, whose presumed index case (source of infection) has TB resistant to INH and Rifampin, should have a referral made to an infectious disease specialist.	14.	Children with a positive Mantoux test and negative chest x-ray and no other symptoms of TB, whose presumed index case (source of infection) has TB resistant to INH and Rifampin, should have a referral made to an infectious disease specialist.	•UNCHANGED•
14.	Prophylaxis with INH should be given for 9 months to asymptomatic children without HIV and 12 months to asymptomatic children with HIV.	15.	Prophylaxis with INH should be given for 9 months to asymptomatic children without HIV and 12 months to asymptomatic children with HIV.	•UNCHANGED•
15.	Children receiving TB chemoprophylaxis should have contact with a clinician at least once every 5 weeks during therapy.	--	Children receiving TB chemoprophylaxis should have contact with a clinician at least once every 5 weeks during therapy.	•UNCHANGED• •DROPPED• due to low validity score from panelists.
16.	All children three years and older who are receiving TB chemoprophylaxis with INH should have a baseline visual acuity test performed or attempted.	--		•DELETED•

Pediatric Quality Indicators

Chapter 19 — Upper Respiratory Infections

	Original Indicator		Modified Indicator	Comments
	(DIAGNOSIS)		**(DIAGNOSIS)**	
	Pharyngitis		**Pharyngitis**	
1.	All patients with sore throat should be asked about presence or absence of fever.	--	All patients with sore throat should be asked about presence or absence of fever.	•UNCHANGED• •DROPPED• due to low validity score from panelists.
2.	All patients with sore throat should be asked about nasal symptoms.	--	All patients with sore throat should be asked about nasal symptoms.	•UNCHANGED• •DROPPED• due to low validity score from panelists.
2a.	•NEW•	--	**Children with sore throat should have their temperature measured.**	Panelists felt that fever is an important element in deciding about work-up and management of pharyngitis. •DROPPED• due to low validity score from panelists.
3.	If a rapid streptococcal test is negative, a culture should be sent within 24 hours.	--	If a rapid streptococcal test is negative, a culture should be sent within 24 hours.	•UNCHANGED• •DROPPED• due to disagreement among panelists.
4.	Diagnosis of GABHS, *N. gonorrhoeae*, or *C. haemolyticum* by gram stain in the absense of culture or rapid test is not appropriate.	--	Diagnosis of GABHS, *N. gonorrhoeae*, or *C. haemolyticum* by gram stain in the **absence** of culture or rapid test is not appropriate.	Absence added because it was a typographical error in original indicator. •DROPPED• due to low validity score from panelists.
17.	If a diagnosis of infectious mononucleosis is made, it should be on the basis of a positive heterophil antibody test or other EBV antibody tests.	1.	If a diagnosis of infectious mononucleosis is made, it should be on the basis of a positive heterophil antibody test or other EBV antibody tests.	•UNCHANGED•
	Bronchitis/Cough		**Bronchitis/Cough**	
5.	The history of patients presenting with cough of less than 3 weeks' duration should document presence or absence of preceding viral infection (e.g., common cold, influenza).	--	The history of patients presenting with cough of less than 3 weeks' duration should document presence or absence of preceding viral infection (e.g., common cold, influenza).	•UNCHANGED• •DROPPED• due to low validity score from panelists.
6.	The history of patients presenting with cough of less than 3 weeks' duration should document presence or absence of fever and shortness of breath (dyspnea).	2.	The history of patients presenting with cough of less than 3 weeks' duration should document presence or absence of fever, and shortness of breath (dyspnea), **and chest pain**	Panelists felt that chest pain was important and should be documented.
7.	Patients presenting with acute cough should receive a physical examination of the chest for evidence of pneumonia.	3.	Patients presenting with acute cough should receive a physical examination of the chest for evidence of pneumonia.	•UNCHANGED•

	Original Indicator	Modified Indicator	Comments
8.	Patients presenting with acute cough and with evidence of consolidation on physical exam of the chest (dullness to percussion, egophony, etc.) should receive a chest x-ray to look for evidence of pneumonia.	4. Patients presenting with acute cough and with evidence of consolidation on physical exam of the chest (dullness to percussion, egophony, etc.) should receive a chest x-ray ~~to look for evidence of pneumonia.~~	Panelists felt that the indicator should be modified because the chest x-ray is used to look for other pathology as well (e.g., tumors).
	Nasal Congestion	**Nasal Congestion**	
9.	If a patient presents with the complaint of nasal congestion and/or rhinorrhea not attributed to the common cold, the history should include: seasonality of symptoms, presence or absence of sneezing, facial pain, fever, specific irritants, use of topical nasal decongestants.	-- If a patient presents with the complaint of nasal congestion and/or rhinorrhea not attributed to the common cold, the history should include: seasonality of symptoms, presence or absence of sneezing, facial pain, fever, specific irritants, use of topical nasal decongestants.	•UNCHANGED• •DROPPED• due to low validity score from panelists.
	Acute Sinusitis	**Acute Sinusitis**	
10.	If the diagnosis of acute sinusitis is made, symptoms should be present for a duration of less than 3 weeks (e.g., fever, malaise, cough, nasal congestion, purulent nasal discharge, ear pain or blockage, post-nasal drip, dental pain, headache, or facial pain).	-- If the diagnosis of acute sinusitis is made, symptoms should be present for a duration of less than 3 weeks (e.g., fever, malaise, cough, nasal congestion, purulent nasal discharge, ear pain or blockage, post-nasal drip, dental pain, headache, or facial pain).	•UNCHANGED• •DROPPED• due to low validity score from panelists.
	(TREATMENT)	(TREATMENT)	
	Pharyngitis	**Pharyngitis**	
11.	Patients with documented or presumed streptococcal infection should be treated with intramuscular benzathine penicillin G or procaine penicillin, oral potassium penicillin V for 10 days, or (if the patient is allergic to penicillin) erythromycin for 10 days. First generation cephalosporins are acceptable for individuals allergic to penicillin.	--	•DELETED•
11.5	•NEW•	5. **Antibiotics should only be prescribed in a patient with nasal congestion and pharyngitis if a rapid strep test or throat culture is obtained, or if there is documentation of other bacterial infections.**	•NEW• Pharyngitis combined with nasal congestion is usually due to a viral infection, so antibiotics should only be given if laboratory diagnosis is attempted.
12.	Tetracyclines and sulfonamides should not be used for treating GABHS pharyngitis.	6. Tetracyclines and sulfonamides should not be used for treating GABHS pharyngitis.	•UNCHANGED•
13.	No antibiotics should be used for a patient with a diagnosis of viral pharyngitis (unless antibiotics were prescribed before culture results were obtained).	-- No antibiotics should be used for a patient with a diagnosis of viral pharyngitis (unless antibiotics were prescribed before culture results were obtained).	•UNCHANGED• •DROPPED• due to disagreement among panelists.
14.	Antibiotics should only be prescribed in a patient with conjunctivitis and pharyngitis if a rapid streptococcal test or throat culture is obtained.	-- Antibiotics should only be prescribed in a patient with conjunctivitis and pharyngitis if a rapid streptococcal test or throat culture is obtained.	•UNCHANGED• •DROPPED• due to low validity score from panelists.

Original Indicator	Modified Indicator	Comments
15. Beta-lactamase-resistant and antistaphylococcal medications (e.g., amoxicillin-clavulanate, narrow-spectrum cephalosporins, dicloxacillin, and clindamycin) should be prescribed in patients who have had four episodes of documented or presumed and treated Strep throat in a one-year period.	-- Beta-lactamase-resistant and antistaphylococcal medications (e.g., amoxicillin-clavulanate, narrow-spectrum cephalosporins, dicloxacillin, and clindamycin) should be prescribed in Patients who have had four episodes of documented or presumed and treated Strep throat in a one-year period **should not have penicillin prescribed for the next episode.**	Panelists felt this indicator should emphasize that the patient should not continue to receive the same medication rather than specify what the patient should receive instead. •DROPPED• due to low validity score from panelists.
16. Aspirin should not be used in children and teenagers with pharyngitis.	7. Aspirin should not be used in children and teenagers with pharyngitis.	•UNCHANGED•
Bronchitis/Cough	*Bronchitis/Cough*	
18. If an antibiotic is prescribed for acute cough, documentation of drug allergies should be in the chart.	--	•DELETED• Duplicate of Ch. 23 #1.
19. If the history documents cigarette smoking in a patient with acute cough, encouragement to stop smoking should be documented.	--	•DELETED• Duplicate of Ch. 2 #21.
Nasal Congestion	*Nasal Congestion*	
20. If nasal decongestants are prescribed, duration of treatment should be for no longer than 4 days.	8. If **topical** nasal decongestants are prescribed, duration of treatment should be for no longer than 4 days.	Wording changed to clarify original indicator.
Acute Sinusitis	*Acute Sinusitis*	
21. Treatment for acute sinusitis should be with antibiotics for 10-14 days.	9. Treatment for acute sinusitis should be with antibiotics for **at least 10 days.**	Panelists felt upper bound did not reflect the range of standard practice.
22. If an antibiotic is prescribed for acute sinusitis, documentation of presence or absence of drug allergies should be in the chart.	--	•DELETED• Duplicate of Ch. 23 #1.
23. In the absence of symptoms of allergic rhinitis (thin, watery rhinorrhea, and sneezing), antihistamines should not be prescribed for acute sinusitis.	10. In the absence of symptoms of allergic rhinitis (thin, watery rhinorrhea, and sneezing), antihistamines should not be prescribed for acute sinusitis.	•UNCHANGED•
24. If symptoms fail to improve after 48 hours of antibiotic treatment, clinical re-evaluation and therapy with another antibiotic should be instituted.	-- If symptoms fail to improve after 48 hours of antibiotic treatment, clinical re-evaluation and therapy with another antibiotic should be instituted.	•UNCHANGED• •DROPPED• due to low validity score from panelists.
25. If the patient does not improve after two courses of antibiotics, referral to an otolaryngologist for a diagnostic test (CT, x-ray, ultrasound of the sinuses) is indicated.	-- If the patient does not improve after two courses of antibiotics, referral to an otolaryngologist **or** for a diagnostic test (CT, x-ray, ultrasound of the sinuses) is indicated.	"Or" added because it was a typographical error in original indicator corrected. •DROPPED• due to low validity score from panelists.
Chronic Sinusitis	*Chronic Sinusitis*	
26. If a diagnosis of chronic sinusitis is made, the patient should be treated with at least 3 weeks of antibiotics.	-- If a diagnosis of chronic sinusitis is made, the patient should be treated with at least 3 weeks of antibiotics.	•UNCHANGED• •DROPPED• due to low validity score from panelists.

cont'd

	Original Indicator		Modified Indicator	Comments
27.	If patient has repeated symptoms after 2 separate 3 week trials of antibiotics, a referral to an otolaryngologist should be ordered.	--	If patient has repeated symptoms after 2 separate 3 week trials of antibiotics, a referral to an otolaryngologist should be ordered.	•UNCHANGED• •DROPPED• due to low validity score from panelists.
28.	If topical or oral decongestants are prescribed, duration of treatment should be for no longer than 4 days.	11.	If topical ~~or oral~~ decongestants are prescribed, duration of treatment should be for no longer than 4 days.	Wording changed to clarify original indicator.
29.	In the absence of symptoms of allergic rhinitis (thin, watery rhinorrhea, and sneezing), antihistamines should not be prescribed.	12.	In the absence of symptoms of allergic rhinitis (thin, watery rhinorrhea, and sneezing), antihistamines should not be prescribed.	•UNCHANGED•

Pediatric Quality Indicators

Chapter 20 — Urinary Tract Infection

[Note: These indicators apply to children <13].

Original Indicator	Modified Indicator	Comments
(DIAGNOSIS)	(DIAGNOSIS)	
1. If an infant or child presents with any of the following symptoms/signs, either a urine culture should be performed or a urinalysis should be performed; if urinalysis is positive, a urine culture should be performed: a. Malodorous urine, abnormal urinary stream, or change in urinary stream in an infant or child. b. Failure to thrive in an infant or child. c. Vomiting associated with fever in an infant. d. Jaundice associated with fever in a neonate. e. Pain/discomfort with urination (dysuria), frequency, urgency, flank pain (unrelated to trauma) in a child. f. Hematuria unrelated to trauma in infant or child. g. Secondary enuresis in a child.	1. If an infant or child presents with any of the following symptoms/signs, either a urine culture should be performed or a urinalysis should be performed; if urinalysis is positive, a urine culture should be performed: a. Malodorous urine, abnormal urinary stream, or change in urinary stream in an infant or child. b. Failure to thrive in an infant or child. -- Vomiting associated with fever in an infant. c. Jaundice associated with fever in a neonate. d. Pain/discomfort with urination (dysuria), frequency, urgency, flank pain (unrelated to trauma) in a child. e. Hematuria unrelated to trauma in infant or child. f. Secondary enuresis in a child.	•UNCHANGED• •MODIFIED• **Dropped (c)** due to low validity score from panelists.
2. In order to diagnose UTI, a positive culture from one of the following methods of urine collection is necessary: – bladder tap, or – catheterization, or – clean catch.	2. In order to diagnose UTI, a positive culture from one of the following methods of urine collection is necessary: – bladder tap, or – catheterization, or – clean catch.	•UNCHANGED•
3. In order to rule out UTI, a negative UA or culture from one of the following methods of urine collection is necessary: – bladder tap, or – catheterization, or – clean catch, or – urine bag.	-- In order to rule out UTI, a negative UA or culture from one of the following methods of urine collection is necessary: – bladder tap, or – catheterization, or – clean catch, or – urine bag.	•UNCHANGED• •DROPPED• due to difficulty in operationalizing "rule out UTI".
4. If the culture shows greater than 100,000 colonies/ml urine of a single organism, then the patient should be diagnosed and treated for UTI.	3. If the culture shows greater than 100,000 colonies/ml urine of a single organism, then the patient should be diagnosed and treated for UTI.	•UNCHANGED•
5. If there is bacterial growth of a single organism with at least 10,000 colonies/ml urine from a catherized specimen, then UTI should be diagnosed and treated.	4. If there is bacterial growth of a single organism with at least 10,000 colonies/ml urine from a catherized specimen, then UTI should be diagnosed and treated.	•UNCHANGED•
6. Growth of 10,000 to 100,000 colonies/ml urine from clean catch should be followed up with a repeat urine culture if the patient has not already been treated.	-- Growth of 10,000 to 100,000 colonies/ml urine from clean catch should be followed up with a repeat urine culture if the patient has not already been treated.	•UNCHANGED• •DROPPED• due to low validity score from panelists.
7. If there is any bacterial growth from a specimen obtained from a bladder tap then a UTI should be diagnosed and treated.	5. If there is any bacterial growth from a specimen obtained from a bladder tap then a UTI should be diagnosed and treated.	•UNCHANGED•
8. Urine culture must be obtained by clean catch, catheterization, or bladder tap before antibiotics are given.	-- Urine culture must be obtained by clean catch, catheterization, or bladder tap before antibiotics are given.	•UNCHANGED• •DROPPED• due to low validity score from panelists.

cont'd

Original Indicator	Modified Indicator	Comments
(TREATMENT)	(TREATMENT)	
9. All infants with a diagnosis of UTI must initially receive intravenous antibiotics.	6. All infants **under 3 months of age** with a diagnosis of UTI must initially receive **parenteral** antibiotics.	Panelists felt this indicator should be restricted to young infants. Parental was substituted to cover both intravenous and intramuscular antibiotics.
10. IV antibiotics may be switched to oral antibiotics if the infant has had at least 3 days without fever, a negative repeat urine culture, and negative blood and CSF culture.	-- **Parenteral** antibiotics may be switched to oral antibiotics if the infant has had at least 3 days without fever, a negative repeat urine culture, and negative blood and CSF culture.	Parenteral was substituted to cover both intravenous and intramuscular antibiotics. •DROPPED• due to low validity score from panelists.
11. Infants with UTI should receive a total of at least 10 days of antibiotics (IV and oral).	7. Infants with UTI should receive a total of at least 10 days of antibiotics (**parenteral** and oral).	Parental was substituted to cover both intravenous and intramuscular antibiotics.
11.5 •NEW•	8. **Children with a diagnosed UTI should be reassessed at 48 hours to determine if there is clinical improvement.**	•NEW• Panelists wanted an additional indicator to assess treatment effectiveness.
12. Infants with UTI should have a repeat urine culture between 48 hours and the end of the fifth day of IV therapy.	9. Infants with UTI **who are reassessed, but are not clinically improved by 48 hours of the initiation of antibiotic therapy,** should have a repeat urine culture between 48 hours and 72 hours of antibiotic therapy. **within 24 hours of reassessment.**	Panelists felt follow-up urine culture not necessary if patient improved. They also wanted to rate a shorter time frame for follow-up. IV changed to antibiotic to allow for therapy that was not just IV.
13. Children with UTI and systemic symptoms such as hypotension, poor perfusion, anorexia, or emesis, should be treated initially with IV antibiotics.	10. Children with UTI and systemic symptoms such as hypotension, poor perfusion, anorexia, or emesis, should be treated initially with **parenteral** antibiotics.	•UNCHANGED• Parenteral was substituted to cover both intravenous and intramuscular antibiotics.
14. If the child is being treated with oral antibiotics, by the fourth day, either (1) antibiotic sensitivities must be determined, or (2) a repeat culture must be sent.	11. If the child is being treated with oral antibiotics **and is not clinically improved** by 48 hours, either (1) antibiotic sensitivities must be determined, or (2) a repeat culture must be sent.	Panelists felt follow-up urine culture not necessary if patient is clinically improved. They also wanted to rate a shorter time frame for follow-up.
15. When antibiotic sensitivities are checked, if the organism is not sensitive to the antibiotic, the antibiotic should be switched to one to which the organism is sensitive within 1 day.	-- When antibiotic sensitivities are checked, if the organism is not sensitive to the antibiotic, the antibiotic should be switched to one to which the organism is sensitive within 1 day.	•UNCHANGED• •DROPPED• due to low validity score from panelists.
16. All children with the diagnosis of UTI should receive at least 7 days of antibiotics.	-- All children with the diagnosis of UTI should receive at least 7 days of antibiotics.	•UNCHANGED• •DROPPED• due to low validity score from panelists.

Pediatric Quality Indicators

cont'd

	Original Indicator	Modified Indicator	Comments
17.	All children with the diagnosis of pyelonephritis should be treated initially with IV antibiotics.	--	All children with the diagnosis of pyelonephritis should be treated initially with **parenteral** antibiotics. •DROPPED• **due to low validity score from panelists.**
18.	A child with four UTIs in a single year should receive prophylactic antibiotics until the reflux has resolved.	12.	A child with four UTIs in a single year should receive prophylactic antibiotics for at least six months.	•UNCHANGED•

Radiologic Work-up

	Original Indicator	Modified Indicator	Comments
19.	Any boy less than 10 years old with a first UTI or with systemic symptoms (and/or who has not had the following study before) should have a VCUG and one of the following within three months of diagnosis: – RUS, or – IVP, or – nuclear medicine renal scan.	13.	Any boy less than 10 years old with a first UTI or with systemic symptoms (and/or who has not had the following studies before) should have a VCUG and one of the following within three months of diagnosis: – RUS, or – IVP, or – nuclear medicine renal scan.	•UNCHANGED•
20.	Any girl less than 3 years old with a first UTI or less than 10 years old with systemic symptoms (and/or who has not had the following studies before) should have a VCUG or IC and one of the following within three months of diagnosis: – RUS, or – IVP, or – nuclear medicine renal scan.	14.	Any girl less than 3 years old with a first UTI or less than 10 years old with systemic symptoms (and/or who has not had the following studies before) should have a VCUG or IC and one of the following within three months of diagnosis: – RUS, or – IVP, or – nuclear medicine renal scan.	•UNCHANGED•
21.	If a child with a diagnosis of UTI remains febrile for more than 48 hours on therapy, or if repeat urine culture is positive despite appropriate antibiotics, the child needs an immediate evaluation for urologic obstruction or abscess with renal ultrasound (RUS), intravenous pyelogram (IVP), or nuclear medicine renal scan.	15.	If a child with a diagnosis of UTI **is not improving in 48** hours on therapy, **and** repeat urine culture is positive despite appropriate antibiotics, the child **should have an** evaluation for urologic obstruction or abscess with renal ultrasound (RUS), intravenous pyelogram (IVP), or nuclear medicine renal scan **within 24 hours.**	Panelists felt both conditions should be met before referral is required. Wording revised to provide a time-frame for "immediate."
22.	Children who have a VCUG or IC following a UTI should be on prophylactic or therapeutic antibiotics continuously from the beginning of therapy for the UTI until the time of the study.	--	Children who have a VCUG or IC following a UTI should be on **continuous antibiotics** (prophylactic **should follow** therapeutic antibiotics) ~~continuously~~ from the beginning of therapy for the UTI until the time of the study.	Panelists felt the wording needed to be modified to clarify the intent of the indicator (that the patient would switch to prophylactic antibiotics when the therapeutic course was complete). •DROPPED• **due to low validity score from panelists.**

Vesicoureteral Reflux (VUR)

	Original Indicator	Modified Indicator	Comments
23.	Children diagnosed with Grade II or higher VUR should be on prophylactic antibiotics until the reflux has resolved.	--	Children diagnosed with Grade II or higher VUR should be on prophylactic antibiotics until the reflux has resolved.	•UNCHANGED• •DROPPED• **due to low validity score from panelists.**
24.	Children with VUR should have annual monitoring with VCUG or nuclear cystogram.	16.	Children with VUR should have annual monitoring with VCUG or nuclear cystogram.	•UNCHANGED•

cont'd

	Original Indicator		Modified Indicator	Comments
25.	Children with high grade (Grade IV or higher) VUR or other anatomic abnormalities, such as posterior urethral valves, abnormal urethral implantation, or horse-shoe kidney, should be referred to a urologist.	17.	Children with high grade (Grade IV or higher) VUR, **obstructive symptoms,** or other anatomic abnormalities, such as posterior urethral valves, abnormal urethral implantation, or horse-shoe kidney, should be referred to a urologist.	**•UNCHANGED•**
26.	Children with obstructive symptoms should be referred to a urologist.	--		**•DELETED•** Merged with original indicator #25.
27.	Children with VUR or other anatomic abnormalities who also have hypertension, decreased renal function, failure to thrive, or other related signs, should be referred to a pediatric nephrologist for treatment of renal insufficiency and hypertension.	18.	Children with VUR or other anatomic abnormalities who also have hypertension, decreased renal function, failure to thrive, or other related signs, should be referred to a pediatric nephrologist for treatment of renal insufficiency and hypertension.	**•UNCHANGED•** "Failure to thrive, or other related signs" removed due to word processing error.

Pediatric Quality Indicators

Chapter 21 — Vaginitis and STDs

Original Indicator		Modified Indicator		Comments
(DIAGNOSIS)			**(DIAGNOSIS)**	
Vaginitis			**Vaginitis**	
1.	In adolescent girls presenting with complaint of vaginal discharge, the practitioner should perform a speculum exam to determine the source of discharge.	1.	In ~~sexually-active adolescent girls~~ **adolescent girls who are having vaginal intercourse and who** present with a complaint of vaginal discharge, the practitioner should perform a speculum exam to determine the source of discharge.	Panelists felt that for adolescents who have not had vaginal intercourse, the differential diagnosis of vaginal discharge is more limited and does not require a speculum exam.
2.	At a minimum, the following tests should be performed on the vaginal discharge: normal saline wet mount for clue cells and trichomads; KOH wet mount for yeast hyphae.	2.	At a minimum, the following tests should be performed on the vaginal discharge: normal saline wet mount for clue cells and trichomads; KOH wet mount for yeast hyphae.	•UNCHANGED•
3.	A sexual history should be obtained from all women presenting with a vaginal discharge. The history should include: a. No. of sexual partners in previous 6 months. b. Absence or presence of symptoms in partners. c. Use of condoms. d. Prior history of sexually transmitted diseases.	3.	A sexual history should be obtained from all women presenting with a vaginal discharge. The history should include: a. No. of sexual partners in previous 6 months. b. Absence or presence of symptoms in partners. c. Use of condoms. d. Prior history of sexually transmitted diseases.	•UNCHANGED•
4.	If three of the following four criteria are met, a diagnosis of bacterial vaginosis or gardnerella vaginosis should be made: pH greater than 4.5; positive whiff test; clue cells on wet mount; thin homogenous discharge.	4.	If three of the following four criteria are met, a diagnosis of bacterial vaginosis or gardnerella vaginosis should be made: pH greater than 4.5; positive whiff test; clue cells on wet mount; thin homogenous discharge.	•UNCHANGED•
Cervicitis			**Cervicitis**	
5.	Routine testing for gonorrhea and chlamydia trachomatis (culture and antigen detection, respectively) should be performed with the routine pelvic exam in all adolescent girls.	5.	Routine testing for gonorrhea and chlamydia trachomatis (culture and antigen detection, respectively) should be performed with the routine pelvic exam in all adolescent girls.	•UNCHANGED•
PID			**PID**	
6.	If a patient is given the diagnosis of PID, a speculum and bimanual pelvic exam should have been performed.	6.	If a patient is given the diagnosis of PID, a speculum and bimanual pelvic exam should have been performed.	•UNCHANGED•
7.	If a patient is given the diagnosis of PID, at least 2 of the following signs should be present on physical exam: - lower abdominal tenderness - adnexal tenderness - cervical motion tenderness.	7.	If a patient is given the diagnosis of PID, at least 2 of the following signs should be present on physical exam: - lower abdominal tenderness - adnexal tenderness - cervical motion tenderness.	•UNCHANGED•
7.5a	•NEW•	8.	**If a patient has symptoms of urethritis, he should be tested for both chlamydia and gonorrhea or receive proper treatment for both.**	•NEW• Panelists requested additional indicators for males and resubmission to them for final review.
7.5b	•NEW•	9.	**If a patient has evidence of asymptomatic urethritis, he should be tested for both chlamydia and gonorrhea or receive proper treatment for both.**	•NEW•
Genital Ulcers **STDs—General**			**STDs—General**	

cont'd

	Original Indicator		Modified Indicator	Comments
8.	If a patient presents with genital ulcer(s) of any cause, HIV testing should be recommended.	10.	If a patient presents with **any STD**, HIV testing should be **offered**.	All STD's indicate possible HIV risk. Wording changed to clarify original indicator.
	STDs—General			
9.	If a patient presents with any sexually transmitted disease (gonorrhea, chlamydia, trachomatis, herpes, chancroid, syphilis) a non-treponemal test (VDRL or RPR) for syphilis should be obtained.	11.	If a patient presents with any sexually transmitted disease (gonorrhea, chlamydia, trachomatis, herpes, chancroid, syphilis) a non-treponemal test (VDRL or RPR) for syphilis should be obtained.	•UNCHANGED•
	(TREATMENT)		(TREATMENT)	
	Vaginitis		**Vaginitis**	
10.	Treatment for bacterial vaginosis should be with metronidazole (orally or vaginally) or clindamycin (orally or vaginally) per the CDC recommendations.	12.	Treatment for bacterial vaginosis should be with metronidazole (orally or vaginally) or clindamycin (orally or vaginally) ~~per the CDC recommendations~~.	•UNCHANGED• Deleted "per CDC recommendations" because of difficulty in operationalizing.
11.	Treatment for *T. vaginalis* should be with oral metronidazole in the absence of allergy to metronidazole.	13.	Treatment for *T. vaginalis* should be with oral metronidazole in the absence of allergy to metronidazole.	•UNCHANGED•
12.	Treatment for non-recurrent (three or fewer episodes in previous year) yeast vaginitis should be with topical "azole" preparations (e.g., clotrimazole, butoconazole, etc.) or fluconazole.	14.	Treatment for non-recurrent (three or fewer episodes in previous year) yeast vaginitis should be with topical "azole" preparations (e.g., clotrimazole, butoconazole, etc.) or fluconazole.	•UNCHANGED•
	Cervicitis		**Cervicitis**	
13.	All women treated for gonorrhea should also be treated for chlamydia per the CDC recommendations.	15.	All women treated for gonorrhea should also be treated for chlamydia ~~per the CDC recommendations~~.	•UNCHANGED• Deleted "per CDC recommendations" because of difficulty in operationalizing.
	PID		**PID**	
14.	Patients with PID and any of the following conditions should be hospitalized: - appendicitis, - ectopic pregnancy, - pelvic abscess is present or suspected, - the patient is pregnant, - the patient is an adolescent (under age 18), - the patient has HIV infection, - uncontrolled nausea and vomiting, - clinical follow-up within 72 hours of starting antibiotic treatment cannot be arranged, or - the patient does not improve within 72 hours of starting therapy.	16.	Patients with PID and any of the following conditions should be hospitalized: - appendicitis, - ectopic pregnancy, - pelvic abscess is present or suspected, - the patient is pregnant, - ~~the patient is an adolescent (under age 18),~~ - the patient has HIV infection, - uncontrolled nausea and vomiting, - clinical follow-up within 72 hours of starting antibiotic treatment cannot be arranged, or - the patient does not improve within 72 hours of starting therapy.	Wording deleted because the sample is already restricted to adolescents.
15.	Total antibiotic therapy for PID should be for no less than 10 days (inpatient, if applicable, plus outpatient).	17.	Total antibiotic therapy for PID should be for no less than 10 days (inpatient, if applicable, plus outpatient).	•UNCHANGED•
	Genital Ulcers		**Genital Ulcers**	
16.	All patients with genital herpes should be counseled regarding reducing the risk of transmission to sexual partners.	18.	All patients with genital herpes should be counseled regarding reducing the risk of transmission to sexual partners.	•UNCHANGED•

Original Indicator	Modified Indicator	Comments
17. In the absence of allergy, patients with chancroid should be treated with Azithromycin, Ceftriaxone, or Erythromycin.	19. In the absence of allergy, patients with chancroid should be treated with Azithromycin, Ceftriaxone, or Erythromycin.	•UNCHANGED•
18. In the absence of allergy, patients with primary and secondary syphilis should be treated with benzathine penicillin G (IM).	20. In the absence of allergy, patients with primary and secondary syphilis should be treated with benzathine penicillin G (IM).	•UNCHANGED•
19. If a patient has a primary ulcer consistent with syphilis, treatment for syphilis should be initiated before laboratory test results are received.	21. If a patient has a primary ulcer consistent with syphilis, treatment for syphilis should be initiated before laboratory test results are received.	•UNCHANGED•
STDs—General	**STDs—General**	
20. Sexual partners of patients with new diagnoses of gonorrhea, chlamydia, chancroid, and primary or secondary syphilis should be referred for treatment.	22. Sexual partners of patients with new diagnoses of *T. vaginalis*, gonorrhea, chlamydia, chancroid, and primary or secondary syphilis should be referred for treatment.	*T. vaginalis* added because it was inadvertently omitted from original indicator.
(FOLLOW-UP)	(FOLLOW-UP)	
PID	**PID**	
21. Patients receiving outpatient therapy for PID should receive a follow-up visit within 72 hours of diagnosis.	23. Patients receiving outpatient therapy for PID should receive a follow-up visit within 72 hours of diagnosis.	•UNCHANGED•
22. All patients being treated for PID should have a microbiological re-examination (e.g., cultures) within 10 days of completing therapy.	24. All patients being treated for PID should have a microbiological re-examination (i.e., cultures) within 10 days of completing therapy.	•UNCHANGED•
Genital Ulcers	**Genital Ulcers**	
23. Patients receiving treatment for chancroid should be re-examined within 7 days of treatment initiation to assess clinical improvement.	-- Patients receiving treatment for chancroid should be re-examined within 7 days of treatment initiation to assess clinical improvement.	•UNCHANGED• •DROPPED• due to low validity score from panelists.
24. Patients with primary or secondary syphilis should be re-examined clinically and serologically within 6 months after treatment.	25. Patients with primary or secondary syphilis should be re-examined clinically and serologically within 6 months after treatment.	•UNCHANGED•
25. •NEW•	26. **Patients with a sexually transmitted disease should have a follow-up visit within 4 weeks of the diagnosis.**	•NEW• Panelists felt a follow-up indicator was needed because of the importance of assessing treatment effectiveness and providing additional risk prevention counseling.

Chapter 22 — Well Child Care

[Note: This section was reorganized. The panelists voted on some of the original indicators but also asked for modifications in the full set to reduce the emphasis on the newborn exam and to broaden the coverage of anticipatory guidance topics. They requested a resubmission for final review. Note: The original and new indicator columns do not match.]

Original Indicator	•NEW• Indicator	Comments
1. Within 24 hours of birth, every child not admitted to a neonatal intensive care unit should have a physical examination that determines and documents all of the following:		
	History and Anticipatory Guidance	
a. whether the anterior fontanelle is normal;	1. The mother's pregnancy and delivery history (e.g., length of pregnancy; illnesses; use of medications; use of alcohol, drugs, or tobacco during pregnancy; complications) should be documented by the end of the first month of life.	Modified from original indicator #7.
b. whether jaundice is present;	2. Discussion of feeding and nutritional issues should be documented at least once during the first two months of life.	•NEW• Panelists requested the addition of feeding and nutrition indicators.
c. whether a red reflex is present;	3. Discussion of transition to foods other than breast milk or formula should be documented at least once during the first six months of life.	•NEW• Panelists requested the addition of feeding and nutrition indicators.
d. whether the palate is intact;	4. Discussion of age-appropriate injury prevention (per TIPP) should be documented at least twice during the first year of life.	Modified from original indicators #17-20.
e. whether heart rate and rhythm are regular, whether a murmur is present;	5. Discussion of age-appropriate injury prevention (per TIPP) should be documented at least once a year during the second-sixth year of life.	Modified from original indicators #17-20.
f. whether femoral pulses are normal;	6. Discussion of age-appropriate injury prevention (per TIPP) should be documented at least once every other year during the seventh-twelfth year of life.	Modified from original indicators #17-20.
g. whether respiratory rate is normal;	*Physical Examination*	
h. whether lung sounds are normal;	7. Before discharge from the hospital, the newborn's weight should be documented.	Modified from original indicator #2.
i. whether abdominal exam is normal, including normal bowel sounds, absence of enlarged liver and spleen, and absence of abnormal masses;	8. The child's weight should be documented at least four times between the end of the first week and the end of the first year of life. This information must either be plotted on a growth curve or be recorded with the age/gender percentile.	Modified from original indicator #8.

Original Indicator	•NEW• Indicator	Comments
j. whether genitals are normal, whether testes are descended;	9. The child's weight should be documented at least twice during the second year of life. This information must either be plotted on a growth curve or be recorded with the age/gender percentile.	Modified from original indicator #8.
k. whether the anus is patent;	10. The child's weight should be documented at least once a year during the third-sixth year of life. This information must either be plotted on a growth curve or be recorded with the age/gender percentile.	Modified from original indicator #8.
l. whether hips are dislocated;	11. The child's weight should be documented at least once every other year during the seventh-twelfth year of life. This information must either be plotted on a growth curve or be recorded with the age/gender percentile.	Modified from original indicator #8.
m. whether evidence of a possible a neural tube defect is present (e.g., sacral dimple, sacral mass, hair tuft, and pilonidal sinus tract);	12. Before discharge from the hospital, the newborn's height should be documented.	Modified from original indicator #3.
n. whether there are the proper number of fingers and toes and the extremities are formed normally;	13. The child's height should be documented at least four times between the end of the first week and the end of the first year of life. This information must either be plotted on a growth curve or be recorded with the age/gender percentile.	Modified from original indicator #9.
o. whether the child moves all four extremities;	14. The child's height should be documented at least twice during the second year of life. This information must either be plotted on a growth curve or be recorded with the age/gender percentile.	Modified from original indicator #9.
p. whether tone is normal;	15. The child's height should be documented at least once a year during the third-sixth year of life. This information must either be plotted on a growth curve or be recorded with the age/gender percentile.	Modified from original indicator #9.
q. whether the Moro reflex is normal.	16. The child's height should be documented at least once every other year during the seventh-twelfth year of life. This information must either be plotted on a growth curve or be recorded with the age/gender percentile.	Modified from original indicator #9.
2. Weight should be documented.	17. Before discharge from the hospital, the newborn's head circumference should be documented.	Modified from original indicator #4.
3. Length should be documented.	18. The child's head circumference should be documented at least four times between the end of the first week and the end of the first year of life. This information must either be plotted on a growth curve or be recorded with the age/gender percentile.	Modified from original indicator #10.
4. Head circumference should be documented.	19. The child's head circumference should be documented at least twice during the second year of life. This information must either be plotted on a growth curve or be recorded with the age/gender percentile.	Modified from original indicator #10.
5. Screening for congenital hypothyroidism should have been done by the seventh day of life.	20. Heart rate should be documented during the first 24 hours of life.	Modified from original indicator #1e.
6. Screening for phenylketonuria should have been done after 24 hours of age and before two weeks of age.	21. Respiratory rate should be documented during the first 24 hours of life.	Modified from original indicator #1g.

Pediatric Quality Indicators

Original Indicator	•NEW• Indicator	Comments
The following criteria apply to well child care for infants and children.		
7. An inquiry should be made about the mother's pregnancy and delivery history (e.g., length of pregnancy; illnesses; use of medications; use of alcohol, drugs, or tobacco during pregnancy; complications) by the end of the first month of life.	22. A heart examination (in addition to heart rate) should be documented during the first 24 hours of life.	Modified from original indicator #1e.
8. The child's weight should be measured at least four times during the first year of life. This information must either be plotted on a growth curve or be recorded with the age/gender percentile.	23. Examination of the femoral pulses should be documented during the first 24 hours of life.	Modified from original indicator #1f.
9. The child's length should be measured at least four times during the first year of life. This information must either be plotted on a growth curve or be recorded with the age/gender percentile.	24. An abdominal examination should be documented during the first 24 hours of life.	Modified from original indicator #1i.
10. The child's head circumference should be measured at least four times during the first year of life. This information must either be plotted on a growth curve or be recorded with the age/gender percentile.	25. The newborn's feeding pattern should be documented before discharge.	•NEW• Panelists requested the addition of feeding and nutrition indicators.
11. If a boy has been circumcised, a follow-up examination of his penis should be conducted during the first month of life.	26. A hip examination should be documented at least once during the first two months of life.	Modified from original indicator #11 and #14.
12. The child's umbilicus should be examined after the newborn exam during the first month of life.	27. A heart examination should be documented at least once between 72 hours and two months of life.	Modified from original indicators #1e and #13.
13. The child's heart and femoral pulses should be examined at least once after the newborn exam during the first month of life.	28. A lung examination should be documented at least once during the first two months of life.	Modified from original indicator #1h.
14. A child's hips should be examined at least four times during the first year of life.	29. An abdominal examination should be documented at least once between the end of the first week and two months of life.	Modified from original indicator #1i.
15. A child should be checked for strabismus between the end of the second month of life and the end of the sixth month of life.	30. Examination of the femoral pulses should be documented between the end of the first week and two months of life.	Modified from original indicator #1f.
16. A child's deep tendon reflexes should be examined at least once during the first year of life.	31. A neurologic examination (e.g., tone, reflexes) should be documented at least once during the first two months of life.	Modified from original indicators #1m, 1o, 1p, 1q and #16.
17. An inquiry about use of a car seat should be made by the end of the first month.	32. A genital examination (e.g., descended testes) should be documented at least once during the first 2 months of life.	Modified from original indicators #1j and #11.
18. An inquiry about use of a car seat should be made between the end of the sixth month and the end of the first year.	33. A physical examination should be documented at least twice during the second six months of life.	•NEW• The panel felt that routine physical examinations were important indicators of quality.
19. Child-proofing the home should be discussed by the end of the seventh month of life.	34. A physical examination should be documented at least twice during the second year of life.	•NEW• The panel felt that routine physical examinations were important indicators of quality.
	35. A physical examination should be documented at least once a year during the third-sixth year of life.	•NEW• The panel felt that routine physical examinations were important indicators of quality.

cont'd

Original Indicator		•NEW• Indicator		Comments
20.	The number for a poison center should have been given by the end of the seventh month of life.			**•NEW•** The panel felt that routine physical examinations were important indicators of quality.
		36.	**A physical examination should be documented at least once every other year during the seventh-eleventh year of life.**	
21.	A hemoglobin or hematocrit should be checked between the first outpatient visit and the end of the 18th month of life.			Original indicator #22. **•DROPPED•** because time window is too long for operationalization.
22.	Hearing should be screened by an audiometer by the end of the fourth year of life.	--	Hearing should be screened by an audiometer by the end of the fourth year of life.	Modified from original indicator #23.
23.	If the child fails to hear the stimulus at two frequencies in one ear, he/she should be referred to an audiologist within one month.	37.	**If the child fails to hear the stimulus at two frequencies in one ear further evaluation/work-up should be ordered within one month.**	Modified from original indicator #24. **•DROPPED•** because time window is too long for operationalization.
24.	Vision should be tested by the end of the fourth year of life.	--	Vision screening should be performed by the end of the fourth year of life.	
			Laboratory Screening	
		38.	Screening for congenital hypothyroidism should have been done by the seventh day of life.	Original indicator #5.
		39.	Screening for phenylketonuria should have been done after 24 hours of age and before two weeks of age.	Original indicator #6.
		40.	**A hemoglobin or hematocrit should be checked by the end of the 18th month of life.**	Modified from original indicator #21.

-548-

Chapter 23 — Medications

[note: There is no text chapter corresponding to these indicators.]

Original Indicator		Modified Indicator		Comments
2.	The chart should have a clearly specified place to mark medication allergies.	1.	The chart should have a clearly specified place to mark **all** medication allergies.	Wording changed to clarify original indicator. Order changed from indicator #2 to indicator #1.
3.	All allergies found in the chart must be listed in the allergy list discussed in the preceding indicator.	--	All allergies found in the chart must be listed in the allergy list discussed in the preceding indicator.	•**UNCHANGED**• **DELETED because of operationalization difficulties.**
1.	At the time someone is prescribed a medication, there should be a notation in the chart stating what medications, if any, the person is allergic to.	2.	**When** prescribed a medication, **the patient's allergy status** should be a **recorded** in the **progress note and/or on the designated allergy list.**	Wording changed to clarify original indicator. Order changed from indicator #1 to indicator #2.
4.	People with an allergy to a medication should only receive it if they have a notation in their chart stating why.	3.	People with an allergy to a medication should only receive it if they have a notation in their chart stating why.	•**UNCHANGED**•